DISCARD
D0764055

BIOGRAPHICAL DICTIONARY OF MEDICINE

BIOGRAPHICAL DICTIONARY OF MEDICINE

Jessica Bendiner and Elmer Bendiner

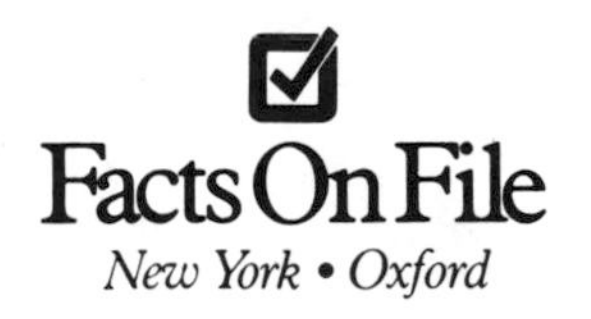

Facts On File
New York • Oxford

Biographical Dictionary of Medicine

Facts On File, Inc.
460 Park Avenue South
New York NY 10016
USA

Facts On File Limited
Collins Street
Oxford OX4 1XJ
United Kingdom

Library of Congress Cataloging-in-Publication Data

Bendiner, Jessica.
Biographical dictionary of medicine / Jessica Bendiner and Elmer Bendiner.
p. cm.
Includes bibliographical references.
ISBN 0-8160-1864-2
1. Physicians—Biography—Dictionaries. I. Bendiner, Elmer. II. Title.
[DNLM: 1. Physicians—biography. WZ 112 B524b]
R134.B455 1990
610'.92'2—dc20
DNLM/DLC
for Library of Congress 89-23604

British CIP data available on request from Facts On File.

Composition by Facts On File, Inc.
Manufactured by The Maple-Vail Book Manufacturing Group
Printed in United States of America

10 9 8 7 6 5 4 3 2 1

This book is printed on acid-free paper.

Contents

Introduction

The *Biographical Dictionary of Medicine* is designed as a guide to the huge cast of characters involved in the history of medicine. It describes the players who have taken the stage at one time or another in this epic drama that has spanned several millennia. It includes ancient herbalists, battlefield surgeons of the Renaissance, alchemists and anatomists—those skilled geographers of the human body—and the many people who have participated in the great explosion of biological science and technology in the nineteenth and twentieth centuries.

Though the book is indeed a dictionary in the sense that the entries are arranged alphabetically for ready reference, its conciseness does not approach that of a standard dictionary. Rather, the entries attempt to give the reader at least the flavor of the life and times, difficulties and achievements of each biographical subject.

Of course, not every player can get equal billing. The choice of whom to include and how much of the limited space available to devote to each subject is the result of careful consideration by the authors, who assume full responsibility for such decisions, knowing that not all readers will agree in every case. The prime criteria used for selection are the importance and influence of the candidate in the history of medicine, the likelihood that a student will require a summary biography, and the interest such a life may have for the thoughtful inquirer who may wish to spend a little time among great, or at least interesting, people.

To locate the people described in the context of world history, the reader is invited to consult the chronology at the end of the book. If, as hoped, readers wish to delve more deeply into the life and work of a particular character, they may find suggestions for further reading in the bibliography.

Finally, the authors hope that through this book, these men and women will, in a limited sense, live again for millions who, in one way or another, have surely benefited from their legacies.

BIOGRAPHICAL DICTIONARY OF MEDICINE

A

John Abernethy 1764–1831

John Abernethy gained widespread recognition in his own lifetime as one of the most important and distinguished surgeons of the early nineteenth century. He gained his reputation in part because of an aggressive eccentricity, and in spite of a blunt, often rude bedside manner.

At fifteen Abernethy was named apprentice to a surgeon at London's St. Bartholomew's Hospital, where in eight years' time he became an assistant surgeon. It was then that he began a lecture series on anatomy for students, presented in his own home. The governors of the hospital were so struck by Abernethy's dramatic abilities and his impact on the students that they built an auditorium on hospital grounds so he could expand his lectures and his audience. Among his fans was ROBERT LISTON, the surgeon, who seems to have assimilated some of Abernethy's overbearing temperament as well as his teachings.

Abernethy's discourses on anatomy, physiology and surgery were greatly influenced by his private and classroom studies with JOHN HUNTER, who was considered the reigning master in the field of surgery. Abernethy stunned the medical community while performing Hunter's operation for the cure of aneuryism by managing to successfully tie the patient's iliac artery, a distinct advance beyond Hunter's original technique.

Patients flocked to Abernethy's consulting rooms to encounter his boorishness and great disdain. He went so far as to send one patient, whom he deemed a hypochondriac, on a long journey to Scotland in search of a fictitious "Dr. Robinson."

Later in life Abernethy withdrew from surgery and developed a rather shortsighted view of medicine. He insisted that the root of all disease was a disorder of the digestive system, and that the basis of all cure would be therefore be an alteration of one's diet. While his theories were oversimplified, they did encourage the British medical community to consider not only the symptoms but the life-style of a patient.

Robert Adams 1791–1875

Irish surgeon and pathologist Robert Adams is remembered in association with the celebrated Dublin school of medicine. A popular lecturer and practitioner, Adams played an important role in the development of clinical investigation in the mid-nineteenth century, most notably in the areas of internal medicine and cardiology.

In 1827 he published a monograph entitled *Cases of Diseases of the Heart, Accompanied with Pathological Observations,* which included a number of significant findings. Adams reported the relationship of pericardial adhesion to muscular hypertrophy (the presence of dense fibrous tissue between the pericardian and the heart) the overgrowth of a muscle, due to enlargement of individual cells); and associated the heading of tissue in the coronary vessels with angina.

Based on clinical observation of a 68-year-old cardiac patient, Adams described a syndrome in which cerebral symptoms and attenuated pulse occurred in association with the approach of heart block. Dublin physician WILLIAM STOKES confirmed the pathology several decades later as a syndrome characterized by attacks of unconsciousness, slow pulse, and occasionally convulsive seizures or uncontrollable giddiness. Acknowledging prior clinical reports, the syndrome is now called Adams-Stokes disease, and occasionally Morgagni-Adams-Stokes disease, in reference to the findings of Italian anatomist GIOVANNI BATTISTA MORGAGNI, which preceded those of Adams.

Emphasizing the value of postmortem examination, Adams correlated clinical and pathological observations in cases of pneumonia, hernia, joint disease, ulcers, apoplexy, vascular disorders, and rheumatic gout. Adams himself suffered from this last condition, which he described in 1857 in a popular work entitled *A Treatise on Rheumatic Gout, or Chronic Rheumatic Arthritis of All the Joints.*

A native of Dublin, Adams was apprenticed to leading Irish surgeon William Hartigan and to George Stewart, surgeon-general to the British army. In 1832, after receiving a medical degree from Dublin University, he served on the surgical staffs at Jervis Street and Richmond Hospitals in that city. Adams was instrumental in the organization and establishment of the Peter Street School of Medicine, later breaking that affiliation to found the Richmond School of Medicine and Surgery (subsequently renamed Carmichael School of Medicine and Surgery).

An esteemed figure in the Irish medical establishment, Adams was elected president of both the Royal College of Surgeons and the Dublin Pathological Society. At the age of seventy he was appointed regius professor of surgery at Dublin, accepting the position of surgeon to the queen in that same year.

Edgar Douglas Adrian, First Baron Adrian
1889–1977

Preeminent physiologist of the early twentieth century, Edgar Douglas Adrian is remembered for his pioneer research on the mechanisms of the nervous system, most notably in the investigation of nerve impulse transmission. Elaborating on the pioneer studies of CHARLES SHERRINGTON, Adrian established fundamental principles of stimulus response and nerve fiber activity. His ground-breaking investigation of the physical and electrical basis of nerve function brought important advances to the modern understanding of sensation, perception and neural activity.

Throughout his distinguished career as a research physiologist, Cambridge professor, Trinity College master, university chancellor and president of the Royal Society (1950–1955), Adrian was showered with honors. These included the Order of Merit in 1942 and the 1932 Nobel Prize for Physiology or Medicine, which he shared with Charles Sherrington.

Born in London, Edgar Adrian was granted a science scholarship at Trinity College, Cambridge, where he received a medical degree in 1915. After serving a tour of military duty in the British Army Medical Corps, he returned to Cambridge, establishing a lifelong association with Trinity College.

In 1913, while still an undergraduate, Adrian launched his earliest research on the physiology of the nervous system. In collaboration with Keith Lucas, Adrian conducted a pivotal study on nerve impulse transmission that formed the basis of a critical principle known as the "all-or-none law."

Several years earlier Sherrington had noted that the strength of a nervous response might vary with the location of the stimulus, as well as the frequency of stimulation at the same location. With these observations in mind Adrian sought to analyze the underlying mechanism of nerve response by identifying the functional units in physical terms.

To examine the activity of a nerve impulse he adapted the principles of radio wave reception to create a remarkably sensitive recording device called the triode amplifier. Designed to register the electrical discharges of the nerve fibers, Adrian's system could detect the minute fluctuations in voltage as individual nerve fibers responded to controlled electrical stimuli.

By the 1920s Adrian's research had firmly established the all-or-none law, which states that the intensity of any response is determined by the frequency of stimulation, rather than any supposed difference in the "weight" or "strength" of a nervous impulse. In fact, Adrian showed that the magnitude of nerve impulses is invariable, so that the individual units of the sensory or motor signal carry no information as to the content or size of the message. Any sensory or motor impulse is conveyed as a sequence of indistinguishable transmission units, to be evaluated in terms of the frequency of signals and intervals. Adrian found that to heighten the intensity of a response, impulse frequency must be increased, either by dispatching more individual signals at a faster rate or by recruiting more nerve fibers to carry a larger load of message units at a time.

Within this digital system of communication sensory distinctions are determined by the nature of the fiber transmitting the impulse. It might be said that the experiences of light and sound are subjective interpretations of the same impression. The occasional unreliability of the system serves to illustrate the concept of interchangeable "information bits." When mechanical pressure is applied to the eyeball, the stimulus is experienced at the retina. The optic nerve then dispatches the impulse to the brain, delivering a false impression of light.

Focusing later investigations on the electrophysiology of nerve impulse, Adrian pioneered the study of brain waves and developed the use of electroencephalography in clinical and experimental research on epilepsy and brain lesions. His published works include *The Basis of Sensation* (1928), *The Mechanism of Nervous Action* (1932), and *The Physical Basis of Perception* (1947).

Fuller Albright 1900–1969

"As with eggs, there is no such thing as a poor doctor, [they] are either good or bad," declared Fuller Albright, who disdained mediocrity throughout his wide-ranging career in the exploration of metabolism and endocrinology.

Albright's research studies of glandular function and dysfunctions included an investigation of the diagnosis and treatment of hypo- and hyper-parathyroidism.

A group of four small exocrine glands arranged in two pairs, the parathyroids are attached to the thyroid gland on either side of the trachea in the base of the neck. Parathyroid hormone, synthesized and secreted by the parathyroid glands, is necessary for the metabolism of calcium and phosphorus and serves an important function in neuromuscular excitation and blood clotting.

Albright demonstrated the role of age, disuse, dysfunction of the gonads and corticosteroids (a group of hormones produced in the adrenal cortex), in the development of osteoporosis bone fragility due to a loss of bone tissue. He proposed the use of anabolic steroids in the treatment of osteoporosis and, anticipating the subsequent attention to steroids in the 1980s, he initiated the first quantitative studies of steroid levels in urine. Albright also introduced a method for measuring urinary gonadotropins and significantly advanced the understanding of the "adreno-genital syndrome," a hyperfunction of the adrenal gland that causes drastic abnormalities in male and female sexual development.

Albright also established the procedure of medical D & C (the dilatation of the cervix, and curettage, or scraping, of the lining of the uterus) as an alternative to surgical treatment for metropathia hemorrhagica, or uterine hemorrhage. Under his supervision the Ovarian Dysfunction Clinic at Massachussetts General Hospital became recognized as an influential center for the treatment of reproductive disorders in both men and women. It was there that Albright developed hormone replacement therapy for women undergoing menopause, establishing fundamental principles of endocrinology that would later be applied in the invention of oral contraceptives.

Distinguished for his theoretical insight as well as for his rigorous standards in experimental methodology, Albright is also noted for his contributions in renal medicine. Elucidating the role of hormones in the formation of various types of kidney stones, he advocated diagnosis and treatment of the underlying metabolic factors rather than the more complacent approach of removing the stones surgically.

When Albright graduated from Harvard Medical School in 1924 he obtained a series of prestigious research fellowships allowing him to conduct studies in industrial and clinical medicine at the university in association with Massachussetts General Hospital. After forty years as a member of the Harvard faculty Albright retired as Professor of Medicine Emeritus in 1961, but his career had been effectively terminated five years earlier when drastic surgery for advanced Parkonsonism left him incapacitated and unable to communicate.

Alcmaeon of Crotona c. 535 B.C.

Although he never practiced as a physician, Alcmaeon of Crotona is regarded as one of the earliest pioneers of medical science. Thought to be a student of the legendary PYTHAGORAS, Alcmaeon is recognized for his influential studies in natural philosophy, biology and anatomy, and most notably for his development of a comprehensive doctrine of the pathological and physiological aspects of internal disease.

Citing his extensive research on sensory perception, many scholars credit Alcmaeon as the originator of experimental psychology. He is also noted as the first to perform an animal dissection, initiating the practice during his investigation of the anatomy and physiology of the eye. Exploring the interaction between sense organs and the brain, Alcmaeon sliced through an eyeball in the hope of finding what he imagined would be a connecting channel between it and the brain.

Although HIPPOCRATES undoubtedly perpetuated the practice of animal dissection in the century that followed, many historians believe that Aristotle was the first to apply the method as a systematic research procedure. It was not until the beginning of the third century B.C. that human dissection and vivisection were reportedly introduced by Alexandrian physicians HEROPHILUS and ERASISTRATUS.

Alcmaeon was born in Crotona in Magna Graecia, a Greek colony in southern Italy, where, in addition to the principles of Pythagorean doctrine, he was taught pathology and anatomy by some of the leading physicians of his day. Drawing on his knowledge of natural philosophy and his observations in clinical medicine, Alcmaeon developed an influential doctrine of pathology and physiology in which health is defined as a balance of opposing forces or sensations, such as wet and dry, hot and cold, sweet and sour; while disease is seen as the consequence of excessive power, or "monarchy," held by one of these forces. Within this philosophical concept of illness Alcmaeon classified disease in terms of origin, depending on whether the cause was environmental, nutritional or behavioral.

Humbly acknowledging the hypothetical nature of his precepts, as well as the limitations of human perception, Alcmaeon referred to his teachings as an "opinion about the invisible."

Alexander of Tralles 525–605

With the collapse of political and social order following the fall of the Roman Empire, Western civilization entered an "Age of Faith" in which scientific study and observation were overshadowed by metaphysical and religious doctrine. The Byzantine Empire, however, fostered a revival of the Greek tradition in architecture, art and science during the sixth century.

Greek physician Alexander of Tralles was celebrated as an independent and innovative thinker, best known for his monumental work entitled *Twelve Books on Medicine.* Completed in the last years of his life, the twelfth and final volume, entitled *Concerning Fever,* contains a number of important insights into the characteristics and diagnostic interpretation of fevers. Although many of his prescriptions may now be characterized as magic potions, Alexander is noted for the accuracy of his clinical observations and analyses, as well as the clarity and simplicity of his prose. Long after his death his books were widely read in Latin and Arabic translations.

After extensive travels through Greece, Italy, Spain and Gaul, Alexander settled in Rome, where he established a medical practice. Drawing from clinical experience, he developed theories based on direct observation rather than relying on the widely trusted doctrines of HIPPOCRATES, GALEN and other medical luminaries of the past.

Alexander of Tralles is noted for his application of finger pressure in the diagnosis of edema, an excess of fluid under the skin, and ascites, an excess of fluid in the abdominal cavity. He was also an early practitioner of palpation as a means of diagnosing an enlarged spleen.

Hattie Elizabeth Alexander 1901–1968

In collaboration with immunochemist Michael Heidelberger, Hattie Elizabeth Alexander discovered a cure for meningitis, an inflammation of the membranes surrounding the brain, which was one of the most frightening diseases of her time. Alexander first witnessed the heartbreaking casualties of meningitis after her graduation from Johns Hopkins Medical School, when she interned at the Babies Hospital of Columbia-Presbyterian Medical Center in New York. In 1930 there was no effective treatment for this disease, which was considered 100% fatal in infants. Known also as meningococcal disease, part of its terror was due to the fact that death could occur as rapidly as ten hours after the onset of symptoms. After several years of bacteriologic research Alexander and Heidelberger were able to isolate an antibody that led to the development of a serum that could cure meningitis.

Alexander continued her research while director of Columbia-Presbyterian Medical Center's microbiological laboratory contributing valuable data concerning the transmission of genetic characteristics. She was named president of the American Pediatrics Society in 1965 and held the post until her death from cancer in 1968.

Edgar Allen 1892–1943

A leading authority on the mechanisms of sex hormones, Edgar Allen is best known for his discovery of estrogen and its role in the female reproductive cycle.

Investigating the origins and development of the ovum in 1923, Allen observed that females do not possess a full complement of ova at birth but instead accumulate them by continual production in the germinal epithelium, a layer of cells that eventually cover the internal and external surfaces of the gonad. Noting a cyclical process of development and decay in the follicles surrounding the ova, Allen hazarded that the ovarian follicles might be the controlling factor in the menstrual cycle. Seeking to confirm his suspicions, Allen, in collaboration with noted biochemist EDWARD A. DOISY, performed a series of experiments using fluid extracted from the ovarian follicle. It was found that repeated injections of the substance induced a series of cellular changes that replicated the early stages of a normal menstruation. When the substance was withheld the subject entered a later menstrual phase.

Born in Colorado and raised in Rhode Island, Edgar Allen attended Brown University, where he received a doctorate in biology in 1921. His thesis, published the following year, presented a detailed description of the cellular changes in primary and secondary sex organs over the course of a complete reproductive cycle in a female mouse.

In 1923, as professor of anatomy at the University of Minnesota, Allen conducted his landmark study of estrogen. Later appointed dean of the medical school and director of the university hospital, Allen remained at Minnesota for ten years before returning to the East Coast. Accepting the chair of anatomy at the Yale School of Medicine, he retained that position until his death at the age of fifty-two.

Allen presided over the American Association of Anatomists and the Association for the Study of Internal Secretions, also serving as a trustee of the Scientific Advisory Committee of the International Cancer Research Foundation. In recognition of his significant role in the advancement of modern endocrinology he was made a member of the French Legion of Honor in 1937 and was awarded the prestigious Baly Medal of the British Royal College of Physicians in 1941.

Al-Nafis (Ibn Al-Nafis or Al-Qarashi) c. 1205–1288

Although thirteenth-century Arabic physician Al-Nafis was the first to describe the circulation of blood passing from the right ventricle of the heart and through the lungs, his observations were never assimilated into Western medicine. It has been suggested that his works were known to some European anatomists of the Renaissance, but it was not until the twentieth century that historians discovered the medical legacy left by Al-Nafis, in which he significantly challenged GALENIC doctrine, particularly on pulmonary function.

Consisting of three hundred volumes, of which eighty were published, *Kitab al-Shamil fi 'l-Sina'a al-Tibbiyya* (*A Comprehensive Treatise on the Art of Medicine*) is a compilation of the teachings of Al-Nafis written when he was in his thirties. The entire work was thought to have disappeared until 1952, when a single volume was found among the Islamic manuscripts of the Cambridge University Library.

Other manuscripts have since been found at Stanford University and in libraries in Baghdad and Damascus. The rediscovered sections, as yet unpublished, are said to contain material of significant interest on the surgical techniques and methodology developed by Al-Nafis, as well as guidelines for postoperative care and the responsibilities of surgeons, nurses and other members of the hospital staff.

Born in al-Qurashiyya, near Damascus, Al-Nafis studied at Nuri Hospital, the region's most distinguished center for medical education and treatment.

Attaining the rank of *ra'is al-atibba* (master of medical practice), he was appointed personal physician to the sovereign ruler al-Zahir Baybars al- Bunduqdari, who reigned from 1260 to 1277.

The earliest known writings of Al-Nafis are his commentaries on anatomy, reproduced in an anthology compiled by Ibn Sina, one of his disciples. Despite the fact that, as a follower of Islam, he was not permitted to desecrate the body of any animal, his physiological insights are noteworthy, particularly in the discovery of secondary circulation:

> This is the right cavity of the two cavities of the heart. When the blood in this cavity has become thin, it must be transferred into the left cavity, where the pneuma is generated. But there is no passage between these two cavities, the substance of the heart there seems impermeable. It neither contains a visible passage, as some people have thought, nor does it contain an invisible passage which would permit the passage of blood, as Galen thought...It must, therefore, be that when the blood has become thin, it is passed into the arterial vein [pulmonary artery] to the lung, in order to be dispersed inside the substance of the lung, and to mix with the air. The finest parts of the lung are then strained, passing into the venous artery [pulmonary vein] reaching the left of the two cavities of the heart...

Al-Nafis also wrote extensively on jurisprudence, religious law, logic, and philosophy. One essay, a fantasy concerning a population spontaneously generated on a desert island, describes the rediscovery by "independent reasoning" of the main principles of Islamic and scientific law.

Another manuscript by Al-Nafis, entitled *Sharh Tabi'at al-Insan li-Buqrat* (*Commentary on Hippocrates's Nature of Man*), was discovered in Damascus in 1933. Other recently discovered writings include commentaries on *Aphorisms* and *Epidemics* (two texts by Hippocrates), as well as a physician's reference manual and a treatise on ophthalmology.

Alois Alzheimer 1864–1915

Bavarian neurologist Alois Alzheimer is best remembered for his description of the form of mental deterioration that now bears his name. Generally appearing in mid-maturity, Alzheimer's disease, or presenile dementia, is characterized by progressive loss of speech and memory, along with intellectual disturbances that eventually lead to complete loss of all mental ability.

In postmortem examination of victims of this condition Alzheimer noted a loss of cells in all cortical layers except the motor cortex and a degeneration of neurofibrils, the filaments found in and around nerve cells. In advanced cases of the disease autopsies reveal condensed clumps of these filaments between the nerve cells, now known as "Alzheimer's baskets."

Born in the town of Marktbreit, Alzheimer studied at the universities of Aschaffenburg, Tübingen, Berlin, and Wurzburg, where he was granted a degree in medicine in 1887. His doctoral thesis, on the wax-producing glands of the ear, was based on experimental research performed in the laboratory of noted Swiss physiologist and histologist R.A. VON KÖLLIKER.

Joining the staff at Frankfurt's Irrenanstalt Asylum as a clinical assistant, Alzheimer worked closely with distinguished neurologist Franz Nissl (1860–1919). At Nissl's suggestion Alzheimer embarked on an extensive investigation of the pathology of the nervous system. The two developed a long and productive partnership in which Nissl's energetic and imaginative enthusiasm was complemented and shaped by Alzheimer's powers of deduction as well as his advanced techniques in experimental histology. His staining method for the detection of Negri bodies, a definitive indicator of rabies, is known as "Alzheimer's stain."

Published between 1904 and 1918, the six volumes of the *Histologic and Histopathologic Studies of the Cerebral Cortex* were the result of Alzheimer's and Nissl's exhaustive study of normal and abnormal structure in the central nervous system. Among Alzheimer's notable contributions are discussions on alcoholic delirium, dementia praecox (psychoses of psychological origin), brain tumors, epilepsy, Huntington's chorea and general paralysis.

Appointed director of the Irrenanstalt Institute in 1895, Alzheimer continued research on a wide range of subjects, including clinical studies of manic depression and schizophrenia. Distinguishing the clinical characteristics of arteriosclerotic atrophy of the brain from those associated with senility and other forms of mental degeneration, he noted such symptoms as loss of pupil reflexes, increase in tendon reflexes, and alternating moods of euphoria and depression. At a cellular level he reported the degeneration of the smaller cerebral blood vessels, a process now referred to as "Alzheimer's sclerosis."

Leaving Frankfurt in 1902, he joined Nissl at Heidelberg, later accompanying him to Munich, where, in 1908, Alzheimer joined the staff of the Psychiatric Institute as professor and director of the clinic's anatomical laboratory.

In 1912 he left Frankfurt to accept a similar position at the Psychiatric and Neurologic Institute of Breslau. Though troubled by rapidly declining health, Alzheimer devoted the last three years of his life to research and clinical practice. His death at the age of 51 was the result of heart failure and uremia.

Dorothy Hansine Anderson 1901–1963

Leading pathologist and pediatrician Dorothy Hansine Andersen discovered a previously unrecognized disease, which she named cystic fibrosis. A hereditary condition appearing in infancy or early childhood, cystic fibrosis is a disorder of the exocrine glands in which a thick mucus is produced, clogging glandular ducts in the pancreas, lungs and intestines. As secretions of the glands are blocked from exiting, they accumulate and eventually cause swellings and cysts. Andersen discovered that all victims of cystic fibrosis die in childhood, generally as a result of respiratory tract infection.

In 1938, after presenting her report at a joint meeting of the American Pediatric Society and the Society for Pediatric Research, Andersen set out to establish a diagnostic test for cystic fibrosis. Gaining the necessary education in advanced biochemistry on her own, she established that enzyme analysis would reveal the presence of the disorder. To obtain a reliable indicator of the disease, she developed a technique for extracting fluid from the duodenum (the first part of the small intestine).

Andersen continued to study the nature of cystic fibrosis in the early 1940s at the Babies' Hospital at Columbia Presbyterian Medical Center. Her published articles included studies on the genetic aspects of the disease and reports on the use of chemotherapy in treating respiratory infections in cystic fibrosis patients. When the research team at Babies' Hospital observed consistently high levels of salt in the sweat of cystic fibrosis patients, the discovery gave rise to a simple diagnostic test, replacing Andersen's original method of detection.

Born in Asheville, North Carolina, Dorothy was prematurely thrust into adulthood when her father died in 1914. Barely an adolescent, she took on the full responsibility of caring for her invalid mother. Dorothy brought her north to St. Johnsbury, Vermont, and attended her until her death in 1920.

Enrolling at Johns Hopkins Medical College two years later, she showed early promise in her first major research studies, conducted in the laboratory of celebrated anatomist FLORENCE SABIN. Andersen's first two papers, reporting on the anatomy of specific organs of the reproductive system, were published in *Contributions to Embryology*.

She received a degree in medicine in 1926, completing a surgical internship at Strong Memorial Hospital in Rochester. Despite her impressive record, the hospital stuck to its policy barring women from appointment in the surgery and pathology departments, and Andersen was forced to seek employment at another institution. Accepting a post as assistant in pathology at the College of Physicians & Surgeons of New York's Columbia University, Andersen embarked on her study of the role of glands in the female reproductive cycle.

In 1930 she was appointed to Columbia's medical faculty as an instructor in pathology, and five years later she joined the staff at Babies' Hospital. It was there that she began her celebrated collection of infants' hearts showing various congenital defects. With the development of open-heart surgery in the following decades, Andersen was called upon as a leading authority on cardiac anatomy and embryology. Incorporating her infant heart collection into a training program for cardiologists, Andersen's program became a required course for surgeons at Babies' Hospital as well as at a number of other medical institutions.

In 1952 Andersen took over as chief of pathology at Babies' Hospital, becoming one of the center's most controversial figures. Detractors cited her unconventional and somewhat disorganized style, condemning her interest in athletics and carpentry as "unladylike." She was staunchly defended, however, by her many supporters, who admired Andersen's great generosity with her time and talent as well as her contributions to medicine.

Appointed full professor in 1958, she spent the last years of her life studying cystic fibrosis in young adults.

Andersen died of lung cancer in 1962 and was posthumously awarded the distinguished service medal of the Columbia Presbyterian Medical Center.

Elizabeth Garrett Anderson 1836–1917

The first British woman to be licensed as a physician, in 1870, Elizabeth Garrett Anderson is celebrated not only for her active medical career but also for the tenacity she showed in its pursuit. Although in 1849 ELIZABETH BLACKWELL became the first woman to receive a medical degree, and Pennsylvania established Women's Medical College the following year, England had not yet followed the American lead. Garrett's perseverance in challenging the prevailing attitudes toward women in British medicine paved the way for those who were to follow.

Elizabeth Garrett entered Middlesex Hospital as a nursing student, but she surreptitiously attended clinical courses, obtaining top grades. At the brink of fulfilling the necessary requirements for a change of degree, she was dismissed from the school without official explanation.

Following rejection from Oxford, Cambridge and the University of London, Garrett decided to pursue a degree from the Society of Apothecaries. She fulfilled her apprenticeship with Joshua Plaskit but was refused official candidacy from St. Andrews College and Edinburgh University in Scotland. She continued studying wherever she was allowed, such as in classes given by SIR JAMES SIMPSON, a renowned physician and an avid supporter of women's rights.

With a polite but persistent approach Garrett fulfilled all her educational requirements and returned to Middlesex to present her application for licensing to the

Society of Apothecaries. When they refused to allow her to take the qualifying examination her father threatened a lawsuit. The Society relented, and Garrett became the first woman licensed by the Society, which meant her name was entered into the Medical Register as an officially sanctioned physician.

By 1870 Garrett had developed an extensive private practice, established a clinic known as St. Mary's Dispensary for Women, received a full medical degree from the University of Paris and married the wealthy James Anderson. She was instrumental in the establishment, in 1874, of the London School of Medicine for Women and was its dean for twenty years. Through a bureaucratic oversight she was admitted to the British Medical Association, which did not officially accept women until 1892.

After her husband's death in 1907 Anderson was elected mayor of Aldeburgh, achieving another first for women in Britain. Her commitment to the advancement of women as patients, professionals and citizens lasted until her death on December 17, 1917, and her work advanced the careers of many of the women who were soon to follow in her footsteps. Elizabeth Garrett Anderson's daughter Louisa carried on the family tradition, both by organizing hospitals in France during World War I and writing her mother's biography, published in 1939.

Virginia Apgar 1909–1974

Dr Virginia Apgar is best known for having introduced a series of measurements, taken immediately after a baby's birth, to evaluate the infant's heart rate, muscle tone, respiratory effort, color and muscle irritability. These five factors are each given a score from 0 to a normal of 2, with a total ranging from 0 to 10. A score of seven or less indicates an immediate problem. Until the introduction of the Newborn Scoring System, or Apgar Score, newborns were sent to the nursery immediately after delivery and only later examined by a nurse or doctor. With the information now taken one minute after delivery and again five minutes later, doctors can detect any abnormalities and possibly avert an infant's death. In particular, pulmonary or circulatory distress may be corrected if discovered at this early time.

Virginia Apgar was one of the first women graduates of Columbia University and began a promising career as a surgeon at Columbia Presbyterian Medical Center. She found it difficult, however, to be a woman in the predominantly male field of surgery, and after two frustrating years of practice she turned to anesthesiology. That field had long been relegated to the domain of nursing, and it was Apgar who established it as a separate medical specialty. In 1938 she was appointed director of anesthesiology at Columbia Presbyterian Medical Center and was granted the first full professorship in that field, thereby officially establishing anesthesiology as a separate discipline of medical study.

Apgar worked as administrator, practitioner, researcher and author (*Is My Baby Alright?*), and in 1959 she was named director of the National Foundation-March of Dimes. She continued her research on the prevention of birth defects and participated energetically and effectively in foundation fund-raising until her death in 1974.

Werner Arber 1929–

Exploring the interaction between bacterial cells and bacteriophages, Swiss microbiologist Werner Arber discovered certain defensive enzymes within the bacterial cell that ward off attacks by the bacteriophages. These came to be called "restriction and modification enzymes."

In the late 1950s Arber became intrigued by the phenomenon of host-induced variation. Research studies by Giuseppe Bertani, Salvador Luria and others had confirmed the fact that invading bacteriophages not only cause mutations in their bacterial hosts but undergo debilitating mutations themselves.

In 1962 Arber, along with research partner D. Dussoix, demonstrated that some strains of bacteria contain substances called "restriction enzymes" or endonucleases, which serve to prevent infection by breaking apart the DNA molecule of the invading bacteriophage, thereby rendering it inactive. By 1968 Arber confirmed that it is upon recognition of specific nucleotide sequences in the phage DNA that the endonuclease cleaves the DNA molecule.

Examining the aftermath of a thwarted bacteriophage infection, Arber and his colleagues noted that a small fraction of phage genes survive and will grow normally if introduced into another bacterial cell. This observation led to the discovery of another strain-specific bacterial enzyme that recognizes the same nucleotide sequences as those detected by the restriction enzyme. Terming these "modification enzymes," Arber and his laboratory team found that these substances act as chemical shields, protecting the bacterial DNA against the destructive effects of the restriction enzyme. They concluded that these modification enzymes also act on a small portion of the invading bacteriophages before they can be destroyed.

The first series of restriction enzymes discovered by Arber belonged to a class, later identified as type I, in which the splitting of the DNA occurs at random locations. Subsequent studies by HAMILTON SMITH and DANIEL NATHANS revealed a type II restriction enzyme, which characteristically severs the invading strand of DNA at a strain-specific site. Providing a biochemical key to the nucleotide sequences of DNA, this second class of restriction enzymes opened up new avenues in genetic research.

Werner Arber was born and raised in Switzerland, where he studied microbiology at the Swiss Federal Institute of Technology in Zurich and at the University of Geneva. After receiving his doctorate in 1958 he spent one year as a research associate in medical microbiology at the University of Southern California. Returning to join the faculty at the University of Geneva in 1960, Arber was appointed extraordinary professor of molecular genetics five years later, at the age of 36. He currently serves as professor of molecular biology at the University of Basel.

Introducing a fundamental principle of molecular biology, Arber's discovery of restriction enzymes launched a series of revolutionary studies that gave rise to the development of genetic engineering. The 1978 Nobel Prize for Physiology or Medicine was awarded to Arber, along with fellow microbiologists Daniel Nathans and Hamilton Smith, in acknowledgment of the importance and far-reaching implications of their independent studies of host-controlled restriction and modification.

Aristotle 384–322 B.C.

Fifteen hundred years after the death of Aristotle, the most renowned of ancient Greek scholars, Bacon, heralding the dawn of modern scientific thought, declared: "If I had my way, I should burn all the books of Aristotle, for the study of them can lead to a loss of time, produce error, and increase ignorance."

Seventeenth-century pioneers of the new science railed against Aristotle's millennial reign as the unassailable master of thought because they recognized that despite his glorified reputation—or because of it—Aristotle had contributed significantly to the stultification of intellectual development.

Aristotle's all-encompassing authority was upheld for nearly two thousand years, influencing Christian and Islamic philosophies and establishing a royal dogma in cosmology, physics, chemistry, biology and medicine. Elaborating on EMPEDOCLES's concept of four basic elements (earth, air, fire and water), Aristotle developed a theory of disease based on four "humors" (designated as blood, phlegm, white bile and black bile) and four "qualities" (cold, hot, moist and dry). These principles were accepted and applied to physiology, pathology and clinical medicine until the early 1700s, even though contradictory evidence was available long before then.

It has been said that Aristotle's greatest disservice to science was his total reliance on the power of pure reason. To determine the speed of falling objects he tested a leaf and a stone, an experiment of limited validity from which he concluded that objects of greater weight fall faster than objects of lesser weight. Two thousand years later Galileo was met with considerable resistance when he proved otherwise. When Aristotle finally lost his title in the scientific revolution, observation began to take precedence over theory. In 1662 the Royal Society was incorporated as the Royal Society of London for Improving Natural Knowledge, adopting as its motto a line from Horace: *Nullius in verba* ("words are of no account").

Aristotle's investigations in the biological sciences, and particularly embryology, were somewhat better grounded than were his pronouncements in physics, mainly as a result of his methods of observation. Considered the first to conduct systematic animal dissections, he repudiated the concept that fetuses are miniature, preformed adults, and that their sex is determined by the position in the womb. On the whole, however, Aristotle's biological teachings are based on incomplete investigation or misguided information. Declaring medicine a theoretical science, Aristotle, along with Plato, his mentor, is often blamed for the disassociation of medicine from the physical sciences, as well as the class distinction between physicians and surgical practitioners.

Born in Stagira, Aristotle was the son of noted physician Nicomachus, who served in the royal court of Greek Macedonia. When Aristotle was orphaned at the age of seventeen he was sent to Athens to study at Plato's academy, where he joined in intellectual dialogues with Plato and Socrates for the next twenty years. After Plato's death Aristotle traveled through Greece and Asia Minor until 342 B.C., when he accepted a position as tutor for Alexander, the thirteen-year-old son of the king of Macedonia, who grew up to become Alexander the Great.

At the age of 52 Aristotle left for Athens to establish the Lyceum, an institute for education and research where he conducted an exhaustive and systematic investigation of plants and animals. It is based on these studies that he derived the voluminous collection of biological information and misinformation that led to the construction of his *Scala Naturae* ("Scale of Being"). Classifying organisms by their degree of complexity, Aristotle's hierarchical organization of the living world established the principle of a natural order that is perhaps his greatest contribution to science, even though the order he suggested seems far from what modern science could find useful.

Salvino Armato 1245–c. 1300

Although the question remains open to speculation, many historians are convinced that the first pair of eyeglasses was created by Salvino Armato, an Italian physicist and glassmaker. There is evidence to suggest that a comparable device may have existed in ancient China or Greece, but it is widely believed that the first pair of corrective eye lenses appeared in Europe sometime between 1280 and 1290. Disputing Armato's priority in the invention, some references suggest that the idea originated with the English scientist and philosopher Roger Bacon (1214–1294).

A noted scientist with advanced training in optical physics, Armato impaired his sight in the year 1280 during a series of light refraction studies in which he acted as his own experimental subject. Armato is thought to have trained himself as a glass craftsman in order to fashion a pair of lenses that would compensate for his visual defects.

The crude but effective result was an unattached pair of thick glass circles with biconvex surfaces, held in place only by facial muscles and sheer will. For centuries eyeglass wearers struggled with various cords and leather straps, but it was not until the eighteenth century that the refinement of a rigid frame was developed.

As word spread of the remarkable device that would alleviate failing vision by simple magnification, the art of making eyeglasses took hold, catering to nobility and the clergy. The optician's practice was still a long way off, however, as the correction of vision remained outside the scope of the medical profession throughout the Middle Ages. The customer determined his own prescription by selecting a suitable pair of lenses from the collection of the local glass craftsman.

Over the next century the rounded circles of glass became known as *lenticchie*, the Italian word for "lentil," which would later serve as the root for the word "lens." Functioning essentially as magnifiers, these "glass lentils" were of no use in correcting the problem of nearsightedness, in which the eye cannot form a focused image of objects beyond a certain distance.

To correct nearsightedness the lenses must be made of concave glass so that the light rays will diverge slightly, causing distant objects to appear closer to the eye. Introduced in the fifteenth century, these lenses were rarer and far more expensive than convex eyeglasses, but money was certainly no object for the extravagant and extremely nearsighted Cardinal Giovanni de Medici. When he became Pope Leo X he commissioned Raphael to paint his portrait with his glasses on his nose, thus initiating the first depiction of concave lenses in art.

Asclepios (variations: Aesculapius, Asclepius, Asklepios)

> They came to him with ulcers the flesh had grown, or their limbs mangled with the gray bronze, or bruised with the stone flung from afar,
> or the body stormed with summer fever, or chill; and he released each man and led him
> from his individual grief. Some he treated with guile of incantations,
> some with healing potions to drink; or he tended the limbs with salves
> from near and far; and some by the knife he set on their feet again.
> But even genius is tied to profit. Someone
> turned even Asclepios with a winning price, showing the gold in his hand,
> to bring back from death a man
> already gone. But Kronion, with a cast of his hand, tore life from the hearts of both men
> instantly, and the shining thunder dashed them to death.
> With our mortal minds we should seek from the gods that which becomes us,
> knowing the way of the destiny ever at our feet.
>
> [Pindar, *Pythian*, 3.1–68 ASKLEPIOS [Richmond Lattimore])

Asclepios was worshipped in ancient Greece as the god of medicine, although, for a healer of mankind, his origins and his fate were not as noble as one might suppose. He was the son of Apollo and Koronis; before giving birth, his mother was murdered by his father in a fit of jealous rage. Apollo managed to save their unborn child, however, and he delivered him into the care and tutelage of Cheiron, the good Centaur. It was there that Asclepios learned the fundamentals of medicine and perfected his skills in the art of healing. He is referred to as a deified hero or a heroized god, depending on the account. His wife is alternately known as Epione (Soother of Pain) or Xanthe. Homer mentions two sons, Podaleiros and Machaon, both surgeons, and other authors refer to his daughters, Hygieia (Health), Iaso (Healing), Panakeia (Cure-all), and to a child-deity, Telesphoros (Convalescence).

His enthusiasm for healing brought about an unfortunate end for Asclepios. He was asked by Artemis to restore to life her beloved Hippolytos, and was offered an enormous sum of money as inducement. Unfortunately for Asclepios, his talents were great enough to accomplish the task, thereby enraging Zeus, who, with a bolt of lightning, banished Asclepios to the netherworld.

In 420 B.C. the worship of Asclepios was introduced in Athens, where temples, called Aesclepieia, were erected and spread throughout Greece. These were more like sanatoria than traditional places of worship, and they became models for later hospitals and medical schools.

Oral instruction in the medical arts was offered, as well as treatment for the sick, all provided by the temple priests, or Asclepiads. Drugs were administered and surgery performed, but more often patients were treated to baths, massage, fresh air, sunlight, pure water, good food and large doses of religious and magical ritual. A cure for blindness was said to be effected by giving the patient a special tablet on which he should cast his eyes. The patient's joy at recovering his sight must have been tempered by the fact that on the tablet was written an order to donate a large sum of money to the temple.

It is difficult to determine what proportion of medicine could be found in the practices of the Asclepiads or to know how much of the ills that were treated were psychologically based. Infertility, impotence, headache and skin disease were among the more common ailments that were "cured." It should be mentioned that the Aesclepieia refused entry to the dying, and to pregnant women, who were put in the care of midwives.

It is said that Rome imported the deity in 295 B.C. to defend itself against the stubborn plague that was decimating the population. A temple was built in his honor, and his name was corrupted into Aesculapius.

Eugene Aserinsky 1921–
Nathaniel Kleitman 1895–

Among the earliest pioneers in the field of sleep research, physiologist Eugene Aserinsky and physician Nathaniel Kleitman collaborated on the first systematic investigation of the patterns of neural activity in sleep. Launched in 1953, their influential study established a scientific basis for the recurring period during sleep that is characterized by rapid eye movements.

Commonly referred to as "REM sleep," the phenomenon had been observed even in Ancient Egypt, but Aserinsky and Kleitman were the first to recognize the behavior as an indicator of complex neurological activity. Rejecting the prevailing notion of sleep as a passive state brought on by an absence of stimulus, they speculated that the eye movements reflected a series of mental events occurring as part of a regular pattern of sleep.

As their suspicions were confirmed experimentally Aserinsky and Kleitman discovered that, in humans, sleep alternates between two distinct phases; a period of dreaming in which rapid eye movements and occasionally limb movements occur, and a dreamless phase in which there is little sensory or muscular activity. In subsequent studies by Michel Jouvet, Stephen LaBerge, Graeme Mitchison and FRANCIS CRICK it was established that a certain amount of REM sleep was required in humans, as well as in almost all animals having some form of neocortex. Despite the explosion of sleep and dream research in the three decades since Kleitman and Aserinsky introduced the notion of sleep patterns, REM sleep remains an elusive subject. It is still referred to occasionally as "paradoxical sleep," denoting the phenomenon of dreaming, in which a portion of the cortex is fully activated despite the absence of sensory input.

A native of New York City, Aserinsky was a fellow at the University of Chicago when he met Kleitman in 1951. Focusing mainly on the behavioral patterns and neural functions associated with dreaming, Aserinsky introduced the first objective techniques for experimental sleep research.

Kleitman, concerned mainly with the physiology of sleep, devised methods of "dream measurement," including studies of conditioned reflexes and diurnal cycles of body temperature. Born in the town of Kishinev, near Odessa in southern Russia, Kleitman was twenty years old when he arrived in the United States. After attending the College of the City of New York and Columbia University he completed his doctoral studies in physiology and pharmacology at the University of Chicago. The author of *Sleep Characteristics* (1937) and *Sleep and Wakefulness* (1939), Kleitman worked at the Naval Medical Research Institute in Bethesda, Maryland, while also serving as professor of physiology at the University of Chicago.

Avenzoar (abu-Marwan abd al-Malik ibn Abu'l-Ala Zuhr) 1094–1162

Born at the turn of the twelfth century in Seville, Spain, Avenzoar ranks among the most influential Islamic physicians in history. His family, the Zuhrs, produced a number of important physicians, including Avenzoar's daughter and granddaughter, as well as his father, Abu'l-Ala Zuhr, a Jewish physician recognized for his contributions to the advancement of medicine in the Middle Ages.

Like AVICENNA and RHAZES, Avenzoar worked as medical supervisor of a hospital, where he had the opportunity to observe patients over extended periods of time, tracking the progression of countless diseases. Noted for his clinical acumen, he was the first physician to observe and describe a number of pathological conditions, including diseases of the uterus, cancer of the stomach, and pericarditis. Although he lacked a foundation in chemistry, his writings, particularly on pharmacology and nutrition, are still relevant today. Perhaps most notable, however, was Avenzoar's rejection of many of the doctrines that had been reverently embraced and passed down through the centuries. Prevailing Arabic medical practices generally followed the methods established by the Greeks and Romans. Avenzoar rejected many of the doctrines of ARISTOTLE and Avicenna, questioning some of GALEN'S teachings as well. Condemning the use of astrology and other mystical principles commonly applied in conventional Arabic medicine, Avenzoar stressed clinical practice based on experience and observation rather than textbook and tradition.

Translated into Hebrew and Latin, Avenzoar's writings, documenting his rational, practical teachings, were influential throughout medieval Europe.

Averroës (Averrhoes, also Abul-al-Walid Muhammad ibn-Ahmad ibn-Rushd) 1126–1198

Averroës was an Islamic physician and philosopher who exerted enormous influence on the development of civilization among Christians and Jews as well as within his own culture. Initiating centuries of controversy among Western scholars, his interpretation and commentaries on Aristotelian philosophy also contributed to the establishment of a major Islamic religious sect known as the Mutazlites.

The Mutazlites, upheld the neo-Platonic view that truth can be derived from reason rather than faith, an approach considered heretical by both Islam and Christianity. Repudiating the notion of personal immortality, Averroës also maintained that in death the soul merged with the universe; for such heresies he was banished from North Africa. With the assistance of his celebrated student Maimonides Averroës sought refuge in a Jewish community in Spain, where he taught in hiding for many years. When the Jews were later expelled from Spain, Averroës' philosophical doctrine was spread throughout Europe.

Integrating the scholarship of Arabs, Iranians, Turks, Muslims, Christians and Jews, Islamic science had been established as a powerful international force since the middle of the eighth century, drawing from the rich and varied traditions of Greece, Persia, India and China. Guided by the belief that the quality of knowledge is determined by the quality of human nature, Islamic philosophy placed great importance on a fundamental understanding of mankind as obtained through psychology and medicine. The philosopher-physician therefore held a position of authority, as seen in the great respect accorded to Averroës, Rhazes, and Avicenna. Attempting to organize and systematize the scientific knowledge available, all three produced compendiums of medical information and observations. Averroës's work was widely read in Latin translation under the title *Colliget* (*Collected Works*).

The son of a Muslim magistrate, or *cadi*, Averroës was born in Cordoba, Spain, where he himself served as a cadi. He was also an influential teacher at Cordoba's university, bringing rationalism and pantheism to the study of law and medicine as well as philosophy. Averroës also served as cadi at Seville and in Morocco.

After a long period of exile Averroës was pardoned for his heresies by the accession of a new and more tolerant caliph. Restored to his position of privilege, Averroës remained in Morocco until his death in 1198.

Oswald Theodore Avery 1877–1955

Oswald Avery played a pivotal role in one of the major advances in the history of medicine. In 1944, after years of experimentation, Avery announced his discovery that the vehicle of genetic inheritance was deoxyribonucleic acid, or DNA.

Avery, born in Nova Scotia, Canada, was the son of an evangelical minister. Commanded by the divine voice of "The Master in His Providence," Oswald's father moved his family to the Lower East Side of New York City to follow his calling at the Mariners' Temple on Henry Street. An uninspired student, Oswald graduated from Colgate University in 1900, earning his degree in medicine from the Columbia College for Physicians and Surgeons. He practiced briefly as a physician but was demoralized by the limited effectiveness of clinical medicine.

While serving as associate director at the Hoagland Laboratory in Brooklyn Avery began investigating the chemical composition of pathogenic bacteria. In 1913 SIMON FLEXNER invited Avery to participate in the pneumonia research being conducted at the Rockefeller Institute under his supervision. Avery, who was to remain at the Institute for thirty-five years, made his first observations on the chemical aspects of biological specificity in 1917.

The prevailing notion among the scientific establishment was that nucleic acids were undifferentiated, inert substances, and that agents of biochemical change were most likely to be some form of protein. As early as 1936 Avery began to suspect otherwise, while investigating the remarkable findings of British bacteriologist Frederick Griffith. In an experimental study of the different forms of pneumococci Griffith had injected mice with a mixture of two pneumocoaccal types, one a "rough-shaped" (R) colony of live, nonvirulent pneumococci, the other a "smooth-shaped" (S) colony of formerly virulent but now dead pneumococci. Griffith reported that although the injection should have been harmless, many of the mice died. An examination of their blood revealed only live virulent S colonies of pneumococci. Once injected, the nonvirulent microorganisms had been transformed into the virulent strain with which they had been mixed. The phenomenon was compounded by the fact that, in laboratory cultures, the newly recovered S colonies produced successive generations of virulent S colonies of pneumococci.

Along with the rest of the scientific world, Avery recognized the enormous impact of this discovery. Reproducing Griffith's work in his own laboratory, he set out in search of "the transforming principle." In 1944, after satisfactorily proving to himself and his colleagues that his findings were valid, he published an article in the *Journal of Experimental Medicine* entitled "Induction of Transformation by a Deoxyribonucleic Acid Fraction Isolated from Pneumococcus Type III."

Avery's demonstration that DNA is the vector of genetic information led to a flood of innovative research in the fields of microbiology, epidemiology, histochemistry and molecular genetics. His work influenced the major breakthroughs of the next few decades, most notably the discovery of the crystalline structure of DNA, announced in 1953 by JAMES WATSON and FRANCIS CRICK.

Avicenna (Ibn Sina) 980–1037

An Islamic philosopher and scientist of Persian origin, Avicenna exerted a far-reaching and enduring influence on the development of medicine with his monumental body of writings.

It is reported that he was a child prodigy who mastered the Koran before he was ten years old and challenged the precepts of ARISTOTLE and GALEN while still a young student in Baghdad. When he was twenty-one he published the first of his writings, the *Kitab ash-Shifa* ("The Book of Healing"), a massive encyclopedia of philosophic and scientific knowledge and the first of his major written works.

Avicenna's most celebrated text is his medical encyclopedia, entitled *Kitab al Qanun fi't-tibb* ("The Canon of Medicine"), which was such a comprehensive and definitive reference that it formed the basis of European medical classification and university curriculum until the mid- seventeenth century. A rigorously organized compilation of clinical, pathological and postmortem observations, the Canon describes an astonishing number of morbid conditions, with detailed discussions of symptoms, causes, diagnostic methods, prevention, cures, and theoretical commentary.

Julius Axelrod 1912–

Julius Axelrod was a member of the team that discovered norepinephrine (sometimes called noradrenalin), a hormone involved with the transmission of impulses in the sympathetic nervous system. He shared the 1970 Nobel prize for Physiology and Medicine with his colleagues ULF VON EULER and Sir Bernard Katz for this important research.

After growing up in poverty Axelrod was refused admission to American medical schools because of a prevailing quota on Jewish applicants. He pursued chemical pharmacology instead, obtaining a master's degree in 1941, and in 1955 he became chief of the Pharmacology Division of the National Institute of Mental Health. Axelrod's research in the areas of neurophysiology and neuropharmacology helped lay the groundwork in the ongoing search for cures for schizophrenia and hypertension.

B

Joseph François Felix Babinski 1857–1922

The second half of the nineteenth century witnessed many important discoveries in the field of neurological medicine, but it was not until the very end of that era that the French neurologist Joseph Babinski described a foot reflex, now considered a vital part of any neurological examination. Known today as "Babinski's sign", the reflex may signal brain or spinal cord disease, usually organic hemiplegia (paralyses affecting only one side of the body). When one side of the sole is stroked from heel to toe, the big toe extends upward and the other toes fan out. The reflex is normal only in infants, and in that case it is known as the plantar reflex. "Babinski's sign" also refers to a reflex of the forearm and indicates a lesion of the spinal cord.

Babinski also conducted research with the Viennese pharmacologist Alfred Frohlich, and together they identified the endocrine disorder adiposo-genital dystrophy, known also as Babinski-Frohlich disease. The condition is marked by metabolic disturbances, obesity, and changes in secondary sex characteristics.

Karl Ernst von Baer 1792–1876

Considered one of the founding fathers of modern embryology, Karl von Baer originated theories of developmental biology that greatly advanced scientific understanding of the processes of fertilization and evolution. Directly influencing the work of such eminent scientists as THEODOR SCHWANN and Charles Darwin, von Baer introduced the germ layer theory, based on the concept of epigenesis, an idea first introduced by WILLIAM HARVEY in 1651.

Born at Piep, in Estonia, von Baer studied in his own country at the University of Dorpat, and later at the University of Wurzburg in Germany. After teaching at Wurzburg and at Konigsberg, in 1834 he joined the faculty at the University of St. Petersburg in Russia.

The advent of improved achromatic lenses in the early nineteenth century made possible von Baer's historic observation of the mammalian ovum and his discovery of the notochord, a primitive axis of the fetal body. In 1827 Von Baer dissected a follicle removed from the ovary of a dog, which was a milestone in the study of fertilization and the science of embryology.

Von Baer's detailed studies of the stages of developmental process corroborated the doctrine of epigenesis. In opposition to the notion of "pre-formation," this theory maintains that a structureless cell develops by the successive formation and addition of physiologically differentiated tissues not present in the fertilized ovum. With Christian Heinrich Pander (1794–1865), Karl von Baer introduced the "germ layer theory," suggesting that heterogeneous structural layers, or "germ layers," in the embryo eventually give rise to "adult" forms. Maintaining that all animal life developed from one germ, a single common form, von Baer argued that generalized structure developed into specialized structure.

In his two-volume work, entitled *Uber Entwickelungs geschicte der Thiere* (On the Developmental History of Animals), Von Baer asserted that the embryo of a chick, for example, passes from an archetypal animal form common to all vertebrates, to a more specialized form common to birds, and finally to the form specific to chickens. This view contradicted the theory of "recapitulation," a popular biological doctrine of the time, which was based on the belief that ontogeny, the pattern of embryological development, imitates phylogeny, the developmental pattern of the animal's species.

Although he was to oppose aspects of Darwin's doctrine, von Baer provided insight and observation that was greatly instrumental in the formulation of the theory of evolution. Two embryological structures carry von Baer's name: "Baer's cavity," the opening beneath the blastoderm, and "Baer's vesicle," the ovarian follicle containing the ovum.

Sara Josephine Baker 1873–1945

Sara Josephine Baker, a pioneering medical investigator, was born in 1873 to a well-to-do family in Poughkeepsie, N.Y. Like many women of her time and station, she assumed that she would attend college and be married soon after graduation. Her life took a dramatic turn, however, when her brother and father both died the year that Baker turned sixteen. It is not known whether her father's death from typhoid fever served as her inspiration to pursue a medical career, but this she did despite the opposition of family and friends.

Baker received her degree from the Women's Medical College in New York, but her new practice did not attract many patients. In 1901 she took a job as a New York City medical inspector and was placed in "Hell's Kitchen" to inspect tenement dwellers for contagious diseases such as dysentery, influenza, smallpox, and typhoid fever. Her fieldwork was grueling but enlightening, and she gained the distinction of tracking down

"Typhoid Mary," the cook who was responsible for spreading the disease to a number of households in which she worked. The intrepid Baker was soon appointed assistant commissioner of health, but the fact that she was a woman immediately prompted her all-male staff to resign. Her dedication was persuasive, however, and she convinced them to return, gaining ever more respect as she designed innovative programs to improve public health.

Preventive medicine was a new concept at the turn of the century, and it was Baker who saw the urgent need for educating the public in matters of hygiene, nutrition and infant care. She instituted a program of free milk distribution, created a baby formula that mothers could easily make at home, licensed midwives and offered a program called the "Little Mothers' League" that provided health information for children caring for their younger siblings. In discovering the dangers of the current style of infant clothing, Baker devised an alternative design that opened all the way down the front. She also invented a safe and sanitary means of packaging the eye-drop solution used to prevent gonorrheal infection in babies.

Baker's commitment to child health care produced dramatic results: By the end of her tenure, New York had the lowest infant mortality rate in the United States and Europe. Baker helped found the Federal Children's Bureau and Public Health Service, which led to today's Department of Health and Human Services. Many of her programs were adopted throughout the country and eventually throughout the world.

Baker represented the United States on the Health Committee of the League of Nations from 1922 to 1924 and was president of the American Medical Women's Association in 1935–36. She was also a member of the suffragette delegation that obtained Woodrow Wilson's endorsement of the Nineteenth Amendment. Continuing to work and write until her death in 1945, she published many books and articles, including an autobiography called *Fighting for Life*.

David Baltimore 1938–

"My life is dedicated to increasing knowledge," said microbiologist David Baltimore. "We need no more justification for scientific research than that. My motivating force is not that I will find a "cure' for cancer. There may never be a cure as such. I work because I want to understand."

For his ground-breaking investigation of how viruses radically alter the nature of normal cells, Baltimore was awarded the 1975 Nobel Prize for Physiology or Medicine, which he shared with Howard Temin and RENATO DULBECCO.

Following the revolution in molecular biology during the late 1950s (see FRANCIS HARRY COMPTON CRICK), a fundamental tenet of the new genetic doctrine held that hereditary information is transferred in a specific sequence, passing from DNA to RNA to proteins. In May 1970, Baltimore and Temin presented the results of independent studies, each demonstrating that genetic information can also travel in reverse, transmitting a message from RNA to DNA.

Because the need had not yet presented itself, scientists ignored the possibility of a reversed flow of information until 1964, when Howard Temin dared to contradict scientific doctrine. Based on his investigations of animal cancers, Temin suggested that when a tumor-causing virus enters a cell, the RNA of the virus makes DNA copies of itself, thereby causing the host cell to become cancerous. Because the idea was widely interpreted as a violation of the "central dogma" of genetics, it was scornfully dismissed by most of the scientific establishment, with the notable exception of David Baltimore.

A 26-year-old doctoral student, Baltimore had "no experience in the field and so no axe to grind," as he later recalled. Launching an investigation of the Rauscher murine leukemia virus, he explored Temin's suggestion that some viruses carry a particular enzyme allowing them to duplicate their own RNA in the DNA of their host cell. The theory was confirmed simultaneously by Baltimore and Temin, who announced their findings within days of each other at conventions a thousand miles apart, in New York and Texas, respectively.

Born in New York City, Baltimore studied chemistry at Swarthmore College and the Massachussetts Institute of Technology. Transferring to the Rockefeller Institute (now Rockefeller University), he joined with molecular biophysicist Richard Franklin in investigating RNA growth in animal viruses.

After receiving his doctorate in 1964 Baltimore served a year as postdoctoral fellow at Albert Einstein Medical College in New York, then joined the research staff at the Salk Institute for Biological Studies in California. It was there that he first met Dulbecco, a distinguished pioneer in experimental technique who would serve as mentor to both his fellow Nobel laureates at different points in their careers.

Continuing his investigation of RNA virus replication, Baltimore returned to M.I.T. in 1968 as associate professor of microbiology. For more than four years he had focused his research on the viral group that includes the poliovirus and the Mengo virus, following an assumption that all RNA viruses shared a basic biological similarity, but by 1970 a number of significantly different genetic systems had been reported. Shifting his attention to the variations in these systems, Baltimore began a classification process, distinguishing RNA viruses according to their particular needs for replication.

It was in the course of investigating the radical transformation of cells infected by a tumor-causing virus that Baltimore discovered evidence of what would later be termed "reverse transcription" and "reverse transcriptase enzyme"—the essential ingredient in the process.

A month after their independent demonstrations, Baltimore and Temin published a report of their findings in the June 27, 1970 issue of *Nature*, a British scientific journal. Almost immediately reverse transcription became a prime focus of research in virology, oncology, genetics, pharmacology and molecular biology. Their work had given rise to a surge of optimism in cancer research, but both Baltimore and Temin remained skeptical of the theory of viruses as the cause of cancer in humans.

Baltimore became a full professor at M.I.T. in 1972 and a year later was granted a lifetime research professorship by the American Cancer Society. Distinguished by then as one of the country's leading scientists, Baltimore had become increasingly concerned about the potential dangers of recombinant DNA technology, a powerful and rapidly developing genetic research technique that offered the promise of immeasurable gains for humanity as well as the threat of devastation.

Calling for a demonstration of responsibility on the part of the scientific community, Baltimore joined with ten other molecular biologists to campaign for "autoregulation" in genetic engineering research. At press conferences and in open letters the distinguished group of scientists urged a temporary ban on certain experimental practices, warning that recombinant DNA techniques made it possible to create "new types of infectious DNA elements whose biological properties cannot be completely predicted in advance."

Strongly opposed to the development of new weapons of biological warfare, Baltimore brought attention to the moral and ethical considerations of genetic engineering. "This is a challenge we must meet," he declared. "Many of us grew up with the question of the moral correctness of the atomic bomb." He also expressed concern that the identification of what he called "subtle genetic factors in the makeup of human beings" could erode our "basic concepts of equality."

In February 1975 an international conference was held at the Asilomar conference center in Southern California to establish guidelines for the voluntary regulation of recombinant DNA experimentation. "Many are looking to this meeting for guidance," Baltimore declared in his opening address. "If we don't provide it, we'll have left a serious void." By the following year a Recombinant DNA Advisory Committee was established by the National Institutes of Health to regulate safety standards in federally funded genetic research. The committee elected Baltimore to its board in 1979.

In addition to serving as editor of the *Journal of Virology* and the *Journal of Molecular Biology*, Baltimore is a member of the American Academy of Arts and Sciences, the National Academy of Sciences, the American Society for Microbiologists, the American Association for the Advancement of Science, and the Pontifical Academy of Science. In 1982 he was appointed director of the Whitehead Institute for Biomedical Research, where he has contributed significant advances in genetics, virology and immunology, most notably in the development of synthetic vaccines.

Sir Frederick Grant Banting 1891–1941

When Frederick Banting and his assistant, Charles Best, began to study the mysterious "insular spots" on the pancreas they took the first great step toward a discovery that would save the lives of millions of diabetics.

Through experimental research they determined that these spots on the pancreas, the "isles of Langerhans," secrete a substance that regulates the metabolism of glucose. Diabetes, the condition in which a patient is unable to transform sugar in the blood into fuel, was considered a fatal disease of the pancreas. At the time of Banting's experiments, one consistent but baffling phenomenon had been observed. The insular spots on the pancreas were noticeably shriveled in the bodies of diabetics but of normal size in those who had died of other causes. It was Banting who sensed that the solution to the problem of diabetes lay buried in this fact.

Born on a farm near Alliston, Ontario, Banting was so eager to serve his country in World War I that he left medical school in 1915 to enlist as a private. He was ordered to return and complete his medical education at the University of Toronto. The following year he reenlisted, as a certified doctor, in the Canadian Army medical corps of the 44th battalion. When he returned home, he joined the Toronto Children's Hospital as a surgical resident.

Determined to open up a private practice, Banting moved to London, Ontario, where he had little success in attracting patients. In a desperate attempt to supplement his income, Banting took the position of part-time lecturer in pharmacology at Western Ontario Medical School, although he felt ill-equipped for the job. Keeping one step ahead of his students, he secured all the information he could on diabetes in preparation for an upcoming lecture. His reading inspired him to propose a research experiment to his superior, Professor J.J.R. Macleod.

Assisted by Charles Best, a recent medical graduate with expertise in chemistry, Banting extracted the substance produced in the isles of Langerhans. When he injected the extract into a dog dying from diabetes, he saw an immediate effect: The sugar in the animal's blood decreased, producing a dramatic improvement in its condition. Rejoicing at the discovery of this remarkable "elixir," Banting and Best named it isletin, meaning "island chemical," and set about refining its application for human patients.

Taking the pancreatic glands from among the rejected organs of slaughtered cattle, Banting extracted the isletin and found that it kept diabetic dogs alive. His next step was to experiment on his friend and colleague, Joe Gilchrist, who was in the final, painful stages of the disease. The success of this experiment brought widespread attention to Banting's discovery. Professor Macleod presented a report on the substance to the Association of American Physicians, changing the name chosen by Banting and Best to its Latin version, insulin.

Macleod took over supervision of the research project while Banting and Best continued to develop and refine their technique of treatment. Because the delicate balance needed for proper sugar metabolism was difficult to determine, mistakes were likely to be dangerous. Excessive doses of insulin could lower sugar levels to such a point that the patient might suffer violent shock and convulsions. If not treated immediately, this condition, known as insulin shock, can cause death in a short period of time. The purification of insulin for clinical use was ultimately accomplished by another member of Macleod's group, James B. Collip.

When, in 1922, he and Macleod were jointly awarded the Nobel Prize for Medicine, Banting immediately sent half of his prize money to Best and Macleod gave half of his share to Collip, thus acknowledging the importance of their assistants' participation. In recognition of Banting's contribution to medicine the Canadian government endowed him with an annuity of $1,500.00 and established the Banting Research Foundation to carry on his work. An institute in Toronto was founded in his honor in 1930, and in 1934 Banting was named a Knight Commander of the Order of the British Empire. The following year he was made a fellow of the Royal Society.

Banting modestly accepted the flood of honors, never allowing his fame to interfere with the continuation of his work. He pursued other areas of medical research, producing valuable findings on the cortex of the adrenal glands, silicosis and cancer.

When World War II began, Banting's research studies in the field of aviation medicine had already begun to capture the attention of his colleagues. At the age of 48 he enlisted in military service once again, this time as a major. Banting chaired a committee established to coordinate medical research being done in England and in Canada. He also helped organize the supply of blood for transfusions in military hospitals.

To help dive-bomber crews better endure rapid and drastic altitude changes, the Royal Air Force requested Banting's assistance. Bound for England, Frederick Banting was killed in a plane crash in February, 1941.

Robert Bárány 1876–1936

Robert Bárány's investigation of the interior structure of the ear led to important advances in diagnostic technique and internal surgery. By studying the functions of the inner ear and its interaction with the cerebellum Bárány was able to devise diagnostic tests for diseases of the inner ear, and he became the first to treat otosclerosis, one of the leading causes of deafness.

Born and educated in Austria, Bárány joined the faculty at the University of Vienna in 1909 as a lecturer on diseases of the ear. In March 1915, while in charge of an Austrian field hospital at Przemysl, Bárány was taken prisoner by the Russians. It was in a prisoner-of-war camp in Siberia that he learned that he had been awarded the 1914 Nobel Prize for medicine in recognition of his pioneering studies of the inner ear.

After his release Bárány was invited to join Uppsala University in Sweden. In 1917 he became a Swedish subject and took over directorship of the Ear, Nose, and Throat Clinic at Uppsala. He also taught otology at the university, remaining there until his death in 1936.

Bárány was particularly interested in the balancing apparatus of the inner ear, and his work led to important discoveries in the etiology of seasickness. Through extensive experimentation Bárány conclusively traced its cause to a disturbance of the endolymph in the semicircular canals.

Bárány's written works include *Physiologie und Pathologie des Bogengang-Apparats beim Menschen (Physiology and Pathology of the Apparatus of the Inner Ear in Humans).*

Christiaan Neethling Barnard 1922–

On December 3, 1967, South African surgeon Christiaan Barnard made history when he performed the first human-heart transplant operation at Groote Schuur Hospital in Cape Town. His patient, Louis Washkansky, died of pneumonia eighteen days later, but the transplant was considered a medical milestone. Barnard's second patient, Philip Blaiberg, lived for 594 days, and in the five years that followed more than a hundred heart transplants were performed around the world.

Barnard was lionized by the press, but the heart-transplant procedure stirred great controversy in the medical establishment. Its detractors pointed out that although the design of the operation was technically feasible, it was medically unsound because it did not solve the immunological problems of transplantation. By 1977 nearly all heart recipients had died, mainly due to the body's rejection of the transplanted organ. Today, scientific progress has made this less of a problem.

The son of a Dutch Reform minister, Barnard was born at Beaufort West and studied medicine at the University of Cape Town. After receiving his degree in 1952 he pursued advanced training at the University of Minnesota, studying under OWEN H. WANGENSTEEN and C. WALTON LILLEHEI, two of the leading authorities in cardiac surgery. Barnard completed the intensive five-year program in under three years, obtaining his doctorate in surgery in 1958. It has been suggested that the intensity of his academic diligence and professional ambition was due in part to a progressive condition of arthritis that imposed a time limit on his career as a surgeon.

Returning to Cape Town, Barnard was appointed director of surgical research at Groote Schuur Hospital, where he designed several artificial heart valves and developed techniques for surgical transplantation. Handicapped by the long-threatening arthritis, he abandoned surgical practice in 1983 at the age of sixty.

Murray Llewellyn Barr 1908 –
Ewart George Bartram 1923–

In 1949 Murray Barr and Ewart George Bartram demonstrated that there is a small piece of chromatin at the edge of the nucleus in all human female cells. This has come to be known as the Barr body or extra X chromosome of females. It is this X chromosome that allows doctors to determine the sex of an unborn baby through amniocentesis. While in the womb fetuses shed epithelia, or layers of cells, into the surrounding amniotic fluid. In amniocentesis a needle punctures the abdominal wall and extracts samples of amniotic fluid. If the cells in this fluid contain Barr bodies, the fetus must be female.

James Barry 1797–1865

Dr. James Barry practiced as a medical officer in the British army and enjoyed a reputation as an impressive marksman as well as a skilled surgeon. His fifty-year medical career won the respect of colleagues and patients, but the autopsy performed after his death revealed an astonishing secret: James Barry was a woman. The War Department and the Medical Association were embarrassed by Barry's successful masquerade and the prejudices that had made it necessary for a woman who wanted to pursue a medical career in the nineteenth century.

Bartholin (Bartholinus)
Kaspar 1585–1629
Thomas 1616–1680
Kaspar 1655–1738

The Bartholins were a family of distinguished Scandinavian physicians whose medical tradition began with Kaspar Bartholin in 1585. Born in Malmo, Sweden, the extraordinary range of Kaspar's interests led him to attend all of the most prominent universities in Scandinavia. In 1611 he wrote an anatomy textbook entitled *Institutiones Anatomicae*. He refused professorships in anatomy, philosophy and Greek, but, settling in Copenhagen, he became a professor of medicine in 1613 and of theology in 1624.

Kaspar Bartholin's son Thomas was born in Copenhagen but traveled extensively as a student and teacher of medicine, anatomy, philology, and mathematics. His best-known work is his study of the lymphatic system, in which he confirmed Pecquet's discovery of the thoracic duct, one of the two major trunks from which the lymph drains into the bloodstream. He disliked the life of a traveling lecturer, and in 1661 retired to the countryside. It was there that his library and many of his unpublished manuscripts were destroyed by a devastating fire.

Thomas Bartholin's son Kaspar became a professor of physiology at Copenhagen and is credited with the discovery of an accessory duct of the sublingual salivary gland, as well as the pair of glands located in the vagina, now known as the glands of Bartholin.

Clara Barton 1821–1912

Clara Barton, who was to become a model of heroic nursing and the founder of the American Red Cross, began her professional life as a schoolteacher in her native Massachussetts at the age of eighteen. In 1854 she left teaching to become a clerk at the U.S. Patent Office. When the Civil War began several years later, Barton initiated a program to send supplies to the soldiers and soon joined their ranks as a nurse, tending to patients both in army camps and at the front.

Barton's compassion and efficiency earned her a reputation as the "Angel of the Battlefield." Word of her devotion reached Abraham Lincoln, who, in 1865, enlisted her aid in tracking down missing prisoners. Her thorough search led to the identification of thousands of the dead at Andersonville Prison.

In 1870 Barton was attending a conference in Europe when the Franco-Prussian War broke out. She spent the next three years working for the International Red Cross behind German lines. When she returned to the United States she organized the American National Red Cross, officially established in 1881. The following year she campaigned strenuously for President Chester A. Arthur to sign the Geneva treaty that provided for care of the wounded on the battlefield. Clara Barton presided over the American Red Cross until 1904. During her tenure she continually strove to improve the standards of nursing education and practice, stressing the need for the Red Cross to lend support during natural disasters as well as during wartime.

William Bateson 1861–1926

In his inaugural address to the Third Conference on Hybridization and Plant Breeding in 1906, the English zoologist William Bateson stated:

> I suggest for the consideration of this congress the term Genetics, which sufficiently indicates that our labors are devoted to the elucidation of the phenomena of heredity and variation: In other words to the physiology of descent, with implied bearing on the theoretical problems of the evolutionist and the systematist, and application to the practical problems of the breeder, whether of animals or of plants.

Actually, Bateson first used the word "genetics" in a letter written a year earlier, to describe the subject of his current investigations. It was, however, his inaugural address that launched a revolutionary new discipline, assuring Bateson's place in history as one of the founding fathers of genetics. In 1908 Cambridge University made him the first professor of genetics. Three years later, with English biologist and colleague R.C. Punnett (1875–1967), he founded the *Journal of Genetics*, serving as editor until his death in 1926.

A passionate scientist whose interests ranged from zoology to the collection of Oriental art, Bateson, along with Dutch biologist Hugo de Vries (1845–1935) and American zoologist Thomas Hunt Morgan, is largely responsible for the rediscovery and reinterpretation of GREGOR MENDEL'S now-historic plant-breeding experiments. Modifying Mendel's hybridization theory to apply to animals as well as plants, Bateson argued that variation and heredity were not opposing phenomena but different expressions of the same basic principles of evolutionary theory.

As a leading spokesman for Mendelian genetics, Bateson published a classic treatise on the subject in 1909, entitled *Mendel's Principles of Heredity*. Departing from the rigid precepts of Darwinian doctrine, Bateson joined the earliest proponents of Neo-Darwinism, a newly emerging movement that also included Punnett and Morgan. Attempting to adjust and expand Darwin's inadequate theory of small random variations, Bateson and his colleagues called forth Mendel's demonstration of hybrid breeding. Known as the conservation of genetic variance, this fundamental principle of evolutionary mechanism asserts that male and female reproductive cells contain hereditary "units" or genes, and that each parent contributes one unit of genetic information to determine a particular inherited characteristic in the offspring. Reevaluating the relative importance of natural selection as an agent of evolution, some Neo-Darwinists suggested that acquired traits were the manifestation of intention and creativity in the evolutionary process.

Neo-Darwinism was not widely accepted until after Bateson's death. In his treatise on Mendel he referred to the intellectual atmosphere surrounding any discussion of the evolution of the species as "marked by the apathy characteristic of an age of faith."

Born in Whitby, England, Bateson spent most of his childhood in Cambridge, where his father had been appointed master of St. John's College. Bateson later attended St. Johns, becoming a fellow of the college in 1910.

Ignoring the need for training in mathematics, physics or chemistry, Bateson studied morphology and zoology, with extensive reading of classic literature. The turning point of his life came in May 1900 when he read Mendel's report, thirty-four years after it first appeared. Devoting the rest of his career to the development and popularization of Mendelian theory, Bateson suffered from chronic financial difficulties, which forced him to depend on the support of the Evolution Committee of the Royal Society.

Bateson's extraordinary imagination and insight did not prevent him from committing a glaring error in scientific judgment. Dismissing the role of chromosomes in the transfer of heredity, he offered various alternative theories which were unanimously rejected. As more and more geneticists appeared on the scene Bateson was gradually outpaced in the scientific discipline he had created.

Recognized nonetheless as a leading authority on genetics and evolution, he was awarded a great many honors for his distinguished contributions, including the Darwin Medal in 1904, the Royal Medal in 1920, and a trusteeship at the British Museum in 1922.

After two years at Cambridge Bateson accepted the offer to become the first director of the John Innes Horticultural Institution at Merton College, Oxford. Supervising the development of the center until his death in 1926, Bateson served as president of the British Association for the Advancement of Science in 1914. His son, anthropologist Gregory Bateson (1904–1980), was recognized for his distinguished studies of culture and personality, notably in collaborative research with his wife, Margaret Mead, on the art and culture of Bali.

Gaspard Laurent Bayle, 1774–1816

During his brief medical career, French physician Gaspard Laurent Bayle contributed significantly to the advancement of modern pathology and clinical medicine, most notably with his study of pulmonary phthisis, an infectious disease now referred to as tuberculosis of the lung.

In his classic reference *Research on Pulmonary Phthisis*, published in 1810, Bayle introduced the notion of tuberculosis as a specific disease, rather than a morbid process of wasting away or devastation resulting from a previous illness, as it was commonly viewed. Noting that the development of tubercles, the nodules formed by the tubercle bacillus, could occur before any symptoms appeared, he also established that tubercles are area-specific. The study distinguished a number of different forms of the disease, such as tuberculosis of the ovaries, tubercular laryngitis, lymphadenitis (inflammation of the lymph nodes), enteritis (inflammation of the intestine) and acute "miliary tuberculosis," a term coined by Bayle and still used to describe the presence in the body of lesions resembling millet seeds.

As the first accurate description of tuberculosis pathology, Bayle's report had an immediate impact on clinical practice as well as a broader effect on medical research and nosology (the study of disease classification). Although his investigations were elaborated by French physician RENÉ LAËNNEC, who distinguished additional forms of the disease and introduced a number of diagnostic techniques, the mechanism of tuberculosis was not clearly understood until the 1880s.

Bayle was born in Vernet, a mountain village in the region of Haute-Provence. With the luxury of financial independence, Bayle casually pursued careers in theology, law and local politics before turning to medicine as his chosen profession. At twenty-seven he received his medical degree from the École de Medécine in Paris, and, after joining the staff at the prestigious Hôpital de la Charité in 1807, he was appointed physician to Napoleon's household and the royal infirmary. A member of the Parisian Society of the Faculty of Medicine, Bayle served for several years as personal physician to the Emperor.

In addition to his extensive investigation of tuberculosis, Bayle also pioneered the study of cancer pathology, most notably in the area of lung and liver. That research was compiled by his nephew and published posthumously as *Treatise on Cancer*. The two-volume report appeared in 1833, seventeen years after Bayle's death from tuberculosis at the age of 42.

George Wells Beadle 1903–

George Wells Beadle taught biology at the California Institute of Technology from 1931 to 1936, and it was there, in T.H. Morgan's* laboratory, that he began his genetic research on the fruit fly, *Drosophila*.

In 1937, at Stanford University, Beadle met E.L. TATUM, with whom he collaborated on the research that was to win them both a place in the history of science. Beadle and Tatum's work on the bread mold *Neurospora crassa* demonstrated that every gene is responsible for the structure of a particular enzyme that in turn produces a specific chemical reaction. This one-to-one relationship between gene and chemical reaction in the cell is known as the "one gene–one enzyme" theory, and it is for the establishment of this concept that they were awarded the Nobel Prize in 1958 (shared with JOSHUA LEDERBERG). In the 1960s, when the relationship between gene and enzyme was examined at a molecular level, Tatum and Beadle's schema was replaced by the concept of "one gene–one polypeptide."

Beadle was chairman of the biology department at Stanford University from 1946 until 1961, when he joined the University of Chicago as chancellor. With his wife, Muriel, he wrote *The Language of Life* (published in 1966), a discussion of the relationship between genes and the basic chemistry of the cell.

Clifford Whittingham Beers 1876–1943

Mental hygiene is a phrase, as well as a movement, that came into prominence at the beginning of the twentieth century largely due to the courageous efforts of C.W. Beers. He was born in New Haven, Connecticut, where he graduated from Sheffield Scientific School, but by 1900 Beers was suffering from severe mental illness. From 1900 to 1903 he was confined in a number of institutions.

This experience inspired him to write an autobiographical account of his life in confinement, *A Mind that Found Itself*, published in 1908. The book served as a means of educating a public generally misinformed on the subject of mental illness. Beers led a crusade to improve understanding worldwide, and the eloquence and candor of his autobiographical account rallied support in political as well as medical circles.

He dedicated his life to the reform of existing conditions and treatment of the mentally ill, and to the search for preventive measures. In 1909 he founded the National Commission for Mental Hygiene and served as secretary for the American Foundation for Mental Hygiene from 1928 to 1939. In 1930 Beers organized the first International Congress for Mental Hygiene.

Emil von Behring 1854–1917

At the end of the nineteenth century Emil von Behring shed a bright new light on the body's mechanism of resistance to disease, introducing the term "antitoxin" for a substance manufactured by the body in response to the introduction of a toxin or poison. Working in ROBERT KOCH'S laboratory at the University of Berlin, von Behring and his colleague SHIBASABURO KITASATO observed that, in the presence of a foreign substance, agents known as "antibodies" were summoned by the body to counteract the effect of the foreign agent, or "antigen."

In 1888 A.E.J. YERSIN and P.P.E. Roux had isolated the specific toxin produced by the diphtheria bacillus. On the theory that specific antibodies acted against specific toxins, von Behring sought an antidote in antitoxic sera obtained from an animal injected with the bacillus of a particular disease. In 1891, using the antitoxin method, he successfully treated a child suffering from diphtheria, a common and dreaded disease with a high mortality rate due to damage to the heart, kidney and larynx. In the following year Von Behring and Kitasato had similar success with their antitoxin procedure in the treatment of tetanus.

Von Behring's achievement led the way to specific treatments for specific infections, a great step beyond the more generalized medical measures of rest and improved nutrition. PAUL EHRLICH coined the term "passive immunization" to differentiate von Behring's antitoxin treatment from EDWARD JENNER'S system of vaccination introduced a century earlier. Known as "active immunization," Jenner's technique involved the stimulating of antibody production by introducing small amounts of the antigen.

Von Behring and Kitasato observed that in addition to providing antibodies to fight off the disease, the sera of animals immunized against diphtheria and tetanus had other therapeutic and prophylactic effects. By 1894 antitoxin treatment of diphtheria was widespread, finally controlling this major childhood disease.

Von Behring, a native of West Prussia, joined the Marburg Hygiene Institute as professor of bacteriology in 1895, eventually taking over as director. For his enormous contribution to the advancement of medicine von Behring carries the distinction of receiving the first Nobel Prize in Medicine, awarded in 1901.

Martinus Willem Beijerinck 1851–1931

The founding father of virology was a Dutch botanist named Martinus Willem Beijerinck, who first recognized a filterable virus as the cause of infectious disease.

Born in Amsterdam, Beijerinck was the son of a freight clerk for the Holland Railway Company. His enthusiasm for plants began at fifteen, when he entered and won a student botany contest organized by the Netherlands Agricultural Society. Gathering one hundred and fifty different specimens, Beijerinck identified each one by its Dutch and Latin names as well as the date and place he found it.

Despite this newfound passion, he was enrolled in a three-year training program in chemistry at the Delft Polytechnical School. After graduating in 1874 he taught chemistry at a small-town agricultural school in Warffum until the following year, when the death of his mother, followed by his own bout with typhoid fever, temporarily suspended Beijerinck's career.

He recovered by the end of 1876 and found new and much more satisfying employment at the Agricultural High School in Wangeningen, where he was given his first opportunity to teach botany and conduct research on various plant diseases. It was there that Beijerinck first learned of the contagious tobacco plant disease that would later admit him to the secret world of viruses. With little background in bacteriology, however, his initial investigations revealed no clues to the cause of the disease.

A man of highly critical and frequently antagonistic temperament, Beijerinck resigned from Wangeningen over unresolvable personal conflicts with students and faculty. The tempting offer of a new laboratory and a much higher salary convinced him to leave the academic world, so in 1885 he joined the staff at the Netherlands Yeast and Spirit Works at Delft to embark on his new career as an industrial scientist.

Over the course of the next decade Beijerinck earned a distinguished reputation among agricultural scientists and bacteriologists, in particular for his discovery of several strains of bacteria responsible for the formation of root nodules in leguminous plants.

Encouraged by his success, Beijerinck resumed his search for the cause of tobacco mosaic disease, but again he found no sign of bacteria in the culture dishes or under the microscope. With all his attention directed toward the study of plant disease, Beijerinck contributed little to the advancement of yeast production, and, in fairness to his employer, he felt obliged to resign.

He accepted a position at the Delft Polytechnic School when, after lengthy and elaborate negotiations, he was granted a new house, a new laboratory, and a salary higher than that of the director. Beijerinck conducted a great number of biological investigations over the course of the next twenty-six years, but by far the most significant of these was an investigation he had already attempted twice before.

In 1897 he once again sought the microorganism responsible for tobacco mosaic disease, but this time he discovered that the disease was apparently transmitted by a fluid after it had passed through a "bacteria-tight" filter. Concluding that the toxin was in the form of an infectious fluid, he published a short article in 1898 entitled *Contagium vivum fluidum* (*Contagious Living Fluid*). The word virus—from the Latin meaning "slime" or "poisonous juice"—was introduced by Beijerinck to refer to a cell-free filtrate as a cause of disease, initiating the term "filterable virus."

Ignoring the possibility of a virus particle, Beijerinck retained his belief in a living, infectious fluid up until his death. In 1913 he wrote, "The existence of these contagia proves that the concept of life...is not inseparably linked up with that of structure...In its most primitive form, life is, therefore, no longer bound to the cell."

Although few bacteriologists took seriously his notion of life in a fluid form, the discovery of the filterable virus attracted considerable attention throughout the scientific community. In 1925 pioneer microbiologist Felix d'Herelle pointed out the magnitude of Beijerinck's contribution: "All biology rested, still rests, upon the fundamental hypothesis that the unit of living matter is the cell. Beijerinck...freed himself from this dogma, and proclaimed the fact that life is not the result of a cellular organization, but derives from another phenomenon..."

Georg von Bekesy 1899–1972

A leading authority on aural physiology, Georg von Bekesy was awarded the Nobel Prize for Physiology or Medicine in 1961 for his investigation of the "physical mechanics of acoustic stimulation." Bekesy's anatomical and physiological studies of the inner ear elucidated the mechanical processes involved in the interpretation of sound.

The inner ear comprises a delicate network of tubes called the membraneous labyrinth, within which lies the cochlea, a snail-shaped spiral tunnel made of bone. The basilar membrane and the reticular membrane divide the space inside the tunnel into three separate chambers. Also coiled inside the cochlea is the "cochlear duct," which contains the organ of Corti, the receptor organ for hearing. The organ of Corti is made up of specialized auditory receptor cells arranged on the basilar membrane, a structure in the ear.

Bekesy described step by step the process that is initiated when sound vibrations are transmitted to the basilar membrane. Different areas of the basilar membrane respond to different sound frequencies, stimulating different parts of the organ of Corti. Performing a function similar to that of a microphone, the receptor cells respond to this stimulation by producing nerve impulses that vary in accordance with the vibrations' frequencies. Nerve fibers from the receptor cells then transmit this auditory information to the brain.

A native of Budapest, Bekesy received a degree in biophysics from the University of Budapest in 1923. In that same year he was hired by the Hungarian telephone system to study the physics of telecommunications in its research laboratory.

As an employee of the telephone company for almost 23 years, Bekesy conducted an extensive and detailed investigation of the physiology and anatomy of the human ear. During that time he also taught biophysics at the University of Hungary. He gave up both positions in 1946 to join Sweden's celebrated Karolinska Institute as a research professor. In 1949 Bekesy left Europe to accept an invitation from Harvard University, where he became a senior research fellow in its psychoacoustic laboratory and taught there until 1966. Receiving American citizenship in 1956, Bekesy settled in Cambridge, Massachussetts.

His writings include *Experiments in Hearing*, published in 1960, and *Sensory Inhibition*, published in 1967.

Sir Charles Bell 1774–1842

Exploring the functional anatomy of the nervous system, Scottish surgeon and anatomist Charles Bell observed that sensory stimuli and motor impulses travel in separate channels before they reach the spinal cord.

Some historians, however, credit FRANÇOIS MAGENDIE with the discovery, contending that the noted French physician and physiologist presented the first experimental demonstration of that important finding. The dispute has been settled by terming the principle of nerve traffic the "Bell-Magendie law." This describes a sensorimotor division of nervous activity in which the anterior roots of the spinal nerves carry motor impulses and the posterior roots carry sensory information.

The struggle for priority began with Magendie himself, who argued that while Bell had merely noted a functional specificity in peripheral nerves, the more significant finding emerged from his own experimental study, which established the anatomical organization of sensory and motor nerve function. In any case, the formulation of the "Bell-Magendie law" represented a major step forward in the development of neurophysiology.

Born in Edinburgh, Charles Bell was the youngest son of a minister of the Church of England. By the time Charles reached adolescence his oldest brother, John Bell (1763–1820), had begun to establish himself as a prominent surgeon. John also taught private classes in anatomy and invited his younger brother to serve as his laboratory assistant. Although Charles had received little formal education apart from tutoring in art, he took advantage of the educational opportunity, supplementing John's teachings with lectures at Edinburgh University. In 1799 Charles entered the Royal College of Surgeons, earning his degree five years later.

The rival Edinburgh faculty resented the Bells' success as independent medical instructors and conspired to have them barred from practice at the Royal Hospital. Emigrating to England in 1804, Charles established a private surgical practice in London, where he was soon established as a distinguished lecturer on anatomy and surgery.

Combining his abilities as a painter with his knowledge of medical science, Bell produced a popular book for artists and art students entitled *Essays on the Anatomy of Expression in Painting*. First published in 1806, the book presented an anatomical and physiological analysis of facial expressions placed in a context of art history, theory and philosophy.

By 1810 Bell had already begun his systematic study of peripheral nerves, developing his own experimental techniques for correlating anatomical structure and brain function. Emerging from eighteenth-century notions of "irritability" and "sensibility," (respectively, the conscious and unconscious reaction to stimuli) the movement to establish a physiological basis for psychological phenomena focused attention on the organization of the nervous system as a key to an understanding of mental processes. Bell's methodology, even more than his research findings, contributed significantly to the development of neurophysiology and experimental psychology in the nineteenth century, notably influencing Johannes Muller's landmark studies on sensory function.

In 1811 Bell published his *Idea of a New Anatomy of the Brain*, in which he discusses the [functional specificity] of the spinal nerve roots. Primarily intended as a demonstration of [cerebral localization,] Bell's report also asserted that a peripheral nerve is made up of different segments "united for convenience of distribution" but "distinct in office." The specific function of each of these segments, or divisions, is dictated by the particular area of the brain to which it is attached.

In 1812 Bell was appointed resident surgeon at Middlesex Hospital, where he further developed a reputation as an eminent lecturer on surgery and clinical medicine. At the same time he joined the celebrated Great Windmill Street School of Anatomy, founded by WILLIAM HUNTER, serving for more than a decade as co-director and head lecturer. Appointed professor of anatomy and surgery at London's College of Surgeons in 1824, Bell helped to establish the Middlesex Hospital Medical School, becoming the institution's first director in 1828.

In his *Nervous System of the Human Body*, published in 1830, Bell presented a description of sensory and motor function in the cranial nerves. Based on clinical and experimental observations, Bell's study is particularly notable for its discussion of a form of facial paralysis, now referred to as "Bell's palsy," which results from a lesion of the seventh cranial nerve.

Knighted in 1831, Bell returned to Scotland five years later to become professor of surgery at the University of Edinburgh.

Joseph Bell 1837–1911

> A thin wiry dark man with a high-nosed acute face, penetrating grey eyes, angular shoulders, high discordant voice, Dr. Bell would sit in his receiving room with a face like a red Indian and diagnose the people as they came in, before they even had a chance to speak. He would tell their symptoms and even give them details of their past life [sic], and hardly ever make a mistake. [from the autobiography of Sir Arthur Conan Doyle.]

Scottish-born Joseph Bell is recognized as the model for Sir Arthur Conan Doyle's legendary creation, Sherlock Holmes. As fiction's most illustrious detective, Holmes owes a large portion of his remarkable skills of deduction and much of his surly disposition to Dr. Bell, Conan Doyle's mentor and professor of physiology at the Royal Infirmary in Edinburgh.

Conan Doyle recalled the circumstances of Sherlock Holmes's conception: "I thought of my old teacher, Joe Bell, of his eagle face, of his curious ways, of his eerie tricks of spotting details. If he were a detective, he would surely reduce this fascinating but unorganized business to something nearer to an exact science."

Joseph Bell reveled in the elegance of science. He regarded an ability in deductive reasoning as a requirement for the practice of diagnostic medicine, declaring,

> The experienced physician and the trained surgeon every day in their examination of the humblest patient, have to go through a similar process of reasoning, quick or slow according to the personal equation of each, almost automatic in the experienced man, labored and often erratic in the tyro, yet requiring just the same, simple requisites, senses to know facts, and education and intelligence to apply them.

Possessed of a flair for showmanship, Bell astounded students and colleagues with his ability to derive a precise clinical picture from a brief and seemingly superficial consultation. Relying on an enormous store of wide-ranging knowledge, Bell turned his attention to every detail of a patient's appearance and demeanor, drawing medical inferences from the fabric of his clothes, the clay on his shoes, the pattern of his speech, or the pace of his step. In a dazzling display of deductive virtuousity Bell would rapidly correlate all these external clues to obtain details of a patient's personal and medical history.

Joseph was heir to a family tradition of medical distinction, following in the footsteps of noted Edinburgh surgeons John and CHARLES BELL. Appointed fellow of the Royal College of Surgeons, Joseph Bell was for many years an influential professor of surgery at the University of Edinburgh. As consulting surgeon to the Royal Infirmary and the Royal Hospital for Sick Children, Bell presided over the outpatient clinic as an exalted master, surrounded by an entourage of adoring students and assistants. Among these star-struck fans was Conan Doyle, who was both awed and intimidated by his professor's feats of deduction. Singling him out as a prize student, Bell enlisted Doyle as his "outpatient clerk" at the clinic.

Bell's unnerving effect on his students, and notably on Doyle, is reflected in the characterization of the devoted Dr. Watson, who struggled vainly to follow the master's great leaps of deduction, inevitably collapsing into dumbfounded astonishment.

Bell summed up the essence of Holmes's technique in the preface he wrote for an 1893 edition of Doyle's *A Study in Scarlet:* "The importance of the infinitely little is incalculable." As an example of the power of the infinitesimal, Bell cited "those minute organisms which disseminate cholera and fever, tubercle and anthrax."

Baruj Benacerraf 1920–

In honor of his distinguished study of genetic function in pathology and immunology, Venezuelan-born Baruj Benacerraf was awarded the 1980 Nobel Prize for Physiology or Medicine, which he shared with fellow immunologists GEORGE SNELL and JEAN DAUSSET. The committee hailed Benacerraf's research for providing "the possibility of analyzing the background of the varying ability of different individuals to mobilize an immune response to infections."

Born in Caracas, Benacerraf attended Columbia University in New York and completed graduate training at the Medical College of Virginia in 1945. He served as research supervisor at the National Center for Scientific Research in Paris until 1956, when he returned to the United States to join the faculty at the New York University School of Medicine. It was there, Benacerraf has said, that his prizewinning research originated in 1962. He continued his immunological investigations at the National Institutes of Health between 1968 and 1970, and since then at the Harvard University Medical School, where he was named to the Fabya Chair of Comparative Pathology.

Recognized as the leading authorities of transplant immunology, Benacerraf, Snell and Dausset conducted independent investigations of the nature of antigens, the mechanisms of the immune system, and the transplantability of human organs. For more than twenty-five years they explored what is known as "histocompatibility," the ability of the cells of one tissue to survive in the presence of cells of another tissue. Their combined research established the existence of a genetically determined complex of antigens that regulates the body's rejection of foreign substances. Investigating the genetic bases of cancer, infectious disease and other pathologies, Benacerraf contributed a major advance in the development of immunologic medicine with his discovery of specific genes that control the body's immune-response.

Currently serving as chairman of the Department of Pathology at Harvard, Benacerraf is also associate editor of *The American Journal of Pathology* and contributes to a number of other scientific publications, including *The Journal of Experimental Medicine* and *The Journal of Immunology and Immunogenetics*.

Paul Berg 1926–

A pioneer in the controversial branch of biochemistry known as genetic engineering, Paul Berg conceived the experimental technique of "gene splicing." Berg discovered that the gene of any living organism could be extracted from its chromosome and returned to its original position, or recombined into the string of genes of another organism.

He reasoned that if a gene, which contains chemical instructions for the cellular production of a specific protein, were "spliced" into the genetic sequence of a bacterial cell, the rapidly multiplying bacterium would quickly produce billions of identical cells, each carrying the newly inserted gene. Each such cell would also produce the protein dictated by that gene. Developing the gene splicing technique with an animal cancer virus called SV-40, Berg demonstrated that the spliced genes functioned properly, as did the reproduced copies.

Revolutionizing the field of genetics, Berg's new technique also enabled the mass production of previously scarce substances such as insulin and interferon for use in medical research and practice. In recognition of this monumental contribution to medical science Berg was awarded the 1980 Nobel Prize for Physiology or Medicine, which he shared with WALTER GILBERT and Frederick Sanger.

Credited as the father of the controversial branch of biochemistry known as recombinant DNA technology, Berg took quite seriously the attendant responsibilities of that role. Recognizing the potential dangers of creating and reproducing new microbes, Berg was influential in the establishment of stringent guidelines for maintaining the safety and propriety of genetic engineering research. In 1975 he organized a convention of one hundred scientists from sixteen countries to review the potential hazards and examine possible safety measures.

Paul Berg was born and raised in Brooklyn, New York, where he attended Abraham Lincoln High School. It was there that his scientific curiosity was encouraged by the woman in charge of the school's supply room. She initiated a science club for the students, and Berg credits her with the inspiration for his career.

Graduating in 1948 from Pennsylvania State College, Berg received a Ph.D. in microbiology in 1952 from Western Reserve University (now Case Western Reserve). He conducted postgraduate work at the Institute of Cytophysiology in Copenhagen and at Washington University in St. Louis, where he entered a lifelong association with distinguished biochemist ARTHUR KORNBERG.

Joining the staff at Stanford University in 1959, Berg became professor of biochemistry, later serving as chairman of the department from 1969 until 1974. A Willson Professor at Stanford since 1970, Berg remains associated with the university, living on the Palo Alto campus with his wife and son.

Sune Karl Bergstrom 1916–

As chairman of the Foundation Board of the NOBEL Committee since 1975, Sune Bergstrom establishes guidelines for the deliberations of the panel that chooses the Nobel prizewinners for physiology or medicine.

Bergstrom himself the recipient of a Nobel prize for his research on prostaglandins, has been affiliated for much of his career with Sweden's Karolinska Institute, which was designated by the terms of Alfred Nobel's will to select the medical laureate.

Bergstrom's foremost scientific achievement, initiated in 1947, is his landmark study of prostaglandins, a group of naturally occurring substances that are produced as needed in cell membranes throughout the body. These versatile and highly potent substances play an important role in regulating metabolism, blood pressure, glandular secretion and smooth-muscle activity, among other functions.

By purifying prostaglandins Bergstrom successfully described their chemical structure for the first time. His research further revealed that all of the hormonelike compounds are synthesized from unsaturated fatty acids. In recognition of the importance of his findings Bergstrom was awarded the 1982 Nobel Prize for Physiology or Medicine, which he shared with Karolinska's current president BENGT SAMUELSSON, and with English chemist and pharmacologist JOHN VANE. All three were honored for their separate contributions to the study of prostaglandins.

Bergstrom, a native of Sweden, studied medicine and biochemistry at the Karolinska Institute, receiving doctoral degrees in both disciplines in 1943. Four years later he joined the faculty at the University of Lund, where he began investigating the chemistry of prostaglandins. He left Lund in 1958 to return to Karolinska, where he continued his work as a researcher until 1981. In addition to fulfilling the considerable demands of his position at the Nobel Foundation, Bergstrom serves on the World Health Organization's advisory committee on medical research.

Claude Bernard 1813–1878

In ten tumultuous years, from 1848 to 1858, French physiologist Claude Bernard clarified the process of digestion in a series of brilliant experiments leading to conclusions that have remained valid for over 125 years.

He demonstrated the liver's secretion of glucose and its ability to convert glycogen to sugar even after the organ's removal from the body. He dramatically showed the effects of nerves on metabolism when he made an animal diabetic by inflicting a lesion on the central nervous system. He suggested the neural effects on circulation by demonstrating that a severing of the sympathetic nerve can raise the temperature in an animal's limb. He charted the key function of the pancreas in the digestion of fat. He showed how carbon monoxide suffocates by reacting chemically with hemoglobin and revealed the mechanism by which the poison curare fatally affects the interplay between nerve and muscle.

Bernard's catalog of achievements might well have sufficed to satisfy the life's ambition of most scientists, but his influence exceeded even the number of his discoveries, for he established experimental physiology as a scientific discipline and offered a model of logical precision in research.

Bernard was born in the village of St. Julien in the Jura mountains, not far from Geneva. His father, a singularly unprosperous vintner, managed to send him to a series of church schools that gave the boy a smattering of Latin, Greek, arithmetic and literature. When the family ran out of funds, Claude left school and apprenticed himself to a pharmacist in Lyons.

In his spare time behind the counter of the drugstore he dreamed of being a playwright and produced a script for a short musical in the somewhat overblown style of the period. Encouraged by a small production of his first work, Bernard took his second play to Paris, but a prominent critic told him that, while the play was not bad, the author could look forward to no more than the meager rewards of mediocrity in the theater. It was then that the disappointed Claude Bernard settled for a career in medicine.

He qualified for admission to the Faculté de Médicine in Paris, where his record was less than brilliant until he heard a lecture given by that apostle of scientific experimentation FRANÇOIS MAGENDIE, who was to exercise an enormous influence on Bernard. He taught Bernard the surgical and investigative techniques he would need for his experiments and interested him in the physiology of nerves and digestion, which was to be his primary concern.

Bernard's doctoral thesis—on the function of gastric secretions in the digestive process—was accepted, but he failed the examination that would qualify him for a faculty post at the medical school. With no money left for continued study he faced what to him was the grim prospect of setting up a medical practice in his home town of St. Julien. Instead he married Fanny Martin, the daughter of a wealthy physician in Paris with a dowry fat enough to enable him to stay in Paris and continue his research in physiology. Actually his wife was fiercely opposed to his following such a career, especially when she realized that he was experimenting on dogs. Later she would raise their daughters as fervent antivisectionists, much to the dismay of Claude Bernard.

Meanwhile Bernard, following Magendie's precepts but reaching beyond them, was able, by ingenious surgery, to expose the workings of the pancreas and to reveal its role in the digestion of fat. From there he went on to discover the presence of sugar in the blood of an animal that had gone without solid food for long periods and to show that blood sugar was not dependent on diet alone but was manufactured in the liver.

When postmortems revealed that the quantity of sugar in the blood increased after death, Bernard probed still further and found that so long as the liver is perfused with blood it will continue to make sugar. Though the finding seemed no more than an unexpected curio, Bernard searched for its significance. "Nothing is accidental," he declared. "And what seems to us accident is only an unknown fact whose explanation may furnish the occasion for a more or less important discovery." In this case it led him to discover that the liver makes its sugar from glycogen (animal starch).

It also prompted him to examine the role of nerves in the liver's functioning. When he severed the cervical sympathetic nerve of a rabbit he expected the circulation to slow down, but instead he observed "a striking hyperactivity" and, instead of lower temperatures on the side of the animal's head, an increased warmth. This led him to the discovery of vasoconstricting and vasodilating nerves.

Seeking clues to neural functions by studying the disruptive effects of poisons, Bernard showed that curare did its work by destroying the motor nerves without noticeable effects on the sensory nerves. It was left to a student of Bernard's to refine that observation and show that curare acted on the end plates of the nerves.

Whenever the unexplained presented itself, Bernard would "question nature," as he put it. Puzzled by the bright scarlet color of veins and arteries in a dog asphyxiated by carbon monoxide, he conducted a series of experiments that demonstrated the mechanism of asphyxiation. The carbon monoxide, he concluded, replaces oxygen in the red blood cells, forming the compound carboxyhemoglobin and resulting in asphyxiation.

The series of rapid-fire announcements of far-reaching discoveries established Bernard as a lecturer at the Collège de France, where he shared the platform with his former teacher Magendie. When Magendie retired in 1852 Bernard took over most of his professor's duties, and three years, later, on the death of Magendie, Bernard inherited the full title of professor at the college.

He had been made a Chevalier d'Honneur for his work on the pancreas and given a doctorate in zoology by the Sorbonne after his revelations concerning the liver. He was elected to the Académie des Sciences and served as vice president, later as president of the Société de Biologie. Though he did little original work after 1858, the flood of honors continued with his election to the Académie Française, then to the presidency of the Académie. Finally the Emperor Napoleon III issued a decree appointing Claude Bernard to the Senate—then not a deliberative body so much as an honorary society. It seemed that only his wife remained unconvinced of his greatness, bitterly regretting that he had not become a country doctor and angrily proclaiming that her husband had spent his life practicing vivisection supported by her dowry.

What began as an essay in pamphlet form summing up Bernard's scientific and philosophic views grew in length and profundity until in 1865 it was published as a book under the title *An Introduction to the Study of Experimental Medicine*. The book is still read, quoted and admired. In it he goes beyond the teachings of Magendie to stress the importance of theory. "It is impossible," he wrote, "to devise an experiment without a preconceived idea; devising an experiment is putting a question; we never conceive a question without an idea which invites an answer." Though the book has been cited in defense of many ideologies, it warns of letting any theory degenerate into a dogma.

When on February 10, 1978 Claude Bernard died of nephritis he was mourned by the literary as well as the scientific world. Émile Zola said that he had given him the idea for a literary technique he called "the experimental novel." Others saw in him the champion of idealism, materialism or pragmatism. Though he was claimed by religionists and atheists alike, his only pronouncement on the afterlife was: "When we get to the village we'll see the houses."

For students, as for all experimental researchers, he defined what he called "the science of life" when he wrote, "It is a superb and dazzlingly lighted hall which may be reached only by passing through a long and ghastly kitchen."

Rosalie Bertell 1929–

"The day of being naive about things we can't see or smell or taste is over," Rosalie Bertell has said. As founding president of the International Institute for Public Health in Toronto, Canada, Bertell is recognized as a leading authority on the biological effects of radiation. For her significant contribution to the campaign against the hazards of radiation and toxic waste, Bertell was honored in 1987 with the Right Livelihood Award for outstanding scientific activism.

Bertell was born in Buffalo, New York, where a deeply religious family atmosphere helped to foster her sense of social responsibility and community involvement. After receiving a bachelor's degree in mathematics and physics from D'Youville College in 1951, Bertell entered the Carmelite order of nuns, and for the next five years worked as a manual laborer, "learning how to raise food, dig irrigation ditches, and thread pipe." At the age of twenty-five she suffered a serious heart attack, which forced her to seek a less strenuous form of service with the Gray Nuns of the Sacred Heart, a teaching order in Philadelphia.

In 1959 Bertell completed doctoral studies at Catholic University, where she earned a degree in mathematics and biometry—the mathematical analysis of biological data. Accepting a research position in epidemiology at Roswell Park Memorial Cancer Institute in Buffalo, New York, Bertell began an investigation of the geographical distribution of leukemia and the role of environmental health hazards in the incidence of the disease. Based on a three-year study of leukemia rates in three states, Bertell's findings implicated low-level radiation from X rays as a significant factor in at least 12% of the cases.

Alarmed by statistics that indicated the significant health hazards of radiation, Bertell became a leading spokesperson in the campaign against a proposed nuclear plant to be established near Buffalo.

In the years that followed she dedicated herself to the investigation of national and international standards for the control of radiation levels to counter what seemed to be a general disregard of public health and safety. Established in the early 1950s, the International Commission on Radiological Protection, independent of public health authority, continues to determine safety levels for radiation and radioactive waste. Although the limited test-ban treaty of 1963 banned above-ground detonation of nuclear weapons, Bertell found the levels of radiation emitted in underground testing to be a continuing hazard to public health and the environment.

In 1978 Bertell left Roswell Park to establish a public interest group in Buffalo called the Ministry of Concern for Public Health. Following the nuclear accident at Three Mile Island in 1979, Bertell joined a panel of scientists in Washington, D.C. to challenge the official statements released by the government on levels of radiation emissions in the Harrisburg area and along the Susquehanna River and to demand a Congressional investigation.

Bertell's organization later moved its headquarters to Toronto, where it became the International Institute for Public Health. In addition to demanding that governments take responsibility for informing the public and providing protection against nuclear health threats, the institute also seeks to hold utility companies responsible for any negligence in the operation of nuclear plants. In the early 1980s Bertell was involved in the successful campaign to limit the toxic effects of uranium mines in New Mexico that had caused a significant increase in the rate of birth defects among the local Navajo Indians.

"This little earth is just too small and fragile and polluted," Bertell declares. "We're seeing the death of the old system and the birthing of a global consciousness. Either we learn, or we go the way of the dinosaurs."

Charles Herbert Best 1899–1978

Charles Best was a 22-year-old undergraduate student at the University of Toronto when he was hired to assist FREDERICK BANTING in an experimental animal study on diabetes and the internal secretions of the pancreas. Soon accepted as an equal partner, Best helped to develop a means of isolating insulin, the active principle that controls blood sugar.

By extracting the pancreatic secretions from dogs Best and Banting obtained a preparation of insulin that served as an effective replacement for a deficiency of the hormone in humans. Their discovery saved the lives of many millions who suffer from diabetes, a complex and chronic metabolic disorder caused by deficient secretion of insulin or the inability of insulin to function normally in the body.

Citing the discovery of insulin as an outstanding contribution to medical science, the 1923 Nobel Prize for Physiology or Medicine honored Banting and John Macleod, the head of the laboratory where the work had been performed, but the committee failed to recognize Best's participation. The outraged Banting protested the inequity of the award and shared his cash award equally with Best.

Born in West Pembroke, Maine, Best had received his bachelor's degree only weeks before he and Banting completed their insulin experiment. Best continued graduate training at the University of Toronto, earning his degree in medicine in 1925.

After obtaining a doctorate in physiology from the University of London in 1929, he returned to Canada to join the faculty at the University of Toronto, later serving as associate director of the Connaught Laboratories.

In 1941 he took over as director of the Banting and Best Department of Medical Research at the University of Toronto, where he conducted significant studies on the mechanism and treatment of diabetes and other forms of metabolic disorder. Best is distinguished as the first to introduce a coagulant for the treatment of thrombosis (the formation of a blood clot within a blood vessel) and is also noted for the discoveries of choline, a vitamin that prevents liver damage, and histaminase, the enzyme that breaks down histamine.

Best's published works include *The Living Body* (with N.B. Taylor, rev. ed. 1946), *The Physiological Basis of Medical Practice* (4th ed. 1946), and *The Human Body and Its Functions* (3d ed. 1956).

Marie François Xavier Bichat 1771–1802

Hailed as the "father of histology", Xavier Bichat brought a new perspective to medicine by introducing the notion of specific tissue types as fundamental units of anatomy. Rather than viewing the human body as a collection of visibly recognizable objects related by function, Bichat shifted his focus down to a substructure of various material textures and revealed a new order of pathological infiltration.

Classifying membranes as fibrous, mucous or serious, he described how these three types combine to form twenty-one distinct "compound membranes." Bichat charted the distribution of these tissue types throughout the body and showed that even in anatomically separate organs, tissues of similar physical and chemical characteristics respond similarly to pathogenic as well as therapeutic stimuli. Rejecting all but the most direct and tangible evidence, he pursued his investigations without a microscope to avoid the imposition of an artificial intermediary.

France was at the brink of revolutionary upheaval when Bichat was born in the tiny village of Thoirette-en-bas, where his father was a country doctor and apprehensive member of the bourgeoisie. When the Bastille fell in 1789 Bichat was sent to Lyons to study at the seminary of Saint Irenaeus, while across the country intellectual establishments were being toppled as relics of the ancien régime.

At twenty Bichat enrolled at the Hôtel-Dieu in Lyons to embark on a medical education. Although the law of March 2, 1791 abolished academic requirements for all professions, the faculty at Lyons maintained a disciplined training program in surgery, anatomy and physiology. Recruited for military service in the republican army, Bichat served briefly at a military hospital in Bourg before he escaped to Paris in the fall of 1794.

He moved in with his uncle, aunt and cousins and entered into apprenticeship with the renowned Pierre-Joseph Desault, chief of surgery at the Hôtel-Dieu. More than 100 students and interns would follow Desault each day as he made his rounds, but Bichat was soon singled out for his enthusiasm and diligence. France's most distinguished surgeon became mentor, patron and surrogate father to Bichat, who was invited to live with Desault, his wife and their teenage son.

By the end of 1794 France's political convulsions were subsiding, and medical schools and licensing requirements were reestablished. At 24 Bichat with his extensive training as well as his elite status as Desault's protégé, distinguished himself as a prominent member of the new medical establishment.

After Desault's death in 1795 Bichat assembled the fragments of his mentor's unfinished manuscript and published them with a tribute to Desault and five new articles of his own. Recognized as a major contribution to surgical literature, the *Journal de Chirurgie (Journal of Surgery)* ensured Bichat's professional standing as well as his distinction as heir of the great Desault.

With the reestablishment of formal medical education in France came the resurgence of medical societies. Asserting their commitment to a revival of professional standards, Bichat and his colleagues established the *Société d'Emulation*. In 1800 he was appointed by Napoleon to serve as secretary on a newly created medical advisory board, and in that same year Bichat published his *Traité des membranes (Treatise on Membranes)*.

His discussion of the anatomy of tissue was so well received that he was asked to produce an expanded version that would include his other theoretical concepts in medicine and biology. Appearing in 1801, Bichat's *Anatomie générale appliquée à la physiologie et à la médicine (General Anatomy Applied to Physiology and Medicine)* was a critical success, although some objected to his liberal borrowing of ideas, and occasionally even words, from the works of PHILIPPE PINEL, THEOPHILE DE BORDEU and others without crediting his sources.

Before embarking on the organization of *Anatomie générale*, Bichat published *Recherches physiologique sur la vie et la mort (Physiological Aspects of Life and Death)*. The treatise presented a refinement of the vitalist distinction between life and "nonlife" which infers that living beings are not governed by the laws of physics and chemistry. Bichat proposed a further distinction between the life processes of growth and reproduction and the conscious life force that allows for self-awareness and interaction with the environment. To support his theory Bichat cited the results of what seems a ruthless experimental investigation in which he drowned, burned, poisoned and smothered a great number of animals.

The critical acceptance of *Recherches physiologiques*, followed by the greater success of his *Anatomie générale*, reinforced Bichat's reputation as a teacher and firmly established him as one of France's leading medical authorities by the time he was thirty-one.

On July 8, 1802 he was standing at the top of a flight of stairs when suddenly he staggered, lurched forward and tumbled down the steps. Within two weeks Bichat was dead, and even after an autopsy the cause of his fall remained a mystery. His body was placed in the standard type of unmarked grave used to hold the remains of postmortem subjects, but Bichat's skull was preserved and kept as a treasure by his disciple Philibert Joseph Roux. Forty-three years later a ceremonial parade through the streets of the city conveyed Bichat's skull and exhumed bones to a Paris cemetery.

James Whyte Black 1924–

For his innovative approach to pharmacological research, Scottish-born James Whyte Black was awarded the 1988 Nobel Prize for Physiology or Medicine, which he shared with American pharmacologists Gertrude B. Elion and George H. Hitchings. Internationally recognized as a pioneer in the development of twentieth-century pharmacology, Black integrated modern advances in cellular biology into the science of drug development.

As senior pharmacologist at Imperial Chemical Industries Ltd., Black was responsible for the development of propranolol, the first drug designed to block the actions of naturally produced chemicals that contribute to high blood pressure and heart disease. It was in 1958 that he introduced the first "beta-blocker," a synthetic drug designed to inhibit the excitatory effects of certain body chemicals by preventing their access to "receptor sites."

In recent studies conducted at the Medical College in Georgia, American biochemist Raymond Ahlquist had suggested that epinephrine and norepinephrine, secreted in the adrenal glands and sympathetic nerve endings, transmit their chemical signals to two types of receptors, known as alpha and beta. These signals, causing an increase in heart rate and a strengthening of muscle contractions, are received at beta receptor sites located in the heart muscle. Based on Ahlquist's theory of chemical receptors, Black set out to create a new chemical compound that would reduce high blood pressure and alleviate the pain of angina by blocking the effects of *epinephrine* and *norepinephrine* at the receptor sites where their signals would normally be received.

Black later participated in the development of cimetidine, a drug designed to block the effects of histamines. At the time, no available antihistamine drug could effectively prevent histamines from stimulating acid secretion in the stomach, a major factor in the development of peptic ulcers. Working at the pharmaceutical laboratory of Smith Kline & French, Black sought to create a substance that would prevent the stimulation of acid production by blocking the histamine signal. Applying Ahlquist's theoretical principle to another type of receptor, Black developed a chemical that would compete with the histamines for access to their signal receiver, known as the H-2 receptor.

A native of Uddingston, Scotland, James Black received a medical degree from the University of St. Andrews in 1946. After more than a decade as a university lecturer Black joined the research staff at Imperial Chemical Industries in 1956. He has since served as director of biological research at Smith Kline & French Laboratories and as head of the Therapeutic Research Division at Wellcome Research Laboratories in Kent.

In recognition of his far-reaching contribution to pharmacological medicine, Black was awarded knighthood in 1981. Affiliated with London's King's College Hospital Medical School since 1973, he served as visiting professor at Albany Medical College in New York in 1986 and is currently a member of the faculty at the Rayne Institute of the University of London. Much of his research is conducted under the auspices of the James Black Foundation, an experimental facility funded by Johnson & Johnson.

Elizabeth Blackwell 1821–1910

The first woman in the United States to receive a medical degree, Elizabeth Blackwell was a curious mixture of progressive, feminist philosophy and rigid Victorian instincts. A staunch defender of the rights of women, blacks and the poor, she achieved her goal to"commit heresy with intelligence." Though she devoted much of her career to such innovations as medical education for women, free health care for the poor, and preventive medicine with particular attention to environmental conditions, Blackwell retained an intolerance for such "passing fads" as bacteriology and the practice of vaccination and exhibited a particularly disdainful aversion to romantic love and sex. These lapses were far outweighed, however, by her contributions to medical practice and the advancement of women.

Elizabeth was one of five children born to Samuel and Hannah Blackwell, religious dissenters and political liberals who raised their family with a strong reverence for civil liberties. Her younger sister Emily followed in Elizabeth's footsteps, later joining her in medical practice. Their sister Anne became a journalist, and brothers Henry and Samuel were actively committed to the crusade for women's rights.

Elizabeth was 11 years old when her family emigrated from Bristol, England to New York. After fire destroyed the family sugar refinery the Blackwells were emigrants once more, this time settling in Cincinnati, Ohio, an intellectual center known as the "Rome of the West."

In 1844 Elizabeth, who, as she later admitted, had "been always foolishly ashamed of any form of illness," was urged by a family friend to consider a career in medicine. The idea appealed to Blackwell despite her prudishness, or perhaps because of it. She wrote: "Other circumstances forced upon me the necessity of devoting myself to some absorbing occupation...I became impatient of the disturbing influence exercised by the other sex...I felt determined...to become a physician and thus place a strong barrier between me and all ordinary marriage."

Although women were generally accepted as nurses and midwives and a few practiced medicine without benefit of formal training, the notion of a woman enrolling in medical school was unheard of. Blackwell's appeals to colleges and private physicians were almost universally discouraged. Some misguided supporters suggested she disguise herself as a man, but Blackwell's goals were for other women as much as for herself. She finally convinced the Geneva Medical College in upstate New York to admit her after the entire student body agreed to accept her application.

Seeking clinical experience between semesters, she served at the syphilis ward of the Blockley Almshouse in Philadelphia, and in January of 1849 Elizabeth Blackwell became the first woman to be awarded a medical degree. The news was met with mixed reactions in America and in Europe. Returning to England after graduation, she was treated as a celebrity, but British doctors politely suggested she obtain further clinical experience in France.

The French, too, were reluctant to welcome Blackwell, advising her to enters La Maternité, an internationally respected school of midwifery. Seizing the opportunity to study an aspect of women's medical problems, Blackwell enrolled in the summer of 1849. While treating a young child suffering from "purulent ophthalmia," now recognized as a symptom of gonorrhea, Blackwell was accidently splattered with contaminated solution from a syringe. The accident caused her to lose an eye.

Fitted with a glass eye, Blackwell returned to England, where she was invited to study at St. Bartholomew's Hospital in London under the guidance of James Paget•, distinguished for his egalitarian views as well as for his skill as a pathologist. Blackwell remained at St. Bart's until 1851, when she returned to New York to establish her own practice. The radical notion of a woman doctor was met with various and extreme forms of resistance, including threats of mob violence. She delivered a series of lectures, advertised as "The Laws of Life with Special Reference to the Physical Education of Girls," which later appeared in book form.

Turned down for a job at the City Dispensary, a public health clinic, Blackwell resolved to take matters into her own hands. In 1853,with the financial backing of Quaker friends and supporters, she rented a room near Tompkins Square on New York's Lower East Side and founded what would later become the New York Dispensary for Poor Women and Children.

Emily Blackwell, meanwhile, was discovering that what breakthroughs her sister had achieved had scarcely altered prevailing attitudes toward women seeking a medical education. She eventually persuaded the board of admissions at Cleveland Medical College (now Case Western Reserve University), to accept her and subsequently to grant her a medical degree in 1856.

By 1857 Drs. Emily and Elizabeth Blackwell, along with German midwife Marie Zackrzewska, were working together at the New York Dispensary in its more spacious location at 64 Bleecker Street. Despite much opposition from politicians and the public, the hospital gradually gained acceptance. At the end of 1858 Elizabeth Blackwell returned to England to lecture on the advances gained by women in medicine in the United States. It was in that year that Blackwell became the first woman to be registered by the London Medical Council.

Blackwell returned to New York as the country teetered on the brink of the Civil War. Soon filled beyond capacity, the Infirmary became a haven for southern refugees and northern black women, who were the targets of riots and lynch mobs in New York City.

At the outbreak of war the Blackwells had begun training nurses to serve on the battlefront, with the intention of eventually establishing a medical school for women. The New York Infirmary became an accredited medical college in 1864, when it was granted the authority to award a degree in medicine to its graduates.

Under the auspices of the Infirmary Blackwell initiated an outreach program in which doctors were sent to care for poor patients in their homes, advising them on matters of hygiene, preventive medicine and home safety. One appointee who was to visit more than 10,000 homes during her nine years as director of the program was Rebecca Cole, a graduate of the Woman's Medical College of Pennsylvania, and the country's first licensed black woman doctor.

Elizabeth Blackwell returned to England again in 1869 to assist in the foundation of the London School for Women. She remained an active and tireless crusader until her death at the age of 90.

Alfred Blalock 1899–1964

Vascular surgeon Alfred Blalock is widely known for his contribution to the development of the "blue baby operation," a technique usually performed in the first weeks or months of life to correct a congenital heart condition known as "pulmonary stenosis." The characteristic blue tinge in the skin of affected infants is due to insufficient oxygen in the blood.

In the late 1930s HELEN TAUSSIG determined that the condition involves a malformation of the pulmonary artery that limits blood flow to the lungs. Under normal circumstances, oxygen-poor arterial blood is transported by the pulmonary artery from the heart into the lung, where it renews its supply of fresh oxygen and then exits as oxygen-rich venous blood by way of the pulmonary vein. Taussig discovered that in the abnormal circulatory system of "blue babies," the venous and arterial blood mix, impeding the oxygenation of the blood. In 1941 Blalock and Taussig launched their collaboration at Johns Hopkins University, where, three years later, they introduced the surgical technique now known as the Blalock-Taussig Method.

Born in Culloden, Georgia, Blalock graduated from Johns Hopkins Medical School in 1922. After completing his surgical internship and residency Blalock joined the faculty at Vanderbilt University School of Medicine, where he was appointed professor of surgery in 1938. Three years later he returned to Johns Hopkins to serve as director of the department of surgery at the medical school as well as surgeon-in-chief at the university hospital.

By that time he had completed extensive research on the physiology of stress and shock, with particular attention to blood circulation and blood pressure. Demonstrating that surgical shock results from the loss of blood, Blalock introduced the practice of blood or plasma transfusions to compensate for that loss. Appointed chairman of the "Shock Committee" in Washington, D.C., Blalock recognized the urgent need for advanced medical knowledge in these areas as the United States entered World War II. He offered the support of the Committee as well as his professional encouragement to pioneer researchers ANDRÉ COURNAND and HOMER SMITH.

In his own investigations, Blalock was exploring the possibility of a relationship between high blood pressure and hardening of the arteries by conducting a series of experimental studies on dogs. To increase the pulmonary blood pressure of his subjects, he devised a surgical procedure for diverting the systemic blood vessels into the lungs. Although the results of the operation were inconclusive with respect to the central question of his investigation, Blalock's surgical innovation provided the solution to a completely different problem.

By artificially conducting unoxygenated blood back into the lungs, the operation served to correct the circulatory malfunction in "blue babies." Blalock and Taussig conducted experimental studies with animals to modify and refine the procedure, and in 1944 they performed the first "blue baby operation" on a human patient. Although the infant died nine months later, subsequent trials demonstrated the effectiveness of the technique, which soon became widely accepted. Serving to prevent many thousands of deaths that would otherwise have been inevitable, the Blalock-Taussig operation also paved the way for further advances in corrective surgery on congenital defects and cardiac surgery for infants and children.

Konrad Emil Bloch 1912–

Early in his academic career Konrad Bloch discovered the steps in the natural formation of cholesterol. Bloch's research was a great stride toward improving the treatment of various coronary and circulatory diseases, notably atherosclerosis, a painful condition resulting from deposits of cholesterol in the blood vessels.

Bloch began his studies at the Technische Hochschule in Munich during the years Hitler was rising to power. AS a Jew in Germany, the future Nobelist faced mounting dangers. In 1936 he fled to the United States, where, two years later, he was awarded a degree in biochemistry from Columbia University. He served on the faculty at Columbia and later at the University of Chicago, until in 1954 he became the first professor of biochemistry at Harvard.

In 1964 Bloch shared the Nobel Prize for Physiology and Medicine with FEODOR LYNEN for their work on the mechanism of cholesterol and fatty acid metabolism.

Baruch Samuel Blumberg 1925–

For his contribution to the battle against infectious viral disease, Blumberg was awarded the 1976 Nobel Prize for Physiology or Medicine, which he shared with DANIEL CARLETON GAJDUSEK.

To investigate the relationship between ethnic background and pathological response, medical anthropologist Baruch Blumberg embarked on a study of more than 100,000 individuals from diverse populations, including natives of Surinam and Malaysia and the Eskimos of Baffin Island. Blumberg was examining the blood serum samples of a hemophiliac patient and an Australian aborigine when he stumbled on an immunological clue that led to the discovery of the "Australia antigen," the basic component of the hepatitis-B vaccine.

In 1963 Blumberg and his colleagues observed an "allergic" reaction in the hemophiliac's blood when they introduced a blood sample from the aborigine. Over the course of numerous transfusions the hemophiliac had apparently received an antibody against a factor in the aborigine's blood—later determined to be a part of the hepatitis-B virus. Occurring separately from the virus, the "Australia antigen" does not cause the disease, but it does stimulate the production of antibodies, thereby granting immunity to the host.

Blumberg was born and raised in New York City, where he received a medical degree in 1951 from the College of Physicians and Surgeons at Columbia University. After obtaining a doctorate in biochemistry from Oxford University he returned to the United States to accept the appointment as chief of the Geographic, Medicine, and Genetics Division of the National Institutes of Health.

Following his landmark discovery Blumberg was appointed associate director at the Institute for Cancer Research in Philadelphia as well as professor of medicine, human genetics and medical anthropology at the University of Pennsylvania.

At New York University Medical Center Saul Krugman launched the development of an Australia antigen vaccine, and in 1982 it was approved as safe and effective for commercial distribution.

James Blundell 1790–1843

In the early nineteenth century obstetricians were ill-equipped to deal with the demands of a difficult delivery. Severe hemmorhaging was a frequent occurrence, often proving fatal to the mother. James Blundell's sense of helplessness in the face of this problem inspired him to investigate the possibility of borrowing blood to restore his patients' losses, leading to the development of blood transfusion.

Throughout history blood has been invested with great power and mystery. The ancient Romans considered it therapeutic to drink or even bathe in the blood of the strong. In 1666 RICHARD LOWER succeeded in transferring blood directly from one dog to another, and there followed a great many misguided attempts to use animal blood in humans. The incompatibility of the proteins in the blood of different species had not yet been understood. Doctor Richard Leacock of Barbados suspected that animal blood might be ineffective and even harmful to human patients, and he shared his suspicions with Blundell. Blundell then conducted numerous experiments on dogs, proving conclusively the restorative powers of a blood transfusion to a fatally wounded dog. His consistently negative results when transferring the blood of one species to another established a basic principle of blood transfusion, the notion of incompatibility.

In 1818 he performed a transfusion of human blood on an incurably ill patient who survived fifty-six hours after the operation. Blundell felt encouraged enough by his observations to pursue the practice further when opportunities presented themselves. In an 1829 edition of *The Lancet* Blundell described a successful transfusion achieved with an improvised instrument comprising a funnel and pump, which he called an "impellor." He went on to devise a "gravitator," which used the force of gravity to propel the blood into the vein of the patient.

In the course of his lifelong research Blundell also demonstrated that the introduction of a few air bubbles into the bloodstream was not fatal, as had been previously assumed. Blundell's work steered the medical community toward an effective procedure of transfusion and led to the next great leap in the field of blood transfer, the invention in 1853 of the hypodermic syringe by Alexander Wood.

Hermann Böerhaave 1668–1738

In the humanistic tradition of the Renaissance man, Hermann Böerhaave embraced all disciplines, from music, languages and classical literature to mathematics, chemistry, botany, medicine and anatomy. Although many of his medical ideas and hypotheses have been disproved over the last two centuries, his contribution to medicine as a teacher and anatomist have survived the centuries. Perhaps his most important legacy rests in the contributions of the many people directly inspired by his instruction. It is almost entirely due to his spellbinding abilities as a teacher that the University of Leyden in Holland replaced Padua as the center of medical education in the first part of the eighteenth century. (In 1734 WILLIAM BULL attended the university, becoming the first American to be graduated from a medical school.)

Böerhaave's students spread his wisdom throughout Europe, and many universities adopted his teaching methods and curricula. Among his admiring students was Bernhard Albinus, with whom he arranged the reissuing of the works of VESALIUS.

Böerhaave had strong convictions about the requirements of medical education and particularly emphasized bedside instruction, drawing from the teachings of HIPPOCRATES and THOMAS SYDENHAM, whom he particularly admired. He also encouraged students to follow a patient's corpse through autopsy in order to better understand the correlation between symptoms observed and the physical evidence of disease. His autopsies greatly refined the anatomic ideas of his day. (The sweat glands are still known by physicians as "Böerhaave's glands.")

Böerhaave himself was as popular and sought-after a physician as he was a teacher, and his practice served as an additional teaching tool for his students. He was the first to regularly use thermometry in patient examination and encouraged his students to include this important element in their own practices. He published a great many texts, including *Institutiones medicae* (1708), *Aphorismi* (1709), *Index Plantarum* (1709) and *Elementa Chemiae* (1731).

Théophile de Bordeu 1722–1776

Considered by many historians to be the founder of modern endocrinology, French physician Théophile de Bordeu looked upon the organs of the body as quasi-independent entities, thus defining human life as the sum of many "little lives."

Based on clinical observations of the secretions of the organs and glands, most notably the stomach, heart, and brain, Bordeu asserted that the maintenance of health requires proper blood levels and proportions of these substances. His identification of these fluids as originating in organs or glands was in itself a considerable advance over the widely held view tracing these substances to muscle.

Born in the village of Izeste in the south of France, Théophile de Bordeu studied medicine at Montpellier, as had his father and grandfather. After graduating in 1743 Bordeu stayed on at the university for a year of postgraduate studies before taking a job as clinical examiner at La Charité hospital in Paris. His first major work, entitled *Recherches anatomiques sur les articulations des os de la face (Anatomic Research on the Articulation of the Bones of the Face)* gained him the respect of the medical establishment, as well as a membership in the Royal Academy of Sciences.

Returning to Bearn in 1749, Bordeu accepted a position at the mineral baths of Aquitaine, eventually becoming superintendent of the spa, as well as a leading advocate of balneotherapy (the use of baths to relieve pain and improve circulation)—particularly in the mineral waters of the Pyrenees (see PRIESSNITZ). His thoughts on the techniques and medical significance of mineral water treatments are included in his *Journal de Barèges (Journal of Barèges)* and *Recherches sur les maladies chroniques (Research on Chronic Illnesses)* (1775).

Bordeu returned to Paris in 1752 with the intention of opening a medical practice. In compliance with the local statute requiring all physicians in the capital to hold a degree from the Paris Faculty of Medicine, Bordeu re-entered medical school, earning his second degree in 1754. While attending the Paris Faculty he published *Recherches anatomiques sur les differentes positions des glandes et sur leur action, (Anatomic Research on the Different Positions of the Glands and Their Action)* his first important study of the anatomy and function of glands and glandular secretions.

After obtaining the necessary credentials Bordeu accepted a position as attending physician at La Charité, where he quickly established a large following of patients and admirers. His success, however also fostered resentment among a group of influential Parisian physicians, who arranged to have his name dropped from the city's medical roster, effectively terminating his practice in 1761. After a three-year struggle Bordeu was officially reinstated. He quickly regained his popularity, claiming among his patients a number of notable Parisians, including the king's favorite, Madame du Barry.

In 1767 he completed a third research study, entitled *Recherches sur le tissu muqueux, ou L'Organe Cellulaire (Research on Mucus Issue, or The Cellular Organ* in which he discussed the environment of the organs with regard to the role of mucous tissue in nutrition and the mechanisms of exchange between organs and tissues. The phrase "*l'organe cellulaire*" refers to a model of perforated homogeneous material, as described in ROBERT HOOKE'S *Micrographia* (1665). In the eighteenth century the term "tissue" was introduced into anatomic writing from the French word *tissu*, meaning woven cloth (from the Latin *texere*, "to weave"). Discussing the function as well as the textural and structural qualities of body tissue, Bordeu was among the first to treat this connective material as a significant anatomical entity.

An innovative and influential clinician, Bordeu is also noted for his contribution to semiology, the systematic study, interpretation and treatment of symptoms. His significant contribution to the advance of diagnostic and prognostic examination includes the introduction of a technique for taking the pulse, now widely adopted, in which the practitioner applies the tips of four fingers to a hollow area in the wrist below the base of the thumb. As reported in *Recherches sur les crises (Research on Fits)* and *Recherches sur le pouls par rapport aux crises (Research on the Pulse in Connection with Fits)* Bordeu's thoughts on symptomatology and associated studies on pulse were honored by the distinguished philosopher and critic Denis Diderot (1713–1784), who included these two monographs in his celebrated *Encyclopedie*, a compendium of the most important writings of the Age of Enlightenment.

Amédée Borrel 1867–1936

Microbiologist Amedee Borrel was among the first to suggest that a virus may be a prime agent of cancer. He proposed the theory in 1903, five years after BEIJERINCK'S discovery of the filterable virus, at a time when a number of diseases, including yellow fever and rabies, had been found to be the result of viral infection. Noting the rapid proliferation of normal cells following a virus infection, Borrel suspected that cancer's chaotic cell growth might be caused in some cases by a virus. His suggestion, however, was generally ignored, and it was not until Danish virologists Wilhelm Ellerman and Oluf Bang discovered that a particular form of leukemia was caused by a virus that Borrel's hypothesis was confirmed five years later.

In the course of a distinguished research career spanning almost half a century, Borrel explored nearly all of the major areas of microbiology, investigating tuberculosis, lung disease, tetanus and the plague, as well as the cytology and parasitology of tumors, the cultivation of tissues, serum therapy, immunization, filtrable viruses and bacteriophages. Despite the wide range of his interests, however, all of Borrel's studies were aimed at a common target: the mystery of cancer.

In 1891 he completed medical training at the University of Montpellier, delivering his doctoral thesis on the anatomy and pathology of epithelioma, a cancer of the skin and mucous surfaces. The distinctive style and insight of Borrel's research attracted the attention of celebrated Russian bacteriologist ELIE METCHNIKOFF, who invited him to join the faculty and research staff at the prestigious Institut Pasteur in Paris.

Equipped with only a regulation optical microscope, Borrel made one of the earliest virus sightings in 1904 when he observed a virus carried by chickens that was later identified as the fowlpox virus. Assuming that the various "poxes" were all modified versions of human smallpox, Borrel and others failed to distinguish fowlpox virus as a separate disease.

As the number of sightings mounted virologists sought to define what they were seeing. Were the clumped masses they observed under the microscope single viral units or conglomerations of many viruses within a single cell? The question was settled in 1929 when C. Ernest Goodruff and ERNEST GOODPASTURE used the newly invented electron microscope to show that those irregular-shaped clumps could be broken into as many as twenty thousand particles, or bodies, all of which function as infective agents. The viral clusters—or "inclusion bodies"—are composed of tiny, granular agents of infection known as "elementary bodies." In the fowlpox virus these minute particles are called "Borrel bodies." As further acknowledgement of his outstanding contribution to the advancement of virology, Goodpasture paid personal tribute to Borrel by introducing the term *Borreliota* ("little particles of Borrel") as the classification of a genus of microorganisms that includes all pox viruses.

A noted authority in the fields of tropical medicine and hygiene, Borrel traveled frequently in West Africa, where he became a founding member of the Société de Pathologie Exotique et de ses filiales de l'Ouest Africain et de Madagascar (Society of Exotic Pathology and Its Affiliates in West Africa and Madagascar). During World War I he volunteered his services in the campaign to vaccinate African troops against pneumococcal pneumonia.

Retaining a lifelong association with the Institut Pasteur, Borrel spent his last years in Strasbourg, where he served as director at the Institut d'Hygiene et de Bacteriologie as well as professor of medicine at the university.

Jean-Baptiste Bouillaud 1796–1881

In the first half of the nineteenth century Paris was a world center of clinical medicine and Jean-Baptiste Bouillaud was recognized as one of its leading figures. Cited as the model for Docteur Horace Bianchon in Balzac's *Comédie humaine,* Bouillaud was known throughout Europe as the practitioner who had attended Napoleon III and the venerable French surgeon GUILLAUME DUPUYTREN. From his deathbed Dupuytren had selected Bouillaud to preside over his imminent postmortem examination.

Bouillaud was born in Garat, a small town in southwestern France near Angoulême. Growing up in poverty, he was greatly influenced by his uncle, a surgeon-major in the French army, who offered encouragement and financial support for a career in medicine. Enrolled at the University of Paris, Bouillaud interrupted his studies to join the troops of Napoleon during the Hundred Days following his escape from Elba in 1815.

Returning to Paris, Bouillaud studied surgery under Dupuytren, experimental physiology under FRANCOIS MAGENDIE, clinical medicine under François Joseph Victor Broussais (1772–1838), and cardiology under JEAN NICOLAS CORVISART. Following Bouillaud's presentation of his doctoral thesis on the diagnosis of aneurysms of the aorta, he received his degree in medicine from the University of Paris in 1823.

As an intern at the Hôpital Cohin Bouillaud assisted in a study on cardiac disorders which appeared in two volumes as *A Clinical Treatise on Maladies of the Heart.* Published in 1824, the impressive report launched his reputation for probing and insightful investigation, most notably in the area of cardiac disorders. An exhaustive study of congenital heart disease, Bouillaud's study described the pathology of the endocardium, a term he introduced to indicate the membrane lining the heart. The study also related the appearance of pancarditis, a general inflammation of the heart, to a prior condition of acute rheumatic fever. The association of endocarditis and pericarditis had been suggested earlier, by celebrated physician EDWARD JENNER and others, but it was Bouillaud's precise physical measurements and statistical analyses that provided confirmation and elucidation of this finding.

Recognized for his contributions in other areas of clinical medicine, Bouillaud published a number of distinguished monographs on neurological topics, including his *Clinical Studies to Demonstrate That Loss of Speech Corresponds with Lesions of the Anterior Lobes of the Brain, and to Confirm (Francis) Gall's Opinion on the Seat of Articulate Language* (1825) and *Clinical Studies Tending to Refute Gall's Opinion on the Function of the Cerebellum and to Prove that this Organ Coordinates Equilibrium and Ability to Stand and Walk* (1827).

Among the important concepts established in these essays is the clinical distinction between loss of speech resulting from an inability to recall and use words and sentences, and that resulting from an inability to control the movements required for speech. In their original presentation, Bouillaud's assertions on cerebral localization were incomplete, and they were generally rejected until his studies were modified and expanded in 1861 by his son-in-law, French physician Simon Aubertin.

In 1831 Bouillaud joined the staff at Paris's Hôpital de la Pitié in 1831, also serving as professor of clinical medicine. Despite a reputedly abrasive and arrogant manner, he achieved considerable success in the medical establishment. At the age of 52 he was named dean of the medical faculty at the University of Paris, and in 1862 he became president of the Academy of Medicine. Five years later Bouillaud presided over the first International Medical Congress, and in 1868 he was made commander of the Légion d'Honneur.

Daniele Bovet 1907–

Swiss pharmacologist Daniele Bovet is most widely recognized for his fundamental contribution to three major advances in his field. The first of Bovet's landmark achievements was the introduction of an antihistamine, which brought relief to millions of allergy sufferers. The second was his development of sulfa drugs, which involved further investigation of how substances interact and interfere with invading microorganisms in the body. Although antibiotics are now the more common means of treating bacterial infection, sulfa drugs are still used for that purpose in many parts of the world and are also of value in specific diseases, such as diabetes and leprosy, and in combination with other drugs. Bovet's third area of pharmacological innovation was the study of curare and its derivatives. He found that in small doses, and in conjunction with general anesthesia, it could be used to induce a relaxation of the muscles that was extremely beneficial in some surgical operations.

Bovet was born in Switzerland and studied pharmacology at the University of Geneva. After receiving his doctorate in 1929 he joined the research staff at the renowned Pasteur Institute in Paris, where he later became head of the Laboratory of Therapeutic chemistry. It was at the Pasteur Institute that Bovet conducted his most famous research.

In 1947 Bovet emigrated to Italy and became affiliated with the Instituto Superiore de Sanita in Rome. For his enormous contributions to the advancement of pharmacology, Bovet was awarded the Nobel Prize in Physiology and Medicine in 1957.

Throughout his career Bovet wrote extensively on microbiology, endocrinology and toxicology. He is also recognized for his study of the relationship between mental illness and the brain's chemistry.

John Boyd Orr, First Baron Boyd Orr 1880–1971

John Boyd Orr spent his career fighting world hunger and malnutrition, working with institutions such as the United Nations to bring about worldwide changes in public health.

Born and educated in Scotland, Boyd Orr founded the Rowett Research Institute in Aberdeen in 1922 and served as director until 1945, during which time he began a journal, *Nutrition Abstracts and Views,* which drew attention to the universal problem of malnutrition. As editor of the journal, Boyd Orr statistically correlated poverty, improper nutrition and poor health. While presenting a frightening picture of the present and potential crises of malnutrition, Boyd Orr recommended ways of reconciling the interests of agriculture and public health. He proposed a number of programs for increasing food production throughout the world, expanding the science of nutrition and presenting it as a crucial part of the solution to the problem of world hunger. Inspired by his work, the League of Nations established its Committee on Nutrition. In 1935 Boyd Orr was knighted to honor his work on world hunger.

Boyd Orr taught agriculture at the University of Aberdeen from 1942 to 1945, then left teaching to become the first director of the United Nations Food and Agriculture Organization. He was by then convinced that an adequate food supply was an essential step toward achieving world peace, and he was tireless in his fight to eliminate food shortages. As a means of achieving a universal food policy based on human need, uninfluenced by commercial and political interests, he advocated a system of world government. For his humanitarian concerns and achievements Boyd Orr was awarded the Nobel Peace Prize in 1949 and was named a baron in that same year. His writings include *Food Health and Income* (1936), *Food and the People* (1944), *Food; Foundation of World Unity* (1948), *The White Man's Dilemma* (1952), *Feast and Famine* (1957), and *As I Recall* (1966).

Zabdiel Boylston 1679–1766

In early eighteenth-century Boston Zabdiel Boylston was known as a skilled and responsible medical practitioner, despite the fact that he lacked the formal qualifications of a degree. (He had trained privately under his father, Dr. Thomas Boylston, and noted physician John Cutter.) In 1721 Boylston ensured himself both historical distinction and the outrage of his contemporaries by introducing smallpox vaccination in the United States (see EDWARD JENNER).

Fourteen years earlier Onesimus, a member of one of the Guramantese tribes of Africa, was brought to America as a slave to work for one of Boston's Puritan families. When the family presented him as a gift to their clergyman, Cotton Mather, the most renowned of all New England Puritans, Onesimus described to the minister a common practice of prophylactic medicine in Africa that involved introducing a weakened form of a disease into the body for the purpose of protection against the disease in its contagious form. Mather, an enthusiast of the sciences and the first American to become a fellow of the Royal Society, discovered subsequent references to this technique, known as inoculation, in a paper published by the Royal Society reporting the practice in Constantinople.

On April 15, 1721 a ship from the West Indies docked in Boston Harbor, importing the first cases of smallpox to Boston. Within months the disease was rampant, and on June 6 Mather distributed his "Address to the Physicians of Boston," encouraging them to inoculate their patients. Scornfully dismissed by the city doctors, Mather sent a description of the inoculation procedure to Boylston two weeks later, concluding with the recommendation that "If upon mature deliberation you should think it advisable to be proceeded in, it may save lives that we set a great value on."

Convinced of both the soundness of the technique and the urgency of the problem, Boylston launched the campaign, beginning with his sons Thomas and John, two slaves, and several of his patients. (He did not inoculate himself, since he had already had smallpox and was hence immune to the disease.)

As news spread of Boylston's practice the public voiced widespread opposition to inoculation, which appeared to have struck a particularly emotional chord among the citizens of Boston. Encouraged by the continued health of his patients, Boylston continued to perform inoculations in the face of increasingly violent public reaction. Inflammatory newspaper articles, open letters and pamphlets attacked both Boylston and Mather, who was the target of a hand grenade tossed through the window of his study. When Boylston continued his activities after an ordinance was passed prohibiting inoculations, angry mobs attacked him in the street and surrounded his home.

Boylston and Mather defended themselves in a series of joint pamphlets, the first appearing in September 1721. Referring to the report from Constantinople, the first monograph was entitled *Some account of what is said of Inoculation or Transplanting the Small Pox By The Learned Dr. Emanuel Timonius, and Jacobus Pylarinus...Answer to the scruples of many about the Lawfulness of this Method*. Boylston described his observations in a number of subsequent articles, reporting in February 1722 that of the 241 patients inoculated only six had died, four of whom had contracted smallpox before their inoculation.

Most Bostonians remained unconvinced, and in 1724 Boylston left for London to prepare a book based on his findings. Although he did not perform inoculations during his stay in England, he was well received as a lecturer at the Royal College of Physicians and at the Royal Society, where he was elected to membership at the beginning of 1726. Completed later that same year, his *Historical Account* is distinguished as a systematic and thorough clinical report on inoculation, as well as the first medical study to be presented by an American.

Boylston returned to Boston in the winter of 1726, administering smallpox inoculations intermittently during periods when the disease threatened to become epidemic. Retiring from medical practice in his sixties, he returned to the farm in Brookline, Massachussetts, where he had spent his childhood. He raised thoroughbred horses until his death after a long bout with lung disease.

On his tombstone the inscription reads: "...Through a life of extensive beneficence, he was always faithful to his word, just in his dealings, affable in his manners; and after a long sickness, in which he was exemplary for his patience and resignation to his Maker, he quitted this mortal life, in a just expectation of a happy immortality."

James Braid 1795–1860

James Braid was a pragmatic and skeptical surgeon who launched medicine's most precarious discipline, the practice of hypnotism. Although it was FRANZ MESMER who actually discovered hypnotic technique, his work was not generally taken seriously, and many of his ideas proved to be misguided. Braid not only coined the phrase "hypnotism" (from the Greek *hypnos*, meaning sleep), but he also developed a sound technique for inducing the phenomenon and brought it to the attention of J.M. CHARCOT and his students at the Salpetriere, the distinguished hospital in Paris for the mentally ill.

With the same reservations as many of his peers, Braid attended a public demonstration of "mesmeric treatment" given by a Swiss who billed himself as a "magnetizer." Braid did not believe in the magnetism the demonstrator claimed to exude, but he was stunned by the obvious power he exerted over his patients. It was their sleeplike trance that fascinated Braid, and, through his own research, he discovered that such a state could be induced by having a patient fix his gaze on a stationary or slowly oscillating object.

In 1843 he published *Neurypnology*, an influential book in which he repudiated Mesmer's fanciful theories of "magnetic fluid" and attributed the effects of hypnosis to the psychological suggestion exercised by the hypnotist. Enthusiastically received in England and France, Braid's doctrine eventually spread throughout the medical community. Before the end of the century it gave rise to Freud's revolutionary application of hypnosis in psychoanalysis.

More than contributing a respectable name to a technique discredited by most of his profession, Braid placed hypnotism in a scientific context and recognized a medical, therapeutic potential in a process that is still being questioned and explored today.

Louis Braille 1809–1852

> I am blind. Now poses the question: How can I arrange to see? How is it possible for me to read that which has been set down by the seeing? About history? About art? About medicine? About politics? About women and men? About me? About the mystery of love and birth? In short, how is it possible for me to take my place in the world as part of the world?
>
> —from the diary of young Louis Braille

Until the introduction of Braille's system of reading and writing, the blind were generally isolated from society, enjoying little chance for gainful employment or social interaction. The "Braille method," requiring only the sense of touch, granted the blind access to education, creative expression, and the status of fully participating members of society.

On the centenary of his death Helen Keller wrote: "Braille was, I believe, among the forerunners of unimagined changes in society and the views which cement it. For he wrought his will through an invention so to mold the world of the blind that today their spirit and mind are different...His invention of a dot system as a tool for their education was a means by which their intellectual release was effected."

In 1809, at the height of the Napoleonic empire, Louis Braille was born in the village of Coupvray, not far from Paris. The son of a harnessmaker, Louis was three years old when he was blinded while playing with an awl in his father's shop. The accident resulted in sympathetic ophthalmia, a severe inflammation of the eye often characterized by an infection of the uveal tissue in both eyes.

With the hardships imposed by Napoleon's levies on bread, cows, mares, hay and other essentials of rural life, Simon René Braille was not able to enroll his son in school until 1822. Louis was thirteen when he was brought to Paris to attend the Institution des Jeunes Aveugles (The Institute for Young Blind People). He found the staff gentle and affectionate, but Braille soon recognized that the existing methods of education for the blind were sorely deficient.

Valentin Hauy, the founder of the institute, had introduced the first system of embossed type for the blind, using regular upper-case lettering. Although he continued to modify the characters to make them more distinguishable to the touch, Hauy's basic premise was to keep the system as close as possible to traditional lettering and language. A second system, developed by Charles Barbier, introduced the use of lines and dots in combination, but the various configurations took up too much space, making it cumbersome to follow with one's fingertips. In contrast to Hauy, Barbier rejected the notion of traditional rules of grammar, spelling and phonetics, severely limiting the system's educational potential.

Adapting the idea of a coded alphabet in relief, Braille devised a system of six dots that could be combined in sixty-three different configurations, providing sufficient symbols for letters, punctuation marks, numbers and mathematical symbols. Braille, who was a dedicated musician, later added modifications that provided for musical notation.

By 1829 Braille had become a teacher at the Institut des Jeunes Aveugles, and it was in that year that he formally presented his ideas to M. Pignier, the school's director of studies. Impressed by the efficiency and scope of Braille's system, Pignier incorporated it into the teaching methods at the institute. The first pamphlet in embossed "Braille" was published later that year, and by the time the first edition was placed on display at the Paris Exposition of Industrial Products in 1834 the system had already changed the lives of hundreds of grateful students at the institute.

Suffering from pulmonary tuberculosis, Braille was on leave from the school when his friend Pignier was replaced by M. Dufau, a new headmaster who opposed the idea of an alphabet for the blind. Insisting that Braille's method of teaching the blind would only decrease their chances for assimilation into society, Dufau also recognized that seeing teachers would object to using a system that eventually could be taught by the blind.

Jean Gaudet, the school's assistant director, strongly supported Braille, however, and composed a fifteen-page pamphlet in his defense, entitled "Account of the System of Raised Dots for Use by the Blind." Published in 1844, Gaudet's analysis and testimonial convinced even Dufau of the value of the Braille system.

Since his premature death from tuberculosis at the age of 43 Braille has been internationally acclaimed for his enormous contribution to the welfare of the blind. The Louis Braille Foundation for Blind Musicians continues to honor his memory, and the Braille method has been adopted in schools throughout the world.

Pierre Fidèle Bretonneau 1778–1862

A dedicated physician and distinguished botanist, Pierre Bretonneau is best known for his epidemiological research, particularly in the study of typhoid and diphtheria. Bretonneau seized the opportunity to investigate diphtheria during an epidemic that devastated his native Tours between 1818 and 1820. His research formed the basis of a treatise published in 1821 in which Bretonneau named diphtheria, distinguishing the disease from scarlet fever.

Based on his observations of a typhoid epidemic in Chenonceaux, Bretonneau differentiated this disease from typhus, also describing the role of contact in the spread of the epidemic. Foreshadowing the revolutionary findings of LOUIS PASTEUR, Bretonneau proposed the notion of morbid specificity in 1855, suggesting that communicable diseases are caused by specific reproductive agents. Although he did not successfully isolate or identify these agents, Bretonneau's germ theory of disease was confirmed within the next decade by Pasteur, Émile Roux and others.

Although his father was a noted surgeon, Pierre-Fidele received almost no formal education as a child, learning to read on his own at the age of nine. At seventeen he was enrolled at the École de Santé in Paris, where he studied under celebrated physician JEAN NICOLAS CORVISART. Failing his final examinations, Bretonneau took a job as a public health officer in Chenonceaux, where he established a distinguished reputation for his skill and sensitivity as a medical practitioner. Offered the position of chief medical officer at the Tours Hospital, Bretonneau took the doctoral examinations, receiving his medical degree in 1815.

Bretonneau accepted the hospital post, taking on additional duties as director of the École de Santé at Tours. Identifying diphtheria in 1819, he published an analytic description of the disease two years later, noting the initial inflammation of the tonsils and possible subsequent involvement of the ear, nose and throat. Bretonneau also observed that certain symptoms, including fever and asphyxia, would occur regardless of the localization of the disease. These findings led him to understand that the duration and severity of some symptoms are functions of the specific type of inflammation rather than the kind of tissue in which the disease is located.

In an effort to prevent the fatal condition of asphyxia due to inflammation of the larynx, Bretonneau developed the tracheotomy, a surgical procedure in which blockage of the larynx is bypassed by an incision made in the trachea, or windpipe. His first successful operation, performed in 1825 on a four-year-old girl, was made possible in part by Bretonneau's invention of the double cannula, an instrument designed to close the trachea immediately after incision in order to prevent blood from entering the organ.

Retaining his prestigious positions at the hospital and at the École de Santé, Bretonneau pursued a wide range of other interests, including sculpture, painting, engineering, entomology, botany and horticulture. He established a celebrated botanic garden and produced a widely respected monograph on plant grafting.

In 1838 he abandoned his administrative duties, choosing to dedicate the remainder of his career to medical practice among the poor. After the death of his wife, twenty-five years his senior, Bretonneau remarried, at the age of seventy-eight, a girl of eighteen.

Richard Bright 1789–1858

English physician Richard Bright is best remembered for his outstanding contribution to the study of kidney disease. A prominent member of the faculty at Guy's Hospital in London, Bright, along with Thomas Addison, Astley Cooper and THOMAS HODGKIN, helped to usher in a new era of clinical medicine while developing one of Britain's most distinguished medical institutions.

With a spirit of inquiry that was both systematic and meticulous, Bright navigated the transition to modern clinical practice by combining old medical traditions with progressive ideas. "For my part I am very fond of seeing," he wrote during his first years as a medical student, and throughout his career Bright would rely on his remarkable powers of observation in research and practice.

Born to a wealthy family in Bristol, Bright entered medical school at the University of Edinburgh when he was nineteen but dropped out after the first year to serve as geologist, botanist, zoologist and staff artist on an expedition to Iceland with Sir George Mackenzie.

Bright resumed his medical education in 1810 at Guy's Hospital, where he trained for two years, and then returned to Edinburgh to graduate in 1813. Later that year he enrolled at Cambridge, but restlessness and boredom soon drove him to take off again, this time on a grand tour of Germany, Austria and Hungary. An account of Bright's observations and experiences, accompanied by his own illustrations, was published in 1818 as *Travels from Vienna Through Lower Hungary: With Some Remarks on the State of Vienna During the Congress in the Year 1814.*

Bright decided to settle down as he entered his thirties, obtaining a license from the London College of Physicians and then joining the staff at Guy's Hospital as an assistant physician. He was appointed full physician in 1824 and also became a professor of medicine and anatomy.

Suspicious of medical theories or philosophical frameworks, Bright dealt only with the "facts of observation" in his practice, gathering information from clinical, laboratory, and postmortem investigations. From a mass of data he would seek meaningful patterns, or, as he put it, "such facts as seem to throw light upon each other," in order to identify clinico-pathological correlations.

In an outstanding demonstration of the process, Bright published a study on kidney disease in 1827 that is considered a masterpiece of clinical literature. Following the course of illness in 100 patients, he recorded the meticulous details of "morbid appearance" in life, in death and after dissection and then correlated chemical, pathological and clinical phenomena to identify a new disease pattern known as "Bright's disease." The pattern was later shown to be characteristic of a large group of distinct disease entities associated with albuminuria and edema, including arteriolar nephrosclerosis, diabetic nephropathy, or lupus nephritis.

Through the efforts of Bright and his talented colleagues, Guy's Hospital gained distinction as one of Britain's most prestigious medical schools. Bright's influence was felt most notably in his advancement of clinical research and education. *Guy's Hospital Reports*, the journal he helped to establish, announced the success of Bright's clinical training program in 1837: "Each student who has passed three months in the clinical wards is ready to admit that that period has proved the most profitable portion of his medical education...Under the guidance of the experienced physicians, the student is instructed how to make observations upon the sick, and to interpret the signs of disease..."

In addition to numerous research papers, critical treatises and biographical studies, Bright's published works include *Reports of Medical Cases Selected with a View of Illustrating Symptoms and Cure of Diseases with a Reference to Morbid Anatomy* (2 vols., 1827–1831) and *Elements of the Practice of Medicine* (with Thomas Addison, 1839).

Pierre Paul Broca 1824–1880

Paul Broca's landmark demonstration of cerebral localization was one of the earliest attempts at a scientific examination of the relationship between mind and brain. A distinguished anthropologist, surgeon and neuroanatomist, Paul Broca discovered that aphasia, a condition characterized by difficulties in expressing speech, could be traced to damage of a particular portion of the brain's left hemisphere. Despite the fact that his findings were later judged to be simplistic and in some cases inaccurate, Broca's work was a milestone in the study of cerebral neurology. Although centers for mental functions cannot be clearly delineated, Broca proved conclusively that areas of the brain are specialized in their control of mental activities, and that the two hemispheres of the brain are neither identical nor mirror images of each other, as was commonly thought.

In presenting his findings to the Paris Anthropological Society in 1861, Broca exhibited the brain of M. Leborgne, an aphasic patient known in the literature as Tan Tan, a nickname derived from the only phrase Leborgne was able to speak. Tan Tan's comprehension was unimpaired, and he communicated with gestures and facial expression, but he had lost his ability to speak or write. In a postmortem Broca found a damaged area approximately the size of a golf ball in the left hemisphere of Tan Tan's brain.

Many were convinced by Broca's demonstration, although his findings were resisted by some who distrusted his anatomical observations and by others who warily recalled the misguided theories of FRANCIS GALL. Ten years later German neurologist Karl Wernicke (1848–1905) related other forms of aphasia to identifiable regions of the left hemisphere of the brain, further confirming the theory of cerebral localization. Pointing out the many complex mechanisms involved in the function of speech, modern proponents of a holistic view of the brain maintain that all areas must work in concert to successfully achieve mental function. It has nonetheless been clearly demonstrated that damage or inhibition of specific portions of the brain will cause a disturbance in corresponding mental functions.

The term "convolution of Broca," or "Broca's area," refers to the section of the brain he identified as the center for speech function. It is the third convolution of the left frontal lobe. Broca lent his name to a number of other anatomical and medical terms, including "Broca's aphasia," a condition in which the patient cannot write or speak fluently or coherently but retains his abilities to comprehend and even sing. "Broca's fissure" is the fold surrounding the lower left convolution of the frontal lobe; "Broca's plane" refers to the plane of vision; "Broca's pouch" is the sac located in the labia majora, also known as the pudendal sac; and "Broca's space" identifies a section of the inner olfactory lobe of the brain.

Paul Broca was born at Sainte-Foy-le-Grande, a small town near the south Atlantic coast of France. He was educated in Paris, earning degrees in surgery, pathology and anthropology. In addition to his distinguished work as a clinician, Broca held concurrent professorships at the Faculty of Medicine of Paris and at the Anthropological Institute.

As founder of the Anthropological Society in 1859, Broca was a pioneer in the study of anthropology at a time when the discipline was discounted by the scientific establishment and opposed by the government and a number of religious factions. Broca contributed significantly to the advancement of human anthropology, establishing brain and skull ratios and other methods of classification based on physical characteristics. In 1872 he founded France's first anthropological journal, *Revue d'Anthropologie*. He is also noted for extensive research on ancient surgical practices.

Benjamin Collins Brodie 1783–1862

Philosopher, writer, statesman and physician, Benjamin Brodie was among the outstanding surgeons of nineteenth-century London. A distinguished member of the staff at St. George's Hospital, Brodie was called in to attend an operation for removal of a skin tumor performed on King George IV.

Somewhat less flamboyant than his contemporaries William Fergusson• and James Paget•, Brodie established his reputation as a generous and compassionate practitioner. Opposing the prevailing practice of indiscriminate amputation, Brodie advocated milder, more innovative forms of treatment, particularly in cases of joint disease.

Brodie devoted much of his attention to the study of localized nervous afflictions, delivering a series of lectures on hysterical pain and other manifestations of a disordered nervous system. "Brodie's knee" came to refer to a condition of stiff knees frequently observed in hysterical patients. The term now denotes a particular form of chronic inflammation in the knee joint, also known as "Brodie's disease."

Born at Winterslow Rectory in Wiltshire, England, Brodie received part of his medical training at the celebrated Hunterian School in London. He continued his studies at St. George's Hospital, where he later became chief surgeon.

Brodie produced an autobiographical work, which was included in a three-volume collection of his writings published in 1898. His son, Benjamin Collins Brodie (1817–1880), became a distinguished chemist, noted for the discovery of graphitic acid.

Michael Stuart Brown 1941–

In 1973 molecular geneticist Michael Brown and his colleague JOSEPH GOLDSTEIN discovered the existence of cholesterol-seeking receptor cells responsible for extracting cholesterol particles from the bloodstream. These low-density lipoproteins, or LDL's are cholesterol-carrying particles which must be drawn into the cells before the cholesterol can be broken down.

Seeking the genetic component in high blood cholesterol levels, Brown and Goldstein determined that patients with a hereditary predisposition to this condition were deficient in LDL receptors or lacked them altogether.

Their research also revealed that as cells take in lipoproteins the production of new LDL receptors is inhibited, so that when the body is overloaded with cholesterol, normal cholesterol metabolism may be impeded. The arteries may thus become clogged with excess cholesterol—a condition that can result in strokes, heart attacks and hardening of the arteries.

By describing the LDL receptor cells as essential to cholesterol metabolism, Brown and Goldstein opened the door to new methods of treatment and prevention of diseases related to the accumulation of fatty cholesterol. Their contribution was acknowledged in 1985 with the award of the Nobel Prize for Physiology or Medicine.

A native of New York City, Brown received his medical degree in 1966 from the University of Pennsylvania. During his internship at Massachusetts General Hospital in Boston he became friends with Goldstein, who was also completing his internship. In 1968 Brown joined the research staff of the National Institutes of Health, where he was assigned to study the chemistry and pathology of the digestive system.

Brown and Goldstein were reunited in Dallas in 1971 at the Southwestern Medical School of the University of Texas, where Brown had accepted a position as assistant professor. It was at Southwestern that their successful partnership was launched, resulting in the landmark discovery of LDL receptors. Brown and Goldstein later resumed their collaboration in an attempt to decipher the genetic code for the LDL receptor. They have also conducted joint research in an effort to develop safe and effective drugs for use in lowering blood cholesterol levels.

In 1977 Brown was appointed director of the Center for Genetic Diseases in Dallas, where he continues to teach and conduct research.

William Tillinghast Bull 1849–1909

As director of the the Chambers Street Hospital in lower Manhattan, American surgeon William Bull introduced a number of significant advances in surgical techniques, particularly in procedures for emergency operations. While still a young man Bull gained distinction as one of the country's leading surgeons, most notably for his development of the laparotomy, a surgical incision in the abdominal wall. Bull pioneered the use of the technique for the treatment of gunshot wounds, in which severe damage to the intestines or other abdominal organs often required immediate repair by suture.

Born in Newport, Rhode Island, William Bull was heir to one of the oldest Anglo-American families, dating back to Henry Bull, twice governor of the colony, and one of the nine original members of the Roger Williams settlement of Newport (then Aquidneck). Bull graduated from Harvard College in 1869, receiving a degree in medicine from the New York College of Physicians and Surgeons in 1872.

After completing his surgical internship at Bellevue Hospital Bull left for Europe to supplement his medical education at distinguished clinics in Paris, London, Vienna and Berlin. In 1875 he returned to New York to take over as director of the New York Dispensary, joining the staff at Chambers Street Hospital two years later.

Establishing a distinguished reputation both for himself and for the hospital, Bull contributed significantly to advancing surgical treatment for injuries to the chest and abdomen. In the 1870s the mortality rate among patients treated for gunshot wounds of the abdomen was a grim 87% but the figure had dropped below 65% by the time Bull left Chambers Street in 1888.

In addition to improved operating techniques, Bull owed a large measure of his distinguished surgical record to an advanced knowledge of antisepsis. One of JOSEPH LISTER's leading exponents in the United States, Bull exhorted all surgical practitioners to adopt the use of disinfectants and sterile surgical instruments and supplies.

Serving as attending or consulting physician at the Hospital for the Ruptured and Crippled, Woman's Hospital, New York Hospital and St. Luke's Hospital, he was appointed professor of surgery at the College of Physicians and Surgeons in 1889.

Other notable contributions to surgical practice include Bull's recommendations for treating hernias, described in a number of published works, including an article coauthored with William B. Coley entitled *Observations on the Mechanical and Operative Treatment of Hernia at the Hospital for the Ruptured and Crippled* (1893). Also noted for his clinical study of breast cancer, Bull published a report in 1894 entitled *Cases of Cancer of the Breast Treated by Radical Operation, with a Report of 118 Cases*].

Diagnosed with a severe form of cancer of the neck in 1908, Bull died in February of the following year at the age of sixty.

Denis Burkitt 1911–

Combining the perspectives of a surgeon and an epidemiologist, Denis Burkitt conducted important investigations of cancer pathology and its geographical distribution that led to the discovery of the first virus to cause cancer in humans. A leading authority on the epidemiological aspects of cancer, Burkitt confirmed the dietary theories of T.L. Cleave, which associated the use of refined carbohydrates with the spread of certain kinds of disease.

In the late 1960s Burkitt's studies of disease distribution patterns revealed a correlation between a diet low in cereals, grains, fruits and vegetables—all food groups containing fiber—and a higher incidence of diseases such as appendicitis, diverticulitis, hiatus hernia and cancer of the colon.

Examining the relationship between dietary fiber and disease, subsequent research indicated that cancer-inhibiting effects vary with both the specific form of the disease and the particular type of fiber. Most recent studies suggest a chemical factor linking bowel disease with the interaction between the immune system and the brain, suggesting that the introduction of a virus might trigger the disease by intervening in this system.

Born in Enniskillen, Ireland, Burkitt obtained his medical degree in 1935 from Trinity College in Dublin. During World War II he served as an army surgeon, receiving his discharge in 1945. That same year he left for Africa, where he spent more than twenty years as a surgeon at the Makerere College Medical School in Uganda.

Among his patients were a great many children who exhibited tumors in a number of specific locations, including the kidneys, liver, testicles and bones. Noting that a great many of these young patients had tumors in two or more of these areas, Burkitt suspected that rather than representing different forms of cancer, as was popularly believed, these tumors were all of one type, merely manifesting themselves at characteristic locations. In the late 1950s he conducted further clinical studies indicating an association between the age of the child and the site of the tumor.

Mapping the distribution of this particular form of lymphoma in Africa and New Guinea, Burkitt found by far the highest incidence of the disease in hot and humid areas, suggesting the possibility of an insect vector in the transmission of an environmental agent. Until this century it was widely believed that malignant tumors were the result of a mysterious metabolic process, rather than any external cause. Notable exceptions include references throughout history to the dangers of tobacco and studies in the mid-nineteenth century of lung cancer in miners and bladder cancer in aniline workers. Introducing the first experimental evidence of a cancer-causing virus in animals, microbiologist FRANCIS PEYTON ROUS demonstrated in 1911 the transmissibility of a form of sarcoma between birds.

It was more than half a century before noted English virologists M.A. Epstein and E. Barr discovered the virus responsible for "Burkitt's tumor," now referred to as "Burkitt's lymphoma." The causative agent, known as the "EB virus," was later implicated in infectious mononucleosis as well as nasopharyngeal cancer, the most common form of the disease in Southeast Asia.

Burkitt's lymphoma proved particularly responsive to chemotherapy, suggesting that, in addition to the effectiveness of the cytotoxic drugs, the high rates of survival might also be due to biological mechanisms acting against the remaining malignant cells. Based on his clinical observations at Makerere, Burkitt's investigations contributed to research developments in cancer, chemotherapy and immunology.

Sir Frank MacFarlane Burnet 1899–1985

One of the twentieth century's leading virologists, Sir Frank MacFarlane Burnet formulated the theory that made it possible to overcome the immunological obstacles to tissue and organ transplants.

The ability to resist disease depends on the ability of the body's immunological system to produce antibodies in the presence of foreign substances, or antigens. Immunological tolerance is defined as the failure to develop an immune reaction when exposed to a substance that would normally be antigenic. A compatibility between the body and its own immunological system must develop at birth so that the animal will not respond to its own body tissues as antigenic.

Working independently, Australian-born Burnet and British biologist PETER MEDAWAR investigated the mechanisms of the immunological system, focusing on the earliest stage of development. Both scientists discovered that tolerance to a particular substance could be induced in a newborn by exposing the infant to it before his immune system became fully developed. In recognition of the far-reaching implications of their findings, Burnet and Medawar were jointly awarded the Nobel Prize for Physiology or Medicine in 1960.

Originally proposed by noted immunologist Lewis Thomas, the concept of immunologic surveillance was developed by Burnet as a means of explaining the body's tendency to reject transplanted tissues and organs. Arguing that this negative response to a foreign substance is an unfortunate offshoot of an essential protective mechanism, Burnet suggested that the rejection of variant forms of normal tissue cells reflects a natural defense against cancer. Based on the evidence that many incipient cancers never develop to become clinically threatening, Burnet and others contended that under normal conditions an immunological system of surveillance guards against tumor growth.

Although it has been found that tumors grow more rapidly when the immunological system is disrupted or damaged, the accuracy of Burnet's theory has yet to be determined. Regardless, Burnet's insights and explorations have launched significant studies in the fight against cancer.

Burnet's numerous and diverse achievements also include the discovery of several different strains of the poliomyelitis virus and the isolation of the microorganism responsible for Q fever, (Q for query), an acute illness found throughout the world and generally characterized by respiratory infection and high fever. The disease is caused by a rickettsial organism now referred to as *Coxiella burnetti,* in homage to its discoverer.

Burnet also made important advances in the study of influenza and the development of an immunization against that disease. Recognized for his pioneer study of the multiplication of bacteriophages, Burnet also introduced a laboratory technique for cultivating viruses in living chick embryos.

Born at Traralgon in Victoria, Australia, Burnet was a resident pathologist at the Royal Melbourne Hospital before coming to England for a year as a Beit fellow at the Lister Institute in London. He returned to Australia in 1928 as assistant director of the Walter and Eliza Hall Institute at the Royal Melbourne Hospital. In 1944 he took over as director of the institute, accepting a professorship at the University of Melbourne that same year. Lecturing at major universities throughout the world, Burnet gained international distinction for his groundbreaking research. He received a knighthood in 1951 and was awarded the Order of Merit in 1958. Permanently based in Australia, he served as director at the Walter and Eliza Hall Institute for nearly twenty- five years.

Burnet published an autobiography in 1968 entitled *Changing Patterns.* Other written works include *Natural History of Infectious Disease* (3rd edition published in 1962), *Viruses and Man* (2nd edition published in 1955), and *Credo and Comment* (1978).

C

Albert Calmette 1863–1933

A disciple of LOUIS PASTEUR and Émile Roux, bacteriologist Albert Calmette is best known for his work with Camille Guérin which led to the first vaccine against tuberculosis. In 1908, working together at the newly founded Pasteur Institute in Lille, Calmette and Guérin developed a strain of tubercle bacillus of such low virulence that even alive it could be safely used in a vaccine.

Noting the similarity between the human and bovine forms of tubercle bacilli, Calmette and Guérin experimented with a strain of bovine bacillus initially isolated by ROBERT KOCH in 1882. Known as BCG (Bacillus Calmette-Guérin), their newly developed strain was effective in producing tuberculosis immunity in humans and cattle.

Born in Nice, Calmette joined the medical corps of the French navy in 1883. After six years of travel in naval service he arrived in Paris, where he enrolled in a course in microbiology designed by Émile Roux and ALEXANDRE YERSIN at the Pasteur Institute. Pasteur himself was so impressed with Calmette's dedication and talent for microbiology that he asked him to organize a branch of the Pasteur Institute in Saigon in 1891. It was as supervisor of the Saigon research laboratory that Calmette began his research on snake poison, becoming one of the first to investigate the injection of blood serum from immune individuals in the treatment against animal venom. In 1894 he introduced the first anti-snakebite serum.

Calmette returned to France two years later, taking over directorship of the Pasteur Institute at Lille. In addition to his collaborative research on tuberculosis, Calmette explored a number of other public health problems, including ancylostomiasis or hookworm disease.

In 1919 Calmette became assistant director at the Pasteur Institute in Paris, where he founded a separate department for the study of tuberculosis. After its introduction in 1921 the anti-tuberculosis BCG vaccine was threatened with scandal when a group of children in Lubeck died after being inoculated. Calmette, Guérin and the BCG were vindicated when it was established that the lethal batch of vaccine had been improperly prepared.

The BCG vaccine, administered shortly after birth, has been given to more than 50 million children throughout the world under the auspices of the World Health Organization. It was not adopted in the United States until 1940, and in Great Britain in 1956. By the mid-1940s therapeutic drugs were developed to combat tuberculosis, most notably streptomycin, an antibiotic introduced by S.A. WAKSMAN in 1944.

Calmette's written works include *Les venins, les animaux venimeux et la serotherapie anti-venimeuse (Venoms, Animal Venom and Anti-Venom Serotheraphy)* (1907), *Recherches experimentales sur la tuberculose (Experimental Research on Tuberculosis)* (1907–1914), *L'infection bacillaire et la tuberculose chez l'homme et chez les animaux (Bacillary Infection and Human and Animal Tuberculosis)* (1920) *La vaccination preventive par le BCG (Preventive Vaccination by BCG)* (1927).

Walter Bradford Cannon 1871–1945

Walter Cannon had not yet graduated from Harvard Medical School when he attracted the attention of the scientific community in 1897 by using X rays in a physiological examination. Cannon had devised a mealy substance made from bismuth subnitrate which was of such high atomic density that it was impenetrable by X ray. Feeding the bismuth meal in gelatin capsules to animal subjects, he used fluoroscopic technique to track its passage through the alimentary tract. Once the meal was ingested, the subject's intestinal system appeared as a white image against a black background.

Cannon presented the results of these experimental observations in *The Mechanical Factors of Digestion*, published in 1911. Causing widespread sensation within the scientific community, Cannon's landmark demonstration yielded the first photographs of an internal organ as it functioned within the body.

By the time he received his medical degree Cannon was already a member of the Harvard faculty. A versatile and innovative thinker, he proposed that medical education incorporate the " case system" as it is used in the study of law.

Cannon's career at Harvard spanned nearly half a century, during which time he produced a significant body of research focused largely on the nervous system and related phenomena. Noting the effects of strong emotions on gastrointestinal function, Cannon became intrigued by the function and mechanism of the sympathetic nervous system, a division of the autonomic nervous system. As the trigger for a number of physiological responses, including dilation of pupils, constriction of blood vessels and increase in heart rate, the sympathetic nerves help prepare the body for "fright, fight or flight."

In 1915 Cannon published *Pain, Hunger, Fear, and Rage,* describing the body's functioning in an emergency. As a member of British and American shock committees during World War I he conducted extensive studies of hemorrhagic and traumatic shock cases among wounded soldiers, presenting his findings in a treatise entitled *Traumatic Shock.*

In 1926 Cannon introduced the term homeostasis, describing the body's ability to stabilize internal physiological functions. Based on the work of French physiologists CLAUDE BERNARD and C.R. Richet, as well as on his own studies of metabolic hormone regulation, the autonomic nervous system and the physiological bases of hunger and thirst, Cannon's homeostatic theory states that under moderately variable external conditions an organism strives to maintain a stable internal environment. This process of continual internal readjustment is accomplished primarily by the regulation of a number of hormones, most notably a substance Cannon named sympathin, now known as either adrenaline or epinephrine. Presented in a popular and accessible work entitled *Wisdom of the Body* (1932), the principle of homeostasis has had far-reaching implications throughout medicine.

The establishment of a "normal" range of internal biochemical variations has enabled the development of a great many diagnostic tests, including the testing of blood sugar levels for diabetes and hypoglycemia testing. Homeostatic principles formed the basis of biofeedback theory and were applied broadly by Cannon and fellow Harvard physiologist L.J. Henderson (1878–1942) to political and social philosophy. Reflecting his commitment to the universality of science and the family of man, Cannon's functionalist approach led him to participate in the establishment and direction of a number of international medical organizations.

Investigating the concept of homeostasis and the physiological effects of emotion, Cannon established that the generation of emotions occurred in the limbic system of the brain. This was a startling assertion in 1929, when it was generally believed that emotions were the result of a stimulation of physical sensation, a theory that suggests that a person feels happy because he has been made to laugh, and that he feels fear because he is running away.

Pursuing his study of the chemistry of impulse transmission in the sympathetic nervous system, Cannon discovered that even under normal non-stressful conditions the nerves produce a substance similar to adrenaline. Working with Arturo Rosenblueth, Cannon suggested the existence of two different "sympathin" compounds of opposing functions—one excitatory, one inhibitory. These hormonal substances are now known as adrenaline and noradrenaline, or epinephrine and norepinephrine.

Cannon retired from Harvard as professor emeritus in 1942. That year he published a provocative article entitled *Voodoo Death* in which he discussed magical voodoo phenomena in physiological terms. Lending credence and dignity to a subject that was usually dismissed in scientific discussions, Cannon accepted the premise that voodoo magic can work and sought to explain its effectiveness as the result of "...shock induced by prolonged and intense emotion." He suggested that a voodoo attack could have drastic effects on the sympathicoadrenal system of the victim, causing a profound drop in blood pressure and an interruption of oxygen flow to vital organs. Concluding that the death of a victim cursed by voodoo is a psychosomatic event "due to shocking emotional stress—to obvious or repressed terror," Cannon's scientific insight on "psychotransference" and other magical phenomena is acknowledged by physiologists as well as by such notable anthropologists as Claude Levi-Strauss (1908–).

Published in the year of his death, Cannon's influential autobiography, *The Way of an Investigator,* is an inspirational account of an imaginative and fruitful career in science.

Alexis Carrel 1873–1944

French-born biologist and experimental surgeon Alexis Carrel devoted much of his career to the development of organ transplantation and the prolongation of the life of tissues. He is celebrated for introducing a number of important innovations in cardiovascular technique, including most notably a method of suturing blood vessels end to end to produce a watertight joint without compromising the width of the channel. Enabling surgeons to connect a vessel to a transplanted organ, the procedure is applicable to small or large veins and arteries.

Many of Carrel's methods were eventually incorporated into clinical practice in transplantation and heart surgery, although it took several decades for medical technology to catch up with his ideas. For his contribution to vascular ligature and the transplantation of organs, Carrel received the Nobel Prize for Physiology or Medicine in 1912. A naturalized citizen of the United States by then, he became the first American to win the award in that category.

Carrel was born at Ste. Foy-les-Lyon, a small town near Lyons in central France. Educated at the University of Lyons, he obtained his medical degree in 1900 at the age of 27. After four years of postgraduate studies in experimental surgery he left Lyons to launch his career in the United States.

In 1906 he joined the staff of the Rockefeller Institute for Medical Research (now Rockefeller University), where he was to produce the most important work of his career. Becoming a member of the prestigious institute in 1912, he retained the professional association for more than 25 years.

Early in his career, Carrel embarked on a collaboration with famed aviator Charles A. Lindbergh (1902–1974) to produce an artificial or mechanical heart that could sustain a variety of tissues and living organs outside the body. keep. The apparatus was a germ-proof perfusion pump that was designed to permeate the organ with a constant supply of blood. Monitoring the long-term results of the experiment, Carrel kept alive tissue from the heart of a chicken for more than 30 years. With Lindbergh he published a report of their research in 1938, entitled *The Culture of Organs*.

Carrel also collaborated with noted English chemist HENRY DRYSDALE DAKIN in an effort to develop a treatment for wounds during World War I. The result was "Dakin's", or the "Carrel-Dakin" solution—a 5% solution of sodium- hypochlorite for the irrigation and sterilization of deep wounds.

Carrel continued to explore techniques of cardiovascular surgery, transplantation and transfusion throughout his long and productive career at Rockefeller University. In 1939 he returned to France, where he spent the last five years of his life. He died in Paris at the age of 71.

Edith Cavell 1865–1915

Edith Cavell, who dedicated her life to the advancement of nursing, is celebrated by many as a martyr to the cause of compassion even in war. Following her death, memorial services throughout the world paid tribute to her, and in St. Martin's Place, London, a statue was erected in honor of her courage and devotion.

As first matron of the Berkendael Medical Institute in Brussels, Cavell was granted permission by the Germans to continue her work during World War I and to establish the institute as a Red Cross hospital. Devoted to the care of wounded soldiers, regardless of their political affiliation, Cavell was accused of harboring Allied soldiers at her hospital and "conducting soldiers to the enemy." She was placed in solitary confinement for nine weeks under suspicion of espionage, a capital offense. Denied legal counsel, Cavell confessed to helping Allied soldiers escape to the neutral territory of the Netherlands and admitted that, with her assistance, many had arrived safely in England.

Struggling to defend Cavell against the injustice of German military law were Brand Whitlock, the United States minister in Brussels, and Sadi Kirchen, a Belgian lawyer engaged by Cavell's friends and supporters; but by most accounts, her conviction was a foregone conclusion. She was arraigned with thirty-five other prisoners before a court-martial tribunal in which proceedings were conducted in German.

On October 8, 1915 she was found guilty of aiding the escape of Allied prisoners and was sentenced to death, although there was no evidence of treason or espionage. Cavell went before a firing sqaud at dawn less than four days later.

She was born in Norfolk, England, the eldest daughter of the vicar of Swardeston. After attending a small school in Somerset Cavell left England to continue her education on the Continent. Subsidized by a small inheritance, she traveled through Europe, visiting hospitals and training centers for nurses. She became interested in a free clinic in southern Germany and donated a substantial endowment for the purchase of medical equipment and supplies.

Returning to England in 1895, she joined the staff at London Hospital as a nursing intern and within two years was placed in charge of an emergency typhoid clinic in Maidstone.

In 1906 she returned to Belgium to help develop a modern school for nursing in Brussels, where training was limited mainly to the Catholic religious orders. Working with Dr. Depage, director of the Berkendael Medical Institute, Cavell introduced the English system of nursing care and training, and the clinic soon became Belgium's leading hospital and educational facility for nurses. Officially recognized by the state, the institute was granted government funds for expansion shortly before war broke out.

In addition to serving as first matron at Berkendael, Cavell undertook the organization of St. Gilles Hospital, also in Brussels. In August 1914 Depage joined the effort to organize a network of military hospitals, leaving Cavell in charge of the institute. Within months Belgium fell to the Germans, and all French and British troops were ordered to leave the country. Soldiers who had been separated from their units relied on the Belgian underground for protection and a means of escape. Edith Cavell offered these military refugees all resources available for their return to safety.

Aulus Cornelius Celsus (also Aurelius Cornelius Celsus) c. 14–37 A.D.

Much of our knowledge of Alexandrian and Roman medicine of the first century has been gleaned from the eight volumes surviving of a larger encyclopedia written by Cornelius Celsus. Although neither physician nor scientist, Celsus endeavored to include in his work all available knowledge, covering the areas of politics, law, philosophy, science, agriculture and medicine. Little remains of his work beyond the eight books he wrote in 30 A.D. entitled *De Medicina*—an extensive and detailed study of the history, philosophy and practice of medicine.

De Medicina was exceptional not only for its enormous scope but also because it was one of the few scientific or intellectual works of its time written in Latin. Though influential at the time it was written, his great work was ignored for centuries because Celsus did not choose the more intellectually acceptable Greek language. *De Medicina* was rediscovered during the Renaissance by Pope Nicholas V and later became the first medical writing to be printed in movable type, in Florence in 1478.

Although he was not a medical practitioner, Celsus's descriptions of pathology and surgical techniques are considered perceptive and precise. He was the first to identify the cardinal symptoms of inflammation: *rubor* (redness), *tumor* (swelling), *calor* (heat) and *dolor* (pain). His discussions of wounds, amputations and hernias are vivid and astute. His writing on surgery is astonishingly modern, including descriptions of a reconstruction of the nose, surgical treatment for hernias, and techniques for the removal of tonsils and goiters.

Celsus's approach to medicine drew largely from the philosophies of HIPPOCRATES and Asclepiades, stressing mild, sensible treatment and a sympathetic bedside manner. He wrote: "The physician of experience is recognized by his not at once seizing the arm of his patient as soon as he comes to his side, but he looks upon him and as it were sifts him first with a serene look, to discover how he really is: and if the sick man manifests fear, he soothes him with suitable words before proceeding to a manual examination."

Since the rediscovery of *De Medicina*, scores of subsequent editions have been published in continued acknowledgment of Celsus's ever-applicable wisdom. The work was translated into English in 1756 by James Grieve, and a second translation, by W.G. Spencer, appeared in 1935.

Sir Edwin Chadwick 1800–1890

A staunch advocate of the "utilitarian" doctrine of Jeremy Bentham (1748–1832), which taught that the individual's greatest happiness depends on the happiness of others, Sir Edwin Chadwick enthusiastically joined the British movement for public health reforms in the mid-nineteenth century. Beginning with improvements in England's Poor Act in 1834, Chadwick went on to lead the campaign for passage of the Public Health Act of 1848, which formally established a governmental board of health. Chadwick's treatise *Inquiry into the Sanitary Conditions of the Labouring Population*, published in 1842, brought about significant advances in public health legislation.

Collecting and analyzing vital statistics, Chadwick correlated mortality rates with living conditions. Although he mistakenly believed that diseases could be caused by "miasmas" (noxious emanations) that lingered in garbage, in impure water and in inefficient drainage systems, the concept of "filth diseases" was used persuasively by Chadwick in to initiate important environmental reforms in housing, water supply and sewage systems. An ardent promoter of Chadwick's environmental programs, FLORENCE NIGHTINGALE contributed her own statistical findings to support his cause.

Born in Manchester, Chadwick worked for many years as aide to Bentham before passing the bar in 1830. In 1833, as assistant poor-law commissioner, Chadwick submitted a report that established the principles of a system of government inspection. After the reforms of 1834 he was named secretary of the new Poor Law Board. A compilation of his works, published in 1887, is entitled *The Health of Nations*.

Ernst Boris Chain 1906–1979

Ernst Chain, whose work as a biochemist led to the lifesaving therapeutic use of penicillin, was a Russian Jew born in Germany. He had almost completed his education at the Friedrich-Wilhelm University in Berlin when he was forced to emigrate to England as Hitler was rising to power in 1933. His work at Cambridge University caught the attention of HOWARD FLOREY, who invited him to join the department of Pathology at Oxford. It was there that Chain began lecturing on chemical pathology in 1936.

Chain and Florey were both interested in the ten-year-old findings of ALEXANDER FLEMING on the inhibiting effects of penicillin on bacteria. This phenomenon had been observed even before Fleming's experiments, but no thought had yet been given to a therapeutic use for penicillin. As time went by, however, the devastation of World War II created a pressing need for aggressive medical care of wounds and trauma. Although sulfa drugs had proved to be an enormous boon to medicine, their side effects, particularly on the blood and kidneys, were a disturbing drawback. Penicillin seemed as if it could be an improved alternative, as it was harmless to anything save the bacteria that it destroyed. Chain and Florey's work, which consisted of extracting and purifying penicillin, confirmed the drug's enormous therapeutic potential as an antibiotic (antibacterial) agent.

Chain, Florey and Fleming shared a Nobel Prize in 1945 for launching the widespread use of antibiotics that was to save the lives of millions.

In 1951 Chain became director of the International Research Center for Chemical Microbiology at the Istituto Superiore de Sanita in Rome. He remained for ten years and then returned to London to resume teaching biochemistry at the University of London.

Chang Min-chueh 1908–

Recognized as an authority on reproductive biology, Chang Min-chueh advanced modern understanding of the principles of embryology, fertility and the process of fertilization. Chang's research findings were fundamental to the development of oral contraceptives, artificial insemination and *in vitro* fertilization.

Born in T'ai-yuan, China, Chang was educated at Tsinghua University in Peking and at Cambridge, where he received his doctorate in 1941. Arriving in the United States in 1945, Chang joined the research staff of the Worcester Foundation in Shrewsbury, Massachusetts, where he continues to conduct research on the physiology and endocrinology of mammalian fertilization. Since 1961 he has also served as professor of reproductive biology at Boston University.

A research biologist for nearly half a century, Chang performed the pivotal studies on ovulation in mammals that gave rise to the development of progesterone as a chemical method of inhibiting ovulation (see GREGORY PINCUS).

In 1951 Chang discovered the phenomenon now known as "capacitation," establishing that "a period of time in the female tract is required for the spermatozoa to acquire their fertilizing capacity." Six years later he identified a "decapacitation factor" in the seminal fluid, removable only by centrifugation.

In a dramatic experiment conducted in 1959 Chang used rabbit eggs fertilized *in vitro* and transplanted them into the uterus of a female deer. Continuing along similar experimental lines, he performed variations and refined versions of the experiment over the course of the next decade.

In acknowledgment of his distinguished research, Chang was honored with the Ortho Award in 1950, the Albert Lasker Award in 1954 and the Ortho Award and Medal in 1961.

Jean-Martin Charcot 1825–1893

By creating a unified scientific framework for the study of mental and physical disorders, French pathologist Jean-Martin Charcot helped to lay the foundations of modern psychiatry and neurology.

The internationally acclaimed master clinician ventured into the unexplored territories of neuropathology to identify and describe a wide range of disorders. The array of eponyms that mark his discoveries includes Charcot's joint (a joint disease originating in the nervous system), Charcot's syndrome (amyotrophic lateral sclerosis), Charcot's fever (intermittent hepatic fever) and Charcot's sign (a motion of the eyebrow in peripheral facial paralysis).

A major portion of his work was unsigned, however, and although he enjoyed the privileges and power of worldwide renown, Charcot's reputation faded from public memory in the years after his death. It was more than half a century later that scholars rediscovered the magnitude of his contribution.

"To take from neurology all the discoveries made by Charcot would be to render it unrecognizable," declared JOSEPH BABINSKI, one of many distinguished scientists to have studied under Charcot. Undoubtedly the most celebrated of his disciples was SIGMUND FREUD, who hailed Charcot as one of "the greatest of all physicians and a man whose common sense is of the order of genius."

In the 1870s Charcot launched what would become a landmark investigation of the nature and clinical manifestations of hysteria, a disorder characterized by abnormal emotional response, as shown in unusual sensory, circulatory, intestinal, or other responses. In addition to describing various forms of paralysis, contractures, rythmic choreas, anorexia, mutism, spasms and stuttering, he identified the dermatologic, respiratory, cardiac and gastric expressions of hysteria. He also delineated the characteristics of what he called the "major crisis of hysteria," now referred to as catatonic schizophrenia. Recognizing that mental activity could produce physiological symptoms, Charcot explored the possibility of curing such symptoms by implanting thoughts or suggestions. He studied and taught hypnosis and conducted experimental research on the correlation between hysteria and hypnotic states.

Above all, Charcot cast out the demonic associations and mythological interpretations that had defined hysteria for centuries. By applying scientific discipline he repudiated the many unfounded (though firmly held) beliefs that still prevailed in the late nineteenth century. Derived from the Greek word *hustera*, meaning womb, the term hysteria is itself a product of the fanciful assumption that it is caused by ovarian malfunction in sexually frustrated women. Though he left hysteria its misbegotten name, Charcot effectively shattered that superstition along with many others.

The son of a Parisian carriage maker, Charcot began his medical training at the age of 19 at Salpêtrière, in Paris, one of the largest and most prestigious medical facilities in all of Europe. By the time he was 37 he had become a prominent member of the hospital staff and faculty, serving as a chief of services, attending physician and professor of clinical medicine.

The Salpêtrière was part of a system of public health care and organized charity that was founded in the 1600s by Vincent de Paul, a renowned French priest who was eventually canonized in 1737. The dedicated activist, who is said to have inspired the revival of French Catholicism, expressed ideas that were far ahead of his time. "Mental disease is not different from bodily disease," he declared, "and Christ demanded of the humane and powerful to protect, and the skillful to relieve, the one as well as the other."

Such unorthodox principles were absent from the code of operations at the Salpêtrière, however, as it quickly gained notoriety across the continent as a wretched warehouse of human suffering. It was not until the end of the eighteenth century that humanitarian and scientific reforms were initiated by PHILIPPE PINEL to provide proper care and treatment for the mentally ill.

Nevertheless, when Charcot began his work at the Salpêtrière seventy years later he found a mass of patients in undifferentiated states of misery, with little or no hope of relief. There were over 5,000 "displaced bodies and souls," Charcot wrote, "a pandemonium of infirmities." With the help of his distinguished colleague and friend Edmé Félix Alfred Vulpian (1826–1887) he set out to evaluate each individual case, observing systems, conducting laboratory tests and consulting with other medical authorities such as Guillaume Duchenne, whom Charcot considered his "master in neurology."

The monumental undertaking was accomplished by means of a system of clinical investigation that became widely known as "Charcot's method." Relying mainly on visual scrutiny and deep concentration, Charcot would contemplate a patient in silence, observing reflexes and sensory responses, then examine another patient and compare the two, then return to the first and repeat his observations over and over until the nature of the disorder became clear.

Freud reported Charcot's contention that "the greatest satisfaction a man can experience is to see something new, that is, to recognize it as new," and described how

> he constantly returned with repeated observations to the subject of the difficulties and value of such 'seeing.' He wondered how it happened that in the practice of medicine men could only see what they had already been taught to see; he described how wonderful it was suddenly to see new things—new diseases—though they were probably as old as the human race; he said that he often had to admit that he could now see many a thing which for thirty years in his wards he had ignored.

It was through such deliberation that Charcot produced significant studies in neuropathology, including, most notably, his delineation of amyotrophic lateral sclerosis, a degenerative disease of the central nervous system that is characterized by rapidly progressive atrophy of the muscles. Identified as Charcot's disease, the rare and fatal form of paralysis has borne a second eponym since 1939, when it gained tragic publicity as Lou Gehrig's disease.

Charcot also discovered and meticulously described what he called *sclérose à plaques*, now known as multiple sclerosis, and asserted, "The spinal form of the disease is far from rare, and without doubt there are a large number of cases still diagnosed very loosely in medical practice as chronic myelitis, which really belong to the domain of multiple sclerosis, and because of this, the incidence of this disease will tend to increase as its diagnosis reaches a higher level of accuracy."

Charcot left a profound impact on the development of modern medicine not only through his own achievements as a clinical scientist, but through his powerful influence on the lives and thinking of his colleagues and students. Freud was not yet thirty years old when he arrived at the Salpêtrière as a young physician from Vienna in October 1885. He was awed by Charcot and deeply impressed by his teachings on cerebral localization, genetic predisposition to mental disorders and the role of trauma. It was Charcot who drew Freud's attention to psychopathology and the study of hysteria during five months of intensive study that would continue to reverberate throughout Freud's prodigious career. He conceded to Charcot the "glory of being the first to elucidate hysteria" and freely acknowledged the powerful influence of Charcot's thinking on his own.

Distinguished as one of the leading intellects of his day, Charcot became the nucleus of a group that included not only the leading lights of science, but the most celebrated figures of literature, politics and society. His most gifted disciples would be invited to attend the weekly gathering in Charcot's salon where they might meet LOUIS PASTEUR, Leon Gambetta, Edmond de Goncourt or noted author Alphonse Daudet, a friend and neighbor who described Charcot's appearance at age 60 as "half- Danteish and half-Napoleonic."

Five years later Charcot suffered his first anginal attack at a New Year's Eve supper ushering in 1891. The physician who examined him told Charcot he had only two and a half years to live. The man who had long recognized the interaction between mind and body died of a heart attack in the summer of 1893, within days of the date he had been given.

John Charnley 1911–1982

As the originator of the "Charnley procedure," British orthopedic surgeon John Charnley brought relief to many thousands of arthritis sufferers throughout the world with his invention of an artificial hip. Facing widespread opposition from the surgical and orthopedic establishment, he labored for nearly two decades on the development of a viable mechanical substitute for the hip and a safe and practical method of surgical implantation.

Charnley was born in the village of Bury in Lancashire, where his father worked as a pharmacist. Completing his medical training at the University of Manchester, he enlisted for military service in the early months of World War II. He treated wounded soldiers during the evacuation of British troops from Dunkirk and was later dispatched to Egypt, where he performed surgery on the battlefield at El Alamein.

Sir Henry Platt, medical advisor to the British forces and a leading orthopedic surgeon, saw great promise in the young surgeon with a mechanical bent and offered Charnley a position in the orthopedics division. Within months Charnley made the decision to pursue a career in orthopedics, and after the war he studied under Platt at the University of Manchester. Joining the staff at Wrightington Hospital of the neighboring town of Wigan, Charnley launched his first independent research on the physiological effects of arthritis on the knee joints. In 1948 he found that he had pitted himself against his entire profession with the announcement of his radical new surgical technique for fusing the bones of the knee into a single solid structure. "People were against the whole idea," he recalled later with amusement. "They thought it was unphysiological."

Prosthetics, the practice of replacing a body part with an artificial device, dates back to at least 600 B.C. with the invention of the wooden leg, and it is believed that the first metal hand was constructed in the mid-1500s. Since then the eyes, limbs, organs, teeth, skin, blood and bone have all proved to be replaceable, but the creation of an artificial hip presented Charnley with a particularly complex set of medical and mechanical problems.

The hip is the area of articulation between the pelvis and the leg in which the rounded upper end of the thighbone, or femur, fits tightly inside the hollowed area at the bottom of the hipbone, or ilium, to form what is called a "ball-and-socket joint." When a degenerative disease causes the breakdown of bone tissue, the surfaces of the joint become rough and irregular, so that when the ball of the femur rubs against the hip socket even the slightest pressure can be extremely painful.

Predating Charnley's invention, various replacement hips had been developed, including two fashioned from stainless steel. Unsafe, unreliable and uncomfortable, the metal ball was attached to the femur with a screw, which would gradually loosen and eventually come unfastened. In addition, the steel hip squeaked with every step. Realizing that the body's natural fluids could not adequately lubricate the steel, Charnley conducted exhaustive studies on the physics and chemistry of lubricants, adhesives, plastics, and the principles of tribology (the science of wear).

Settling on a high-density polyethylene and a form of cement used in dentistry, Charnley performed the first clinical tests of a prosthetic hip in November 1972 at Wrightington Hospital in England. The mechanical success of the hip replacement was remarkable, but the extent of exposed areas required by the surgery resulted in a number of serious infections. Seeking to reduce bacteria levels to a minimum during surgery, Charnley devised an enclosed operating table with a system of ventilation and specially designed gowns for all attending medical personnel. These measures effectively reduced the rate of infection to a manageable level, and by 1976 Charnley's procedure had helped more than 9,000 patients to walk without crutches.

Internationally acclaimed for his outstanding contribution to orthopedic medicine, Charnley was knighted by Queen Elizabeth in 1977. Among the tributes honoring his achievement, the Albert Lasker Award for Medical Research acknowledged Charnley in 1974 for having "restored normal living to tens of thousands of patients throughout the world."

Guy de Chauliac 1290–1370

Guy de Chauliac has been celebrated for centuries as an enlightened anatomist and surgeon, far in advance of the medical establishment of his day.

Named for the town of his birth in Auvergne, France, Chauliac studied at the universities of Toulouse, Boulogne, and, lastly, Montpellier, where he received a master's degree in medicine in 1325. After serving as canon of Lyons, Rheims and Mende he was appointed private physician to popes Clement VI, Innocent VI, and Urban V, eventually gaining the title of *capellanus*, or papal clerk. In the course of his duties in Avignon, which was the papal see until 1378, Chauliac established a relationship with Petrarch (1404–1374), the renowned Italian poet and humanist.

In spite of his professional obligation to the papacy, Chauliac advocated a separation between medicine and theology, expressing a degree of sophistication that would not become popular for several centuries. Asserting the responsibilities and resources of the physician, he railed against "the sect of women and many idiots who place patients afflicted with any disease in the hands of the saints, doing this because "The Lord has given me what pleases Him.'"

Chauliac produced a collection of classic reference texts on anatomy and surgery that would serve as standard physicians' manuals until the seventeenth century. Chief among these is the *Inventorium sive collectorium in parte chirurgiciali medicine*, widely referred to as *Chirurgia* or *Chirurgia magna*. First appearing in 1363, this monumental work of seven volumes contains sections on surgical technique and methodology as well as discussions on anatomy, diet and the history of medicine and surgery. Chauliac also provided a biographical encyclopedia, describing the careers of many of the notable physicians and surgeons who preceded him, and including references from GALEN, HIPPOCRATES, ARISTOTLE, RHAZES AVERROËS AVICENNA, along with selected contemporaries of the mid-fourteenth century.

Chirurgia is particularly valuable in its report on the plague, furnishing descriptions of the epidemics of 1384 and 1360 at Avignon and distinguishing between the pneumonic form of the disease, in which there is extensive involvement of the lungs, and the bubonic form, which is marked by swelling of the lymph nodes. Revealing the limits of his enlightenment, Chauliac's study of the plague concluded that it was due either to a particular astrological configuration or to the vengeful efforts of the Jews, who he claimed were seeking to poison the entire human race. Despite these less-than-scientific vagaries, he did observe the infectious nature of the disease, advocating therapies of air purification and enriched diets for plague victims.

Debating Chauliac's status as a medical pioneer, some historians cite his misguided ideas on the treatment of infection, most notably his belief in the theory of "laudable pus," which views pus as an essential element in the healing process. Other scholars judge him less harshly, admiring the acuity of his scientific perception in the context of medieval medicine.

William Cheselden 1688–1752

"If I have any reputation in this way I have earned it dearly," wrote William Cheselden about his career as a celebrity surgeon, "for no one ever endured more anxiety and sickness before an operation, yet from the time I began to operate all uneasiness ceased and if I have had better success than some others I do not impute it to more knowledge but to the happiness of mind that was never ruffled or disconcerted and a hand that never trembled during any operation..."

English surgeon William Cheselden is best remembered for his innovations in surgical technique for lithotomy, the surgical removal of bladder stones. On March 27, 1727 he introduced the practice of "lateral lithotomy," in which the stones are removed through an incision in the perineum, the region between the urethral opening and the anus. A vast improvement over the previously used supra-pubic approach (from above the pubic arch), the procedure was soon adopted throughout Europe, and within a year mortality rates for bladder stone removal had dropped from 50% to less than 10%. Lateral lithotomy was practiced for more than two centuries before it was superseded by "lithotrity," the mechanical crushing of bladder stones.

By all accounts a masterful practitioner, Cheselden was celebrated for his precision and dexterity, and most notably for his speed (a highly desirable virtue in the days before anesthesia). Reports vary slightly, but his average time for executing a lateral lithotomy was probably somewhere between 30 and 90 seconds.

Born in Somerby, Leicestershire, Cheselden was given a classical education in Greek and Latin before he began his surgical apprenticeship in Leicester at the age of fifteen. He continued studies in London under noted anatomist William Cowper (1666–1709) and at St. Thomas's Hospital under James Ferne, an English surgeon and specialist in lithotomy.

By the time he was 23 Cheselden was lecturing on anatomy at St. Thomas's, and in eight years time he became one of the institution's chief surgeons. By then he had also gained distinction as an author for his *Anatomy of the Human Body* (1713), which endured as a standard reference until the end of the century.

Shortly after Cheselden's impressive demonstration of lateral lithotomy Queen Caroline appointed him court physician, and in less than a year he caused another surgical sensation. Introducing his latest surgical innovation, Cheselden restored a blind man's vision by means of "iridotomy," a treatment for certain types of blindness in which a surgically created opening functions as an "artificial pupil."

In addition to his *Anatomy of the Human Body* Cheselden produced a second classic reference work in 1733 entitled *Osteographia, or the Anatomy of the Bones.* The book, which includes illustrations by the engraver G. Van der Gucht, is a comprehensive atlas of osteology that has been praised for its scientific accuracy as well as its artistic merits.

Despite his professional enthusiasm, Cheselden's versatility and wide-ranging interests led him beyond the scope of surgery and medicine to become a patron of boxing, an amateur artist and most notably a distinguished draftsman, whose designs include the Surgeons' Hall in the Old Bailey, Old Putney Bridge and Fulham Bridge in London.

As further assurance of Cheselden's status as a legendary figure of medicine, Alexander Pope includes his name in the following couplet:

> I'll do what Mead and Cheselden advise,
> To keep these limbs and to preserve those eyes.

Albert Claude 1898–1983

Nobel laureate Albert Claude is acknowledged as one of the founding fathers of modern cell biology. Recognizing the potential of the electron microscope, Claude was the first to use the instrument for cellular observation. (The electron microscope uses a stream of electrons controlled by magnetic fields, allowing far greater magnification and depth of focus than a compound microscope, which is limited by the powers of lens and light.) By devising a method of protecting the cells from the onslaught of electrons created by the microscope, Claude was able to make the first detailed observations of cellular structure.

Although his parents were both American citizens, Claude was born and raised in Longlier, Belgium. As a child Albert dreamed of becoming a doctor, but before he could finish secondary school he was forced to abandon his studies for a job as an apprentice draftsman at a steelworks. A volunteer for the British Intelligence

Service during World War I, Claude was cited by Winston Churchill, then Britain's Minister of War. In recognition of his meritorious war record the Belgian government allowed Claude to enroll at the University of Liege even though he had not yet graduated from secondary school. In 1928 he was awarded a degree in medicine.

Claude came to New York in 1931 at the invitation of the Rockefeller Institute for Medical Research (now known as Rockefeller University). As a member of the institute's research staff Claude introduced his innovative application of the electron microscope, in the process giving rise to the exciting new discipline of cell biology.

Claude devised various techniques for cellular examination and analysis, notably the use of centrifuges to separate cellular components. He identified a number of subcellular structures, including mitochondria, the source of energy for many cell functions. In 1933 Claude achieved the first isolation of a cancer virus, characterizing it as a ribonucleic acid (RNA) virus. Working with distinguished colleagues GEORGE EMIL PALADE and CHRISTIAN DE DUVE, Claude went on to describe many of the fundamental constituents of a cell. Among other discoveries, this distinguished team of scientists identified the form and structure of ribosomes (the site of protein synthesis) and lysosomes, important to the digestion and removal of dead cells. Claude compiled his "submicroscopic" observations in the first detailed description of cellular anatomy, published in 1945.

Naturalized as an American citizen in 1941, Claude left the United States seven years later to become chief of Belgium's Jules Bordet Institute. In addition to his duties as director, Claude served as head of the cytology department at the Free University of Brussels until 1969. Although he stepped down from his post at the Jules Bordet Institute in 1972, Claude remained an active member of the scientific community. Retaining an association with the University of Liege, he founded a center for the advancement of cancer research in Brussels. His enormous contribution to medicine was acknowledged with a number of distinguished awards, the most prestigious of these being the 1974 Nobel Prize for Physiology or Medicine, which he shared with colleagues George Palade and Christian de Duve.

Stanley Cohen 1922–

Stanley Cohen was hailed as "the father of growth factor research" by the Endocrine Society when it granted him the prestigious Koch Award in 1986 for his discovery and investigation of "epidermal growth factor." Later he was given the Nobel Prize for Physiology or Medicine, which he shared with his colleague, Italian biologist RITA LEVI-MONTALCINI.

Cohen first became aware of the presence of "epidermal growth factor" in the 1950s while studying the effects of nerve growth factor on infant mice. Several years earlier Levi-Montalcini and noted biologist Viktor Hamburger had pioneered the study of nerve growth factor, establishing the material as a key element in the stimulation of nerve cell growth and in the organizational process of the nervous system. By secreting this substance, a target cell attracts the axon of an immature nerve cell, inducing the formation of synapses that connect the nerve cell axon with the target cell.

Observing the first stages of growth and development in newborn mice injected with nerve growth factor, Cohen noted that his precocious infant subjects opened their eyes considerably earlier than normally developing mice. Noticing a premature appearance of teeth as well, Cohen was puzzled by the fact that these phenomena occurred in developmental processes unrelated to nerve growth. Friend and colleague Graham Carpenter recalled the early stages of Cohen's research, saying that "people used to sort of laugh when he started talking about something that caused mice to open their eyes...but Stan has always been very focused on what he wanted to know."

Recognizing the profound logic and complexity of developmental processes, Cohen reasoned that a factor powerful enough to alter the course of those processes might provide valuable biological insights. Over the course of twenty-five years of exhaustive research he isolated the "epidermal growth factor" and established a complete chemical analysis indicating the composition, amino acid sequence and three-dimensional structure of the molecule.

Studying the biochemical mechanisms of growth, Cohen discovered a protein on the cell's surface that acts as a receptor, registering and responding to the chemical signals of the growth factor. He then established that protein and growth factor enter the cell together, altering cellular processes from within.

Cohen was born and raised in the Flatbush section of Brooklyn, New York, where his father, a Russian immigrant, worked as a tailor. Graduating from Brooklyn College in 1943, Cohen attended Oberlin College and the University of Michigan, receiving a doctorate in biochemistry in 1948. After several years of pediatric research at the University of Colorado he joined Viktor Hamburger's growth factor research project at Washington University in St. Louis, where he and Levi-Montalcini began their collaboration.

In 1959 Cohen accepted a position at Vanderbilt University in Nashville, Tennessee, where he was later appointed professor of biochemistry and American Cancer Society Research professor. In recognition of his contribution to medicine he was presented with the General Motors Cancer Foundation Award in 1982, and four years later, amid the many other prestigious honors bestowed on them in 1986, Cohen and Levi-Montalcini accepted the Albert Lasker Award and the Nobel Prize.

As Cohen had anticipated, the study of growth factors has begun to uncover vital clues in the understanding of brain function, cancer formation and various developmental processes of the body. In a more immediate application, Cohen's epidermal growth factor enables the laboratory culture of human skin tissue for use in research and in the treatment of severe burns.

Ferdinand Julius Cohn 1828–1898

Recognized as one of the founding fathers of bacteriology, noted botanist Ferdinand Cohn was the first to define and name *bacteria*, describing them as motile cells without walls. Influenced by the findings of LOUIS PASTEUR, Cohn published a landmark treatise entitled *Untersuchungen über Bacterien*, the first systematic investigation of bacteria. The three-volume work, published in 1872, elucidated their life cycle, classifying the organisms into genera and species. Cohn identified four categories of bacteria differentiated by characteristics of external form and specific fermentative activities.

Cohn further expounded his methods of classification three years later in a second series of *Researches on Bacteria*, in which he also presented his discovery of spores, the reproductive bodies that detach from the parent to produce an offspring. Describing various types of spore, including bacterial, Cohn observed that spore production could only occur in the presence of air. He also noted that bacteria could survive even in temperatures of extreme heat. These discoveries eventually allowed Cohn, Pasteur and noted English physicist John Tyndall (1820–1893) to finally put an end to the theory of spontaneous generation, which held that living creatures could be spawned by inanimate matter.

Cohn was born to a Jewish family living in Breslau (now called Wroclaw) in Poland. A child prodigy, Ferdinand could read and write by the time he was two years old. He entered the University of Breslau at fourteen, but, despite four years of distinguished achievement, the school refused to grant him a degree because of his religious background. Transferring to the University of Berlin, where he studied under the distinguished German physiologist J.P. Müller, Cohn was granted his doctorate in botany the following year, at the age of nineteen.

Throughout his career Cohn grappled with anti-Semitism, compounded by his liberal leanings during the revolution of 1848. Unable to find work elsewhere, Cohn returned to Breslau to teach. He was eventually granted a professorship in botany at the university, and in 1866 he founded the first institute for plant physiology. In association with the institute he established *Beiträge zur Biologie der Pflanzen* (*Contribution on Plant Biology*) a journal that would serve as the voice of the newly emerging discipline of bacteriology.

Cohn's early interest was in microscopic algae and fungi. Introducing significant improvements in the construction of microscopes, he discovered cilia in zoospores (asexual spores produced by algae and fungi), protein crystals in potatoes and, most notably, demonstrated that the protoplasmic material of plants and animals is essentially identical. Noting contractility in plant tissue and sexuality algae, Cohn was the first to maintain that bacteria are plants rather than animals.

A well-respected and influential teacher, he is acknowledged for his support and encouragement of bacteriologist in training ROBERT KOCH. Cohn is credited with arranging for the publication of Koch's important study of anthrax.

Sir Astley Cooper 1768–1841

Astley Cooper was noted for his vigor and enterprise, qualities which were at least as important as his surgical skills in gaining him a reputation as the medical paragon of his day. His father, a clergyman, sent Astley at an early age to apprentice with his grandfather, a noted surgeon in Norwich. At sixteen he was dispatched to London to study with Henry Cline, an important surgeon at St. Thomas's Hospital, who encouraged him to attend the popular lectures being offered by the eminent JOHN HUNTER. Both surgeons recognized great talent and dedication in the young student, and by 1789 Cooper gained professional status as lecturer on anatomy at St. Thomas's Hospital. In that same year his financial status was also considerably improved by his marriage to the very wealthy Anne Cock.

In the years that followed Cooper was selected to lecture on anatomy at the College of Surgeons and was appointed surgeon at the prestigious Guy's Hospital. In his students' memoirs Cooper's charm and grace are often recalled, as well as his insight and intelligence. It is perhaps this combination of gifts that inspired such great confidence in his students and patients and insured him an extensive and highly successful private practice. By 1806 he was earning more than £15,000 a year, an enormous sum for that time, exceeding even the income of the prime minister. Cooper's assistant in his consulting office is said to have padded his own income considerably by showing preferential treatment to patients waiting in line to see the doctor.

In 1802 Cooper published an essay on the loss of the eardrum that gained him the Copley Medal of the Royal Society, of which he became a fellow in 1805. Cooper's reputation spread to the court, so that in 1820 he was asked to remove a sebaceous cyst from the head of King George IV. The king rewarded him with a baronetcy.

In 1825 Astley Cooper had decided to pass his post of lecturer at St. Thomas's Hospital to his nephew, Bransby Cooper. The governors of the hospital, who did not consider this position inheritable, appointed another lecturer. Sir Astley was so enraged that he created the now-famous medical school at Guy's Hospital, as much to challenge St. Thomas's as to console his nephew. In retaliation, St. Thomas's Hospital took possession of the teaching materials and specimens that Cooper had left behind in his lecture rooms. Sir Astley promptly furnished Guy's with a new and improved collection.

Through delicacy and discretion Cooper's reputation remained intact, and in 1827 he was named president of the College of Surgeons. The following year he became sergeant-surgeon to the king, and in 1830 he was made vice president of the Royal Society. His writings, which, though outdated, still command respect, include *Hernia* (1804–1807), *Dislocations and Fractures* (1822), *Anatomy and Diseases of the Breast* (1829–1840), and *Anatomy of the Thymus Gland* (1832). His immortality is also assured by the number of anatomical structures and surgical procedures that still bear his name.

Hazel Corbin 1895–1988

Hazel Corbin dedicated much of her life to a crusade for improved conditions and practices in childbirth and child care. For half a century she led a campaign to study prevailing and alternative health care methods and disseminate findings to physicians, nurses and parents. An influential advocate of nurse-midwifery, Corbin fought to establish certification programs at a number of prestigious universities, including Columbia, Yale and Johns Hopkins.

Born in Nova Scotia, Corbin emigrated to the United States during World War I, enrolling in Brooklyn College School of Nursing. Although her intention was to enlist as an army nurse, Corbin's first job was at New York's Maternity Center. The first health- care facility of its kind, the center was established by the Women's City Club in an effort to reduce the particularly high infant mortality rates in some areas of New York City. Serving as a field nurse, Corbin saw firsthand the poor conditions, inconsistent standards and widespread ignorance in the medical approach to childbirth.

In her capacity as director of the Maternity Center Association, which had been formally established in 1918, Corbin demonstrated effective methods of maternal and infant care at Maternity Center clinics, emphasizing the importance of the father's role in family health. She helped to establish classes for fathers as early as the 1930s.

Along with her support of midwifery Corbin encouraged the practice of natural childbirth, teaching that "When any woman has her baby naturally, she cooperates with the forces at work within her body and does the job by her own efforts, with or without assistance to help her along."

In 1965 Hazel Corbin retired from the Maternity Center Association. The following year she received the Martha May Eliot Award of the American Public Health Association in recognition of her lifetime of work in service to public health. In 1968 the Maternity Center Association awarded her their highest honor, the Medal for Distinguished Service.

Carl Ferdinand Cori 1896–1984
Gerty Theresa Cori 1896–1957

Czech-born biochemists Carl and Gerty (Gertrude) Cori are best known for their ground-breaking research on carbohydrate metabolism and the mechanisms of energy production and utilization. The distinguished husband-and-wife research team formally launched their collaboration in 1923 with the publication of their joint report on the roles of adrenaline and insulin in the conversion of liver glycogen to glucose.

For nearly twenty years the Coris pursued the investigation of carbohydrate metabolism in animals, elucidating the enzymatic mechanism involved in the formation of glucose and its regulation by hormones. By the early 1940s they had identified the enzymes involved in the formation and breakdown of the glycogen molecule and, as a result of those findings, were able to produce the first batch of synthetic glycogen.

In 1947 the Coris received the Nobel Prize for Physiology or Medicine, which they shared with Argentine physiologist Bernardo Houssay. The award included an ancillary honor for Gerty Cori, who was the first woman to win a Nobel Prize in Medicine and the third to win one in any science.

Carl Cori and Gerty Theresa Radnitz were both born in 1896 in Prague, and it was there that they met twenty years later as first-year medical students at the German University (also known as Ferdinand University). They graduated together in 1920, married that summer, and by the end of the year were settled in Vienna, where Gerty Cori conducted research on metabolic function at the Karolinen Children's Hospital.

Two years later the Coris emigrated to the United States, adopting American citizenship in 1926. Working both independently and in collaboration, they served for nearly a decade as research biochemists at the Institute for the Study of Malignant Diseases in Buffalo, New York. The couple moved to St. Louis, Missouri in 1931 to join the medical faculty at Washington University, where Carl Cori was appointed professor in pharmacology and biochemistry. In 1947 Gerty Cori became professor of biochemistry, a position she retained until her death ten years later. Carl Cori retired at the age of seventy-one to serve as visiting lecturer at Massachussetts General Hospital in Boston.

Allan Macleod Cormack 1924–

The development of modern "CAT scans" is owed in large part to the pioneering work of Allan Cormack. Born in South Africa, Cormack studied physics and engineering at the University of Cape Town, completing his graduate work at Cambridge University in England. He returned to Cape Town in 1956 to work at Groote Shuur Hospital as a medical physicist, and it was there that he began his studies in X-ray technology. He continued his studies the following year as a physics professor at Tufts University in Massachussetts. Cormack began a series of analyses of the X-ray absorption rates of different kinds of human tissue. These results laid the foundation for the development, in 1973, of computerized axial tomography, or "CAT scan". This technique of X-ray photography permits a "slice" or cross-section view of the human body that offered far more detailed information than had been available by previous noninvasive techniques.

For his important contribution to the field of radiology Cormack was awarded the 1979 Nobel Prize for Physiology or Medicine, which he shared with Godfrey Hounsfield.

James Leonard Corning 1855–1923

In 1885 American neurologist James Corning introduced the technique of spinal anesthesia, launching the practice of local numbing of specific areas of the body without loss of consciousness. Unlike general anesthesia, which blocks sensation by inhibiting the function of various nerve centers in the brain, local or regional anesthesia acts on the nerves or nerve tracts, preventing the transmission of impulses to the brain from that particular area.

Less than forty years before Corning devised his spinal anesthesia, William Morton had introduced his revolutionary "painless surgery" at Massachussetts General Hospital in Boston. In that time pharmacology rapidly developed as an independent scientific discipline, particularly in Germany and France, where pioneer pharmacist-chemists had discovered and isolated a number of plant alkaloids, including atropine, colchicine and, most notably, cocaine.

In 1884 ophthalmic surgeon Carl Koller (1857–1944) applied cocaine to the eye as a topical anesthetic, and American surgeon WILLIAM HALSTED investigated the possibilities of using cocaine as a systemic anesthetic by injecting it directly into the nerve trunks. At the same time, Corning was experimenting with various pharmacological substances, and he had demonstrated that subcutaneous injection of cocaine produced a prolonged numbing effect in a localized area.

Born in Stamford, Connecticut, Corning was eighteen when he entered the University of Heidelberg in 1873. He completed his training in neurological medicine five years later at the University of Wurzburg and returned to the United States to serve as consulting physician at a number of hospitals in New York City.

In 1885 Corning published an article in the *New York Journal of Medicine* entitled "Spinal Anaesthesia and Local Medication of the Cord," in which he reported physiological and clinical observations of "a procedure in therapy which, as far as I am aware, possesses the merit of novelty." Basing his findings on experimental animal studies, he determined that

> it is not necessary to bring the [anesthetic] substance into direct contact with the cord; it is not necessary to inject the same beneath the membranes...since the effects are entirely due to the absorption of the fluid by the minute vessels. On the other hand, in order to obtain these local effects, it is necessary to inject the solution in the vicinity of the cord, and, secondly, to select such a spot as will insure the most direct possible entry of the fluid into the circulation about the cord...

He suggested that "it was highly probable that, if the anaesthetic was placed between the spinous processes of the vertebrae, it [the anaesthetic] would be rapidly absorbed by the minute ramifications of the veins...and, being transported by the blood to the substance of the cord, would give rise to the anaesthesia of the sensory and perhaps also of the motor tracts of the same."

Noting that sensation can be effectively blocked in a particular area of the body without the application of general anesthesia, Corning pointed out the relatively brief recovery period and insignificant aftereffects of localized medication. He suggested, "The therapeutic advantages afforded by such local medication would seem to be great in a large number of morbid conditions of the cord" and concluded his report by stating: "Whether the method will ever find an application as a substitute for etherization in genito-urinary or other branches of surgery, further experience alone can show. Be the destiny of the observation what it may, it has seemed to me, on the whole, worth recording."

Corning's published writings include *Brain Rest* (1883), *Brain Exhaustion* (1886), *Local Anesthesia* (1886), *Hysteria and Epilepsy* (1888), *A Treatise on Headache and Neuralgia* (1888) and *Pain in its Neuropathological and Neurotherapeutic Relations* (1894).

Jean-Nicolas Corvisart, Baron Corvisart des Marets 1755–1821

Among the first physicians in France to reject the traditional examination techniques of passive observation and brief questioning of the patient, Jean-Nicolas Corvisart developed a comprehensive and systematic approach to diagnosis that helped to establish clinical medicine in France.

"I do not believe in medicine," declared Napoleon, "but I do believe in Corvisart." After only one interview the first consul of the republic became Corvisart's most famous patient and an influential supporter of modern clinical practices.

Viennese physician Leopold Auenbrugger (1722–1809) was an early pioneer of a new approach to medical practice, introducing the concept of "percussion" in 1761. Using one finger to tap sharply against another on the surface of the body, Auenbrugger elicited sounds from various parts of the body to determine the size and shape of internal structures as well as the presence of fluid inside the body cavity. He introduced the percussion technique in a short treatise entitled *Inventum Novum* (*New Invention*), which was quickly dismissed by the few interested professionals who read it.

It was nearly half a century before Auenbrugger's idea was rediscovered by Corvisart, who recognized its significance and translated the pamphlet from Latin into French. Now considered a basic part of medical examinations, the practice of percussion first gained acceptance as a diagnostic technique when it was popularized by Corvisart. As a side benefit to clinical practice, Auenbrugger's procedure required the physician to touch the patient's body and observe different areas of exposed skin, initiating a more direct and thorough examination than was commonly performed.

Shortly before Corvisart's death clinical investigation took another major step forward with RENÉ LAËNNEC'S introduction of "auscultation"—an offshoot of percussion in which the sounds of the abdomen, heart, lungs and other organs are studied as an aid to diagnosis.

Corvisart was born in the tiny village of Dricourt in the Ardennes, where his father was a "retired" attorney who had been exiled from Paris by Louis XV. It was not long, however, before the family was allowed to return to the capital, where Corvisart studied at the College Sainte-Barbe and completed his medical training in 1782 at the Faculté de Médecine.

Distinguished as a promising but irreverent student, he applied for a position at the Hôpital des Paroisses, but his reputation did not appeal to Mme. Necker, founder of the hospital and wife of the minister of finance. She rejected Corvisart's candidacy as a physician on the pretext that he refused to wear a wig.

Appointed to serve the poor at Saint-Sulpice, he earned a meager 300 francs in his first year as a physician, but in time he was offered residency positions at the celebrated Hôpital de la Charité. Over the course of the next several years Corvisart gained a distinguished reputation at la Charité as both a clinician and a teacher.

In 1794 a new faculty position was specially created for him at la Charité, establishing Corvisart as the first professor of internal clinical medicine. Maintaining his practice as a clinician, Corvisart also took over as supervising editor of the *Journal de médicine, chirurgie et pharmacie* (*Journal of Medicine, Surgery and Pharmacology*). He was appointed professor of clinical medicine at the École de Médecine and later at the Collège de France, and in 1806 he published his *Essais sur les maladies organiques du coeur et des gros vaisseaux* (*Essays on Organic Diseases of the Heart and Blood Vessels*). A pioneer investigation of the diseases of the heart, Corvisart's magnum opus is considered by some to be the first formal treatise on cardiology.

As first consul of the republic, Napoleon chose Corvisart as his personal physician in 1801. When Napoleon became emperor seven years later Corvisart was named first physician of the court and abandoned all other professional responsibilities to serve him and his family.

Cosmas and Damian c.225–278 A.D.

Cosmas and Damian were twin brothers of Arabian parentage who became the first Christian saints to be invoked for relief from disease. As practicing physicians at Aegaea in Cilicia they would offer medical care without charge in order to bring in converts to Christianity. Diocletian condemned the twins to die, but it is said that angels intervened to save them from being drowned at sea, burned at the stake and stoned to death. Cosmas and Damian were finally beheaded, a scene memorialized in a fifteenth- century painting by Fra Angelico.

Celebrated for delivering miracle cures in life and after death, Cosmas and Damian were depicted by other painters of the fifteenth and sixteenth centuries, notably Ambrosius Francken and Fernando del Rincon. Rincon illustrated the twin saints' most renowned miracle, the transplant of a dead man's leg to replace the gangrenous limb of a church sacristan. The operation is said to have taken place in a church that now bears their names at the edge of the Forum in Rome.

André Frédéric Cournand 1895–1988

Internationally recognized for his contribution to the field of cardiology, physician and physiologist Andre Cournand was a key figure in the development of cardiac catheterization. Cournand and his long-term collaborator DICKENSON RICHARDS became interested in studying cardiac function while investigating pathology of the respiratory system. To determine the effects of various forms of treatment on the cardiopulmonary system of a patient with lung disease, Cournand and Richards needed a means of analyzing the blood transported from the tissues into the heart.

As early as 1847 noted physiologist CLAUDE BERNARD had referred to "heart catheterism," later describing techniques of right-heart and left-heart catheterization similar to those performed today. By the turn of the century many thousands of animal experiments had been performed, but it was not until the work of WERNER FORSSMANN in 1929 that human heart catheterization received any notice. The subject of much controversy and ridicule, Forssmann's demonstration was primarily intended as a method for direct injection of drugs into the heart. In the 1930s cardiac catheterization had been effectively used in pulmonary angiography (X-rays of the pulmonary arteries) by Dr. G. Ameuille, a former teacher of Cournand's at the Sorbonne, but his work, too, was dismissed by the medical establishment.

It was not until the following decade that Cournand and Richards refined and developed the technique of cardiac catheterization for use as a safe and reliable method of measuring healthy and diseased heart functions, diagnosing heart disease, and determining the advisability of surgery.

A native of Paris, André Cournand began his medical studies at the Sorbonne in 1914. After only a few months he interrupted his work at the university to enlist in the military. He served on ambulance duty and later as an auxiliary battalion surgeon until he was wounded in August 1918. Returning to Paris, he resumed his studies at the Sorbonne the following spring. After receiving his medical degree in 1930 Cournand decided to spend a year in the United States.

After three months at the Trudeau Sanatorium in upstate New York he joined the staff at Bellevue Hospital in New York City, where he was offered a full-time position in research. It was in 1932, after he had become chief medical resident of the Columbia Division at Bellevue, that Cournand and Dickinson Richards began their long-lasting collaboration and friendship. Together they would spend over four decades studying cardiopulmonary function in healthy subjects as well as in patients with various forms of pulmonary disease. Their enormously productive partnership was to end only with Richards's death in 1973.

Impressed by the work of Dr. Ameuille, Cournand and Richards set out to develop a procedure for cardiac catheterization, performing extensive animal experimentation between 1936 and 1940. Further refinements were made with the help of George Wright, a resident at Bellevue who conducted experiments with human cadavers to determine suitable catheter lengths.

With the onset of World War II there was little resistance to medical research that might offer relief to the mounting numbers of wounded soldiers. Noted surgeon ALFRED BLALOCK, who was chairman of the "Shock Committee" in Washington D.C., saw the potential value of catheterization in the study of shock and arranged for Cournand and Richards to receive funding for additional research. Cournand was granted U.S. citizenship in 1941.

Demonstrating the advantages and feasibility of catheterization in a wide range of shock conditions, Cournand and Richards won acceptance for their technique by the mid-1940s. They went on to develop a system of respiratory assistance in shock conditions at high altitudes which gave rise to the respiration-assisting devices now widely used by anesthesiologists.

In 1956 Cournand shared the Nobel Prize for Physiology or Medicine with Richards and Forssmann for development of cardiac catheterization. In 1960 Cournand joined the faculty at Columbia University as professor of clinical physiology, becoming professor emeritus of medicine four years later.

Francis Harry Compton Crick 1916–
James Dewey Watson 1928–
Maurice Hugh Frederick Wilkins 1916–

"A Structure for Deoxribose Nucleic Acid," the classic one-page paper that James Watson and Francis Crick contributed to the British journal *Nature* on April 2, 1953, has been called a twentieth-century Rosetta Stone that provided the code for translating puzzling biological observations into the precise language of molecules. In this paper and a second one that followed on May 30 of the same year, Watson and Crick presented a model for the molecular structure of deoxyribonucleic acid (DNA) and showed that this model could explain how living cells reproduce themselves in their own likeness and how evolutionary changes and mutations occur. Laying the foundation of modern molecular biology, the Watson-Crick model, as it came to be known, has been compared in importance to the achievements of Newton, Darwin, and Albert Einstein. Crick and Watson shared credit for the discovery with fellow biophysicist Maurice Wilkins, and the legendary trio were honored for their work in 1962 with the Nobel Prize for Physiology or Medicine.

James Dewey Watson was born in Chicago on April 16, 1928. Something of a child prodigy, he graduated from the University of Chicago in 1947 at the age of 19, his principal interest at the time being ornithology. From his virus research at Indiana University (Ph.D., 1950), and from the experiments of microbiologist OSWALD AVERY, whose studies of the pneumococcus bacteria proved that DNA affected hereditary traits, Watson became convinced that the gene could be understood only after something was known about nucleic acid molecules. While working at the University of Copenhagen, he learned that scientists at the Cavendish Laboratories at Cambridge University were using photographic patterns made by X rays that had been shot through protein crystals to study the structure of protein molecules. In October 1951 he became a researcher at the Cavendish Labs, where he met British biophysicist Francis Crick.

Francis Harry Compton Crick was born in Northhampton on June 8, 1916. He graduated from University College London in 1938 with a degree in physics and began doctorate work but was interrupted by the outbreak of World War II, during which he worked as a physicist developing magnetic mines for use in naval warfare. Stirred by a lecture by Nobel Prize–winning chemist LINUS PAULING, Crick turned to biology and spent two years studying the way magnetic particles move in cells, as well as undergoing a general self-education program in biology and chemistry.

Ten years older than Watson, Crick was a late starter in biology and only received his doctorate after determining the structure of DNA in 1953. He became interested in MAX PERUTZ's pioneering efforts to determine the three-dimensional structures of large molecules found in living organisms and, in 1949, transferred to the Medical Research Council Unit at the Cavendish, which was headed by Perutz.

Soon after Crick met Watson the two were sharing an office and exchanging ideas on the nature and mechanism of DNA. Watson convinced Crick that understanding the three-dimensional structure of DNA would make its hereditary behavior apparent. Their DNA research was conducted very informally, almost as a sideline to their official work, and on at least two occasions Crick was forbidden by Lawrence Bragg, head of the Cavendish Laboratory, from even studying DNA.

At that time it was known that DNA played a central role in the hereditary determination of the structure and function of each cell. A large, complex molecule, DNA was known to be composed of nucleotides, which are simpler molecules of sugar (called de-oxyribose), joined to a phosphate group and one of four nitrogenous bases, either one of the two purines—adenine or guanine—or of the two pyrimidines—cystosine or thymine.

In the late 1940s, using the newly developed science of chromatography, Erwin Chargaff had discovered that in DNA, the number of adenine units was approximately equal to the number of guanine units. Linus Pauling formulated the helical structure for polypeptides (proteins) in April 1951. By the early 1950s, a number of scientists, including Pauling, were investigating the structure of DNA. The myth of a "race" to establish the nature of the molecule, however, seems largely based on James Watson's personal account of the story, *The Double Helix*, published in 1968, and his own ambition.

To back their theories Crick and Watson needed experimental data, which they got from the X-ray diffraction studies of DNA being carried out at King's College, London, by Maurice Wilkins and ROSALIND FRANKLIN. Crick and Wilkins were old friends. They had met in Naples in the spring of 1951 and it was then that he had first seen the X-ray diffraction pattern of crystaline DNA.

Maurice Hugh Frederick Wilkins was born in New Zealand on December 15, 1916. After completing his doctorate in physics at St. John's College, Cambridge, he worked on the Manhattan Project during World War II before turning his attention towards biology. In 1946 he joined the Biophysics Unit at King's College in London.

In 1950, the year he became assistant director of the unit, Wilkins received a sample of DNA in a gel, which he manipulated under his microscope using a glass rod. When he pulled the rod away from the gel he noticed that a thin almost invisible fiber would stretch out between the gel and the rod. He realized that this fiber would be ideal for analysis by X-ray diffraction techniques, and adapted some war surplus radiography machine parts for this purpose.

Working with a research student named Raymond Gosling, Wilkins obtained early experimental data that suggested a helical structure for DNA. There were, however, problems in interpreting the results. Rosalind Franklin, a chemist-turned-crystallographer whose work at the Laboratoire Centrale des Services Chimiques de l'État in Paris had helped to provide the basis for what is now carbon fiber technology, joined Wilkins at King's College in 1951, providing the necessary expertise to continue the work. However, personal animosity developed between Wilkins and Franklin, which slowed their progress, and Wilkins apparently preferred to collaborate with Crick and Watson, sharing information and testing out theories with them.

While Franklin refined the X-ray diffraction studies, Crick and Watson constructed possible spiral models of the structure of DNA out of bits of wire, colored beads, sheet metal and cardboard cutouts. Late in 1951, Watson attended a lecture by Franklin in which she stated that her diffraction studies indicated that DNA molecules are helical and that the probable structure of the helix was with the phosphate-sugar backbone on the outside and the nucleotide bases on the inside. Wilkins either ignored this or retained no memory of it, however, and he and Crick proceeded instead to work on triple helixes, which were incompatible with the data of the King's team.

It was not until July 1952, when Chargaff visited the Cavendish that a major breakthrough was made. Unimpressed by Watson and Crick, who had never read his work, Chargaff explained to them again his rules for the complementarity of the four nucleotide base ratios, pointing out that "it is all published!" Crick also found out at that time from John Griffith, a younger Cambridge Mathematics graduate taking an undergraduate course in biochemistry, that adenine attracts thymine and guanine attracts cystosine. Putting these facts together, he developed a theory of replication. If you have a molecule containing the bases C and T and pull it apart, the C will attract another T, while the T will attract another C, so that you end up with two CT molecules. Applied to the length of a DNA chain, this provided an explanation as to how DNA replicates.

Surprisingly, nothing further happened until January 1953, when, pressured by the news that Linus Pauling was making advances towards discovering the structure, Watson made a visit to King's. There, on January 30, unknown to Franklin, Wilkins gave him a copy of one of her DNA photographs. Watson immediately recognized that the pictures supported the hypothesis that DNA was a double chain. The double helix model was, as Watson quipped, "too pretty not to be true." He returned to Cambridge and the team started building models again. For a few weeks they attempted to produce a double helix with the bases still on the outside.

The arrival of American biochemist Jerry Donohue, a former colleague of Linus Pauling, provided the necessary information for them to realize that hydrogen bonds would produce the bonding of adenine to thymine and cystosine to guanine, backing up Chargaff's work, and filling the last gap in the molecular puzzle. The bases, as Franklin had suggested, lay on the inside of a phosphate-sugar backbone, curled in a double spiral and bridged by the hydrogen bonds. The unwinding of each strand of the double helix provided a template or mold for the production of new DNA.

During the first week of March the Cavendish team constructed their model, matching their theories to the X-ray data and at the end of the month made their announcement to *Nature*. A few weeks later Franklin and Gosling published their own report in *Nature*, though their original work now looked like suplementary data to Crick and Watson's findings.

Neither Crick nor Watson were the real experts in the fields involved in DNA research. Their genius was that of bringing together a number of disciplines to obtain new information not the sole domain of any one of these fields. From this fusion of sciences came a new one, molecular biology, which Crick in particular would proceed to develop. The discovery of DNA is structure and the system of "molecular notation" for transmission of hereditary information earned Watson and Crick worldwide recognition and prompted scores of scientists to go into molecular research. Subsequent studies almost completely bore out the Watson-Crick model.

After receiving his doctorate from Cambridge University in 1953 for work on proteins, Crick pursued his investigation of the genetic code, which he described as "the dictionary between the four-letter language of nucleic acid and the twenty-letter language of proteins." Working with a number of other people, most notably biochemist Sydney Brenner, he studied how the sequence of bases in DNA directed the various amino acids to join the forming protein molecules. Crick discovered that RNA or ribonucleic acid, a single-stranded nucleic acid consisting of repeating nucleotide units also found in cells, was as crucial to the process as DNA.

In a paper entitled "The General Nature of Genetic Code for Proteins," which was published in the December 30, 1961 issue of *Nature*, Crick presented experimental evidence to show that the bases on an RNA strand formed groups of three (known as triplets), each of which designated the position of a specific amino acid on the backbone of a protein molecule; that these triplets did not overlap; that the sequence of bases is read from a fixed starting point; that cell mutation is caused by disruptions in the sequence of the bases and that there must be more than one triplet for some of the twenty amino acids (because the four bases combine to produce sixty-four triplets).

It was this work that finally won Crick, along with Watson and Wilkins, the 1962 Nobel Prize. In the next five years, Crick also helped determine the specific base triplets that code for each of the twenty amino acids normally found in a protein (codons), and the way in which the cell eventually uses the RNA to build proteins.

After spending nearly three decades at Cambridge, Crick resigned in 1977 to join the Salk Institute for Biological Studies in California. He gave up molecular biology to devote his remaining years to brain research and specifically the function of dreams. A devout atheist, Crick wrote a book called *Life Itself: Its Origin and Nature* (published in 1981), in which he speculated that life on earth began when an unmanned spacecraft carrying primitive microorganisms crashed into the sea billions of years ago.

Watson left Cambridge in 1953 to become senior research fellow at the California Institute of Technology. He returned briefly two years later to collaborate with Crick in proposing a structure of viruses, which was confirmed in 1962 by electron microscope studies. In 1955 Watson joined the Harvard faculty, serving as an assistant professor of biology while conducting research on the mechanism of protein biosynthesis. Name an associate professor in 1958, he was granted full professorship three years later. In 1965 he published *Molecular Biology*, a reference work that was to become one of the most widely used modern texts on the subject.

Resigning from Harvard in 1968, Watson assumed directorship of the Laboratory of Quantitative Biology at Cold Spring Harbor, Long Island, New York, a world center for research in molecular biology, where he concentrated his attention on cancer research. He was awarded the Presidential Medal of Freedom in 1977 and was made an Honorary Fellow of the Royal Society in 1981.

George Washington Crile 1864–1943

The triumphs of twentieth-century surgery are owed in large part to George Washington Crile, whose discoveries greatly reduced the hazards of surgical shock. His career was launched by an accident he witnessed while still a medical student: Observing the death of a man whose legs had been crushed by a speeding train, Crile noted remarkably little bleeding but a rapid onset of severe nervous shock. It was this experience that launched his investigation into the nature of shock and its role in precipitating death.

Crile developed and perfected the process of anociassociation, the "nerve block" system of anesthesia used to reduce or prevent surgical shock. The area to be operated on was "shut off" from the patient's brain by a strategic combination of local and general anesthesia, confining the shock and stress of the surgery to a limited area of the body, thereby protecting the brain and nervous system. This technique, also known as conduction anesthesia, was hailed as one of the most important surgical advances since JOSEPH LISTER'S work in the previous century.

Crile was born in Ohio and studied at Ohio Northern University, and in 1887 he received his medical degree from Wooster University (later to merge with Western Reserve University). Over the next ten years Crile taught histology, physiology and surgery at Western Reserve University, regularly taking time off to study the latest medical advances in Vienna, London and Paris. He married Grace McBride in 1900, and together they were to have four children.

Crile served as an army surgeon in the Spanish-American War and in World War I, attaining the rank of brigadier general by 1921. His work as researcher, consultant and director of the U.S. base hospital at Neuilly in France earned him the Distinguished Service Medal from his own government as well as the Legion of Honor from the French and a membership in the Military Division of the Order of Bath from the British. Crile was honored throughout his life with awards and decorations, among them the American Medal for Service to Humanity in 1914, the National Institute of Social Sciences Medal in 1917, and the Lannelogue International Medal of Surgery, presented by the Societe Internationale de Chirurgie de Paris in 1925.

Even before his pioneering research on shock, Crile was well known as a specialist in respiratory surgery. He was among the first to perform a direct blood transfusion (in 1905) and helped to introduce the medicinal properties of adrenaline to the medical community. Throughout his military career Crile maintained his connection with civilian medicine, serving as visiting surgeon at Lakeside Hospital in Cleveland, Ohio from 1911 to 1924. In 1921 Crile and a group of associates founded the Cleveland Clinic. Crile acted as director and used the facilities to carry on experiments in the area of radioelectric energy. Contending that the phenomena of life could be identified in terms of physical principles, Crile declared, "Mind is a product of electricity generated by matter." He developed a theory maintaining that living organisms are "bipolar mechanisms constructed and energized by radiant and electric energy." Crile's experiments were designed to show that animal brains emit shortwave and infrared radiations that cause the brain to eject electrons from its protoplasm. The electric current created by these electrons, Crile claimed, was responsible for all mental activity.

The Cleveland Clinic also served to support experimentation and study in hemorrhage and transfusion, thyroid surgery and the development of the technique of anociassociation.

In addition to his diverse research projects, Crile wrote extensively and frequently delivered his papers to packed houses at scientific gatherings. His wide-ranging interests are reflected in the titles of some of his books: *Surgical Shock; On the Blood Pressure in Surgery; Anemia and Resuscitation; Anoci-Association* (written with William E. Lower); *Origin and Nature of the Emotions; Man Adaptive Mechanism; The Kinetic Drive; The Fallacy of the German State Philosophy*; and *Notes on Military Surgery*. In *A Mechanistic View of Peace and War*, written shortly after his return from France, Crile recorded his impressions of the military experience, describing strife as a basic element in human nature. He contends that "struggle is a biological necessity, and even war is preferable to pusillanimous peace leading to degeneracy."

Also known for his prowess as a big-game hunter, he originated a technique known as the "Crile Shot." Noting that a lion could still run 100 to 150 feet after being shot through the heart, Crile discovered that the animal would be instantly paralyzed if the shot damaged the pneumogastric nerve in the shoulder.

William Cullen 1710–1790

William Cullen would begin his medical lectures at the University of Glasgow by telling his students, "It will be my endeavor to make you philosophers as well as physicians." One of the eighteenth century's most celebrated teachers, Cullen was influential in the careers of many important physicians, notably the distinguished WILLIAM HUNTER, who referred to his mentor as "a man to whom I owe most and love most of all men in the world."

In addition to his contributions as a teacher, Cullen developed important theories on health and disease, emphasizing the critical role of the nervous system. He studied fevers and "irritability"—the physiological capacity to contract when stimulated—relating both to a disability of the nervous system. It was Cullen's theory that "nervous energy" was the basis of life itself.

Repudiating the venerable doctrine of "humours," a theory stressing the importance of body fluids in causing disease, Cullen concentrated his studies on the solid structures of the body. He became one of the earliest proponents of physiological medicine, relating a number of pathological conditions to physiological events.

Along with noted contemporaries Carl Linnaeus and Boissier de Sauvages (1706–1767), Cullen made important advances in the relatively new field of nosology, the study of disease classification. Based on rigorous and precise experimental methods along with extensive clinical experience, Cullen's organized descriptions of diseases are both detailed and clear.

Born in Hamilton in Lanarkshire, Scotland, Cullen was sent to Glasgow University at an early age to study medicine with John Paisley. Greatly influenced by this solemn but gentle physician, the enthusiastic novice also benefited from Paisley's vast medical library. At the age of nineteen Cullen left his mentor to take a job as a surgeon on a merchant ship bound for the West Indies. After six months Cullen returned to London to work as an apothecary's assistant near Covent Garden.

The sudden deaths of his father and elder brother brought Cullen back to Scotland in 1737. He used his small inheritance to enroll at Edinburgh's Medical School, where he had the good fortune to study under Alexander Monro, the first of three generations of celebrated surgeons. After graduation Cullen lectured on medicine at the university while establishing a successful practice as a physician and surgeon. In 1751 he was appointed to the chair in medicine at Glasgow, but he left four years later to join the faculty at the University of Edinburgh, where he held the chairs in chemistry and medicine.

In Edinburgh Cullen established a rigorous schedule, rising at dawn to dictate several hours of research notes to his clerk. At nine o'clock he would begin the rounds of his patients, maneuvering through Edinburgh's narrow and winding streets in a sedan chair. Cullen's afternoons were spent lecturing at the university and the infirmary, where his generous nature and his engaging style of teaching endeared him to his students. He taught in English, unlike most medical lecturers, who insisted on speaking Latin, and he was closely attentive to his student's interests, inviting them into his home and often providing financial assistance to those in need.

Cullen befriended at least one student, however, who responded ungraciously to his kindness. After studying and working under Cullen for several years John Brown grew contemptuous of his celebrated teacher, disdaining the rest of Edinburgh's faculty as well. Brown gave a series of public lectures on "The Practice of Physic," attempting to discredit many of the basic tenets of current medical doctrine. He was particularly critical of Cullen's ideas on nervous energy, denouncing them in favor of his own unfounded theory of "excitability." Life, Brown claimed, was a function of "exciting powers," and accordingly, if a state of moderate "excitability" were not maintained, disease and death would result. It is not known whether Brown's addiction to drugs and alcohol was the inspiration or the result of his theory, but a key feature of his doctrine, known as Brunonianism, was the prescription of stimulants or sedatives, which he deemed to be the only effective means of treating disease. Although Cullen and many others staunchly opposed Brown, his school of though attracted a loyal following of "Brunonians," many of whom suffered and died from opium and alcohol abuse.

Cullen remained active as a celebrated physician and teacher in Edinburgh until his death at the age of eighty. His chief written works include *Synopsis Nosologiae Methodicae* (1769), *Institutions of Medicine* (1772), *Practice of Physic* (1776–1784) and *Treatics of Materia Medica* (1789).

Marie Salomée Sklodowska Curie 1867–1934
Pierre Curie 1859–1906
Frédéric Joliot-Curie 1900–1958
Irène Joliot-Curie 1897–1956

The Curies—Marie and Pierre, the daughter Irène and son-in-law Frédéric—were the discoverers and prophets of atomic radiation as well as its earliest victims. In the process they became the first family of radiology, creating artificial isotopes of enormous significance to twentieth-century clinical medicine and fundamental research. The world paid its tribute to the family with four Nobel prizes—three for Physiology or Medicine, and one for Peace.

Marie Salomée Sklodowska came to Paris from her native Poland in 1891, four years before WILHELM RÖNTGEN would note the ability of certain rays from a cathode tube to pass through supposedly impervious material. He called these rays "X," the algebraic symbol of the unknown. A year later, in 1896, French physicist Antoine Henri Becquerel (1852–1908) observed that uranium constantly emitted rays with the same astonishing capacity to penetrate solids.

Marie was the youngest of six children in a Polish family living under a harsh Russian occupation. Resistance became a family tradition, so that at an early age Marie not only learned to live as a Pole in a Russian world and as an agnostic in an emphatically religious world but also entertained an ambition to work in science, universally recognized as a man's world. While waiting for a chance to escape to France Marie, her three sisters, one brother and fellow students of a similar turn of mind taught themselves the rudiments of science while they dreamed together of their personal escape and the ultimate liberation of Poland.

Marie's sister Bronia was the first to make it to Paris. In 1891 she sent for Marie, who entered the Sorbonne at 24 with only a smattering of French. Nevertheless, in two years time she had won her licentiate, ranking first in the physical science examinations.

At a party celebrating that triumph as well as her departure to Warsaw for a brief holiday, Marie met Pierre Curie, 34 years old, a gentle, dedicated humanist, son of French physician Eugene Curie. Pierre and his brother Jacques had been raised to share an optimistic view of science as the key to progress.

When the boys were in their early twenties they collaborated on a series of experiments culminating in a demonstration that one could generate electricity by subjecting a crystal to stress, or conversely that one could use electricity to modify the facets of a crystal, a phenomenon that came to be known as "piezoelectricity."

When Marie Sklodowska met Pierre he was running a laboratory at the School of Physics and Chemistry, a job that carried little prestige and less remuneration. He had invented a photographic lens, but the royalties were negligible. For their unconventional wedding in the fall of 1895 the bride chose a gown conveniently dark, because she wanted something that would not show the stains of lab work. After enjoying an equally unconventional honeymoon bicycling around northern France they returned to Paris, where Marie was welcomed as Pierre's fellow worker in his laboratory, although the school that employed them both saw no reason to pay her.

In 1896, still at the top of her class in physics at the Sorbonne, Marie chose for her doctoral thesis an exploration of possible sources of radiation other than the uranium already discovered by Becquerel. In the months that followed, however, work was complicated by Marie's pregnancy. She and Pierre kept postponing a holiday on bicycles they had planned, so that when they finally took off for Brest Marie was in her eighth month. They had not gone far when she had to be rushed back to Paris, where Pierre's father delivered his grandchild, Irene Curie, who was to play a vital part in her parents' work as well as in their personal lives.

While a nursemaid attended to Irene her mother went to work in a leaky, drafty storage shed near Pierre's lab, trying to determine the radiation emitted by selected metals as evidenced by electrical charges in the air. Very quickly she found that two uranium ores were sources of radiation as potent as uranium itself, and that thorium was as powerful as uranium, and she began to suspect that radioactivity—a term she herself invented—was a function not of molecular rearrangements, but of the atom itself.

Pierre gave up his own projects to work with Marie on the radiation experiments. When they isolated a new source of radioactivity found in pitchblende—the principal ore of uranium—they reported the achievement to the Académie des Sciences, officially naming it "polonium, from the name of the homeland of one of us."

More exciting still was their discovery of a substance in pitchblende with a radioactivity they finally realized must be 100,000 times that of uranium. It was to be called radium. Madame Curie's doctoral thesis thus proved to be a major scientific event. Pierre followed up by formulating the law determining the rate of decay of radioactive material, thereby suggesting a measurement of time that makes it possible to date archeological and anthropological discoveries.

Though the achievements won Marie her doctorate and attracted a stream of admirers to their little shed, the Curies were as poor as ever. Pierre could not qualify for a full professorship for lack of a prestigious alma mater, and Marie had to teach at a girls' school to make ends meet. Their fame drew to them such luminaries as Paul Langevin, who would later win world acclaim for his work on relativity and ultrasound, the painter Toulouse-Lautrec, the sculptor Auguste Rodin, and the statesman Henri Poincaré.

While the scientific and lay press hailed the discovery of radium, not even the Curies recognized its dangers, even though Pierre's hands were becoming so scarred that he could no longer tie a cravat, and his legs trembled uncontrollably. The Folies Bergères featured a popular dancer who did her act in a radium glow. Marie, too, felt miserable, and her second pregnancy ended in a premature delivery that the infant barely survived, only to die within hours. Even scientists thought it amusing when their breath proved radioactive.

Marie was too fatigued to accompany Pierre when he went to London to receive the Humphry Davy award in 1903. Later that year, when word came that the two Curies and Becquerel were to share the Nobel Prize, they protested that poor health and a heavy schedule made the trip impossible. In addition to their other more serious problems was the dread of the intrusions on their life and work that fame would bring. In the end they went to Stockholm, but with so many misgivings that Henri Poincaré remarked that Pierre, who made the acceptance speech, "rose to glory with the spirit of a whipped dog."

In that speech Pierre warned of the dangers of probing the atom, but he added: "I am among those who believe that humanity will derive more good than evil from these new discoveries."

The Nobel Prize persuaded the French parliament to grant Pierre a full professorship at the Sorbonne and to put Marie in charge of a new laboratory there. For the first time in her life she would be paid a salary for scientific work. In 1904 a second daughter, Eve, was born to the Curies. However, their health, particularly Pierre's, continued to decline. On April 19, 1906 he was crossing a street when, seemingly oblivious to danger, he walked into the path of a horse-drawn wagon. He fell under the wheels, and his skull was crushed.

Marie worked on at the laboratory. With considerable reluctance on the part of Sorbonne officials she was given the professorship that had been created for Pierre and so became the first woman to hold such rank.

In 1910 she gained wide recognition for a two-volume work on radioactivity and for the standard of measurement she devised for that phenomenon, which came to be called a "curie."

Her peace was shattered a year later when Mme. Langevin, in the midst of dissolving her marriage, released to the press a packet of letters that had been exchanged between her husband and Mme. Curie. In the wake of the resulting scandal booing crowds gathered at Marie's door, and Paul Langevin engaged in a duel that ended farcically when both challenger and challenged refused to fire.

The shattering publicity faded somewhat when a second Nobel Prize was awarded to Marie Curie, this time specifically for her discovery of radium and polonium. After the ceremony she collapsed and spent the next two years recuperating in and out of nursing homes.

When the First World War broke out Marie raised money to convert old vehicles into X-ray units, establishing the first frontline radiological laboratories. As director of the Red Cross Radiology Service she was assisted by Irene, barely 18. After the armistice Marie threw herself into a campaign to raise money for her laboratory, although the pain in her hands had grown worse and her sight was failing. Accompanied by Irene and young Eve, she toured the United States in two successful fund-raising drives.

In 1924, while Marie still took a hand in the management of the laboratory and as Irene was about to get her doctorate, a 24-year-old lieutenant of the Anti-Gas Corps and former student of Paul Langevin came by to visit the Curies, whom he had long admired. Frederic Joliot came from a comfortable middle-class Parisian family with a strong tradition of antiestablishment rebellion. Marie hired him, and in time he wooed and won Irene as his wife. She partly explained her consent by saying, "I recognized that if I did not have children, I could not console myself by the fact that I had not made that remarkable experiment while I was still capable of it." The "experiment" resulted in a daughter and a son.

Another great experiment came to absorb the lives of Irene and Frederic Joliot-Curie—the hybrid name conferred on the couple by the press and adopted enthusiastically by Joliot as well as Curie. Continuing where Marie and Pierre had left off, Frederic and Irene transformed an aluminum sheet into a radioactive isotope of phosphorus, thereby making therapeutic radiation readily available. Marie Curie lived long enough to celebrate the creation of the first artificial radioisotope before she died, on July 4, 1934, of leukemia brought on by years of radiation exposure.

When the Joliot-Curies were awarded the Nobel Prize for Physiology or Medicine in 1935 Frederic warned that soon scientists would be capable of bringing about "transmutations of an explosive character, like chemical chain reactions." Actually both Frederic and Irene came close to theoretically envisaging the atomic bomb with all its terrors. When World War II broke out Frederic sealed his paper detailing the possibility of an unlimited chain reaction using uranium. He deposited it with the Académie des Sciences under a provision that it not be opened for ten years.

While Frederic fought in the French Resistance throughout the war, Irene went on working at the laboratory until the Gestapo seemed to be closing in on her. She then fled with her children to Switzerland.

After the war Frederic headed France's first atomic energy commission, designed the nation's first nuclear center, then broke with the government over questions of disarmament and the politics of peace. Irene took her husband's side in the political storm but devoted herself to the Radium Institute until, in 1955, she died of the Curie occupational disease—leukemia. Frederic took up his wife's job at the Institute and campaigned for an international peace movement until 1958, when the years of working with radiation took his life as well.

In 1965 Eve Curie, the younger daughter of Pierre and Marie, followed in the footsteps of her parents and sister to Stockholm for yet another Nobel Prize, though this was not for any scientific achievement. A distinguished journalist and musician, Eve accepted the Nobel Peace Prize on behalf of her husband, Pierre Labouisse, for his work as Director General of UNICEF—the United Nations International Children's Emergency Fund.

James Currie 1756–1805

> ...Art taught by thee shall o'er the burning frame
>
> The healing freshness pour and bless thy name....

These words, written by a Professor Smyth of Cambridge, are taken from the epitaph on James Currie's tomb in Devon, England. They describe Currie's contribution to medicine but do not indicate the remarkable perseverance and resiliency of Currie's character.

As a boy in Scotland, James Currie dreamed of a career in medicine. He knew that to study he would need money, and, encouraged by his family, he set out for America to take advantage of the opportunities offered in the rapidly developing colonies.

At fifteen he was sent to a relative in Richmond, Virginia. Before he could find a trade he fell victim to an unidentified fever. Fortunately, his host was a physician, who nursed him back to health, at the same time encouraging him to pursue a medical career as soon as possible. He set out to return to Scotland in hopes of entering Edinburgh School of Medicine. Soon after his ship set sail, however, it was seized "in the name of the revolting colonies," and all passengers were left stranded on a deserted strip of coast.

His second attempt to return home was thwarted by pirates. After enduring another attack of fever, a bad case of dysentery and devastating hurricane, Currie landed in St. Eustatius in the British West Indies. Drained, both physically and financially, Currie sought to raise money on the island for a business venture that proved as disastrous as his travel plans. Again he was plagued with fever, this time followed by a temporary paralysis. He recovered on the island of Antigua and set sail once more for Europe.

Many hurricanes and several shipwrecks later, Currie arrived in Edinburgh and began a more restful life as a medical student. One autumn afternoon he went walking with some friends in the Scottish countryside. In the course of the day Currie stopped twice to refresh himself by bathing in the rivers, and then, after sundown, stopped to swim once again, this time in the River Tweed. Currie remembered this last dip as particularly cold. To the activities of that afternoon he ascribed the rheumatic fever that affected his heart for the rest of his life. He ignored his own poor health, however, and eagerly began private practice in Liverpool. In 1797 he produced a work that had particular significance to him: *Reports on the Effects of Water, cold and warm, as a Remedy in Fever and Febrile Diseases, whether applied to the Surface of the Body or used as a Drink, with Observations on the Nature of Fever and on the Effects of Opium, Alcohol, and Inanition*. In it Currie announces three rules to follow in the treatment of fevers:

- In the early stages of fever cold water should be poured over the patient's body.
- In the later stages of fever the patient should be bathed in tepid water.
- During all stages of fever the patient should drink large amounts of cold water.

Currie had read in the *London Medical Journal* of the experiences of Dr. William Wright of Jamaica, who had experimented with a kind of "water shock treatment" to reduce fevers in his patients and himself. For centuries cold bathing had been considered a possible treatment for fever, but Currie was the first to systematically observe and record its results. Along with WILLIAM CULLEN, Currie was among the first to use a clinical thermometer in the diagnosis of fevers, thus adding further substantiation to his findings. Unfortunately, his ill wind continued to blow so that after his death, James Currie's name was forgotten as science found new ways to treat fevers.

Harvey Williams Cushing 1869–1939

Hailed as one of the fathers of neurosurgery, Harvey Cushing introduced major advances in surgical and diagnostic technique, most notably for the treatment of brain and pituitary tumors and the management of intracranial pressure. Cushing, who trained under world-renowned medical scientists WILLIAM HALSTED and SIR WILLIAM OLSER, would gain legendary status himself for his monumental contribution to neurosurgery and medical education.

Medicine had been a professional tradition in Cushing's family that had endured for many generations. Following in a long line of general practitioners, his father and oldest brother both became physicians, but Harvey was the first in his family to become a surgeon. Born and raised in Cleveland, Ohio, he was the youngest of ten children and one of seven who lived to adulthood.

At 18 Harvey entered Yale University, graduating four years later with a firm idea of his professional future. Following in his brother's footsteps, he attended Harvard Medical School, where he was awarded the degrees of M.A. and M.D. cum laude in 1895.

During his last year at Harvard Cushing was selected for appointment at Johns Hopkins University to serve as assistant resident in surgery under William Halsted. Though he had been planning to pursue postgraduate studies in Europe, the offer to join such a distinguished faculty was one he could not refuse. At the age of 26 Cushing found himself in the company of some of the most influential medical scientists of his time. Among the leading figures at Hopkins were William Welch, Howard Kelly, and Sir William Osler, who together with Halsted formed a powerful team known as the "Big Four." Three years earlier they had founded the Baltimore Medical School, and though the first class had not yet graduated, their innovative approach to medical education had already begun to attract international recognition and respect.

At the end of his first year at Johns Hopkins Cushing accepted an appointment as instructor in surgery in addition to retaining his position as a resident. In 1898 he served as a military surgeon in the Spanish-American War and returned to experimental research later that year. Seeking to replace ether with a safer and more controllable means of relieving pain, he began to pursue Halsted's study of cocaine and its use as a local anesthetic. By injecting the drug directly into the area of a particular nerve Cushing created a method of "block" anesthesia that he used successfully in a number of major surgical operations.

In 1900 he took a leave of absence from Johns Hopkins to spend the next year on a grand tour of hospitals, laboratories, and medical schools throughout Europe, seeking out the leading minds of medical science. In London he joined CHARLES SHERRINGTON in his cortical mapping experiments, observed neurosurgical operations performed by VICTOR HORSLEY and met with JOHN HUGHLINGS JACKSON at the National Hospital of Paralysis and Epilepsy. At the Thirteenth Annual Medical Congress in Paris he joined GEORGE CRILE, WILLIAM MAYO and John B. Murphy in a meeting that gave rise to the establishment of the Society of Clinical Surgery. Cushing made the rounds of operating rooms and research centers throughout France, Switzerland and Germany, following his pilgrimage to Italy, where he paid homage to the landmarks of medical history at Padua, Bologna, Venice and Pisa.

Returning to Johns Hopkins University in 1901, Cushing resumed his teaching duties and also joined the surgical staff of the neurological clinic. In the years that followed he devoted more and more of his time to neurological surgery as he continued to develop innovative procedures and designs for surgical instruments. He created a technique for relieving the pain of facial neuralgia by operating on a collection of sensory nerves known as the Gasserian ganglion and introduced a number of safety measures for reducing the risk of hemorrhage, most notably the recording of blood pressure during surgery.

In 1908 Cushing turned his attention to the surgical treatment of pituitary tumors, which were then considered inoperable and nearly impossible to detect in a living patient. Roughly the size and shape of a marble, the pituitary is attached to the hypothalamus (at the base of the brain). As the most complex of the exocrine glands, it produces a range of hormones that control major biological functions, including growth and sexual development. Cushing performed the first successful pituitary operation in 1909 when he removed a portion of the gland from a patient who had been sent to him by Dr. CHARLES MAYO.

The following year Cushing left Baltimore to accept an appointment as chief surgeon at the newly established Peter Bent Brigham Hospital in Boston. During World War I he volunteered to serve overseas, where he devised surgical techniques for improving efficiency and speed under combat conditions.

Shortly after his return to civilian life Cushing began to develop a series of intermittent but chronic symptoms that included fatigue, numbness and weakness in the limbs. He continued to practice nevertheless for the next 20 years, performing more than 2000 brain tumor operations by the time he retired from surgery in 1932.

Cushing drew international attention when he performed the first operation by electrosurgery in 1926, in which he succeeded in removing a tumor from the brain by using a high-frequency current that made it possible to cut into tissue with almost no bleeding. He later modified the technique so that it could also stop bleeding from severed vessels by coagulating the blood.

A prolific author, Cushing published a great number of scientific treatises, most notably on the pituitary gland and the surgical treatment of tumors, but much of his later writing is on topics in medical history. His greatest literary distinction came in 1925, when he published *The Life of William Osler*, which was honored with the Pulitzer Prize for medical biography.

After retiring from surgical practice he continued to write and teach, spending his last six years as Sterling Professor in Neurology at Yale University. Following his death in 1939, an autopsy revealed that Cushing had suffered from a brain tumor.

D

Henry Drysdale Dakin 1880–1952

English chemist Henry Drysdale Dakin is best known for the antiseptic solution he developed in collaboration with ALEXIS CARREL. Known as "Dakin's fluid" or "Dakin's solution," the substance is a borate-buffered aqueous solution of sodium hypochlorite, used extensively during World War I as a wound irrigant and disinfectant. Dakin described this and other chemical bactericides in his *Handbook on Antiseptics,* a valuable treatise published in 1917, co-authored by Edward Dunham.

Although Dakin's antiseptic formula would be replaced by other disinfectants by the 1930s, his contribution to the advancement of biochemistry is a lasting one. With German chemist ALBRECHT KOSSEL, Dakin is credited with the discovery of the enzyme arginase. While working at the Lister Institute for Preventive Medicine in London Dakin synthesized the hormone adrenaline. He also demonstrated the principle of enzyme stereospecificity, which states that a particular enzyme, distinguished by its individual structure or atomic configuration, will react with only one specific class of molecule.

His extensive studies on biochemical oxidation, presented in *Oxidations and Reductions in the Animal Body,* were originally published in 1912 and updated a decade later in a second edition. Other research included significant findings in the chemical analyses of proteins, amino acids and fatty acids.

A native of London, Dakin was educated at Victoria University at Leeds, which had been renamed the University of Leeds by the time he received his doctorate in 1909.

His graduate studies at the Lister Institute in 1902, followed by his work with Albrecht Kossel at the University of Heidelberg, were made possible by the award of an 1851 Exhibition Grant. In 1905 Dakin left for the United States to join the staff of one of the few American research facilities devoted to the newly emerging discipline of biochemistry. The privately owned laboratory in New York City was headed by its founder, Christian A. Herter, who also served as editor of the *Journal of Biological Chemistry.* After Herter's death in 1910 Dakin took over his editorial duties as well as the responsibilities of maintaining the laboratory. In 1916 Dakin and Herter's widow were married.

Within two years Dakin and his new wife moved their research facilities to Scarborough-on-Hudson, a quiet rural area some twenty miles from New York City. A distinguished chemist of international repute, Dakin was often visited at his Scarborough laboratory by notables from the international scientific community. He was presented with honorary degrees from Yale and the universities of Leeds and Heidelberg, elected a fellow of the Institute of Chemistry and the Royal Society, made a Chevalier of the Légion d'Honneur and was awarded numerous medals for his achievements in scientific research.

Despite his elevated status, the retiring Dakin maintained a simple and secluded life-style that permitted him to devote most of his time to his work as a researcher. Dakin died in the winter of 1952, one year after the death of his wife.

Sir Henry Hallett Dale 1875–1968

Sir Henry Hallett Dale was a biochemistry student at Cambridge when he first began working with ergot, a parasitic fungus known to stimulate muscle contraction. Dale's pharmacological research, begun on ergot in 1904, spanned several decades and was eventually honored with a Nobel Prize for Physiology or Medicine.

In 1914, five years after graduation from medical school at Cambridge, Dale was made a member of the Royal Society. His interest in the pharmacology of ergot led to a study of histamines, the compounds released in inflammatory conditions and allergic responses. Histamines can cause a widening of blood vessels, a decrease in blood pressure, an increase in gastric secretions, and a constriction of some muscles in the respiratory system. Various forms of histamine shock can result from these effects. Hale's work helped to clarify the complex role of histamine release.

In 1921 Otto Loewi performed a series of experiments with an isolated heart and attached vagus nerve. The heart rate slowed as the vagus nerve endings released a substance later identified as acetylcholine. Dale's work with histamines led him to isolate this substance and examine its ability to slow the heart rate. His work demonstrated that this chemical could transmit nerve impulses, a major advance in the study of biochemistry and endocrinology. It was for this discovery that Dale and Loewi were given a Nobel Prize in 1936.

Dale was widely respected for his innovative research and was showered with honors throughout his life. He was knighted in 1932 and awarded the Order of Merit in 1944. From 1928 to 1942 he served as director of the National Institute for Medical Research in London. He was also president of the Royal Society and of the British Association for the Advancement of Science. Dale served as director of the Davy-Faraday Laboratory at the Royal Institute and taught chemistry there from 1942 to 1946. His most important scientific writings were reprinted in 1953 in *Adventure in Physiology*. The following year he published a personal memoir entitled *Autumn Gleanings*.

Carl Peter Henrik Dam 1895–1976

Danish biochemist and nutritionist Henrik Dam discovered the naturally occurring element required for the process of blood coagulation. Dubbed vitamin K (for the German *koagulation*), the fat-soluble substance permits the liver to synthesize several factors necessary for blood clotting, most notably prothrombin.

Between 1928 and 1930 Dam investigated the mechanism of cholesterol metabolism at the University of Copenhagen. In an experimental study in which he submitted chicks to a variety of restricted and artificial diets, Dam discovered the ability of the birds to synthesize and break down cholesterol. An unexpected side effect of the experiment, Dam noted, was that after two to three weeks on a sterol-free diet supplemented with vitamins A and D, some of the chicks began to hemorrhage. Blood studies indicated delayed or inadequate coagulation, suggesting a dietary deficiency beyond the absence of cholesterol. After experimenting with salt, wheat germ oil and other nutritional elements, Dam discovered that the symptom disappeared with the introduction of cereals and seeds into the chicks' diet.

Further dietary experimentation revealed that the best sources for this essential factor were green leaves and hog liver. Dam announced his discovery of the previously unknown nutritional factor in 1935, naming it vitamin K, not only for koagulation, but because, coincidentally, the letter K was next in line in the alphabetic designation of vitamins.

Vitamin K, found in abundance in leafy green vegetables, liver and bacteria (including intestinal bacteria), has proved a valuable tool in the management of a number of bleeding conditions, including obstructive jaundice, in which the absence of bile diminishes the absorption of the vitamin from the intestine. Inadequate transfer of vitamin K from mother to fetus can result in excessive bleeding during the infant's first week after birth. This tendency can be prevented or alleviated by administering vitamin K to the mother before labor, or to the infant immediately after delivery.

In 1939, at the St. Louis University School of Medicine, a research team headed by biochemist EDWARD DOISY successfully isolated two pure forms of vitamin K, designated as K_1, derived from plant sources, and K_2, derived from microorganisms. For their discovery and chemical analysis of vitamin K Dam and Doisy were awarded the Nobel Prize for Physiology or Medicine in 1943.

Born and raised in Copenhagen, Henrik Dam was educated in his native city at the Polytechnic Institute and at the University of Copenhagen, where he received a doctorate in biochemistry in 1934. By then he had been teaching for more than a decade at the School of Agriculture and Veterinary Medicine and at the University of Copenhagen. He began his study of sterol metabolism in 1932 as a Rockefeller Fellow at the University of Freiburg.

An associate professor at Copenhagen since 1929, Dam retained the post for twelve years, during which he completed the bulk of his research on cholesterol metabolism. Following his discovery of vitamin K Dam initiated an investigation of the nutritional role of vitamin E.

A frequent guest lecturer at universities throughout North America, Dam settled in the United States for several years, conducting research at the Woods Hole Marine Biological Laboratories, the University of Rochester, and the Rockefeller Institute for Medical Research. Pursuing his study of vitamin E, he continued his dietary experiments using chicks and rats in order to evaluate the effects of vitamin E deficiency. His observations included the antioxidant function of vitamin E and the interrelationship between dietary fat and vitamin E deficiency.

Returning to Denmark in 1945, Dam accepted a professorship in biochemistry at the Polytechnic Institute in Copenhagen. In the early 1950s he began studying gallstones, determining that the formation of cholesterol gallstones is most likely to occur in cases where the diet is lacking in polyunsaturated fats and overloaded with simple sugars. Dam found that gallstone formation is also related to proportional concentrations of cholesterol and bile acids, leading him to investigate the possibility of treating the condition by altering the composition of a patient's bile.

Between 1956 and 1963 Dam served as director of the Biochemical Division of the Danish Fat Research Institute. His many published works include articles on the biochemistry of cholesterol, phospholipids and dietary fat, the nutritional function of vitamin E, and various writings on vitamin K, including *The Discovery of Vitamin K, Its Biological functions and Therapeutical Applications,* published in 1946.

Father Damien (Joseph de Veuster) 1840–1889

Belgian missionary Father Damien gained worldwide recognition for his devotion and self-sacrifice as the "leper priest of Molokai." Located in what are now Hawaiian Islands, Molokai was the site of a famous leper colony where more than 800 victims of the disease were quarantined under government regulations. At the time of his death a national magazine printed this tribute to Father Damien's heroism: "His kindness, his charity, his sympathy, and his religious zeal had not long to wait before their influence was felt. Before he reached Molokai the leper settlement was squalid, hideous, almost hellish; now it is a peaceful, law-abiding community, presenting an attractive and, even on some sides, a cheerful appearance."

The seventh of eight children born to Frans and Catherine de Veuster, young Joseph grew up in the tiny Flemish village of Tremoloo in a rural area of Northern Belgium. Raised in a devoutly Roman Catholic environment, Joseph was one of four children to choose a life of religious service. Following his education at the Collège de Braine-Le Compte Joseph traveled to Honolulu as a missionary to replace his brother, who had taken ill. It was there that he was ordained at the age of twenty-four, taking the name Father Damien in commemoration of sainted physician Damian (see COSMAS AND DAMIAN).

In 1873 Father Damien volunteered to serve the lepers of Molokai, where the mortality rate was often as high as twelve deaths a week. Arriving just before Easter, Father Damien immediately turned all his attention to the needs of his new flock. In the eleven years that followed he transformed the lives of the quarantined inhabitants of Molokai, establishing orphanages and a school where children were taught by qualified instructors.

In 1881 Father Damien was named a Knight Commander of the Order of Kalakaua I. His health began to decline in the years that followed, and by 1885 it was clear that he had become infected with leprosy. The following year he wrote, "Having no doubt myself of the true character of my disease, I feel calm, resigned, and happier among my people. Almighty God knows what is best for my own sanctification."

Before and after Father Damien's death rumors had been circulating around Hawaii accusing him of immoral behavior. After Father Damien succumbed to leprosy, Reverend Charles Hyde, a New England Protestant living in Honolulu, addressed a denunciatory letter to California clergyman H.B. Gage stating, "He was not a pure man in his relations with women, and the leprosy from which he died should be attributed to his vices and carelessness." An official post-mortem investigation exonerated Father Damien of any wrongdoing, and, in defense of the leper priest of Molokai, celebrated author Robert Louis Stevenson addressed a six-thousand-word open letter to the Reverend Hyde.

Jean-Baptiste Gabriel Joachim Dausset 1916–

In 1980 the Nobel Prize for Physiology or Medicine was awarded to French immunologist Jean Dausset, whose outstanding achievements, said the committee, "dramatically blaze the trail toward transplantation." Establishing the existence of a genetically determined system of immune response in humans, Dausset is considered a leading pioneer of "transplant immunology," along with GEORGE SNELL and BARUJ BENACERRAF, with whom he shared the Nobel Prize.

Born in Toulouse, Dausset was pursuing scientific studies at the University of Paris and the Pasteur Institute in 1938 when he interrupted his education to serve in World War II. Before he left Paris to fight with the Free French in North Africa Dausset offered all his identification papers to a colleague at Pasteur—a Jewish scientist who survived the war under the name Jean Dausset.

The real Dausset returned to complete his medical training at the University of Paris in 1945. Accepting a fellowship in hematology at Harvard Medical School in 1948, he lived and worked in the United States for the next ten years, embarking on the scientific journey that would culminate in his Nobel Prize–winning immunological discovery.

In clinical investigations of immune response Dausset noted a particularly wide range of reactions among patients who had received multiple blood transfusions. Suspecting that different levels of response might be the result of a specific genetic variation among people, he eventually demonstrated the existence of "histocompatability," or "HLA antigens." These genetically determined cell structures, also known as "transplantation antigens," are responsible for regulating immunological response, and their variation among people accounts for individual differences in susceptibility or predisposition to disease. As more and more information is gathered on the structural and genetic characteristics of these antigens the "histocompatibility-gene-complex" promises to open the door to widescale organ transplantation and even suggests the possibility of preventive medicine through genetic engineering.

In 1958 Dausset returned to Paris, where he served on the medical faculties at the College of France and the University of Paris. Later appointed director of the immuno-hematology laboratory at the Hôpital St. Louis, he was named to the Chair of Experimental Medicine at the College of France in 1977. Dausset's numerous scientific honors include the Scientific Prize of the City of Paris (1970), the Stratton Award of the International Hematology Society (1970), and the Karl Landsteiner Award from the American Association of Blood Banks (1971). His notable published works include *Human Transplantation* (with Felix Rapaport, 1968), and *Histocompatibility* (with George Snell and Stanley Nathanson, 1976).

Described as "one of the great gentlemen of science," Dausset chose for his own motto *Vouloir pour valoir* (a Gallic version of "Seek and ye shall find").

Casimir Joseph Davaine 1812–1882

French microbiologist Casimir Davaine could scarcely have hoped for a greater tribute than that of LOUIS PASTEUR, who told him, "I pride myself for having so often followed up your own learned research."

Davaine was born at St. Armand-les-Eaux, where his father ran a small distillery. Obtaining his medical training in Paris, Davaine studied under P.F.O. Rayer (1793–1867), a distinguished biologist and one of the first bacteriological investigators. After receiving his degree in 1837 Davaine established a successful general practice in Paris and was granted memberships in the Académie de Médecine and the Société de Biologie.

Recognized as one of the earliest pioneers in bacteriology, Davaine presented the first evidence of microorganisms as a cause of disease in 1850, and in the two decades that followed he played a key role in establishing the revolutionary germ theory of disease. His extensive experimental research on plant and animal pathology included most notably a series of groundbreaking studies of anthrax. An infectious and usually fatal disease in farm animals, anthrax was a serious economic concern for European farmers.

In 1851 Rayer observed the presence of "filiform bodies" in the blood of sheep that had died of anthrax, but it was Davaine who discovered, more than ten years later, that anthractic blood does not transmit the disease if the "filiform bodies" are absent.

In 1869 Davaine performed a landmark demonstration of bacteriological infection in which he diluted anthractic blood in distilled water and let it stand for 24 hours. After the bacteria had settled in a layer at the bottom, Davaine injected the overlying liquid into one guinea pig and the bacterial substance into another. While the liquid produced no sign of the disease, the bottom layer infected the animal with anthrax.

More than twenty years after Davaine first suggested rod-shaped "bacteridia" as the cause of anthrax, celebrated German bacteriologist ROBERT KOCH conducted the classic experiments that confirmed the hypothesis in 1876.

Davaine's published works include *Recherches sur la generation des huitres (Research on the Génération of Oysters)* (1853), *Recherches sur l'anguille du blé niellé (Research on the Eel)* (1857), *Mémoire sur les anomalies de l'oeuf (Study of the Anomalies of the Egg)* (1861), and *Étude sur la genèse et la propagation de charbon (Study of the Generation and Propagation of Charcoal)* (1870).

Jacques Daviel 1696–1762

Recognized as a pioneer in the field of optic surgery, French ophthalmologist Jacques Daviel devised a technique for removing the lens of the eye as a treatment for cataracts. His invention of a rounded surgical knife, later known as "Daviel's spoon," permitted the extraction of the crystalline eye lens by an incision in the cornea.

Located behind the iris and the pupil, the lens gradually develops an opacity, or clouding, that is due to a congealing of the proteins that make up the lens fibers. The coagulation of the fibers generally works its way from the outer edges inward, impairing vision when it reaches the area directly behind the pupil. In "Daviel's operation" the clouded lens, or cataract, is removed through the incised cornea without damaging the iris or pupil.

Born at La Barre in Normandy, Daviel studied surgery at the University of Rouen and completed his medical training at the Hôtel-Dieu in Paris in 1716. After serving a tour of duty as a military surgeon he went to Marseilles to treat the victims of a plague epidemic that had just begun a devastating rampage throughout the southeastern region of Provence.

When the epidemic subsided Daviel married and settled down to a practice of ophthalmic surgery and research, conducting experimental studies with animals to refine current methodology and develop new techniques. It was nearly twenty years before his older brother Remy became the first human patient to undergo Daviel's new technique for the removal of cataracts. The surgery was only partially successful, but Daviel continued to perfect the procedure, achieving a large measure of success in hundreds of subsequent operations.

As news spread of his achievement Daviel was summoned to Paris by the Duc de Villars, who arranged for his appointment to the department of surgery at the Hôpital des Invalides in 1748. It was then that Daviel published an official report on his surgical innovation, presenting a detailed study four years later at France's Academy of Surgeons.

Elected to membership in the academy in 1749, he was appointed ocular surgeon to King Louis XV later that year. For the remainder of his life Daviel enjoyed a distinguished reputation, serving as ophthalmic surgeon in the courts of southern Europe. His written works include *Lettres sur les maladies des yeux (Letters on Diseases of the Eye)* (1748) and *Mémoire sur une nouvelle méthode pour guerir la cataracte par extraction (Account of a New Method for Treating Cataracts by Surgical Extraction)* (1755).

Sir Humphry Davy 1778–1829

In 1799 Humphry Davy stated, "As nitrous oxide in its extensive operation appears capable of destroying physical pain, it may probably be used with advantage in surgical operations..." Even though Davy became widely recognized for his identification of chemical elements in addition to other significant achievements in chemistry, little attention was ever given to his prophetic insight. It was forty-five years later that Connecticut dentist Horace Wells introduced medical anesthesia by experimenting in his dental practice with nitrous oxide. When a patient died as a result of taking nitrous oxide Wells lost sight of the value of his innovation. Soon after the tragedy he gave up practice and eventually killed himself in despair, leaving the development of anesthesia to William Morton, Crawford, Long and others.

Born in Penzance, Davy was the son of a well-to-do English gentleman who practiced wood-carving along with other, more cerebral pursuits. At sixteen Davy was apprenticed to a local surgeon, who taught him the rudiments of experimental chemistry. Through a chance encounter with distinguished scholar Davies Giddy Davy soon became acquainted with a number of scientists from various disciplines. Among these was a physician named Thomas Beddoes, who was looking for an assistant to help manage his recently established Pneumatic Institute in Bristol. Beddoes had built a practice based on his own doctrine of "pneumatic medicine," according to which he treated his patients by administering specially developed gases.

Although Davy was reluctant to give up his medical studies, he accepted the position at Beddoes's institute, where he discovered the remarkable properties of "gaseous oxide of azote," also known as nitrous oxide or "laughing gas." In experimenting on himself he seriously injured the mucous membranes of his mouth, but he subsequently used a more refined dosage on others, and soon word spread about the "new pleasure for which language has no name."

The publication in 1799 of his article "Researches, Chemical and Philosophical, chiefly concerning Nitrous Oxide and its Respiration," brought immediate recognition to Davy, who was invited to join the staff of London's Royal Institution as assistant lecturer and director of the chemistry research laboratory.

Davy's career in chemistry progressed rapidly, allowing little time to expand his early ideas on the use of nitrous oxide as a method of dulling pain. Celebrated chemist and physicist Michael Faraday was working as Davy's assistant in 1815, and together they discovered that ether could produce an intoxication similar to that of laughing gas. Thus began the era of "ether frolics," a parlor amusement in which medical applications and hazards were far from the minds of those who participated.

Recognized as the founder of electrochemistry, Davy introduced the notion of chemical affinity as an electrical phenomenon. He isolated a great number of chemical elements, including potassium, sodium, calcium, barium and magnesium. His research also covered agricultural chemistry, and he is noted for his invention of a safety lamp for miners. He was awarded knighthood in 1812, a baronetcy in 1818 and was elected president of the Royal Society in 1820. His many writings include *Elements of Chemical Philosophy* (1812), *On the Safety-lamp* (1818), *Salmonia, or the Days of Fly-Fishing* (1828), and *Consolations in Travel* (1830).

Augusta Marie Klumpke Dejerine 1859–1927
Joseph Jules Dejerine 1849–1917

The husband-and-wife team of Jules and Augusta Dejerine contributed to neurologic literature a monumental two-volume reference work that became a classic—*Anatomy of the Nervous System*. The two, who are celebrated for their individual achievements as well as for their fruitful collaboration, for many years presided together over the Clinic for Nervous Diseases at La Salpêtrière.

Born in San Francisco, Augusta Klumpke was educated at the University of Paris, where she was admitted to the Faculté de Médecine in 1877. Distinguished as the first woman in Paris to obtain a medical internship, Klumpke was completing her course in clinical medicine when she discovered a syndrome of muscular pathology caused by lesions in certain dorsal and cervical nerves. She described the disorder in 1885 in a monograph entitled *Paralysies Radiculaires du plexus brachial du type Klumpke* (*Klumpke's Paralysis of the Network of Nerves in the Arm*), which was honored the following year with the prestigious Prix Godart. (Characterized by atrophy and paralysis of the muscles of the lower arm and hand, "Klumpke's paralysis" is particularly common in infants born in breech presentation.) Augusta Klumpke did not receive her degree in medicine until 1889, a year after her marriage to Joseph-Jules Dejerine, thereby launching a momentous 30-year partnership in neurological research.

Born in Geneva, Switzerland, Dejerine left home at the age of 21 to study medicine in Paris. While training at La Salpêtrière under noted French neurologist Edmé Félix Vulpian, Dejerine served in the auxiliary division of the International Committee of the French Society of Aid to the Military Sick and Wounded, earning the Bronze Cross.

In 1879 he delivered his doctoral thesis on the role of lesions of the nervous system in "acute ascending paralysis," for which he received the Goddard Prize of the Anatomical Society of Paris along with his degree in medicine. In that same year he was appointed director of the clinic at La Charité, where within a few years he was to join the faculty as professor of clinical medicine. While Augusta Dejerine devoted a great part of her career to administrative and clinical duties at La Salpêtrière, the two worked together on a series of influential studies.

By 1885 the team of Augusta and Jules Dejerine was serving jointly as directors of the hospital's neurology clinic. In 1901 Jules was granted a professorship in the history of medicine and surgery, and he later assumed the chair in internal pathology. As consulting physician at a number of hospitals in Paris Dejerine established a distinguished reputation as a teacher, clinician and authority on neurology and internal pathology.

Widely recognized for his exhaustive investigation of the central and peripheral nervous system, Jules Dejerine collaborated with his wife and others to produce an enormous body of written work. Notable among the treatises he authored independently is his *Classification of Diseases of the Nervous System,* which endured for many years as a standard reference.

As evidence of his sizable contribution to neuropathology, Dejerine's name appears frequently in medical nomenclature in association with many of his clinical discoveries. With French physician Louis Théophile Joseph Landouzy (1845–1917) he was awarded the Montyon prize of the French Academy of Sciences for his identification of a condition characterized by atrophy of the muscles of the arm, shoulder and face. Later found to be the result of a nutritional deficiency,the disorder is now referred to as "Landouzy-Dejerine" dystrophy.

Other neuropathological conditions bearing his name include "Dejerine-Sottas disease," a rare form of congenital neuritis, and "Dejerine-Roussy syndrome," a sensory disorder caused either by inadequate vascular function or by damage to the thalamus, an important sensory relay station in the brain. With German physician Ludwig Lichtheim (1845–1928) Dejerine established what is now termed the "Dejerine-Lichtheim phenomenon," a form of expressive aphasia in which the patient is incapable of verbal communication by speech but can indicate the number of syllables in a word by a show of fingers. Acknowledged for his considerable contribution to the study of aphasia and localization of brain function, Dejerine demonstrated that "word blindness" can be caused by lesions in certain areas on the surface of the brain.

In 1910 the French Academy of Sciences awarded its Montyon prize to Dejerine for the second time for his study of radiculitis and other diseases of the spine, conducted in collaboration with French physician André Thomas. Four years later Dejerine was invited to deliver the Hughlings Jackson lecture at a gathering of the Royal Society of London, where he was he was presented with the Moxon medal for his investigation of spinal nerve disorders.

Meanwhile, Augusta Dejerine was gathering honors in her own right for both her scientific achievements and her personal valor. In 1905 the Rescue Society of Bern decorated her for saving a child from drowning. And in acknowledgment of her medical career she was made a member of the Académie de Médecine in Paris and the Academia di Medicina in Turin, Italy. She also served as president and long-standing member of Société Neurologique de Paris.

Both Dejerines were made officers of the French Legion of Honor, and Jules received an honorary commission in the French Territorial Army. Shortly before his death at the age of 68 he volunteered for active service in the neurology unit of an army hospital while World War I was raging.

After the death of her husband in 1917 Augusta Dejerine served on the medical staff at the Institution Nationale des Invalides, a facility established by the French Army for the treatment of spinal cord wounds.

Jules Dejerine's numerous published works include *L'hérédité dans les maladies du système nerveux* (1886), *De l'agraphie* (1891), *Traité des maladies de la moelle épinière* (1902), *Les manifestations fonctionelles des psycholonevreuses* (1911) and *Sémiologie des affections du système nerveux* (1914).

Max Delbrück 1906–1981

German-born physicist Max Delbrück has been hailed as a pioneer in the study of molecular genetics, contributing significant advances in sensory physiology, bacteriology, and virology. In 1939 Delbrück introduced the "plaque technique," a method of producing a pure bacteriophage virus culture, vital for experimental research.

This required the spreading of a layer of bacterial cells on a thin gelatinous plate and covering it with a virus-infected substance. As the bacteria becomes infected the viral particles multiply, and the bacterial cells lyse, or disintegrate, leaving clear sports the size of pinpoints. These tiny holes in the gelatinous surface, known as plaques, vary significantly in size, shape and number, depending on the infecting virus. The particles, representing a single pure viral strain, guarantee the molecular biologist an uncontaminated basis for experimentation.

Delbrück's technique has paved the way for major advances in human genetics and the investigation of genetic diseases. For his contribution to the study of bacteriophage viruses and molecular genetics Delbrück was awarded the 1969 Nobel Prize for Physiology or Medicine, which he shared with ALFRED DAY HERSHEY and Salvador Luria.

Born in Berlin, Delbrück received a Ph.D. in physics from the University of Göttingen in 1930. After studing theoretical nuclear physics as a research assistant in Denmark and Switzerland, he returned to Germany in 1932 to join the staff at Berlin's Kaiser Wilhelm Institute for Chemistry. It was there that he became intrigued with the study of bacteriophages, which prompted the Rockefeller Foundation to offer him a fellowship in biology at the California Institute of Technology when, in 1935, Delbrück became a refugee from Nazi Germany.

He worked in California until 1939, when he joined the faculty at Vanderbilt University, where he developed his revolutionary technique for the investigation of viruses. During his eight years at Vanderbilt Delbrück discovered that genetic material from different strains of virus can combine to create a new and viable virus (observed independently by Hershey). Delbrück also investigated bacterial mutation, discovering, along with Luria, that genetic changes in both viruses and bacterial cells can occur at random. These studies provided valuable clues to the understanding of virus-resistant strains of bacteria and drug-resistant strains of viruses.

Developing an informal collaboration over the years, Delbrück, Hershey and Luria often exchanged ideas and information at Hershey's laboratory at Cold Spring Harbor, Long Island. They came to be known as the "phage group," and the venerable Delbrück was referred to by many as "the Pope." A soft-spoken and dignified figure, he gained the respect and admiration of students and colleagues, one of whom described Delbrück as "our group conscience, goad and sage."

In 1947 Delbrück returned to the California Institute of Technology, where he served as professor of biology until his death in 1981. Internationally acclaimed for his contributions to physical and biological sciences, Delbrück received many honors in addition to the 1969 Nobel Prize. Earlier that year he and Luria shared a biology research award, accompanied by $25,000. Delbrück donated his share to Amnesty International, a human-rights organization that helps political prisoners gain their freedom. As someone who had escaped Nazi Germany, he offered the money to all "prisoners of conscience."

Democritus c.460–370 B.C.

One of the most influential of the group of Greek philosopher-scientists that flourished in the fifth and sixth centuries B.C., Democritus developed the theory that the universe, including the stars, the souls of men and the most insignificant creature on earth, is composed of atoms, a void and nothing more. Known as the "laughing philosopher," Democritus emphasized the importance of happiness and inner peace in maintaining one's health, even in his very materialistic world. He made clear his priorities when he wrote that he would rather discover the demonstration of a single theorem in geometry "than win the throne of Persia."

Using the letters of the alphabet as a metaphor, Democritus described atoms as the elemental units from which all matter is composed. Immutable, homogeneous and qualitatively identical, these individual elements differ only in size, shape and weight. Their constant movement in a universal void causes them to collide and cluster as letters combine to form words, sentences and new ideas. Democritus taught that the apparently qualitative differences in form and matter are a sensory illusion, indicating only the way in which these aggregations affect the observer. True knowledge cannot be achieved through sensory perception, therefore, but rather through thought.

Recognizing physical laws rather than a universal design postulated by metaphysical thinkers such as PYTHAGORAS and EMPEDOCLES, Democritus was one of the earliest proponents of "corpuscular philosophy," a doctrine later expressed by Epicurus (341–270 B.C.) and opposed in ARISTOTLE'S theory of physics. Maintaining that experiential qualities such as heat, sound and color originate in the sensory system, Democritus asserted that the only quantifiable realities of nature are the shape, size and displacement of atoms.

Democritus was born at Abdera, in Thrace. At an early age he left his home to educate himself through travel, collecting the works of many of the great philosophers who preceded him. He drew inspiration from many sources, notably from Anaxagoras (c.500–c.428) and from his mentor Leucippus (c.485–c.350). Over the course of a very long career Democritus produced texts on physics, mathematics, ethics and music. No complete works have survived, but fragments quoted in the writings of Aristotle and others, have been collected and published, notably by Mullach in Germany in 1843.

W. Donner Denckla 1934–

While searching for a better way to measure the biological effectiveness of thyroid hormones W. Donner Denckla stumbled upon a built-in "hormonal self-destruct program" that inspired an entirely new interpretation of the aging process. In experiments with rats Donner observed that although the hormone supply of the blood remained relatively constant, its biological effectiveness nevertheless decreased continuously over time.

Recognizing that the thyroid is involved in all of the body's major systems, Denckla saw a possible key to the aging process in this predictible pattern of decline.

Further experimentation led Denckla to discover that the pituitary gland functioned as a progressive thyroid block. By removing the pituitary gland Denckla observed that thyroid-dependent systems had no age-related decline. He named the thyroid-blocking hormone DECO, an acronym for Decreasing Oxygen Consumption. Further experiments allowed Denckla to restore biological functions in rats to juvenile levels and to hold them there indefinitely. These animals would then die at advanced ages, and very abruptly.

Denckla's studies present a view of evolution and gerontology that is still resisted by many biologists today. He wrote that:

> In natural selection, once the individual has procreated, and allowed progeny to reach maturity, as far as evolution is concerned he can be dispensed with. An animal that is turning over ten or twenty times faster per century than his competitors is obviously going to have twenty times as many opportunities for natural experiments...[Humans] have developed, through language, and later through scientific method, a very large amount of extragenic information that we can use to make successful adaptations to a changing environment. We're the first animal that's ever made successful adaptations to life-threatening situations within a life span or a generation.

Denckla suggests that the presence of all deteriorative illness is evidence of a pathological aging process. In building his "DECO-blocker" he hopes to prolong and improve human life by reducing the vulnerability to disease.

Derek Ernest Denny-Brown 1901–1981

The activity of a single motor neuron was first described in 1929 by neurophysiologist Derek Denny-Brown. Over the course of the next half-century Denny-Brown studied nerve cell function and dysfunction in a wide range of clinical conditions, including concussion, cerebral palsy, Parkinson's disease, and paralytic stroke, which he showed to be the result of a disruption in the flow of blood to the brain.

Denny-Brown launched a series of investigations on the nature of neurophysiological damage from cancer and contributed significantly to the development of a treatment for myasthenia gravis, a chronic and progressive paralysis of the muscles.

Noting a similarity between the clinical picture of the disease and the characteristic effects of poisoning by curare, Denny-Brown's observations prompted the use of anticholinesterases to bring symptomatic relief. Myasthenia gravis has since been classified as an autoimmune disease that causes the organism to produce antibodies against a constituent of its own tissues. In this particular case, the body destroys its own receptors for the neurotransmitter acetylcholine—a chemical substance needed for the transmission of impulses between motor nerve fibers and skeletal muscles. The introduction of anticholinesterase drugs raises the level of acetylcholine at the neuromuscular junctions, thereby strengthening the action of the muscles.

Born in Christchurch, New Zealand, Denny-Brown completed his undergraduate education at the University of New Zealand in 1924 and obtained a Beit Memorial Fellowship to continue studies in physiology at Oxford University.

After receiving his doctorate in 1928 he joined the staff at London's National Hospital for Nervous Disease, where he served as house officer and registrar for nearly a decade. When Harvard Medical School offered him a faculty position in 1939 he eagerly accepted, but professional and personal plans were frustrated by the outbreak of World War II.

As a member of the British Royal Army Medical Corps Denny-Brown served in India and Burma. He attained the rank of brigadier general and was decorated as an Officer of the Order of the British Empire in recognition of his advanced treatment of head and spinal injuries.

After the war Denny-Brown obtained a medical degree from the University of New Zealand and was appointed to the faculty as James Jackson Putnam Professor of Neurology. In 1950 Harvard Medical School renewed its offer, and by the end of that year Denny-Brown and his family had emigrated to the United States. Naturalized as a citizen in 1952, Denny-Brown conducted the major portion of his research in neuropathology and physiology in the twenty-five years that followed, serving as Harvard professor of neurology and chief neurologist at Boston City Hospital.

René Descartes 1596–1650

René Descartes envisioned a universal science that could be applied to all of biological creation. He proposed, "The whole of philosophy is a tree whose roots are metaphysics, whose trunk is physics, and whose branches are the other sciences."

Considered by many to be the first modern philosopher of science, Descartes rejected the premises of scholasticism and aimed for the certainty of mathematical demonstration in all areas of knowledge, even the understanding of knowledge itself. He proceeded from a starting position of universal doubt, postulating a malevolent force that could distort sensory perception and even reason. In doubting everything, however, he could not doubt that he was thinking. "*Cogito ergo sum,*" he declared—"I think, therefore I am." This catchy Cartesian formula expresses the essential element of dualism in Descartes's philosophy—the notion of the conscious human mind as divorced from all other natural elements or processes, and defined in negative terms as that only which is inaccessible to science.

Emphasizing the continuity of physics, chemistry, biology and astronomy, Descartes maintained that since all nature is subject to the rational laws of cause and effect, all physical phenomena can be reduced to quantifiable elements and explained by mathematical laws.

In this rational and mechanistic world, man is the only exception—a divided creature possessing equal parts of spirit and matter. Descartes distinguished the conscious human mind not only by its faculty of knowing, but also by its indivisibility and uniqueness in nature. Because "physical" and "nonphysical" properties are mutually exclusive, he asserted that the two realms can be joined only by the intervention of God. Assigning a physical reality to this union, Descartes located the bridge between body and soul in the pineal gland, an organ located in the base of the brain behind the forehead at the position of the "third eye."

Much has been made of the holes in this theory. "The idea of an immaterial mind controlling the body is vitalism, no more, no less," declared psychologist and neuroscientist Donald O. Hebb in 1974. "It has no place in science." Twenty-five years earlier English philosopher Gilbert Ryle (1900–1976) had contributed a classic phrase to the scientific idiom when he referred to the "ghost in the machine" as a means of exorcising Cartesian dualism in his *Concept of Mind*. Arguing that the mind is a process rather than an object, Ryle described the flaw in Descartes's model as a "category mistake." He compares Descartes to the foreigner on a guided tour of Oxford who is shown the dormitories, the lecture halls, and the library and keeps asking to see the university.

Despite the failings of a dualistic view of man, Descartes's philosophy offered a radical alternative to the traditional reliance on "supernatural" explanations for natural phenomena. In isolating the conscious mind in a metaphysical ivory tower he allowed all other human functions to be considered in mechanical terms.

Descartes proved to himself the existence of God by reasoning that the idea of a perfect being could not have originated from an imperfect being. Satisfied that a perfect God would not deceive, he could then accept the existence of a physical world and his perceptions of it. Although he relied first and foremost on the powers of reason, Descartes conducted extensive experimental research in physics, optics, biology, psychology and physiology, dissecting animals in various stages of development, measuring the weight of air, and observing the phenomena associated with light reflection and refraction.

Often called the "father of analytical geometry," Descartes is most widely known for his contribution to the development of mathematics. In 1637 he formulated the "Cartesian coordinates" and "Cartesian curves," a system of geometry in which the properties of various shapes and curves are expressed in algebraic terms so that they may be considered subject to mathematical laws.

Descartes was born at La Haye, near Tours, where his father practiced law. His mother, who died shortly after giving birth, left her infant son a substantial inheritance, which ensured his financial independence for life.

After several years of study at the Jesuit college at La Flèche, Descartes obtained a degree in law from the University of Poitiers in 1617. Frustrated by the limitations of scholasticism, he renounced the academic life, vowing "no longer to seek any other science than the knowledge of myself or of the great book of the world."

After two years of voluntary military service under Prince Maurice of Nassau he enlisted in the Bavarian army in 1619. It was in the winter of that same year that Descartes reportedly embarked on his quest for philosophical certainty at the age of 23. Nearly ten years later he resigned from military duty to settle in Holland and devote his full attention to the philosophy of science.

In 1637 Descartes introduced his doctrine in a series of essays, the most important of which was entitled *Discours de la Méthode (Discourse on Method)*. Written in French rather than the customary Latin, the revolutionary work included a formulation of the optical laws of refraction, the system of coordinate geometry and his grand design of a universal science. He later published expanded discussions of Cartesian doctrine, including *Meditationes de Prima Philosophia* (1641), *Principia Philosophiae* (1644), and *Traité des passions de l'ame* (1649)

At the age of fifty-three Descartes moved to Stockholm to accept an appointment as philosophy tutor to Queen Christine of Sweden. In accordance with the queen's wishes they met every morning at five o'clock, regardless of the bitter cold outside and inside the castle. Unaccustomed to such hours and the rigors of Swedish weather, Descartes contracted pneumonia and died in February, 1650.

George Frederick Dick 1881–1967
Gladys Rowena Henry Dick 1881–1963

Hailed for their outstanding contributions to the prevention and treatment of scarlet fever, physicians George and Gladys Dick shared a marriage and scientific partnership that spanned nearly fifty years, ending only with Gladys Dick's death in 1963. They met in 1911 as research pathologists at the University of Chicago, where they collaborated on a ten-year investigation of the etiology and immunological mechanisms of scarlet fever.

George Dick had begun studying the disease a year earlier, when he accepted a position at the John R. McCormick Institute for Infectious Diseases, a research facility that had recently been founded by Edith Rockefeller McCormick and her husband in memory of their son's death from scarlet fever. A contagious and often crippling disease usually occurring in childhood, scarlet fever was then endemic to North America and Europe, where the mortality rate often reached up to 25%.

It was suspected that hemolytic streptocococci played a secondary role in the development of the disease, but in 1923 the Dicks established those bacteria as the actual cause of scarlet fever. In the year that followed they demonstrated that the disease's characteristic red rash is produced by a toxin released by the streptococci. By isolating and standardizing that toxic substance they were able to develop the first method of determining susceptibility to scarlet fever. Known as the "Dick test," the procedure involves an injection of a small amount of the toxin under the skin, which indicates susceptibility by causing a small red patch on the skin within 48 hours. In addition, the Dick toxin formed the basis of a technique for producing active immunity in humans, as well as for the preparation of a specific antitoxin in horses.

The son of a railroad engineer, George Dick was born in Fort Wayne, Indiana. After graduating from Rush Medical College in 1905 he served two years as a physician at the iron mines in Buhl, Montana, and then left for Europe to pursue advanced studies in pathology at the universities of Vienna and Munich. Dick returned to the United States in 1909 to join the faculty at the University of Chicago, where he was later named professor of pathology and chairman of the department of medicine, and eventually professor emeritus in 1945. During that time he also practiced internal medicine in Chicago at Billings, Memorial and Wesley hospitals and served as chief pathologist and director of laboratories at St. Luke's Hospital there.

The youngest of three children, Gladys Rowena Henry was born in Pawnee City, Nebraska, where her father, who had served in the cavalry during the Civil War, raised carriage horses and sold grain. Seeking a proper education for their children, William and Azelia Henry moved the family to Lincoln while Gladys was still an infant.

In 1900 Gladys Henry received a bachelor's degree in science from the University of Nebraska and, after several years of graduate study in zoology, entered the Johns Hopkins University School of Medicine. Graduating in 1907, she pursued postgraduate training in hematology, pathochemistry and experimental surgery as an intern at Johns Hopkins and at the University of Berlin.

The Dicks were married in 1914, and after several months on honeymoon in Egypt and the Balkans they returned to Chicago, where Gladys joined her husband on the research faculty at the McCormick Institute. She retained the position until debilitating cerebral arteriosclerosis forced her to retire in 1953.

After announcing their findings on scarlet fever in the *Journal of the American Medical Association* in a series of articles published in 1923 and 1924, the Dicks became the subject of heated controversy in the scientific community when they secured patents in Britain and the United States for their techniques of toxin and antitoxin production. Amid charges of commercialism in the medical press, the League of Nations in 1935 declared that the terms of the patents restricted further research and obstructed the process of biomedical standardization.

Claiming that the measures were not taken for financial gain but to guarantee the quality of the preparations, George and Gladys Dick succeeded in stopping Lederle Laboratories from using allegedly improper manufacturing methods by suing the company for patent infringement. The matter was dropped in the 1940s after the toxins and antitoxins were superseded by antibiotics for treatment and immunization against scarlet fever.

Grantly Dick-Read 1890–1959

British gynecologist Grantly Dick-Read pioneered a system of "natural childbirth" based on the notion that the pain commonly experienced during labor and delivery is mainly the result of tension, fear and ignorance. Developing a set of psychological and physical exercises, Dick-Read promised expectant mothers that they could give birth safely and painlessly without using drugs.

Dick-Read's preparatory sessions combined educational lectures and physical techniques for breathing and muscle conditioning in a program emphasizing relaxation, self-assurance, and an understanding of the physiological aspects of childbirth. His training of mothers-to-be included a preview of the event itself in the form of a fifty-five-minute recording of the sounds of a delivery room, from the murmurs of the doctor and nurse to the cries of joy from mother and baby.

Reflecting on the inadequacies of modern obstetrics, Dick-Read was quoted as saying that he "could never understand why there was such a fuss when a woman was going to have a baby and yet my animal pets had their young without any trouble."

At 24 he entered Cambridge University, receiving a degree in medicine and surgery in 1920. After graduation his experience in his private gynecology practice in London gave rise to the "Read Method of Natural Birth Control," which he described in *Natural Childbirth,* published in 1933. Nine years later he published *Childbirth Without Fear,* which precipitated a controversy of global proportions and provoked antagonism from a large segment of the medical establishment. Translated into ten languages, the book was the center of heated debate for both its medical and sociological principles.

Two years after his *Birth of a Child* appeared in 1947, he closed his Harley Street practice and left for South Africa to establish an international center for the advancement of painless childbirth. Accompanied by most of his London staff, he arrived in Johannesburg in March, 1949 but was denied permission to practice by the South Africa Medical and Dental Council. The decision was reversed several months later, after Dick-Read brought his case before the South African Supreme Court.

Widely published in translation, Dick-Read's notable writings include *Introduction to Motherhood* (1951) and *No Time for Fear* (1955), an account of birthing practices among tribal women in the Belgian Congo. Although less widely known than the natural childbirth techniques of French obstetrician FERNAND LAMAZE, Dick-Read's system is practiced throughout the world, most commonly in the United States.

Johannes Friedrich Dieffenbach 1795—1847

German surgeon Johannes Friedrich Dieffenbach revived the practice of plastic surgery in the early nineteenth century after a long period of prohibition. Considered heretical at various times in history, the practice of surgical repair of congenital or acquired deformities had been opposed by a number of noted surgeons, including FALLOPIO and AMBROISE PARÉ. The church lifted its official ban in 1822, the year Dieffenbach received his degree in medicine from the University of Wurzburg.

Born in Königsberg, Dieffenbach studied theology at Rostock and Griefswald before changing to a career in medicine. After passing the required state examinations in 1824 he was hired as surgical assistant at La Charité Hospital in Berlin. Professional success came quickly, and within five years he was named director of surgery.

Immediately following a divorce from his first wife, Dieffenbach married the wealthy Emilie Friederike Heydecker in 1933. As attending physician and surgeon to the Prussian Prince Protashow he practiced in Paris and Montpelier while pursuing research on a variety of medical subjects.

Dieffenbach is best known for his innovations in plastic surgery technique, notably in the transplantation of facial features, including noses and lips. Among the first to perform eye surgery on a living person, he pioneered the practice of strabotomy. Introduced in 1839, the operation consists of an incision in the tendon of an eye muscle to correct strabismus, an uncontrollable deviation of the eye.

Applying techniques of tendon surgery in the treatment of limb deformities, Dieffenbach developed a number of effective procedures, including tenotomy, the cutting of specific tendons in the repair of a clubfoot. "Dieffenbach's operation" is an advanced method he devised for amputation at the hip. Other achievements include his use of blood transfusion, most notably in the treatment of cholera, as well as extensive experimental research on transplantation of internal organs.

Serving as professor of surgery at the University of Berlin during the last seven years of his life, Dieffenbach was twice honored with the distinguished Monthyon prize from the Institut de France.

Pedanius Dioscorides of Anazarbus c. 60 A.D.

Up to the seventeenth century European physicians cited as an authoritative pharmacological reference the work of Pedanius Dioscorides, a physician of Ancient Greece. His monumental five-volume compendium, entitled *De Materia Medica (On Medicine)*, includes approximately 827 entries on animal, vegetable and mineral remedies.

Book I provides descriptions of trees and shrubs, noting the medicinal properties of botanic liquids, gums and fruits as well as aromatics, oils and salves. Book II discusses animals, animal parts and animal products and also includes some herbs and grains. Books III and IV describe different groups of herbs, roots and seeds, and Book V includes minerals and fermented fluids.

Each entry identifies the origin of the substance and describes its distinguishing characteristics, therapeutic properties, and harmful side effects. Dioscorides also provided clear instructions for the preparation and application of simple and compound drugs, with appropriate notations on perishability and proper methods of storage as well as techniques for detecting fraudulent or deficient prescriptions.

Dioscorides was born in Anzarbus, not far from Tarsus, an educational center and the capital of Cilicia. Based on the few biographical clues available, most historians believe that he received medical training at Tarsus and Alexandria and practiced as a military physician in the Roman army. In that capacity he traveled extensively, acquiring much of his detailed information on plants from firsthand observation. His contact with foreign cultures provided an additional advantage for Dioscorides, enabling him to cite not only the popular Greek names for plants but the terms used in Egypt, Persia, Africa and Gaul, thereby supplying a valuable resource for students of linguistics and cultural anthropology. As a result of the enduring influence of *De materia medica*, the plant nomenclature introduced by Dioscorides forms the basis of both popular and scientific terminology in modern botany.

An unchallenged authority for sixteen centuries, Dioscorides was reprinted, translated, edited, annotated, and imitated continuously. *De materia medica* inspired a great many treatises and reference works, some of which have been mistakenly attributed to Dioscorides, but it is now widely believed that his entire literary effort was consumed in the creation of a single masterpiece—one of the most enduring and influential pharmacopeias in history.

Edward Adelbert Doisy 1893–1986

American biochemist Edward Doisy gained international prominence for determining the chemical nature of vitamin K, a nutritional factor identified in 1935 by

HENRIK DAM. As a group of fat-soluble substances, vitamin K is found in various animal and plant materials, including fish, liver, egg yolk, spinach, cabbage and hempseed. It is required by the body for the production of prothrombin, a glycoprotein involved in the second stage of blood coagulation. As a result, vitamin K is effective in the promotion of blood-clotting and is widely used to prevent hemorrhaging, particularly in cases of obstructive jaundice.

Four years after it was discovered, Doisy isolated vitamin K in two forms of pure crystalline compound: K_1, (from green plants, and K_2, produced by a form of bacterial decomposition. As the first compound to be obtained, K_1 was extracted from alfalfa and then submitted to a process of extraction and repeated adsorptions to eliminate impurities. Doisy used a similar method to isolate K_2 and established the slight chemical difference between these two substances. He then determined their individual structures and later synthesized vitamin K_1. His outstanding achievement was acknowledged in 1943 with the Nobel Prize for Physiology or Medicine, which he shared with Henrik Dam.

Born in Hume, Illinois, Doisy enrolled in the School of Medical Science at Harvard in 1915. He interrupted his studies to serve in World War I and in 1920 obtained his doctorate in biochemistry from Harvard. Doisy returned to the Midwest to accept a position as teaching instructor at the Washington School of Medicine in St. Louis, Missouri, and when he left three years later it was to take over the chair in biochemistry at the St. Louis University School of Medicine.

Barely thirty years old, Doisy initiated a large-scale experimental study of the regulatory factors in the sex cycle of rats and mice. The prime focus of the research was on the active principles in sex hormones, with particular attention to the various forms of estrogen—a general term used to refer to the female hormones produced in the ovaries and, in smaller amounts, in the testes and adrenals.

In 1929, after six years of intensive research, Doisy isolated estrone—the first crystalline steroidal hormone. In six more years of work he succeeded in isolating estriol, a weak form of estrogen, and estradiol, the most powerful naturally occurring female hormone. These substances and other forms of estrogen are now used to treat a wide range of disorders, including menstrual irregularities and cancer of the prostate. Estrogen drugs also form the basis of oral contraceptives and are prescribed to relieve the symptoms of menopause. Gaining worldwide distinction a leading authority on the biochemical nature of estrogenic substances, Doisy later served on the League of Nations Committee on the Standardization of Sex Hormones.

Doisy made his professional home at St. Louis University for over forty years, during which time he also served as director of the department of biochemistry at St. Mary's Hospital. Following his two major contributions and the citation of the Nobel Committee, Doisy continued to distinguish himself as an outstanding investigator, most notably in the study of antibiotics and the metabolism of hormones and bile acids.

Vincent Paul Dole 1913–

In 1988 the Albert Lasker Medical Research Award was presented to American physician Vincent Dole in honor of his contribution to the medical treatment of opiate addiction. In collaboration with his wife, psychiatrist Marie Nyswander, Dole introduced the therapeutic use of methadone for heroin addiction.

Born in Chicago, Illinois, Dole graduated from the Harvard University Medical School in 1939. In 1947 he was appointed physician and research professor at the Rockefeller Institute and Hospital and later joined the medical faculty at Rockefeller University.

In 1959 New York City Mayor Robert Wagner called for the medical research establishment to confront the urgent problem of narcotic addiction, requesting that immediate attention be directed toward the development of effective medical treatment. Over the next four years the Mayor's Advisory Committee on Narcotic Addiction and the New York City Health Research Council determined that the highest research priority was to find "a pharmaceutical substitute for heroin which would enable addicts to function."

The council invited Dole and Nyswander to launch clinical and pharmacological investigations, and by the mid-1960s they determined that methadone hydrochloride removes the addict's preoccupation with drugs and produces remarkable changes in personality and behavior. A synthetic morphine substitute, methadone hydrochloride is an opiate painkiller that works on the same receptor molecules in the brain as do other opiates such as heroin. Dole found that with continued or increasing use of methadone the patient develops an exceedingly high tolerance, not only to methadone, but to all narcotics, so that a "maintenance" dosage of methadone produces no euphoria or other mind-altering effects but effectively blocks the effects of heroin, morphine or other drugs of the same class.

Based on their research, Dole and Nyswander hypothesized that in some addicts, repeated opiate use induces not only a specific drug dependence, but also irreversible metabolic change. Defending the therapeutic effectiveness of methadone maintenance, they argued that in such cases social rehabilitation, no matter how successful, does not remove this underlying and permanent condition. It is this assumption that has been the most controversial element of the methadone maintenance program since it was introduced in 1965.

The underlying medical, legal and sociological issues of the methadone maintenance programs were hotly debated in New York's political circles as well as in the medical community. In the late 1960s and early 1970s many thousands of former heroin addicts were reportedly rehabilitated in programs that had been established throughout the city.

By 1973, enrollment peaked at 35,000, but the anticipated success of the project was never achieved. While Dole's detractors blamed the medical theory of methadone maintenance, others, including Dole and Nyswander, attributed the disappointing results of the program in New York City to a combination of sociological and political factors and the additional burden of federal bureaucracy.

In 1976 Dole pointed out, "No medicine can rehabilitate persons...Methadone maintenance makes possible a first step toward social rehabilitation by stabilizing the pharmacological condition of addicts...But to succeed in bringing disadvantaged addicts to a productive way of life, a treatment program must enable its patients to feel pride and hope and to accept responsibility. This is not achieved in present-day treatment programs...Patients held in contempt by the staff continue to act like addicts, and the overcrowded facility becomes a public nuisance."

In the 1970s and 1980s investigations were aggressively pursued on the sociology, psychology, neurology and biochemistry of drug addiction; but, more than twenty years after its inception, methadone maintenance continues to be the main treatment for opiate addiction in the United States.

Gerhard Domagk 1895–1964

Gerhard Domagk's discovery of the antibacterial action of a chemical dye called Prontosil marked a milestone in the history of medicine. Noting that prontosil, or sulfonamide-crysoidin, successfully cured streptococcal infections in mice, Domagk went on to discover the chemical's antagonistic effects on a wide range of bacteria. Empowering medical science with one of its most important weapons against disease in the days before antibiotics, Domagk ushered in the era of "sulfa drugs."

A native of Brandenburg, Germany, Domagk earned a medical degree from the University of Kiel and taught bacteriology and pathology at Griefswald and Münster universities. He left teaching in 1927 to become director of the I. G. Farbenindustrie Laboratory for Experimental Pathology and Bacteriology at Wuppertal.

In 1932 Domagk made his landmark discovery of the curative properties of Prontosil red, recognizing by 1935 that it was the sulfanilamide component of the Prontosil molecule that was responsible for its chemotherapeutic effect. Until the advent of "sulfa drugs," streptococcal diseases were considered a major threat to public health. These drugs offered relief from such devastating diseases as meningitis, pneumonia, gonorrhea, puerperal fever, and bacteremia, or "blood poisoning." Among the human test cases bearing witness to the drugs' effectiveness were Domagk's daughter and Franklin D. Roosevelt, Jr.

For his important contribution to medical science Domagk was awarded the Nobel Prize for Physiology or Medicine in 1939, but he was prevented by Nazi decree from accepting the honor. Eight years later he was issued a gold medal in lieu of the prize money.

René Jules Dubos 1901–1982

One of the leading medical scientists of the twentieth century, French-born bacteriologist René Jules Dubos helped to elucidate the profound influence of the environment on physiological and immunological characteristics.

Born and raised in the town of St. Brieuc in Brittany, Dubos left home when he was fourteen to study in Paris at the Institut Nationale Agronomique. After obtaining a degree in agricultural sciences he served for several years as a research associate at the International Institute of Agriculture in Rome. In 1924 Dubos emigrated to the United States to study at Rutgers University, where, less than three years later, he completed his doctorate in microbiology and pathology.

Appointed to the research faculty at Rockefeller Institute (now Rockefeller University), Dubos was investigating a particular form of pneumococcus bacterium when he discovered an enzyme in soil bacteria that destroys the starchlike protective shell surrounding the pneumococci. Thus exposed, the pneumococci succumb to the defense mechanisms of the host and are rendered harmless.

Dubos determined that the highly specific antibacterial enzyme is produced only as it is needed by the soil bacterium as a source of energy. Investigating the mechanism of induced enzyme production, he explored the soil for other antibacteriological agents and, in 1939, isolated tyrothricin from the soil bacterium *Bacillus brevis*. Highly effective against a wide range of bacteria, tyrothricin was found to be extremely toxic to red blood and reproductive cells in humans and thus limited in its medical application to topical use in skin ointments

Obtained from microorganisms or produced synthetically, antibiotics are substances that destroy or inhibit the growth of a microorganism. The term, derived from the Greek words *anti* and *bios*, means literally "destructive of life."

In 1938 Dubos became an American citizen and, with the exception of a brief assignment on the medical faculty at Harvard, spent his entire career at Rockefeller University. During World War II he concentrated his efforts on the medical needs of the military, particularly in the area of immunology, but in the postwar period he turned his attention to the nature of tuberculosis and resistance to disease. The role of nutritional, environmental and social factors in the mechanism of infection became the central focus of all his subsequent research.

In the early 1960s Dubos conducted a study of indigenous microbial flora in human and animal hosts, particularly in the gastrointestinal tract. An analysis of the specific physiological effects of various microbial flora found some species to be harmful, while others were shown to serve a specialized and essential function in the growth and health of the host. In later investigations Dubos established an environmental basis for traits that had been assumed to be hereditary, such as body weight or resistance to infection.

Dubos received many notable awards in the course of his long and distinguished career, including the Lasker Award of the American Public Health Association (1948), the Trudeau Medal of the National Tuberculosis Association (1951), the Centennial Award of the Robert Koch Institute (1960), Passano Foundation Award (1960) and the Award for Scientific Achievement from the American Medical Association (1964).

In addition to serving as editor of the *Journal of Experimental Medicine,* Dubos was a prolific and influential author whose technical writings include *The Bacterial Cell* (1945), *The White Plague: Tuberculosis, Man, and Society* (1952), *Biochemical Determinants of Microbial Diseases* (1954) and *The Unseen World* (1962).

Writing for a more general audience in his later years, he published a number of books on the history and philosophy of science, including *Pasteur and Modern Science* (1960), *Dreams of Reason: Science and Utopias* (1961), *The Torch of Life: Continuity in Living Experience* (1962), *Man Adapting* (1965) and *A God Within* (1972).

Dubos explored the social implications of science most notably in *So Human an Animal,* a study of the interplay between environment and inhabitant. Published in 1968, the book was awarded a Pulitzer Prize for General Non-Fiction the following year.

Guillaume Benjamin Amand Duchenne 1806–1875

French physician and neurologist Guillaume Duchenne pioneered the use of electrical stimuli in the treatment of muscle dysfunction, devising the techniques of electro-analysis and electro-therapeutics. Developing methods of neuromuscular analysis by local electrisation, Duchenne described a number of previously unrecognized disorders, including a progressive form of paralysis now known as "Duchenne's paralysis." He also identified tabes dorsalis (also known as "Aran-Duchenne disease"), a degeneration of the spinal cord and related nerves characterized by intense paroxysmal pain, loss of reflexes, and various other functional disturbances of the sexual and digestive organs.

Widely respected among such celebrated colleagues as JEAN-BAPTISTE BOUILLAUD, JEAN-MARTIN CHARCOT, and Armand Trousseau (1801–1867), Duchenne is distinguished as the inventor of the biopsy—a procedure designed to remove and examine living tissue for purposes of diagnosis. The English neurologist William R. Gowers (1845–1915) christened the method "Duchenne's histological harpoon."

The son of a French seaman, Duchenne was born in Boulogne-sur-Mer, a coastal town near Calais. He was educated at Douais and Paris, receiving his degree in medicine in 1831. He went back to his native village to establish a general medical practice, serving the fishermen and sailors of Boulogne; but in 1842, following the death of his first wife and the end of an unfortunate second marriage, Duchenne returned to Paris.

Devoting his efforts to the study and treatment of neuromuscular disorders, he became adept in the newly emerging practices of medical photography and "electropuncture," a neurological treatment involving the insertion of a needle into the tissue for electrical stimulation. Using batteries and an induction coil, Duchenne devised a procedure for stimulating a single muscle fiber at a time, with particular attention to the distinct forms of progressive muscular atrophy. Applying the principles recently introduced by the English chemist and physicist Michael Faraday (1791–1867). Duchenne pioneered the technique of electrotherapy as a system for evaluating the variations in muscular response in individual cases and determining clues to pathological classification.

Although he was never appointed to a staff position at any hospital or university, Duchenne was admired as an outstanding teacher and clinical neurologist in Paris, where his services as a consultant and private practitioner were widely sought after. His achievement, however, was not fully recognized by the medical establishment until several decades after his death, when a monument was erected in Duchenne's honor at the celebrated Salpêtrière, one of the largest and most distinguished hospitals in the world.

Renato Dulbecco 1914–

For his contribution to the understanding of the relationship between viruses and cancer, Renato Dulbecco received the 1975 Nobel Prize for Physiology or Medicine, which he shared with fellow molecular biologists DAVID BALTIMORE and Howard M. Temin. It was their investigation of the cellular mechanism of cancer formation that led Baltimore, Temin and Dulbecco to examine the interaction between viruses and genetic material.

Dulbecco turned his attention to animal viruses in the late 1950s in an effort to describe the genetic steps in the evolution of a cancer cell. Reasoning that the enormous number of genetic and biochemical variables in a single cell would effectively exclude definitive analysis, Dulbecco proposed an experimental method in which a controlled number of specific viral genes are introduced into a cell. The effects on the cell of each gene can then be determined by a process of elimination.

Although the role of viruses in cancer formation is yet to be determined, Dulbecco's line of inquiry contributed significantly to the battle against that disease. His experimental methods and techniques have enabled researchers to investigate the effects of genetic alteration caused by chemical and physical agents.

Italian-born Renato Dulbecco received his medical training at the University of Turin, where he obtained degrees in physics and medicine. He arrived in the United States in 1947, taking a job as research associate in the laboratory of distinguished biologist Salvador Luria, a childhood friend. Also working in Luria's laboratory at the University of Indiana was another scientist destined for celebrity, biologist JAMES DEWEY WATSON. For several years Luria had been developing experimental techniques using bacterial viruses. It was based on this research that Dulbecco would later develop his own techniques using animal viruses.

Dulbecco left Indiana in 1949, spending the next two decades at the California Institute of Technology and the Salk Institute. At C.I.T. he supervised the doctoral thesis of fellow laureate Howard Temin, delivered in 1959; and at Salk another fellow laureate David Baltimore, worked in Dulbecco's laboratory from 1965 to 1968. The three conducted their Nobel Prize-winning studies independently, however.

Dulbecco left for London in 1972, joining the staff of the Imperial Cancer Research Laboratory. He returned to the United States five years later, where he taught at the Salk Institute and the University of California at San Diego until 1981.

Jean-Henri Dunant 1828–1910

Since the Middle Ages efforts have been made to create rules governing the treatment of war prisoners and the wounded, although fair play and humanitarian sentiment are usually early war casualties. In 1859 France and Italy joined forces against the Austrians in a bloody battle at Solferino, in Northern Italy. Jean Henri Dunant, a Swiss banker who passed through the area soon after the fighting had ceased, was horrified by what he saw. Wounded soldiers by the tens of thousands were strewn everywhere, suffering and unattended.

The Austrians had lost the battle, and their military surgeons had been captured, but Dunant managed to convince the French officers to free the doctors so that they might help in caring for the human devastation on all sides. The local Italians were shocked at Dunant's disregard for political affiliation and refused to help. Dunant, who was working feverishly himself to help the wounded, kept pleading with them, crying, *"Tutti fratelli, tutti fratelli!"* ("All brothers, all brothers!").

He wrote of his experience in *Un Souvenir de Solferino* (the English translation of which is entitled *The Origins of the Red Cross*). The book, which pleaded for the creation of an international organization to care for the casualties of war, appeared in 1862 and profoundly inspired the European community. A number of writers took up Dunant's cause, particularly Victor Hugo and Jules and Edmond Goncourt. Gustave Moynier and the Société genevoise d'Utilité publique helped the campaign for world humanitarianism.

Two international conferences were held, one in 1863 and another in the following year. The second conference was the famous one of 1864, in which sixteen countries signed the convention that established the International Red Cross and created a definitive set of rules for the treatment of all wounded soldiers. It declared all hospitals, whether military or civilian, as neutral territory, and all medical equipment and personnel as free from seizure. Dunant gave the Red Cross its insignia, a red cross on a white field (the reverse of his country's flag).

Dunant also contributed a major part of the funding needed to establish the Red Cross, so that by 1867 he was penniless. Little is known of his life in the fifteen years that followed. In 1882 he was discovered, impoverished and ailing, in a small nursing home in Switzerland. In 1901, along with Frédéric Passy, Dunant was given the Nobel Prize for Peace, the first one ever awarded. He donated all of his prize money to charity.

Guillaume Dupuytren 1777–1835

French surgeon Guillaume Dupuytren rose from poverty to immense wealth, international renown, and unrivaled professional eminence during the early part of the nineteenth century. Students and patients from all parts of the world flocked to the celebrated Hôtel Dieu in Paris, where Dupuytren reigned as chief of surgery for more than twenty years.

His career left a lasting impact on surgical and medical science, with contributions ranging from a classification system for burns to the introduction of corrective procedures and surgical devices of his own design, including a cutting forceps, an early form of stomach tube and a splint for treating lower leg fractures. Most widely known for his exhaustive clinical investigations, Dupuytren focused his research on the diagnosis and surgical management of various ruptures, fractures, congenital dislocations and pathologies.

A spellbinding lecturer, he commanded a vast knowledge of anatomy, pathology and clinical and surgical practices, which was highlighted by his dazzling ability for total recall of case histories, clinical studies and medical details of any kind.

Dupuytren's personal and professional manner was marked, however, by a quality of grim intensity that reflected his fierce and unrelenting ambition. He was revered for his outstanding contribution to medical science, and reviled with equal passion for his ruthless and unprincipled character.

In 1832 he published his description of a fracture of the lower end of the fibula attended by rupture of the lateral ligament and dislocation. Introducing the term "Dupuytren's fracture," he ignored the fact that the condition had been identified a hundred years earlier by English surgeon PERCIVAL POTT. Although Dupuytren's term is still part of the medical lexicon, the condition is more commonly referred to as "Pott's fracture."

A year later he used the same tactics, and with greater result, when he reported his findings on fibrosis of the palmar fascia, a deforming hand ailment that had been described previously by noted English physician SIR ASTLEY COOPER. A number of surgical procedures had already been developed by then to correct the condition, which, in fact, had been known for over a century. The ambitious surgeon staked his claim, however, and "Dupuytren's contracture" now may be his most recognizable credit.

Dupuytren was born in the tiny village of Pierre-Buffiere in west central France, where his family struggled to survive on meager means. By the time Guillaume reached adolescence the Dupuytrens recognized their son's extraordinary intellect and refused to allow such gifts to go to waste. Though his parents could provide no financial assistance for his education, they directed him to pursue a career in medicine, and at the age of sixteen Guillaume was sent him off to Paris.

While he stoically endured the next two years of hunger and desolation, Dupuytren plotted his triumphant future. He attended classes at the Charité, the Salpêtrière, the École de Santé, and the Collège de Magnac-Laval, and by the time he graduated, in 1797, he had already caught the attention of the medical community in Paris. Still in his early twenties, Dupuytren steadily continued to gain professional ground, particularly with his introduction of what proved to be a highly successful lecture series on anatomy and pathology.

In 1804 he secured a position at the Hôtel Dieu, presumably as assistant to Pelletan, the hospital's aging and easygoing chief of surgery. His unenviable role as Dupuytren's last remaining rival in Paris was soon apparent as he found himself thrust into a mortal conflict that raged for nearly ten years. In 1814 Pelletan was finally forced to surrender his post to Dupuytren, who ruled as the forbidding "Brigand of the Hôtel Dieu" until his death in 1835. During that time he was appointed chief surgeon to Louis XVIII, who awarded him a baronetcy in recognition of his dedicated service.

Of the thousands who came in contact with Dupuytren in the course of his life, a great number would undoubtedly share the opinion of French surgeon Pierre-François Percy (1754–1825), who rated his colleague "the first of surgeons and the least of men."

Christian René de Duve 1917–

Nobel laureate Christian de Duve is celebrated for his contribution to the study of cell biology. Applying the pioneering methods of ALBERT CLAUDE, de Duve used an electron microscope for his investigations. Among his most significant discoveries are lysosomes, which function, in the words of de Duve, as the "stomachs of the cell."

Working at the Rockefeller Institute for Medical Research (now Rockefeller University), de Duve and collaborator GEORGE PALADE refined Claude's techniques of electron microscopy, using a centrifuge to separate the components of a cell for individual analysis. De Duve would assess the function of a specialized part of a cell by examining the chemical compounds left in the test tube of the centrifuge. After artificially introducing a chemical to a particular organelle, he noted that the substance was not present in the test tube. Suspecting that the chemical had been consumed by a particular subcellular structure, de Duve discovered the lysosome, a tiny sac containing hydrolytic enzymes that, when liberated, assist in the digestion and removal of dead cells. Lysosomes are also involved in the selective destruction of tissues that occurs during various developmental processes, most conspicuously in metamorphosis.

Forced to leave their native Belgium during World War I, de Duve's parents fled to England, where young Christian was born in Thames Ditton, just outside London. As a young man de Duve returned to Belgium, where he completed doctoral programs in medicine and chemistry at the University of Louvain.

Accepting a position at the Nobel Institute in Stockholm, and later at the Carl Cori Institute in St. Louis, de Duve did not return to Louvain until 1962. It was then that he entered a unique professional arrangement, sharing his time equally between the Rockefeller Institute in New York and the University of Louvain. The results proved beneficial to both research centers, promoting cross-national communication among cell biologists.

Stating, "we are sick because our cells are sick," de Duve committed himself to an investigation of the role of defective organelles in various diseases.

In 1974 he shared the Nobel Prize for Physiology or Medicine with Albert Claude and George Palade. The following year de Duve was named president of the International Institute of Cellular and Molecular Pathology.

E

Sir John Carew Eccles 1903–

John Eccles's study of the mechanism of interneuron communication greatly advanced medical understanding of brain function, nervous disorders and kidney and heart disease. Among Eccles's important discoveries is the chemical, rather than electrical, nature of synaptic transmission. Eccles demonstrated that different chemical substances act to excite or inhibit nerve cell activity.

Born in Australia, John Eccles was a research colleague of biophysicist Bernard Katz at the University of Melbourne. He also studied at Oxford, where his mentor was the noted neurophysiologist CHARLES SHERRINGTON.

Eccles was director of the Kanematsu Research Institute in Sydney, Australia from 1937 until 1944, when he became professor of physiology at Otago University. He remained there until 1951, when he transferred to the faculty of the Australian National University at Canberra. While there he published two books: *The Physiology of Nerve Cells* in 1957 and *The Physiology of Synapses* in 1964.

In recognition of his important contributions to the field of neurophysiology, Eccles was made a knight of the British Empire in 1958. His work was internationally recognized in 1963 with the awarding of the Nobel Prize for Physiology or Medicine, shared with Alan Hodgkin and Andrew Huxley.

Eccles emigrated to the United States in 1966 to head the Institute for Biomedical Research in Evansville, Illinois. Two years later he was invited to join the Research Department of the State University of New York at Buffalo, where he has been professor emeritus since 1975. In 1973 Eccles published another book, *The Understanding of the Brain.*

Convinced after more than half a century of study that consciousness does not reside in the synapse, Eccles, a devout Roman Catholic, continues to view the mind and brain as distinct entities and argues for a gospel of dualism in his neuro-philosophical writings.

Constantin Alexander von Economo 1876–1931

In May, 1917 Austrian physician and neurologist Constantin Alexander von Economo published a report identifying epidemic encephalitis, or Encephalitis lethargica, which, since the last months of 1916, had been plaguing Europe. The mysterious epidemic presented itself in a wide range of different manifestations, suggesting possible schizophrenia, disseminated sclerosis, rabies or delirium. Based on an extensive postmortem investigations, von Economo established a pattern of irregular dissemination of the disease throughout the nervous system, with particular concentration in the gray matter of the mid-brain, or mesencephalon. He designated the pathological response as an inflammatory reaction without blood loss or destruction of tissue. To track down the etiological agent he transmitted the disease to experimental monkeys, thereby producing a series of analogous morbid conditions. These studies, published in the early part of 1918, revealed a submicroscopic virus as the cause of epidemic encephalitis, now commonly known as "von Economo's disease."

It is believed that lethargic encephalitis first appeared as much as two thousand years ago, resurfacing unpredictably since then in epidemics of varying proportions and with various characteristics. In all that time, however, the spread of the disease never reached the scale of a pandemic until the winter of 1916, when the world was subjected to a reign of terror that lasted almost a decade. Of the five million victims, more than a third lost their lives, but most of the survivors never truly recovered. Suspended in a zombielike trance, they reminded von Economo of "extinct volcanoes."

Struck by the bizarre condition of somnolence that marked these patients, von Economo launched a massive neurological investigation in order to identify the site of sleep regulation in the cerebral cortex. Based on more than thirteen years of research, his comprehensive atlas of the brain, entitled *The Cyto-Architectonics of the Adult Human Cortex,* was published in 1930.

Born to an independently wealthy Greek family, von Economo grew up in Trieste, which was at that time under Austrian rule. He was dedicated to a career in medicine at a relatively young age but retained a lifelong interest in mechanical engineering and technology, later gaining distinction as an avid balloonist and aviator. As one of the first in his country to hold a pilot's license, von Economo later served as president of the Royal Aero Club of Austria.

After obtaining a degree in medicine from the University of Vienna von Economo continued his training in neurology at the universities of Paris, Strasbourg, Berlin and Munich, where he was a student of distinguished German psychiatrist Emil Kraepelin. Returning to Vienna, he served as assistant to Austrian neurophysiologist JULIUS WAGNER-JUAREGG at the Psychiatric-Neurologic Clinic, where he later became professor of neurology and psychiatry. Von Economo remained on the faculty at the University of Vienna until his sudden death from coronary embolism at the age of fifty-five.

Gerald Maurice Edelman 1929–

An antibody is one of a group of proteins produced in the lymph tissue in response to the invasion of the body by an antigen, or foreign substance.

Once the structure of an antibody had been determined in the 1960s Gerald Edelman produced the first accurate model of the complex, Y-shaped structure of the biochemical unit within a molecule of serum protein.

Edelman received his doctoral degree in biochemistry from Rockefeller University in 1960. Invited to join the faculty, he remained to pursue research on antibodies. His fragmentation and subsequent structural analysis of the gamma globulin molecule was a ground-breaking achievement. In 1972 Edelman shared the Nobel Prize for Physiology or Medicine with RODNEY PORTER for their contributions to the field of immunology.

In the years that followed, Edelman shifted his attention to the study of neuroscience, eventually heading a research program affiliated with Rockefeller University. Basing his work on investigations of the development of brain activity, Edelman theorized that a selective proccess occurs among neurons comparable to the selection mechanism that occurs when species compete in nature. In an interview Edelman stated, "The brain, in its workings, is a selective system, more like evolution than computation...We are part of that complex web of natural selection which has itself evolved a selective machinery called our brain. In each of us there lies...a second evolutionary path during a lifetime: it unites culture with a marvelous tissue in which the hope of survival lies." Edelman optimistically asserts that rather than genetic predestination, chance, adaptation and an accumulation of mental activity determine the development of one's mind.

Antônio Caetano de Abreau de Egas Moniz 1874–1955

In 1935 Portuguese psychiatrist Antônio Egas Moniz performed the first prefrontal lobotomy, a surgical technique designed to relieve symptoms in several forms of mental illness. Also referred to as prefrontal leucotomy, the procedure involved drilling holes through the skull, then severing the nerve fibers connecting the prefrontal cortex from the rest of the brain. Between 1936 and 1955 many thousands of lobotomies were performed on mental patients, particularly in America, where the technique was widely hailed by the psychiatric establishment.

On September 14, 1936 Walter Freeman performed the first lobotomy in the United States, launching what he called Operation Icepick, a crusade against "rebelliousness" that would later become the subject of much political and ethical controversy. The operation, frequently performed by nonsurgical practitioners, was often used to control hostile or hyperemotional patients. Although these "unacceptable" behavioral patterns would often subside after surgery, the patient would in many cases degenerate into a dull, zombielike state. In other cases, "difficult" symptoms would only aggravated by the surgery.

Egas Moniz taught neurology for over thirty years at the University of Lisbon, producing a voluminous amount of written work on various medical topics. In addition, he managed to maintain a political career, actively participating in the Portuguese legislative system from 1903. In 1917 he served as foreign minister in Madrid, and from 1918 to 1919 he was Portugal's secretary of foreign affairs. In that capacity he led the Portuguese delegation to the Paris Peace Conference.

In recognition of his work on the diagnosis of mental disease, and for his development of the prefrontal lobotomy, Moniz was awarded the Nobel Prize for Physiology or Medicine in 1949, which he shared with W.R. HESS. Announcing the award, the New York Times reported: "Surgeons now think no more of operating on the brain than they do of removing an appendix. [Moniz and his colleagues] taught us to look with less awe on the brain. It is just a big organ with very difficult and complicated functions to perform and no more sacred than the liver."

Paul Ehrlich 1854–1915

Distinguished as the father of chemotherapy, German medical researcher Paul Ehrlich is celebrated as a pioneer in the development of modern immunology, embryology, hematology and cytochemistry, but his legendary renown is as the creator of "Dr. Ehrlich's magic bullet"—the first effective treatment against syphilis. When he introduced the arsenic compound, called salvarsan, in 1910, Ehrlich caused an international furor that would surround him for years to come. There were many who still clung to the ancient notion of syphilis as providential punishment for lechery and who were outraged at Ehrlich for protecting "sinners" from their sexually transmitted due. The drama of the controversy established Ehrlich's place in modern folklore, but his monumental contribution to medical science extends far beyond the invention of salversan.

Ehrlich was born into a prominent Jewish family in Prussian Silesia (now in Poland). At the age of ten he was sent to a boarding school in Breslau and later attended the university there as an undergraduate. He studied medicine at the University of Strasbourg and returned to Breslau to complete his training in 1878.

Ehrlich's distinguished academic record earned him an appointment as senior house physician at the prestigious Charite Hospital in Berlin, where his main responsibility was to keep detailed records on the blood cells of patients, providing exhaustive analyses of their morphology, physiology and pathology. During his first year on the job he discovered a new type of blood cell, which he named eosinophil.

In 1882 Ehrlich attended a lecture given by ROBERT KOCH at the Physiological Society of Berlin during which the celebrated bacteriologist announced his discovery of the tubercle bacillus. Koch described its rodlike shape but had yet to find a way to demonstrate the variable presence of the microorganism in tuberculosis patients and was searching for a stain that would render them clearly visible.

Since his days as a student Ehrlich had been investigating the specificity of aniline dyes for distinctive intracellular structures. He had already observed that certain parasitic organisms would stain more readily than human cells and had identified a number of bacteria and protozoa in this manner. Following Koch's lecture Ehrlich focused his efforts on finding an effective stain for the tubercle bacillus and soon developed a procedure using aniline oil that rendered the rods clearly identifiable. His technique made it possible to test routinely for suspected tuberculosis, imparting an immediate clinical value to Koch's discovery. His invention also launched a long and productive collaboration between the two men, and over the next few years Ehrlich would spend much of his spare time with Koch in the tuberculosis wards at Moabit Hospital.

In 1888 Ehrlich contracted tuberculosis himself. He left Germany with his wife and two daughters and spent the next year in Egypt, where he gradually recovered from the disease. Returning to Berlin, he resumed his research in a small laboratory set up in the back of his living quarters. Koch, who had become director of the Institute for Infectious Diseases, offered Ehrlich his own laboratory and later put him in charge of the Institute's newly established antitoxin control center. Ehrlich's research assistant at the center was bacteriologist AUGUST PAUL VON WASSERMANN who would later gain distinction for inventing the first reliable diagnostic test for syphilis.

In the decades that followed, Ehrlich conducted outstanding research studies on bacteriology, endocrinology, hematology and the causes of cancer. By investigating the quantitative aspect of qualitative chemical changes he developed fundamental techniques of scientific measurement and standardization. He discovered the nature of antigen and antibody formation and laid the foundation for the study of isoimmunization—the production of antibodies against an antigen derived from an individual of the same species.

By the turn of the century Ehrlich had achieved international prominence as one of the leading pioneers of medical science. In 1908 he was honored with the Nobel Prize for Physiology or Medicine, which he shared with Russian biologist ELIE METCHNIKOFF.

Cited for his outstanding contribution to the advancement of immunology, Ehrlich played down these achievements in his acceptance speech to discuss instead the direction of his current research in chemotherapy. He defined the science in Latin as *therapia sterilisans magna*, meaning "the complete sterilization of a highly infected host at one blow."

The underlying principle of chemotherapy was Ehrlich's revolutionary concept of a chemical "magic bullet." His work with aniline dyes had shown that certain chemical agents have highly specific biochemical affinities, so that they react only with particular cells or particular components within those cells. He then established that the biological action of such chemicals is determined by their molecular structure and could therefore be manipulated to produce chemotherapeutic tools—"magic bullets." If the dyes achieved their staining effect by somehow binding to the molecules of particular cells, he reasoned, the same biochemical mechanism might be used to achieve a more damaging effect. Taken internally, these chemical agents could be directed to destroy specific microbial targets without endangering normal cells. In establishing the basis for the development of chemotherapy Ehrlich also formulated a fundamental principle of modern pharmacology.

The prime focus of his chemotherapeutic investigations was the search for a "magic bullet" against the spirochete that causes syphilis. In 1909 Japanese bacteriologist Sahachiro Hata came to the institute to work with Ehrlich, who by then had developed and tested some 3,000 compounds. Over the course of the next year Hata and Ehrlich determined that number 606, a compound of arsenic, was both the safest and the most potent.

The sensational announcement was made at the 1910 meeting of the Congress for Internal Medicine in Wiesbaden, Germany. Cries of moral outrage were accompanied by pleas for massive quantities from all parts of Europe. Ehrlich later produced a more effective compound, called Neosalvarsan, which was used until the advent of penicillin in the 1940s.

Christiaan Eijkman 1858–1930

Christiaan Eijkman, a Dutch physician and pathologist, was awarded the 1929 Nobel Prize in Physiology or Medicine (with FREDERICK GOWLAND HOPKINS) in recognition of his important work in the field of nutrition.

Eijkman was sent to the Dutch East Indies as part of a special commission to study the cause of beri-beri, a common disease in Asia which was generally characterized by neurological and gastrointestinal disturbances, appetite and weight loss, fluid retention and heart failure. After serving several years as director of the Pathological Institute of Batavia (Djakarta) in Indonesia he became an army medical officer in 1886 to continue his research at a laboratory connected with the military hospital in Batavia until 1897. In nutritional experiments using chickens Eijkman studied the causes of beri-beri. Observing that the afflicted chickens were fed only kernels of polished rice, Eijkman found that the disease disappeared when the discarded rice hulls were added to their diet.

Among the first to propose the theory of "essential food factors" (see HOPKINS), Eijkman laid the foundation for the discovery of vitamin B, and for the eventual recognition of diseases caused by nutritional deficiencies (see MINOT and WHIPPLE).

Willem Einthoven 1860–1927

Willem Einthoven devised a method to measure and record the electrical current generated by the human heart, producing the universally used electrocardiogram, or EKG. Measuring the electrical activity produced by contractions of the heart had already been suggested by A.D. Waller in 1887, but it was Einthoven who developed a precise and reliable method. Adapting the mechanism of the galvanometer, an existing device designed to measure current electromagnetically, Einthoven's "string galvanometer" was sensitive enough to detect the heart's minute electrical current. Vertically suspended between the two poles of a magnet, a fine thread of platinum or silvered quartz is deflected in response to electrical current.

The son of a Dutch physician, Willem Einthoven was born in Java, which at that time was part of the Netherlands East Indies. After obtaining a degree in medicine from the University of Utrecht in 1885 Einthoven joined the faculty at the University of Leyden, where he remained as professor of physiology until his death in 1927.

The "string galvanometer," also known as "Einthoven's galvanometer," was introduced in 1903. In the eighteen years that followed, Einthoven perfected and expanded his invention so that the delicate movements of the "string" could be recorded on paper. Electrocardiography ushered in a new era of clinical cardiology.

Studying the graphs produced by patients with various heart conditions, Einthoven identified various forms of heart disease by their EKG patterns. For his contribution to clinical and diagnostic cardiology Einthoven was awarded the Nobel Prize for Physiology or Medicine in 1924.

Gertrude Belle Elion 1918–

A research biochemist for more than forty years, Gertrude Belle Elion dedicated most of her career to the comparative study of normal cells, cancer cells, bacteria and viruses. With long-time collaborator GEORGE H. HITCHINGS she investigated the formation and chemical composition of nucleic acids, focusing specifically on purine and pyrimidine.

In early studies conducted at the Wellcome Research Laboratories in Tuckahoe, New York, Elion and Hitchings discovered that a combination of purines was essential for bacteria growth. Seeking a treatment for leukemia, they investigated biochemical methods of inhibiting the rapid increase in white blood cells by impeding the formation of nucleic acids in those cells.

In cooperation with the research staff at New York's Sloan-Kettering Institute (now Memorial Sloan-Kettering Cancer Center), Elion and Hitchings produced an initial series of substances that effectively blocked the formation of nucleic acids but proved too toxic for humans. By the 1950s, however, Elion and Hitchings introduced thioguanine and 6-mercaptopurine, the first effective antileukemia chemotherapy.

In the decades that followed they pursued this approach in the development of drugs for the treatment of other forms of cancer, autoimmune diseases, malaria, rheumatoid arthritis, gout, herpes and a variety of urinary and respiratory tract infections. In 1988 Elion, Hitchings and English pharmacologist JAMES BLACK were awarded the Nobel Prize for Physiology or Medicine in recognition of their work establishing "important principles for drug treatment." Rather than honoring the discovery of any particular drug, the Nobel committee cited the creativity with which the three laureates had approached pharmacological research, stating, "while drug development had earlier mainly been built on chemical modification of natural products, they introduced a more rational approach based on the understanding of basic biochemical and physiological processes."

Born and raised in New York City, Gertrude Elion was encouraged by her parents to pursue a career despite the considerable obstacles encountered at the time by professional women. When she was fifteen Gertrude's grandfather died after a long and painful bout with cancer. Deeply affected by the suffering he endured, she decided to devote her life to medical research.

In 1937, after obtaining a master's degree in biochemistry from Hunter College, Elion began the frustrating search for a job in research. The chemistry laboratory was then a male-dominated province, and although she never lost sight of her goals, Elion turned to teaching high school chemistry as a means of earning a living.

"It was really the war that gave women opportunities to get into the lab," Elion remembers. As thousands of men left the country during World War II the United States was forced to adjust its attitudes toward working women. In 1944 Elion joined the research staff at Burroughs Wellcome as Hitchings's laboratory assistant. Still lacking a doctorate, Elion enrolled in the Ph.D. program at Brooklyn Polytechnic Institute, where she had to take the train from Tuckahoe each night after work.

The hour-and-a-half commute and the demanding academic schedule eventually forced her to choose between a doctorate and her work with Hitchings. She never regretted her decision to stay at Burroughs Wellcome, where her talent and intelligence earned Elion the unreserved acceptance and respect of her colleagues. Recognizing her abilities as a researcher, Hitchings soon invited her to work as his partner, launching a productive and lasting collaboration.

By developing a chemotherapy that blocks nucleic acid formation in pathogenic cells without damaging normal, healthy cells, Elion and Hitchings established a pivotal principle of pharmacology. This approach has made possible a number of important advances in drug research throughout the world, most notably in the development of azidothymidine, or AZT, the first treatment for Aids to gain federal approval. Elion and Hitchings were also directly involved in the discovery of Trimethoprim, a compound used to combat *Pneumocystis carinii* pneumonia, the most common killer of AIDS victims.

Henry Havelock Ellis 1859–1939

British psychologist Havelock Ellis was an early advocate of birth control, sex education and women's suffrage. A powerful and prolific writer, Ellis was an influential figure in the evolution of public attitudes toward human sexuality. With RICHARD KRAFFT-EBING and SIGMUND FREUD, Ellis helped establish the study of human sexuality as a psychological discipline, with classifications and analyses of pathological syndromes and disorders.

The son of an English sea captain, Ellis traveled extensively through South America and Australia before returning to England to study medicine at St. Thomas's Hospital in London. He practiced medicine briefly, then turned to scientific writing and research.

The first volume of Ellis's major work, *Studies in the Psychology of Sex,* appeared in 1897. This landmark survey of human sexuality caused an uproar in England, where Ellis was charged with obscenity. The book, called "filth" by the judge who banned it from Britain, was subsequently published in the United States, although it was legally available only to doctors. Ellis wrote six more volumes, the final one appearing in America in 1928. Among its contributions to the scientific understanding of sexuality, Ellis's book described male-female differences on three levels: primary, referring to sexual organs; secondary, referring to characteristics associated with reproductive function (e.g., breasts and body hair); and tertiary, referring to sexual differences not apparently related to the reproductive process (e.g., precocity, behavioral tendencies, etc.)

Ellis's work was the first strictly analytical treatment of the subject without moral or religious judgment. He openly discussed his own sexuality, including accounts of his marraige to Edith Lees and his other sexual relationships. These included a liaison with Olive Schreiner, a controversial South African writer and feminist.

In 1940 Ellis published *My Life,* a memoir dealing largely with the history of his marraige. Other written works include *A Study of British Genius* (1904), *The Dance of Life* (1923) and *Man and Woman* (1934).

Empedocles 492–c. 432 B.C.

An influential philosopher, physician, poet and political leader, Empedocles was a major figure in the life and thought of Ancient Greece. As a scientist he is best remembered for his theory that all matter is composed of four independent and indestructible elements—earth, air, fire and water.

Although it is unlikely that Empedocles originated the concept, he was the first to formally state the theory in his teachings within a philosophical and scientific framework. Recognizing that even the atmosphere is substance rather than void, Empedocles defined all motion and change as the interaction and interpenetration of elemental particles. He taught that this constant activity was brought about by the presence in all matter, animate or inanimate, of two operational and opposing forces, referred to as harmony and discord, love and hate, affinity and antipathy.

Empedocles saw life as the conjoinment of these four basic elements and death as the inevitable return of all matter to its elemental state. In his cosmology universal life is described as a never-ending approach to perfection from imperfection, continually reducing and reconstructing with the basic elements of matter.

As a physician Empedocles preached the doctrine of PYTHAGORAS, emphasizing the therapeutic value of exercise, a healthy diet and the maintenance of the purity of mind and body. Convinced of the theory of transmigration of souls, he taught that to eat an animal was an act of cannibalism, since any creature might be the reincarnation of a human soul.

Empedocles's theory of the four basic elements foreshadows fundamental principles in physics and chemistry. In his "Theory of Cause" ARISTOTLE expanded Empedocles's doctrine to include aether, a fifth element found only in heavenly bodies.

Empedocles was born in Acragas (now known as Agrigento) in Sicily, an important center for philosophical and scientific thought during the last six centuries before Christ. Although his arrogant and aristocratic air is often described in later commentaries, Empedocles distinguished himself as a democratic leader who rejected the crown of sovereignty when it was offered to him. When the political climate in Sicily shifted from democracy, he and his disciples were forced into exile.

Legend has it that, attempting a godlike disappearance, he died by leaping into the caldron of Mt. Etna to demonstrate his divinity by vanishing without a trace. Unfortunately, it is said, the volcano tossed up his brass slippers, thus ruining the desired effect.

John Franklin Enders 1897–1985

Pioneer virologist John Franklin Enders played a key role in the development of vaccines against poliomyelitis and measles and helped to usher in a new era in viral tissue methodology in 1948 when he demonstrated the growth of a virus culture in nonneural human tissue. Before that time experimental cultivation of viruses had succeeded only in a medium of nerve tissue—a commodity too scarce to assure the supply required even for experimental research, much less the unlimited quantities needed for mass production of a vaccine.

Born in West Hartford, Connecticut, Enders grew up in the privileged environment of an affluent and socially distinguished New England family. His grandfather served as president of the Aetna Life Insurance Company and his father as president and later chairman of the board of Hartford National Bank. With the luxury of lifelong financial independence as his birthright John was freed from the pressures of earning a livelihood but faced instead the uncertainty and confusion of an undefined future.

As an adolescent educated at aristocratic prep schools he cultivated an interest in literature and the arts rather than in science, and at 18 he enrolled at Yale University with only a vague notion of what he might do with his life. Two years later, when the United States entered World War I, he enlisted in the naval reserve as a flying instructor, returning to Yale after his discharge to obtain his bachelor of arts degree in 1920.

For lack of a better idea, he made a halfhearted and ill-fated attempt to enter the real estate business, but it was not long before he rejoined the academic world, this time at Harvard University, where he immersed himself in English literature and Celtic and Teutonic languages.

At the end of four years, after receiving his masters degree and completing his doctoral thesis, Enders began to feel unsatisfied with the professional choice he had made. Living in a boarding house in Brookline, he floundered disconsolately for several months until he became friends with a fellow boarder named Hugh Ward, an Australian medical student who would help Enders to discover his own passion for science. Ward did not awaken that interest directly but introduced Enders to the man who inspired the shape and focus of his life, distinguished bacteriologist HANS ZINSSER. A brilliant and spellbinding lecturer at the Harvard Medical School, Zinsser had inspired many of his students, like Enders, to change the course of their lives.

Enders joined the ranks of devoted disciples almost immediately and permanently, studying under Zinsser during what would be the last 15 years of his mentor's life. By the time Zinsser died in 1940 Enders had married, completed his doctorate in bacteriology and immunology, and been made an assistant professor on the Harvard faculty. In addition to teaching classes at the medical school and the School of Public Health, he was also deeply involved by then in experimental research on the cultivation of viruses.

In 1946 Enders was invited to establish a new infectious disease research laboratory at Boston's Children's Hospital, and by the following year he had joined with fellow virologists THOMAS WELLER and FREDERICK ROBBINS in what proved to be historic collaboration. In early March, 1948 the team succeeded in producing a culture of the mumps virus in a flask containing a mixture of ox blood, chick embryo membrane and other nutrients. They then proceeded along similar lines to attempt to grow the chicken pox virus in a medium of human embryonic muscle and skin tissue.

Toward the end of the month there happened to be a quantity of poliovirus in the laboratory refrigerator, and on March 30 Enders and his colleagues decided on an impulse to include it in the experiment. They poured washings taken from a chicken pox patient into four flasks containing embryonic nonneural tissue and into the remaining four flasks introduced samples of the poliovirus. The chicken pox virus failed to grow, but as a result of the fortuitous last-minute circumstances the team discovered a practical and effective method of obtaining unlimited amounts of the poliovirus.

Almost immediately the achievement was recognized as a major breakthrough in the advancement of modern virology. Celebrated as international celebrities, Enders, Weller and Robbins accumulated an array of awards, medals and honorary degrees that culminated with the award of the Nobel Prize for Physiology or Medicine, which the trio shared in 1954.

Ranked among the leading scientific investigators of his time, Enders approached his work in an earnest and

unassuming manner that earned him the respect and admiration of his peers. "The man has a green thumb for growing viruses," marveled epidemiologist John Gordon, a friend and Harvard colleague. Distinguished microbiologist RENÉ DUBOS
noted, "He had a genius for stating his ideas simply, a genius for not being fooled by empty words—like the word *genius*."

In the early 1950s, when his collaboration with Weller and Robbins had come to an end, Enders moved on to another successful partnership, working with Samuel Katz on the development of a measles vaccine over the course of the next decade. Using Enders's method of tissue culture, they produced an attenuated live-virus vaccine in 1962 that has nearly succeeded in eradicating the disease.

Erasistratus c. 300–250 B.C.

As one of the founders of the Alexandrian school of medicine Erasistratus was among the first to launch a systematic study of anatomy and physiology based largely on experimentation and dissection. Although little remains of his own writings, GALEN'S commentaries suggest that Erasistratus provided accurate descriptions of the structure of the brain, heart and vascular system.

He distinguished between sensory and motor nerves, tracking them both through the nervous system to the brain. He also identified and described the trachea and the epiglottis, explaining the function of the latter during the process of swallowing. Erasistratus is credited with inventing the first catheter as well as the first calorimeter, a device for measuring the amount of heat generated by an individual. He also associated ascites—an abnormal accumulation of protein-rich fluid in the abdomen—with a "hard liver," by which he probably meant hepatic cirrhosis.

Although often linked with HEROPHILUS, Erasistratus differed from his contemporary on their view of the basis of pathology. Rejecting the notion of "humours," Erasistratus developed an inverted theory of circulation (from veins to arteries), proposing that air, transported from the lungs to the heart, transforms itself into a "vital spirit" as it surges through the arterial network. Stressing the notion of *plethora*, or an excess of blood, as the root of all disease, he recommended various forms of therapy depending on the symptoms exhibited.

Opposing the use of purgatives and bloodletting, Erasistratus often recommended fasting, abstinence and exercise. He dismissed the abstract, metaphysical rationale behind many of the frequently prescribed compounds of animal, mineral and botanic substances, advocating instead simple medicines and restricted diets.

Born in Chios, Erasistratus established his practice in Alexandria, where he was to develop an impressive following that continued several centuries after his death in Samos.

Joseph Erlanger 1874–1965

Joseph Erlanger, a pioneer in the field of neurophysiology, was born in San Francisco and went east to study medicine at Johns Hopkins University, obtaining his medical degree in 1899. He taught at the University of Wisconsin until 1910, at which time he accepted a professorship at Washington University in St. Louis. HERBERT GASSER, one of Erlanger's former students, joined the university in 1916, and the two began their collaborative study of the electrophysiology of nerve activity.

Erlanger and Gasser recognized the separate functions of different nerve fibers and developed the cathode-ray oscillograph in order to analyze the transmission of nerve impulses. They were able to demonstrate that the speed of transmission of a nerve impulse varies with the thickness of the nerve fiber that carries it. Erlanger and Gasser's oscilloscope opened up new vistas of research and launched the study of neurophysiology.

In 1937 Erlanger and Gasser published *Electrical Signs of Nervous Activity*, describing their electrophysiological findings. In 1944 they shared the Nobel Prize for Physiology and Medicine for their notable contributions. Erlanger remained at Washington University Medical School for more than four decades and was made professor emeritus of physiology in 1946.

Ulf Svante von Euler 1905–1983

Ulf von Euler was the first person to identify norepinephrine, the hormonal substance essential to the transmission of neural impulses in the sympathetic nervous system. Although norepinephrine had been suggested earlier as a factor in neurotransmission, von Euler conclusively demonstrated its function as a postganglionic sympathetic neurotransmitter.

Born in Sweden, Ulf von Euler was the son of Nobel Prize-winning biochemist, Hans von Euler-Chelpin. After receiving a degree in medicine from the Karolinska Institute in 1930 he stayed on as a member of the Institute's faculty for the next 41 years, pursuing research in several areas of physiology and biochemistry.

Through research begun in 1935 von Euler discovered prostaglandins, a group of substances that are synthesized from fatty acids. These compounds are produced in almost every type of body tissue, but only as needed, for the regulation of blood pressure, pulse, smooth muscle activity, glandular secretion, nerve transmission and a number of other critical biological functions.

Von Euler's definitive identification of norepinephrine, also known as noradrenalin, emerged from experimental research conducted between 1946 and 1948. In acknowledgement of this breakthrough discovery von Euler was awarded the Nobel Prize for Physiology or Medicine in 1970, which he shared with JULIUS AXELROD and Bernard Katz.

Von Euler was president of the Nobel Foundation from 1965 to 1975. His works include *Noradrenaline*, published in 1956, and *Prostaglandins*, written with Rune Eliasson in 1967.

Bartolomeo Eustachi c.1510–1574

Celebrated for his detailed observations of human anatomy, Italian physician Bartolomeo Eustachi produced an impressive series of anatomical writings that included a collection of remarkably modern and accurate illustrations.

Basing his work on experimental dissections performed on fetuses, infants, children and adults, Eustachi described the auditory system, the venous system, the uterus, the adrenal glands, the thoracic duct and the structure and development of the teeth. His treatise, entitled *De renum structura* (*On the Structure of the Kidneys*), presented the first discussion of the structure and function of the kidney, describing for the first time the suprarenal gland, more commonly known as the adrenal. This work, along with *De auditus organis* (*On the Auditory Organ*), *De vena quae azygos graecis dicitur* (*On the Vein that the Greeks Call the Azygos*), and *De dentibus* (*On the Teeth*), was published in 1564 in a collection entitled *Opuscula anatomica* (*Anatomical Treatise*).

It was in this landmark work that Eustachi described the auditory tube that connects the nasopharynx and the middle ear. This structure, now known as the Eustachian tube, permits communication between the inner ear and the external atmosphere so that equal pressure is maintained on either side of the eardrum. The passage can be opened up by swallowing in order to equalize a difference between internal and external pressure. When the tube becomes blocked due to swelling of its mucous membrane lining, the air in the middle ear is absorbed and replaced by fluids that prevent the eardrum from vibrating in response to sound waves.

Eustachi described a number of other auditory structures, including the tensor tympani, the muscle that tenses the eardrum. He also identified the stapedius muscles, although one of these, the stapes, had been previously mentioned by GIOVANNI FILIPPO INGRASSIA and GABRIELE FALLOPPIO, among others.

Born in Ancona, on the eastern coast of Italy, Bartolomeo was the son of Mariano Eustachi, a celebrated local physician. Mariano insisted upon a well-rounded humanistic education for his son, who studied Greek, Hebrew and Arabic in addition to following a course of medical study at the Archiginnasio della Sapienza (Philosophical Institute) in Rome. When he returned to Ancona in 1540 to establish a medical practice his talents were soon noticed by the Duke of Urbino, who requested Eustachi as his personal physician. In 1547 Eustachi accepted the invitation to serve as physician to Cardinal Giulio della Rovere, the duke's brother. Following the cardinal to Rome, Eustachi joined the faculty at the Sapienza as professor of anatomy. His academic position granted him access to cadavers for dissection, making possible his extensive anatomical investigations.

In 1552, with the help of artist Pier Matteo Pini, Eustachi embarked on the creation of a series of anatomical illustrations for a medical treatise. The written work was never published, but 47 copper-plate engravings were produced, eight of which were used in *Opuscula anatomica*. Assumed to be lost for more than 150 years,the remaining 39 plates, along with the eight that had been published, reappeared in the possession of a descendant of Pier Matteo Pini at the turn of the eighteenth century. The entire collection was published in Rome in 1714 in a volume entitled *Tabulae anatomicae Bartholomaei Eustachi quas a tenebris tandem vindicatas* (*Anatomical Illustrations of Bartolomeo Eustachi Rescued from Obscurity*).

The series of plates contains depictions of muscles, bones, the abdominal structure, the thorax and the vascular system. Particularly notable is *Tabula XVIII*, displaying the base of the brain and the sympathetic nervous system. Clarified with numbered references and juxtaposing views of the body from opposite angles, the illustrations present a remarkably detailed depiction of many anatomical structures as well as a broad anatomical perspective.

Although he continued to serve as physician to Cardinal della Rovere, Eustachi was forced to relinquish his post at the Sapienza due to the debilitating effects of severe gout. He died in the summer of 1574 on his way to join the cardinal at Fossombrone, several miles from the village of his birth.

Herbert McLean Evans 1882–1971

Distinguished for pioneer investigations in endocrinology, embryology, physiology and metabolism, Herbert Evans is most widely known as the discoverer of vitamin E.

Born in California, Evans graduated from Johns Hopkins Medical School in 1908. In 1915 he was appointed professor of anatomy at the University of California at Berkeley, and it was there that he conducted a monumental and wide-ranging body of research dealing with chromosomes, pituitary and sex-gland hormones, reproduction and nutrition.

In 1921 Evans launched a series of experimental studies on nutrition that revealed the existence of a dietary element associated with fertility. Evans and his colleagues found that when they fed rats a diet of vitamins A, B, and D all the animals remained healthy, but some could no longer breed. Dubbing the missing nutritional factor vitamin E, Evans discovered that when it was introduced into the diet the rats resumed normal reproductive function.

In 1930 Evans took over as head of the Institute of Experimental Biology at Berkeley, where he later collaborated with noted biochemist Gladys Emerson in the completion of his investigation of vitamin E. Discovering an abundance of the substance in green leaves and cereals, Evans and Emerson successfully isolated the vitamin and produced it in pure crystalline form in 1935.

Although vitamin E has been identified as an essential factor for normal reproduction in rats, its nutritional function in humans and other animals has not yet been firmly established. In subsequent experimental studies Emerson found that when rabbits are fed a diet low in vitamin E they exhibit signs of muscle weakness and deterioration similar to the symptoms of muscular dystrophy.

Tocopherol, the chemical name for the substance, is derived from the Greek words *tokos*, meaning "childbirth," and *pherein*, meaning "to bear." Evans and Emerson later distinguished two types of tocopherol called alpha and beta, noting that the alpha form, found in cottonseed and corn oil, is by far the more biologically active of the two. Evans is also noted for his contribution, with Joseph A. Long, to the discovery of the pituitary growth hormone.

F

Gabriele Fallopio (Gabriel Fallopius) 1523–1562

Gabriele Fallopio is best known for his discovery of the tubes joining the uterus to the ovaries, now known as the Fallopian tubes. His contribution to medicine, however, extends beyond his namesakes to a number of other important anatomical discoveries.

A prize student of ANDREAS VESALIUS at the University of Padua, Fallopio succeeded his mentor as professor of anatomy when Vesalius left to join the court of the Emperor Charles V in 1551. Next in this noble medical lineage was Fallopio's student Fabricius ab Acquapendente, who in turn passed on the mantle of medical scholarship to his brilliant student, WILLIAM HARVEY.

In addition to his formal education at Padua, Fallopio, like many physicians of the Middle Ages, journeyed throughout Europe in search of medical knowledge. From his travels he learned, among other things, the origins of syphilis. He wrote, "For...Columbus, Ferdinand and Isabella ordered a Frigate to be fitted out, and three Pinnaces...with which he arrived at the West Indies...There was found there, 'tis true, most precious gold and great plenty of it was brought from thence, together with abundance of pearls; but there was also a thorn joined to the rose, and aloes mixed with the honey. For Columbus brought back his vessels laden with the French Disease. There the disease is mild, like Itch amongst us, but transplanted hither it is become so fierce, as to infect and corrupt the head, eyes, nose, palate, skin, flesh, bones, ligaments, and at last the whole bowels." Known as the "French Disease" (except in France, where it was known as the "Italian disease"), syphilis is considered by some to have been originally imported into Europe from the West Indies, although some evidence has been advanced to suggest that it existed in Europe before 1492.

Drawing from the teachings of HIPPOCRATES, ARISTOTLE and GALEN, Fallopio studied the nature of growths and swellings. He refers in his writings to "similar and dissimilar parts" of the human body, distinguishing for the first time between benign and malignant tumors. His other clinical studies included the cranial nerves and the bones and organs of the reproductive system. It is likely that Fallopio is responsible for having named the vagina and the placenta, meaning "sheath" and "cake," respectively, although these terms have also been attributed to Aristotle.

Fallopio's collected writings were published in Venice in 1584, twenty-two years after his death.

Jean Fernel 1497–1558

Although many of the important medical advances of the Renaissance originated from the scientific centers of Northern Italy, French physician Jean Fernel is noted for his significant influence, particularly in the areas of physiology, pathology and hygiene. All three terms, of Greek etymological origin, were in fact introduced by Fernel to replace the Latin terms that distinguished medical studies of "natural," "contra-natural," and "non-natural" (or human initiated) phenomena.

Born in Montdidier in northern France, Fernel studied philosophy, astronomy and mathematics at the Collegè de Ste. Barbe in Paris. After receiving a degree in 1519 he lectured independently in Paris, and in addition produced two treatises on astronomy entitled *Monalosphaerium* and *Cosmotheoria*. These and all subsequent published texts were written under the pseudonym Ambianus, presumably referring to the diocese of Amiens, not far from his place of birth.

Becoming increasingly interested in the biological and medical sciences, Fernel gradually sold his collection of astronomy instruments, including an astrolabe of his own design, to pay for formal medical training. He obtained the qualification of *venia practicandi* (health practitioner) in 1530, and within a short time Fernel established a distinguished reputation as one of the leading physicians and medical lecturers in France. His popularity at the court was ensured when he saved the life of Diane de Poitiers, the mistress of the Dauphin.

Appointed physician to the royal family, Fernel was asked to make his permanent residence at the palace at Fontainebleau, but he convinced the crown prince to allow him to live and work in Paris, where he had attained the position of professor of medicine. For much of his life Fernel would find himself torn between his responsibility to the advancement of medicine and his duties as court physician, particularly after the Dauphin became King Henry II.

By 1548 Fernel had completed *De naturali parte medicinae (On the Natural Aspects of Medicine)*, which included the first use of the term *Physiologiae*. Originating from the Greek *phusikos*, meaning "natural" or "physical," the term was defined as the scientific study of the functions of the body, although it was not until WILLIAM HARVEY'S discovery of the circulatory system of the blood that the discipline attained the status of an experimental science. Fernel's discussion of physiology, later elaborated in his monumental reference text entitled *Medicina,* was mainly a presentation of the prevailing theories of humoral medicine, with little mention of such concerns of modern physiology as circulation, respiration and digestion.

Published in 1554, *Medicina* also contained a discussion of therapeutics and a section of several chapters under the heading *Pathologiae,* defined as the study of abnormal functions of the body. In addition to a comprehensive study of Renaissance understanding of diseases and pathological processes, the book included a number of significant observations, including descriptions of appendicitis and endocarditis. Launching a debate that would continue for centuries, Fernel also suggested that although syphilis and gonorrhea were both transmitted through sexual contact, the two might be distinct pathological entities.

As a leading scientist and medical reformer of the Renaissance, Fernel played an important role in the establishment of a practical and clinical basis for medicine, campaigning against the use of astrological predictions, magical cures and rituals of sorcery in the diagnosis and treatment of disease. Presented in the form of a dialogue among three scholars, his notable work, entitled *De abditis rerum causis, (On the Hidden Causes of Conditions)* called for greater emphasis on observation and experience in the interpretation of nature and biological phenomena.

Other notable published works include his *Febrium curandarum methodus generalis (General Methods of Curing Fevers),* a guide to the treatment of fevers, and *Universa medicina (Collected Medicine),* which was completed and published after Fernel's death by Guillaume Plancy, who later wrote *Vita Fernelii; Febrium curandarum methodus generalis,* a study of Fernel's life and work. Celebrated neurophysiologist CHARLES SHERRINGTON also published a biographical work, entitled *Endeavour of Jean Fernel* (1946).

Johannes Andreas Grib Fibiger 1867–1928

A leading figure in cancer research, Johannes Fibiger was among those who did much to bring nineteenth–century science into the twentieth century. Fibiger was born in Denmark but traveled to Berlin to study with the renowed bacteriologists EMIL VON BEHRING and ROBERT KOCH. By 1900 Fibiger had returned to his native country, where he taught pathology at the University of Copenhagen and later headed the university's Institute of Pathological Anatomy.

As a first step toward studying the causes of cancer Fibiger successfully induced the disease in an experimental animal for the first time. He did this by feeding rats with cockroaches carrying *Spiroptera neoplastica,* a parasite. He theorized that the tumors produced in the rats were caused by irritation of the tissue, but this idea has since been disproved. However, Fibiger's experimental cultivation of the disease played an important part in science's ever-increasing understanding of this complex disease. In 1926 Fibiger was awarded the Nobel Prize for Medicine for his achievements in the field of cancer research.

Adolph Eugen Fick 1829–1901

German physiologist Adolph Fick established a principle for determining cardiac output—the rate of blood flow from the heart. Relating the rate of oxygen consumption to the differential between the amount of oxygen in venous and arterial blood, "Fick's law" relies on a relatively simple equation that permits calculation of cardiac output.

As a disciple of ERMANN VON HELMHOLTZ, Ernst Brucke (1819–1892) and Emil du Bois-Reymond, Fick became a leading spokesman for the new breed of physiologists who sought to define all organic function by applying the laws of physics and chemistry. Based on the interpretation of quantitative measurement, this new orientation in physiology sought to evaluate the individual capacities of isolated components of a structure or process, emphasizing causal analysis within constant or controlled conditions.

Fick gained distinction in the more accessible realm of applied science for developing the first widely used contact lens. Dating back to the sixteenth century, the notion of contact lenses originated with Leonardo da Vinci, who described the device in his *Code on the Eye.* Consisting of a short glass cylinder sealed at one end and filled with water, da Vinci's lens relied on the curved surface of the water against the shape of the eyeball to refract light. Four hundred years before modern contact lenses da Vinci recognized the eye's extreme sensitivity to foreign objects and designed his contact lens so that only water came in contact with the surface of the eye.

Noting the irritating effects of almost all solid materials, Fick developed a method of molding glass to follow the curvature of the eye and then polishing the surfaces until all irregularities were eliminated. Introduced in 1877, the first contact lenses were hard, thick pieces of glass designed to cover the entire surface of the eyeball. Because of the thickness of the glass the lenses were difficult to fit and somewhat uncomfortable to wear, but Fick's invention successfully demonstrated that vision could be directed by a corrective lens against the eye without causing damage or chronic irritation.

Soon after the invention of Plexiglas in 1936 the first plastic contact lenses were produced by Theodore E. Obrig, who also perfected a method for individual fitting. Unfortunately, the improved fit inhibited tear circulation, so that the wearer had to remove the lenses and lubricate his eyes every few hours. In the early 1950s, lenses were redesigned to cover only the cornea, and more recent developments include the use of flexible and porous lenses.

Reginald Herber Fitz 1843–1913

Reginald Heber Fitz, a Bostonian physician of the late nineteenth century, is best known for his systematic study of "perforating inflammation of the vermiform appendix," a condition for which he coined the term "acute appendicitis."

A student in Europe of celebrated clinician JOSEPH SKODA and noted pathologists KARL ROKITANSKY and RUDOLF VIRCHOW, Fitz was first and foremost a clinician who based his findings on evidence gleaned from observations of physiological symptoms and post-mortem conditions. Although he was not the first to describe appendicitis, Fitz investigated more than 250 cases, studying the pathology and potential complications of the condition. Emphasizing the vital importance of early diagnosis, he recommended early abdominal examination, stating that "...eventual treatment by laparotomy [abdominal surgery] is generally indispensable," adding that "urgent symptoms demand immediate exposure of the perforated appendix, after recovery from the shock."

Fitz is also recognized for his significant contribution to the understanding of acute pancreatitis, a condition often associated with trauma, infection or alcoholism in which the pancreas becomes inflamed, causing abdominal and back pain, nausea and vomiting. His study, published in 1889, discusses the organ's susceptibility to hemorrhage and describes hemorrhagic, suppurative (pus-producing) and gangrenous pancreatitis. The treatise detailed a series of diagnostic cues, including abdominal pain, tenderness, vomiting, collapse and tympanites, or distention of the abdomen. The combination of these symptoms signals the condition now known as "Fitz's syndrome."

At a time when antibiotics were still unknown, Fitz's observations and recommendations for the early diagnosis and treatment of these conditions increased survival rates significantly.

The dedicated practitioner began life in Chelsea, Massachusetts, a small town just outside of Boston. A graduate of Harvard College at 21, Fitz obtained his medical degree four years later from Harvard's medical school. After one year of study in Vienna and a second year in Berlin he returned to Harvard as an instructor in pathology.

In the decade that followed, Fitz served as head of the pathology laboratory at Massachussetts General Hospital, later becoming visiting physician. At the age of 35 Fitz was appointed professor of pathological anatomy at Harvard, and at 49 he was named professor of medicine. A distinguished member of the Harvard faculty, he held the Hersey chair of the "Theory and Practice of Physic" from 1892 until 1908, when he was named professor emeritus.

The author of more than 100 written works on clinical medicine and pathology, Fitz also wrote, with Horatio C. Wood, *The Practice of Medicine*, published in 1897.

Sir Alexander Fleming 1881–1955

The man who discovered penicillin was a whimsical Scotsman who described his lifelong preoccupation by saying "I play with microbes."

Alexander Fleming was born on an isolated Ayrshire farm on August 6, 1881, the seventh of eight children. The four oldest, ranging from seven to nineteen, were born to the farmer's first wife, who died, and the last four to a second wife the widower took when he was sixty. Though living conditions must have been tight in the little three-bedroom farmhouse, the families seem to have merged harmoniously, with the first family enjoined by their father and second mother to look after their young half- siblings.

After three years of country schooling Alec, then a short, wiry boy of thirteen with a broken nose and an elfin sense of humor, was sent down to London, where one of his older half-brothers had set up shop as an oculist.

Alec went to the Regent Street Polytechnic until he turned sixteen, then took a job doing office chores for a shipping firm that paid him 10 shillings a week. When the Boer War broke out in 1899 he joined the London Scottish Rifle Volunteers. They never went to South Africa, but the group taught Alec to swim and shoot and also offered him congenial comradeship. As the shortest recruit, however, he was often treated as the regimental mascot.

It soon became clear that he was not cut out for business, and he lacked any alternative ambitions until his older half-brother interested him in a medical career. In 1901 he entered the school attached to St. Mary's Hospital in London, where in his freshman year he won a scholarship covering tuition and the cost of books. He majored in obstetrics and undertook to deliver babies not only in the hospital but in the homes of mothers living in the slums of Paddington, St. Mary's neighborhood.

In 1906 Fleming passed with top scores all examinations set by the Royal College of Surgeons and Physicians, becoming thereby a fully documented physician. He was offered a post as assistant to the brilliant and eccentric professor of pathology at St. Mary's, Sir ALMROTH WRIGHT. The two men were in marked contrast. Wright was huge; Fleming was quite short. Wright was dictatorial and fanatic about his work; Fleming never lost his playfulness and artistic flair. To amuse himself and visitors to the lab, Fleming cultivated chromatic bacteria that in 24 hours would blossom into miniature rock gardens or jungle scenes on agar plates. He was delighted when friends had him inducted into the Chelsea Arts Club.

When World War I broke out Wright sent Fleming and a small staff to the front lines in France to study the possibility of vaccinating the troops against infection. The antityphoid vaccine that Wright and his staff persuaded the military to accept is credited with cutting the mortality of that disease by 90%. Fleming also pinpointed the principal organism infecting war wounds as *Clostridium welchii*. During the war he went on leave to marry Sarah Marion McElroy, who, with her twin sister, ran a nursing home on Baker Street.

Back in England Fleming resumed his prewar routines, now enlivened by a wife and a house in the country. In 1921, thanks to a cold, he discovered a propensity of his own nasal mucus to dissolve bacteria with which it came in contact. Discovery of the defensive substance, named a "lysozyme" by Wright, was acclaimed by British journals and reported in the *Proceedings of the Royal Society*.

The climactic accident of Alexander Fleming's life occurred in August, 1928, when he noticed a curious phenomenon in one of the pile of petri dishes that had accumulated in the laboratory sink. In the dish were several colonies of streptococci, but near the edge he saw a colony of mold around which there were only a few small, semitransparent groups of obviously weakening microorganisms. Clearly the mold was destroying the microorganisms with which it came into contact. Where the mold had come from was a complete mystery. Fleming extracted from it a yellow fluid, which, on the suspicion that the mold was related to *Penicillium rubrum*, he called penicillin.

Using techniques developed during his work on lysozyme, Fleming found penicillin to be effective against a wide range of bacilli. When his data suggested that it was excreted from the bloodstream in two hours but could not be effective in under four hours, he assigned only a limited use to his discovery. However, two Oxford professors, HOWARD WALTER FLOREY and ERNST BORIS CHAIN, after twelve years of laborious research, found that the penicillin extract was indeed effective in mice massively injected with streptococci. On May 25, 1940 they announced the dramatic finding that four of the experimental mice had been killed by the streptococci, while four others treated with penicillin survived in good health.

Animal and human trials continued during the early years of World War II until the enormous value of penicillin became an established fact. Honors began to pour in on Fleming. He was knighted in 1944 and, in the following year, shared the Nobel Prize for Physiology or Medicine with Chain and Florey. The acclaim was universal and tumultuous, marked by honors from heads of state and popular demonstrations of gratitude in the streets of the world's major cities.

In 1949 Fleming's wife died, and four years later he married Amalia Voureka, a Greek bacteriologist who had served as translator on his triumphal international tours. On March 11, 1955 he fell ill but declined to consider it an emergency, telling his doctor to "see your other patients first." After assuring his wife that the difficulty had nothing to do with his heart, he keeled over and died. An autopsy provided clear evidence of a blood clot in his coronary artery.

Fleming's ashes are entombed in St. Paul's Cathedral, and a memorial plaque is embedded in the walls of St. Mary's Hospital.

Simon Flexner 1863–1946
Abraham Flexner 1866–1959

The man who organized and led one of the most brilliant assemblages of medical scientists in the United States, and possibly the world, was a brilliant but largely self-taught pathologist who had failed to finish elementary school.

Simon Flexner, who presided over the Rockefeller Institute for Medical Research in its formative years, was the son of a man who fled the anti-Semitism and dismal economic prospects of Europe in the 1850s. After landing penniless in New York, Moritz Flexner headed west, settling in Kansas. There he and his wife, the former Esther Abraham, raised a family of eight children, two of whom were to greatly influence the course of medicine in the United States. Simon, the fourth child, was born in Louisville in 1863, when the nation was wracked by civil war. Abraham, the sixth in line, came along three years later.

By the time he was ten Simon had endured five boring years of elementary school and resolved to have no more of it, a decision that flew in the face of the family's most cherished belief in the pursuit of education. After he dropped out of school he was not conspicuously successful in a string of odd jobs that rarely lasted long, for he was addicted to mischief, harmless but detracting from any impression of seriousness. A dramatic change occurred however, after he recovered from a life-threatening siege of typhoid fever.

When he was fully recovered his oldest brother Jacob found a pharmacist who took Simon on as an apprentice. Part of the agreement provided that the pharmacist send him through a three-month course at the Louisville College of Pharmacy. To the amazement of his family, Simon did brilliantly. After graduating with honors he went to work in the pharmacy Jacob had established, doing the work of a pharmacist and wringing an education out of the physicians whose prescriptions he filled. Jacob's drug store became a salon for the intellectuals of Louisville.

When the journal *Science* published a modest contribution by Simon concerning the presence of sugar in the granular matter found in beehives, he became something of a celebrity in the town, whereupon he announced his ambition to open a pathology lab in the city one day.

Meanwhile, Jacob's pharmacy had subsidized Abraham in an education at the new undergraduate program at Johns Hopkins University in Baltimore. Since Jacob could afford only two years' tuition, Abraham had to finish the four-year course in half the time. He did it by a combination of brilliance and unremitting work, summer and winter without a break. In any case, he came back to Louisville with his bachelor's degree at the age of 19 with news that the renowned William Henry Welch had just been appointed professor of pathology at the medical school that was about to be opened at Johns Hopkins. For Simon this seemed to offer a pathway to the Louisvile laboratory he envisioned. However, even for admission to such a school he needed an M.D.

With the help of the city's doctors Simon was admitted to the newly organized University of Louisville Medical Institute, offering a two-year course of lectures. Simon would later recall that he got his M.D. without having performed a physical examination or listened to a heartbeat.

His brother Abraham, then employed as a teacher, footed the bill for Simon's first year at Johns Hopkins. After that Simon so impressed Welch and his other teachers that he was offered a fellowship completely covering his tuition. Welch was so confident in Simon that he sent him to unravel a mystery in Maryland where an epidemic of what some doctors thought might be spotted fever was taking a heavy toll among coal miners. It was not spotted fever but meningitis, Flexner discovered.

After two years at Johns Hopkins the idea of a Louisville laboratory had given way to loftier ambitions. Welch hired Simon as his assistant, thereby putting him on the faculty at Johns Hopkins, then sent his protege to Europe to study with those in the forefront of pathological research.

When he returned to Baltimore Simon not only resumed his work with Welch as assistant professor of pathology but was appointed resident pathologist at the university's hospital. At age 32 the young man from Kentucky who had won a medical degree from a two-year school of uncertain reputation, but whose subsequent work was described as brilliant, was elected to the American College of Physicians and had been promoted to associate professor of pathology. A full professorship followed soon after.

Other universities then began to bid for Flexner's services until the University of Pennsylvania, the oldest and most respected medical school in the country, offered him the chairmanship of the pathology department. He anguished over the decision until his friends feared for his health, but even Welsh agreed that to refuse such an offer was unthinkable. While the University of Pennsylvania wrestled with a small group of faculty members who opposed Flexner because he was a Jew, Simon undertook a final mission as a Johns Hopkins pathologist.

The United States was then trying to occupy the Philippines against the stubborn resistance of a guerilla army. To report the situation scientifically, Flexner volunteered to lead a team to investigate the medical plight of the troops, who were suffering from malaria, typhoid fever, tuberculosis and a particularly violent form of dysentery that the Flexner team traced to a bacillus subsequently named *Shigella flexneri*.

That mission and the earlier one he had undertaken among Maryland coal miners prompted the federal government to ask him to investigate what seemed to be an outbreak of plague in San Fransisco's Chinatown. The situation called for exquisite tact, since any publicity given to so awesome a menace could panic the entire West Coast, with frightening economic and political repercussions. Flexner proceeded carefully to confirm the diagnosis of plague, then to isolate the patients from the rats, thus limiting and finally controlling the disease. So secret was the story that Flexner communicated with Washington only by code. The government expressed its gratitude when the plague epidemic was ended with neither medical nor political repercussions.

At the University of Pennsylvania Flexner demonstrated his ability not only as a pathologist but as a master manager of scientists, showing an understanding of their needs, their problems and their quirks. That was the talent sought by John D. Rockefeller Sr. and his son John Jr. when they searched for a director of what they hoped would be the American version of the celebrated Pasteur Institute in Paris. Simon Flexner, the Rockefellers decided, could create and inspire the star team they envisioned.

Simon's first step was to scout Europe for the talent he and the Rockefellers needed. He combined his European survey with a honeymoon, for he had married Helen Thomas, a writer and feminist whose forebears had come over with the Puritans. Later generations of Thomases had become Quakers, abolitionists and suffragettes.

The Flexners returned from their year abroad, settled into a home on Madison Avenue in New York City, and began to build what RENÉ DUBOS, one of the early recruits, called a "commonwealth of scholars." In 1906 Simon was called away from his institute to lead another mission, this one against an outbreak of meningococcal meningitis in New York City. Using infected horses as a factory for antiserum, he cut the fatality rate from 75% to 25% "Flexner's serum" remained the standard therapy for the disease until sulfa drugs were developed in the 1930s.

Abraham Flexner, meanwhile, had made a name for himself as an educator in Louisville and had won national attention with the publication of *The American College*, which took a searching look at the deficiencies of higher education. He was then asked by the Carnegie Foundation for the Advancement of Teaching to study the medical schools of the United States and Canada. Out of that survey came the *Flexner Report*, which stirred a revolution in medical training and set the standards that still govern medical education. The Rockefellers subsequently engaged him to design models for new medical schools, and, with Simon's support, Abraham Flexner was named director of the Institute for Advanced Study at Princeton.

When World War I broke out Simon Flexner converted the Rockefeller Institute into a facility for training army doctors in the latest techniques of battlefield surgery. With the coming of peace the Rockefellers called on Flexner to lead yet another mission—to plan the introduction of Western medical education to China, which was steeped in more ancient traditions of healing and recently ravaged by wars and famine. Flexner, who dreamed of creating "the Johns Hopkins Institute of China," made recommendations that led to the founding of the Peking Union Medical College and subsequent Rockefeller philanthropies designed to spread the gospel of Western medicine.

In 1935 Simon Flexner retired after 30 years at the helm of the Rockefeller Institute. During that time the important studies undertaken under his guidance had filled 100 volumes, and the team had grown from 12 to 120 scientists, most of them highly distinguished in their fields.

Simon Flexner, 72 when he relinquished the reins at the Rockefeller Institute, lived another 11 years, receiving a steady flow of the world's encomia until his death in 1946.

Howard Walter Florey, Baron Florey of Adelaide
1898–1968

The discovery of penicillin in 1928 has been described as a happy accident, but it might never have fulfilled its lifesaving potential if, ten years after the report of ALEXANDER FLEMING'S discovery, Howard Florey and ERNST CHAIN had not studied the substance.

Florey was an Australian pathologist who came to Oxford University as a Rhodes scholar. He continued his studies at Cambridge and was asked to stay on as professor of pathology. In 1935 he became head of the Sir William Dunn School of Pathology at Oxford and invited Chain to run the biochemistry department. In 1939, with a grant from the Rockefeller Foundation, they launched their research into the nature and therapeutic potential of penicillin. In the next two years Chain and Florey came to understand penicillin's enormous antibacterial value by isolating and purifying it and evaluating its effectiveness through extensive experimentation with many different strains of bacteria. In 1945 Florey, Chain and Fleming were awarded the Nobel Prize for Physiology and Medicine in recognition of their work with penicillin. The drug's potential impact on public health was evident, but it could not be produced in sufficient quantities in research laboratories. Florey and Chain presented their work in the United States, where the government and the pharmaceutical industry cooperated for mass production.

Florey was invited to join the Royal Society in 1941, and he served as president from 1960 to 1965. He was knighted in 1944 and in 1965 was made a life peer and given the Order of Merit.

Marie Jean Pierre Flourens 1794–1867

After receiving his medical degree from the University of Montpelier at the age of nineteen, physiologist Pierre Flourens embarked on an illustrious career that would bring him recognition as a politician, philosopher, biographer, popular author, professor and, most notably, pioneer in experimental research on the physiology of the nervous system. As permanent secretary and a prominent member of the Academy of Sciences, Flourens cofounded the academy's influential periodical *Comptes rendus*, (*Proceedings*) in association with French scientist and statesman D.F.J. Arago (1786–1853). In a controversial decision the Académie Française elected Flourens a member in 1840.

A protégé of France's celebrated naturalist Georges Cuvier (1769–1832), Flourens won a place for himself in the scientific establishment when he was barely 30. His reports on the nervous system, first noticed by Cuvier, were presented to the Academy of Sciences in 1822 and published in 1824. Flourens's studies are notable as much for their experimental approach as for their significant advances in the physiology of the nervous system.

Using ablation, an experimental technique in which various anatomical structures are surgically removed in order to determine their individual functions, Flourens conducted a systematic investigation of the faculties of the central nervous system.

Flourens classified the major categories of brain function as intelligence, in which he included perception and volition; sensory ability, comprising reception and transmission of impressions; and excitation of muscle contraction. Advancing physiological understanding in all three of these areas, he established the neurological control of respiration, locating the *noeud vital*, or respiratory center, in the brain's medulla oblongata. In experimental studies using pigeons he demonstrated that vision is dependent on activity in the cerebral hemispheres.

Flourens is also noted for his study of the role of the periosteum, the vascular membrane covering the bones, in the formation and development of bone and the notion of coordination. Noting that lesions in the cerebellum cause a "disharmony of movement" or disrupted equilibrium, Flourens discovered a condition characterized by lack of coordination and compulsive head-jerking that occurs in patients with lesions of the semicircular canals of the inner ear. The function of the inner ear in response to gravity and acceleration remained a mystery, however, to be resolved half a century later by Ernst Mach (1838–1916) and Josef Breuer (1842–1925), among others.

Based on his own interpretation of the phenomenon of coordination, Flourens developed a theory that the entire cerebrum is engaged with each and every psychic or perceptual operation. Overreacting against FRANCIS GALL'S fanciful doctrine of phrenology, Flourens mistakenly denied any aspect of cerebral localization of brain function. His opinionated, authoritarian attitude led to a number of other strongly stated errors in judgment, the most glaring of which was his criticism of Charles Darwin's theory of evolution.

From humble beginnings in the small town of Maureilhan, in southern France, Flourens, with the aid of his influential mentor Cuvier, rose to an early prominence. By 1821 the 27-year-old was lecturing on the physiology of sensation at the Cercle Athenée, a distinguished scientific society in Paris. Based on his first experimental studies of nervous function, these presentations brought Flourens to the attention of the Academy of Sciences.

By the time he was made a member of the academy in 1828 Flourens had already been awarded the prestigious Montyon Prize two years in succession. He joined the faculty at the Collège de France as a deputy lecturer that same year, becoming a full professor by 1832. Before Cuvier died in 1833 he designated Flourens to succeed him as permanent secretary of the Academy of Sciences.

In 1838 Flourens was elected deputy for the southern city of Beziers, not far from the town of his birth. After his election to the Académie Française two years later Flourens gradually began to redirect his professional efforts. In the last twenty-five years of his life he devoted his time to writing philosophical and popular works, most notably a series of acclaimed biographies in which he established a historical and scientific context for his subjects.

His biographical works include *Histoire des travaux et des idées de Buffon* (1844) (*A History of the Work and Ideas of Buffon*), *Éloge historique de François Magendie* (1858) (*Historical Enconium on François Magendie*) and *Éloge historique de A.M.C. Dumeril (Historical Enconium on A.M.C. Dumeril)* (1863). Other writings include *Examen de la phrenologie* (1842), *Histoire de la découverte du sang* (1854, 1857, English translation 1859), *De la longévité humaine et de la quantité de vie sur le globe* (1854), *De la vie et de l'intelligence* (1858), *Ontologie naturelle ou étude philosophique des êtres* (1861), and *Examen du livre de M. Darwin sur l'origine des espèces* (1864).

Werner Forssmann 1904–1979

In 1929, when Werner Forssmann was a first-year intern at a hospital in his native Germany, he worked to develop an emergency procedure that would enable physicians to inject a drug directly into the heart of a patient. Forssmann stunned the medical community by testing his new technique on himself. He placed himself behind a fluoroscopic screen, inserted a catheter tube into his arm and pushed the tube through the venous channels into his heart. He then injected a contrast medium in order to X-ray the process.

The performance was daring, although it proved harmless to Forssmann. In fact the procedure itself, minus the X rays, had been tried fifteen years earlier by Bleichroeder, Unger and Loeb and had received little notice. Forssmann's experiment was generally regarded as a stunt, and it was another twelve years before it was given serious consideration. At that time ANDRE COURNAND and DICKINSON W. RICHARDS, working in the United States, recognized and confirmed the value of the procedure. Their research explored its diagnostic value in heart and lung disease and its use in assessing surgical results.

Forssmann served as an army doctor in Berlin until 1945, then practiced privately in a number of smaller cities in Germany. In 1956 he shared the Nobel Prize for Physiology and Medicine with Cournand and Richards, and later he published an autobiography entitled *Experiments with Myself* (English translation published in 1975).

Girolamo Fracastoro (or Hieronymous Fracastorius) 1483–1553.

Celebrated in his lifetime as a poet, classicist, scientist and pathologist, Girolamo Fracastoro is best remembered for his poem, written in 1530, entitled "Syphilis Sive Morbus Gallicus" ("Syphilis or the French Disease"). He took the name "syphilis" from Syphilus, the shepherd hero of his poem. Borrowing from the poetic style of Ovid, Fracastoro's work describes some of the symptoms of the disease as well as its venereal method of transmission.

Fracastoro's contribution to medicine is also to be found in another written work, published in 1546, entitled *De Contagione, Contagiosis Morbis at eorum Curatione (On Contagion, Contagious Diseases, and Their Treatment)*. This treatise, far advanced for its time, anticipated by several centuries the epidemiological findings of PASTEUR and others. Maintaining that infection followed by contagion is the prime cause of epidemic disease, Fracastoro suggested that *seminaria*, or seeds specific to a particular disease, are infective agents, multiplying within the body and transmitted by three basic modes of contagion: through body contact, through intermediary agents (e.g., old clothes) or through air transport.

Fracastoro's formulation of the modern theory of infection is all the more remarkable because it was based on the mistaken assumption that these contagious agents are self-propagating and inorganic. It was physician-philosopher Giralamo Cardano (1501–1576), a contemporary of Fracastoro, who recognized that these *seminaria* might be living organisms.

Born in Verona, Fracastoro studied medicine at the University of Padua, where Copernicus was a friend and fellow student. Returning to Verona after receiving his degree, Fracastoro taught logic at the university while establishing a successful medical practice. His attention to syphilis went beyond poetry, and a detailed clinical study is included in *De Contagione*. Recognizing that the disease is contracted during coitus, Fracastoro described the sequence of symptoms, from the appearance of small pustules on the genitals to a more generalized spread to the mouth, pharynx and scalp. In clinical observations of syphilitic patients Fracastoro referred to syphilitic cachexia, a condition of overall ill health and malnutrition, noting symptoms of fever, loss of hair, inflammation of the bones and pains in the joints. Fracastoro also discussed congenital syphilis, the appearance of the disease at birth. His other observations include reference to "spotted fever," most likely the disease now known as typhus.

In addition to his impressive work as a medical practitioner and researcher, Fracastoro also studied mathematics, astronomy, geology and physics and wrote a treatise on the theory of music.

Rosalind Franklin 1920–1958

In her short life Rosalind Franklin played an important part in the discovery of the structure of DNA, although she received little recognition for her contribution. She was born into a wealthy London family who intended for her the gracious life of philanthropy. Instead she pursued a career in a field where, as a woman, she was fated to meet the most stubborn resistance. She graduated from Cambridge with a degree in chemistry and was awarded a research scholarship. Unfortunately, she was sent to work under the direction of Ronald Norrish, who found it difficult to seriously accept her or her work. In 1947 Franklin transferred to the Central Laboratory of Chemical Sciences in Paris. Her study of molecular structure and crystallography contributed important advances in the field of carbon-fiber technology.

Franklin worked in France until 1950, when she returned to London to continue her research at King's College under the supervision of MAURICE WILKINS. She made a momentous discovery in 1951, when she identified the helical structure of the DNA molecule. Particularly remarkable was an X-ray photograph that she took of a DNA molecule. In 1953 she published a paper containing some of her revelatory findings. Without her knowledge or permission, Wilkins shared a number of her reports with fellow DNA researchers JAMES WATSON and FRANCIS CRICK. In 1953 Franklin left King's College to accept a research position at Birkbeck College, where she began studies in virology. She was forbidden to discuss the work in which she had participated at King's College, although Watson used her X-ray photographs in his grant proposal for further DNA research, and her studies helped steer him to his final double-helix model.

In 1958, at the age of 37, Rosalind Franklin learned that she had incurable cancer. She continued to work until her death later that year. Four years later Crick, Watson and Wilkins accepted the Nobel Prize for their world-famous discovery of the "double helix." As the award is given only to living candidates, Franklin's crucial contributions to that discovery were never officially acknowledged.

Sigmund Freud 1856–1939

"No one who...conjures up the most evil of those half-tamed demons that inhabit the human breast and seeks to wrestle with them, can expect to come through the struggle unscathed," wrote Sigmund Freud, the Austrian neurologist who achieved immortality as the founding father of psychoanalytic theory.

In his struggle to untangle the mysteries of the mind, Freud led an extraordinary journey into the unconscious—a vast but submerged territory, in his view, where emotionally charged and contradictory impulses persist in exile from immediate awareness. Challenging the time-honored traditional definitions of mind and body he disclosed the unconscious process and established the laws by which the concrete, physical world is connected to the world of irrational, emotional phenomena. Freud's revolutionary investigations gave rise to a comprehensive doctrine of human behavior based primarily on the mechanisms of the unconscious and the lasting effects of infantile sexuality.

Freud began exploring the relationship between repressed memories and psychoneurosis in the mid-1880s when he launched his association with Viennese physician Joseph Breuer. Their landmark clinical research established the fundamental principles of psychoanalysis, a term introduced by Freud that refers both to a system of psychopathology and to a form of psychotherapy. Following the dictum that "in mental life nothing which has once been formed can perish," psychoanalysis was designed to help patients gain conscious access to more of their total psychic energy.

"Where Id was, there Ego shall be," declared Freud in *New Introductory Lectures on Psychoanalysis*, published in 1932. "One might compare the relation of the ego to the id with that between a rider and his horse," he explained. "The horse provides the locomotor energy, and the rider has the prerogative of determining the goal and of guiding the movements of his powerful mount towards it. But all too often," he added, "we find a picture of the less ideal situation in which the rider is obliged to guide his horse in the direction it itself wants to go."

Of Jewish parentage, Sigmund Freud grew up in Freiberg, Moravia, then a territory of Austria and now part of Czechoslovakia. His interest in science and medicine developed early in adolescence and was reportedly inspired by Goethe's essay on nature.

Firmly set in his professional goals by the time he graduated from high school, he embarked on his medical education in 1874 at the University of Vienna. The city was to become Freud's permanent home for most of his adult life. After delaying the completion of his training to pursue independent studies in physiology, he was granted his medical degree in 1881. He remained at the University of Vienna as a postgraduate student in neurology until 1885 when he joined the faculty as lecturer in neuropathology.

Supported by a traveling fellowship he took a leave of absence at the end of that year to study in Paris at the Salpêtrière under legendary French neurologist JEAN-MARTIN CHARCOT. A pioneer in the study of hysterical disorders, Charcot had also conducted extensive research on the medical applications of hypnosis. Although Freud would soon abandon the use of hypnosis, he retained a lifelong admiration for his former mentor and frequently acknowledged the profound influence of Charcot's work on the development of modern psychiatry, neurology and neuropathology.

After an inspiring year in Paris Freud returned to Vienna in 1886, and within a few months he and Breuer had embarked on what was to be an historic collaboration.

Freud had learned of Breuer's discovery of the therapeutic effect of drawing out painful memories through hypnosis, and the two joined together to explore the consequences of probing the unconscious. They applied their findings to the development of various cathartic procedures and integrated the series into "a talking cure."

The birth of psychoanalysis was announced in 1893 when Freud and Breuer published their landmark paper, *On the Psychical Mechanism of Hysterical Phenomenon*. Based on extensive clinical observations, they traced the symptoms of hysterical patients to psychological trauma in early life and identified these symptoms as a manifestation of undischarged emotional energy. Their theory, more fully developed two years later in *Studies on Hysteria*, outlined the "cathartic method" of therapy, in which hypnosis was used to unearth buried memories in order to release the pressure of unconscious forces.

Some of Freud's most revolutionary concepts, including the phenomena of repression, resistance and transference as mechanisms of the unconscious, were introduced during the early stage of his career. The medical establishment received his unorthodox doctrine with violent and uncomprehending opposition from the start, and his insistence on infant sexuality and the sexual nature of unconscious forces eventually cost him his partnership with Breuer. Before the end of the century he was forced into isolation, working independently until 1906, when he was joined by Swiss psychiatrists Eugen Bleuler and Carl Jung and a few other forward-thinking colleagues.

The hostility of the professional community intensified in 1900 with his publication of *The Interpretation of Dreams*, a monumental work that has endured after nearly a century to become a major literary classic and one of Freud's most celebrated achievements.

Referring to dreams as "the royal road to the unconscious," Freud was convinced of their vital role in maintaining mental health. He introduced the concept of dreaming as a kind of psychological safety valve, allowing the mind to discharge some of the "forbidden" impulses that crowd the unconscious. These emotionally charged thoughts are given a censored form of expression in dreams, disguising their meaning in symbolic images and extraordinary narrative.

Appointed professor of neurology at the University of Vienna in 1902, Freud began to gather disciples among his students, who formed the original "Psychological Wednesday Society." Developing into the Vienna Psychoanalytical Society in 1908, the group was established two years later as the International Psychoanalytical Association. With Jung as first president, the organization boasted a distinguished membership, including such legendary names as Adler, Steckel, Rank, Ferenczi, Jones and Brill.

In 1905 Freud published *The Psychopathology of Everyday Life* and a year later produced *Three Contributions to the Sexual Theory*. Both books aroused the inevitable denouncements from the medical establishment, and it was not before 1930, when he was awarded the Goethe Prize, that Freud's work began to gain public acceptance.

In 1933, however, psychoanalysis was banned by decree of Adolf Hitler. After the Nazi invasion of Austria, Freud escaped with his family to England to spend the last years of his life in Hampstead. He died there at the age of 83 from cancer of the jaw, a disease that had afflicted him for 17 years.

Freud's vast collection of noted writings includes *Totem and Tabu* (1913, Eng. trans. 1918), an investigation of the origins of religion and morality; *The Ego and the Id* (1923, Eng. trans. 1927), his last contribution to psychoanalytic theory; *Why War?* (coauthored with Albert Einstein and published in 1933); and an autobiographical study (published in 1925 and translated by Strachey in 1935).

G

Daniel Carleton Gajdusek 1923–

To investigate the mechanism of a mysterious disease known as kuru, Daniel Gajdusek spent nearly a year in a jungle village living among the Fore people of New Guinea. A fatal disease of the nervous system, kuru seemed to claim its victims only from this one cannibalistic tribe. In 1957 Gajdusek discovered that the disease was caused by a virus transmitted by the ingestion of human brain tissue. As the practice of cannibalism has waned the disease has virtually disappeared, but Gajdusek's study shed light on the transmission and mechanism of similar slow viruses related to neurological disorders, such as Creutzfeldt-Jakob disease in humans and scrapie in animals. Kuru, which takes from two to twenty years to incubate, is a degenerative neurological disorder that may offer clues to multiple sclerosis and Parkinsonism. For his work on the causes and transmission of infectious diseases Gajdusek received the 1976 Nobel Prize for Physiology or Medicine, which he shared with B.S. BLUMBERG.

Trading tools for the corpses of kuru victims, Gajdusek performed numerous autopsies in search of the roots of the disease, but the key to kuru was only revealed after he came to learn the cannibalistic traditions of the Fore tribe. As part of a ritual believed to ensure the immortality of the deceased by incorporating their virtues into the living, some members of the Fore tribe would eat the bodies of those who died. Gajdusek discovered that in cases where the deceased had been victim of kuru, a far less desirable transmission took place. The slow-acting but deadly kuru virus was passed on through ingestion of infected brain tissue, causing a gradual breakdown of the nervous system in its new victims. Since the women prepared the body for the cannibalistic rite and, in so doing, handled the victim's brain, they were among the most affected by kuru. When they handled children, they transmitted the disease along with their maternal care.

A leading authority on virology, immunology, pediatric medicine, genetics, neurology and anthropology, Gajdusek is widely recognized for his broad range of interests and achievements. Fluent in French, Spanish, German, Slavic and Rumanian, Gajdusek also converses in the less familiar languages of the many peoples he has studied around the world. Born in Yonkers, New York, he received his medical degree from Harvard Medical School in 1946, completing postdoctoral research at the California Institute of Technology. Returning from New Guinea in 1958, Gajdusek joined the Institute of Neurological Diseases and Stroke, a division of the National Institutes of Health.

Over the course of his many research expeditions to the South Pacific Gajdusek has adopted 16 boys, bringing them back to the United States, raising them and arranging for their education. Hearing that he had been awarded the Nobel Prize, he said: "I'll use the money to put the boys through college. At times I've had seven in college, and it's been a bit of a strain."

Galen c. 129–c. 200

For nearly 1,500 years Galen's doctrine remained the incontrovertible authority on medicine throughout many parts of the world. Though his theories were largely ignored in Western Europe during the Middle Ages, it was not until they were revived, and finally challenged in the early part of the 17th century, that medical science could advance beyond the venerable wisdom of Galen.

Born to a wealthy and distinguished family in the Greek city of Pergamum, Galen was launched on an intensive course of education at an early age. He was tutored by his father until he turned 14 and then trained by scholars in philosophy, mathematics, empiricism, natural sciences and Hippocratic doctrine. According to Galen's writings, it was his father who directed him towards medicine, reportedly as a result of a dream in which the great ASCLEPIOS revealed to him the destiny of his son.

Galen pursued his education first at Smyrna, then at Corinth. After more than a decade of study he reached Alexandria, a leading center for anatomy and physiology in the Roman world, representing 300 years of medical tradition.

In the course of his exhaustive training, Galen explored all avenues of medical science and philosophy, traveling far and wide to obtain the broadest possible spectrum of knowledge. He was exposed to a wide variety of clinical practices, physiological theories and medical philosophies, and accumulated extensive information on botany and pharmacology.

After many long years of itinerant study and practice he returned to Pergamum. Widely renowned as a master physician by then, he had also gained prominence in medical science with the publication of his first writings on anatomy and physiology.

From the stream of professional offers that came his way, Galen accepted an appointment as physician and surgeon to the gladiators. The position not only gave him the chance to sharpen his surgical skills in treating a vast array of severe injuries but also provided a unique opportunity to observe muscles, bones, blood flow and other aspects of living human anatomy.

The struggle to keep his patients in optimum health and physical fitness while battling the effects of their brutal life-style prompted Galen to develop principles of diet, hygiene and preventive medicine that would later become integrated into his medical doctrine.

Galen gave up his surgical activities when he left for Rome in 162 A.D. but the early practical experience would later serve as a basis for his outstanding collection of writings on surgical techniques and procedures.

In 169 A.D. Galen's medical authority was officially declared when he was enlisted as physician to the emperor Marcus Aurelius. His new status afforded the privileges of leisure and complacency, but such indulgence was not in his nature. Driven by unrelenting energy and a voracious appetite for knowledge, he continued to study, travel and lecture, debating and demonstrating new theories as his literary output grew to monumental proportions. Though an inestimable number of Galen's manuscripts were destroyed by fire in 192 A.D. the surviving body of his work totals more than 9,000 pages.

He wrote in his native Greek, which was also the language of science. A major part of his work involved the compilation and integration of all existing medical information. Past knowledge was the source of progress, Galen believed, and the work of his predecessors was a key element in his writing and his scientific creativity. Though experimental and direct observation were emphasized, his doctrine was deeply rooted in the historical context of the time and took shape by incorporating and consolidating the traditions of HIPPOCRATES, Plato, ARISTOTLE, and the physicians of Alexandria.

The teleological concept of universal design was a fundamental element in Galen's thinking. Following Aristotle's dictum that "Nature does nothing without a purpose," the theory states that all structures in the body reflect a predetermined function. Galen went a step further to assert that he could identify that function. The principle of divine universal purposiveness was well-suited to both Christian and Islamic faiths and satisfied the scientific needs of the public for many centuries to come.

Another basic concept in Galen's system was the "humoral theory," which posits that the universe is composed of four fundamental substances, or humors, representing the four irreducible elements of earth, air, fire and water. Although the idea is thought to have originated with the Greek philosopher EMPEDOCLES in the fourth century B.C., it is most widely associated with Hippocrates, who presented an exhaustive study of humors in his treatise entitled *On the Nature of Man*.

Enduring in one form or another until the end of the 17th century, the ancient theory had the flexibility to incorporate past and future ideas, ranging from the psychological principles of Plato (427–347 B.C.) to the pharmacological principles of PARACELCUS (1493–1541), and the mechanical principles of RENÉ DESCARTES (1596–1650).

The basic qualities of cold, dry, hot and wet were identified in physiological terms as phlegm, blood, yellow bile and black bile. According to the theory, health is preserved by maintaining the correct proportions of these factors for the individual and the primary cause of disease is an imbalance in the humoral formula. Galen developed the psychological application of the theory, classifying all personalities into four types: phlegmatic, sanguine, choleric and melancholic.

Based on experimental and clinical research, Galen's medical formulation of humoral theory combined Hippocratic doctrine with elements of natural science and philosophy. He claimed that vital humors are created in the living body from inanimate elements found in food and drink. As the nutritive material is transformed into blood in the liver, it is imbued with what he called "Natural Spirit"—an active ingredient that flows out of the liver, passes through the right ventricle and is exhaled through the lungs. A small amount of this substance seeps into the left ventricle, however, to be processed into the more potent "Vital Spirit" and distributed throughout the arterial system. Some of this substance is destined for further refinement in the brain to become "Animal Spirit"—defined by Galen as the principle needed to convert thought into action.

Though his doctrine was fraught with medical misconceptions, the magnitude of Galen's achievement was enormous. Forbidden by law from practicing human dissection, he derived much of his anatomical understanding, and misunderstanding, from experimentation on animals, mainly pigs, dogs and Barbary apes. Despite the limitations, he succeeded in identifying and accurately describing a wide range of physiological and anatomical phenomena.

He differentiated sensory and motor nerves, identified seven (out of 12) cranial nerves, and recognized many of the major structures in the brain, including the hemispheres, cerebellum, corpus callosum and the meninges—the tissue membranes that protect and enclose the brain. He demonstrated that nerves originate in the central nervous system, that veins are connected to the heart, and that arteries contain blood, not air as was widely believed. Much of his research focused on the structure and mechanism of the heart and lungs, and in particular, the nature of pulse, a topic to which he devoted 16 books.

A master of clinical and diagnostic investigation, Galen rose to unrivaled eminence as a physician. Following in the Hippocratic tradition, he was meticulous and exhaustive in his examination of a patient and would proceed with medical treatment only after completing a detailed analysis of the morbid condition. Though he did not record case histories, as Hippocrates had done, Galen recognized the significance and interaction of emotional and environmental factors in his evaluation of a patient's condition.

As a physician, he directed his greatest effort toward the prevention of disease, which he considered the primary duty of his profession. In his view, physical health was a reflection of the natural harmony of the qualities of the body—a condition highly susceptible to disturbance from external forces. To maintain a healthy equilbrium, he recommended various regimens of diet, rest, exercise, massage and hygiene.

In order to cure disease, Galen sought to restore natural balance, mainly with the use of drugs. He developed an elaborate system of therapeutics that involved thousands of different herbs, each possessing one or more of the fundamental principles. The nature and intensity of the symptoms of a particular disease would determine the ingredients in the remedy, which might include cooling substances, such as cucumber seed, for reducing fever, or heat-producing substances, such as pepper, for relieving chills.

Over the course of half a century, Galen produced a vast collection of pharmacological concoctions to be administered either internally or externally as specific treatments, many of which called for a hundred ingredients or more. He devoted several thousand pages of text to the discussion of drug remedies, outlining in exhaustive detail the procedures for gathering and storing herbs as well as instructions for the preparation, usage and indications of each prescription. A central focus of his practice and research, Galen's therapeutic doctrine proved to be one of his most enduring and influential contributions.

Francis Joseph Gall 1758–1828

The theory of phrenology or cranioscopy has long been relegated to the ranks of pseudoscience and often referred to as an example of charlatanism. But when Francis Gall introduced this idea he brought a new and important perspective to neurology. At the basis of phrenology is the notion that mental processes might be localized, and that the brain is made up of different sections governing specific and discrete functions. That principle is now accepted as a basic tenet of brain physiology. While Gall's conclusions were ill-founded and often fanciful, his attention to mental faculties and functioning opened an important door to the study of the human brain.

Gall was born in Germany but settled in Vienna in 1785 to begin private practice as a physician. Though he had studied anatomy of the brain in France and Austria, he became diverted early by a fascination with the variations of the human skull. He evolved his theory of phrenology as a diagnostic tool with which to predict "innate mental character" by observing the size and shape of a patient's head. He broke down human mental function into 33 distinct faculties and identified separate cerebral organs that he correlated with each of these functions. Gall claimed he could assess the power of each separate faculty by the size and expansion of its own governing organ, contending that the outward contours of the skull paralleled those of the underlying cerebrum.

In 1791 he publicly announced these ideas, and in his doctrine Gall determined the existence of a vital force separate from and independent of the soul. His public appearances attracted tremendous interest both in the medical community and outside it, but in 1802 his lectures were suppressed as being subversive of religion. Phrenology was a popular success, but Gall was continually pressured to leave Austria for his irreligious ideas. He soon moved to France, where he was welcomed with honors and acclaim. With the assistance of his favorite student, John Caspar Spurzheim, Gall created and published *Anatomie et Physiologies du Système Nerveux (Anatomy and Physiologies of the Nervous System)* a four-volume work including a complete "atlas of the brain" that appeared in installments from 1810 to 1819. In this book he set forth his doctrine of localization of brain function and also demonstrated the existence of nerve fibers in the white matter of the brain.

Gall lectured for more than twenty years in France and died in Paris, a wealthy and successful man. Spurzheim spread his doctrine to England and America, where phrenology was enthusiastically embraced throughout the next century. George Combe (1788–1858), an Edinburgh lawyer, saw Gall's work as a vital part of mid-nineteenth-century materialist and naturalist thought and further popularized phrenology by using it as a means toward social reform.

Sir Francis Galton 1812–1911

"I do not see why any insolence of caste should prevent the gifted class, when they had the power, from treating their compatriots with all kindness, so long as they maintained celibacy," wrote Francis Galton in 1873, "but if these continued to procreate children inferior in moral, intellectual, and physical qualities, it is easy to believe the time may come when such persons would be considered as enemies of the State, and to have forfeited all claims to kindness."

The astonishing class-angled approach thus expressed by Francis Galton did not overwhelm his scientific talents or obscure his contribution. His career had great impact on the history of medicine, and a number of his ideas and insights have transcended his own biases.

With W.F.R. Weldon (1860–1906) and Karl Pearson (1857–1936) Galton founded a new discipline combining biology and mathematics, which Galton named "biometrics." The intention was to study evolution using statistical methods and to discover ranges, frequencies and distributions of biological traits. These investigations served to support another discipline, eugenics, with implications more social than scientific.

Although expressed somewhat late in Galton's own life, interest in heredity was a family trait. His grandfather was Erasmus Darwin, and his cousin was Charles Darwin. Galton chose to study medicine, first at Birmingham Hospital and then at King's College and Trinity College in London. After graduation he took up life as an explorer and adventurer, traveling to North Africa in 1846 and returning in 1850 to explore as yet uncharted areas of South Africa. He described his experiences in *Narrative of an Explorer in South Africa* and *Art of Travel*. In this period of his life Galton also studied meteorology, publishing his *Meteorographica* in 1863.

It was at this point that Galton turned his attentions to heredity and its many applications. He is credited with introducing the now well-worn phrase "nature/nurture," and he described the contrast between environmental and hereditary factors in his book *English Men of Science; their Nature and Nurture*, published in 1874. Galton also coined the term "eugenics" for the movement that calls for legislative efforts to ensure continued genetic improvement of the race. He described the goals of this crusade as follows:"I conceive it to fall well within his [man's] province to replace Natural Selection by other processes that are more merciful and not less effective. This is precisely the aim of eugenics."

Using his cousin's recently published ideas on natural selection, he began a campaign for eugenic breeding, a recurrent theme in the racist and fascist forces to emerge in later decades.

Galton is also responsible for mathematically stating and expanding the widely accepted though faulty notion of blending inheritance. Galton's Ancestral Law of Inheritance asserts that different traits in parents are merged in their offspring. Therefore an individual genetic trait would gradually become diluted after generations of intermingled genes. Charles Darwin had demonstrated, with various examples of persisting traits, that heredity does not necessarily blend, but Galton referred to the threat of "regression toward a mean" and stood behind his mathematical authority.

Galton's interest in "individual differences" led him to attempt a mathematical analysis of the sensory functions. He assumed that mental ability was based on the rate at which these functions were performed, and he devised intelligence tests that essentially measured perceptual acuity and speed. These indicated little about a subject's intelligence and were soon replaced by a number of other models.

Biometrics later found uses outside the field of genetics, for example as a research tool in clinical experimentation and ecological study. As such it is now considered a legitimate part of statistics, and Galton is credited with pioneering a number of other statistical concepts that are still widely accepted. He also contributed techniques for studying large populations as a whole, a field known as prosopography. This study led to important investigations in the sociology of medicine and biology. In the course of his investigations in heredity Galton also raised interesting points in the area of color blindness, mental imagery, and the value of twins in the study of his favorite contest, nature vs. nurture.

Luigi Galvani 1737–1798

The earliest report of electrical phenomena dates back to 600 B.C., when Thales of Miletus observed the static charge produced by rubbing amber with a cloth; but electrical function in living matter was not contemplated until the late eighteenth century, when Italian physicist and physiologist Luigi Galvani discovered the electrical properties of the nervous system. Best remembered for his role in the discovery of current electricity, Galvani lent his name to a number of terms used in electrical science.

He was born and raised in Bologna, where he pursued doctoral studies concurrently in medicine and philosophy. Receiving degrees in both disciplines in 1759, he embarked on an equally hectic professional schedule in which he divided his time among medical and surgical practices, laboratory research, and teaching at the University of Bologna.

Concentrating in his initial inquiries on various aspects of anatomy, Galvani conducted a number of important investigations over the next ten years, most notably on the structure and pathology of bones and the comparative anatomical structure of the ear in different species of birds.

In the 1770s he shifted the emphasis of his research to animal physiology, with particular attention to the muscles and nerves and the phenomenon of irritability. Inspired by contemporary studies of electrical nerve stimulation, Galvani launched a series of experiments in 1780 using frogs to examine the effects of stimulating nervous tissue by static electricity. His subjects were actually units of dissected parts of frogs, comprising only nerves and muscles of the lower limbs and a spinal cord.

By that time he had settled down as professor-adjunct in anatomy at the university, curator and demonstrator of its anatomical museum and a happily married gentleman of Bologna. Legend has it that he and his wife, Lucia, would regularly hold dinner parties at which Galvani delighted in performing his frog experiments as a form of postprandial entertainment. At one of these soirees he reportedly placed a "frog preparation" on the dining table, wiring one of the feet to the inside of a nearby well and the spinal cord to a metal rod on the balcony. Anticipating the approach of a thunderstorm, Galvani hurriedly called his guests to the table just in time to observe the first flash of lightning and the synchronized muscle twitch of a dissected frog.

Demonstrating that nervous activity in the muscle can be induced by experimental electrical charges, Galvani established the discipline of scientific investigation known as electrophysiology. Unfortunately, Galvani's experimental results began to lead him astray, and by the mid-1780s he had formulated a theory of "animal electricity," which postulated the generation of electricity within nervous tissue. However misguided, the idea inspired Italian physicist Alessandro Volta to invent an electric battery in the process of discrediting Galvani's theory. Volta effectively disproved the existence of animal electricity in 1792, but the notion lingered into the nineteenth century.

Shortly after Lucia died in 1790 Galvani fell on hard times politically, academically and financially. For refusing to sign an oath of loyalty to Napoleon's Cisalpine Republic he was forced to resign from his academic posts. He died alone and impoverished at the age of 61.

Sir Archibald Edward Garrod 1857–1936

Archibald Garrod belonged to a family distinguished in a number of scientific areas. His father was Sir Alfred Baring Garrod, a prominent nineteenth-century English physician and authority on gout. His daughter was the archeologist Dorothy Garrod, who headed a number of expeditions and excavations and is noted as the first female professor at Cambridge (1939). However, Archibald is perhaps the best-known member of the Garrod family, for his pioneer research in the area of inherited metabolic disorders.

Garrod studied at Oxford and in 1920 became the university's regius professor of medicine. He studied rheumatism and the chemical and metabolic nature of a number of rare and congenital abnormalities. In 1902, in a discussion of the disease alkaptonuria, he suggested the idea that every gene precipitates the synthesis of a particular enzyme. This concept, now known as the "one gene—one enzyme theory," was not fully developed until the work of G.W. BEADLE and E.L. TATUM several decades later.

In 1909 his book *Inborn Errors of Metabolism* was hailed as a breakthrough in the field of congenital metabolic disease. It was reprinted in 1923 and again in 1963. The book described a series of inherited biochemical disorders caused by the absence of an enzyme that, in turn, prevented a particular metabolic process from taking place. The result was a specific pathological condition such as alkaptonuria or cystinuria. Ivor Flling (1888–1973) later described this same metabolic process in his analysis of phenylketonuria.

Garrod was knighted in 1918 and acted as vice president of the Royal Society from 1926 to 1928.

Herbert Spencer Gasser 1888–1963

Using a cathode-ray oscillograph, Herbert Spencer Gasser and his mentor JOSEPH ERLANGER demonstrated that the speed of nerve impulses was a function of the thickness of the transmitting nerve fiber. They also described the basic differences between sensory and motor nerves. For this work Gasser and Erlanger were given the Nobel Prize for Physiology or Medicine in 1944.

Gasser was born in Wisconsin and received B.A. and M.A. degrees from the University of Wisconsin before attending Johns Hopkins Medical School. He graduated in 1915 and the following year joined Washington University in St. Louis, where he began the collaboration and research that would win him a Nobel Prize.

Gasser and Erlanger began studying the electrophyiology of nerves, working together in St. Louis until 1931, when Gasser transferred to Cornell University Medical Center to teach physiology. Four years later he was invited to direct the Rockefeller Institute for Medical Research, and he held the post until 1953. In that time Gasser and Erlanger continued their research and, in 1937, published their findings in *Electrical Signs of Nervous Activity*.

John Gibbon 1903–1971

Poet-turned-surgeon John Gibbon introduced the first model of the heart-lung machine, an apparatus designed to perform the functions of the heart and lung in a cardiac patient during surgery.

Gibbon was born in Philadelphia, where for four generations the men of his family had been surgeons. Convinced by his father to follow in the family tradition, John Gibbon abandoned his aspirations as a poet and dutifully attended Princeton University and Thomas Jefferson Medical College, where his father was professor of surgery. After obtaining his degree in 1927 Gibbon left for Boston to serve as a research fellow at Massachussetts General Hospital. It was there that he met a medical technician who would become his wife and research partner.

For nineteen years they worked together to develop a method by which open-heart surgery could be performed without interrupting the patient's flow of blood. Seeking to delegate the functions of the heart and lungs during surgery, the Gibbons devised a "heart-lung machine" in which the patient's blood is "by-passed" or circulated outside the body to be oxygenated and cleansed of carbon dioxide. The apparatus causes the blood to spread out into a thin sheet and pass across stainless steel screens in an atmosphere of oxygen. Christening their machine the "Queen Mary" (in honor of Mrs. Gibbon), the couple achieved success in 1953, when they operated on an eighteen-year-old girl to repair an atrial septal defect, a large hole between the left and right chambers of the heart.

Using the machine in open-heart surgery at Thomas Jefferson University Hospital in Philadelphia, Gibbon and a team of surgeons were able to effectively repair the damaged heart of a patient, who made a complete recovery. Subsequent attempts to use Gibbon's model were unsuccessful, however, and before he was able to perfect the system of oxygenation a simpler and more dependable heart-lung machine was introduced by C. Walton Lillehei* in 1955. Recognized nevertheless as a pioneer in the field of open-heart surgery, Gibbon was one of four American surgeons to receive the Annual Gairdner Foundation International Award in 1960.

Walter Gilbert 1932–

The winner of the 1980 Nobel Prize for Chemistry, molecular biologist Walter Gilbert developed a method for analyzing the chemical composition of the four subunits of DNA (deoxyribonucleic acid). The subunits of DNA, known as bases, are repeated in various combinations many thousands of times along the strands of DNA molecules, formulating a message in a universal genetic code. RNA (ribonucleic acid) translates the encoded message, relaying it to the ribosomes, which produce proteins according to the genetic instructions expressed by the base sequences in the DNA.

Gilbert shared the Nobel Prize with PAUL BERG and FREDERICK SANGER, who, in independent research, had also developed a technique for determining the structure of large segments of DNA. This revolutionary advance enabled the artificial manufacture of a gene for producing any protein for which the chemical structure is known.

As founder and part owner of Biogen, a Swiss-based company specializing in DNA technology, Gilbert recognized the enormous commercial potential in his findings. The capability of mass-producing such substances as insulin or interferon provided what he called "social rewards" as well as the "fun of building a large industrial structure from something I do."

A native of Boston, Massachussetts, Gilbert received his master's degree from Harvard University in 1954. After earning his doctorate at Cambridge University Gilbert returned to Harvard three years later as a post-doctoral fellow. He remained at the university, becoming professor of microbiology in 1968. The recipient of a number of prestigious fellowships and prizes, Gilbert received the Albert Lasker Basic Science Award in 1979.

Sir Harold Deif Gillies 1882–1960

Harold Gillies gained distinction as a pioneer in the development of plastic surgery as a recognized branch of medicine. In 1918 Gillies became the first physician to specialize in this field, later serving as attending plastic surgeon at a number of London hospitals and in service to the Royal Air Force.

The youngest son of amateur astronomer Robert Gillies, Harold and his five brothers were raised in Dunedin, New Zealand. Robert received his medical education at Cambridge, completing a clinical internship at the celebrated St. Bartholomew's Hospital, where he developed an interest in otorhinolaryngology, the study of the physiology and pathology of the ear, nose and throat.

Notorious for spirited antics and practical jokes, Gillies rarely resisted an opportunity to deflate pomposity, a pleasure frequently provided by his colleagues. He may have inherited this waggish spirit from his granduncle, the poet-artist Edward Lear. Gillies's enthusiasm was expressed in a wide range of other nonscientific interests that he avidly pursued throughout his life. A world-class golfer, he won the St. George's Grand Challenge Cup in 1913. He also distinguished himself as a cricket player, a noted fisherman, and a respected artist whose oil paintings were exhibited during his life and posthumously at several London galleries.

In 1915, as a member of the Royal Army Medical Corps, he was sent to France, where he was deeply impressed by the advanced techniques of reconstruction skillfully performed by French and German surgeons. Later that year Gillies convinced British authorities to organize a government-sponsored center for reconstructive surgery, which was established in the southern village of Aldershot. Appointed director of the facility, Gillies gained valuable experience in the medical care and reconstructive treatment of burns, limb injuries and various congenital deformities.

In 1918, at the end of the war, when most of Gillies's staff left Aldershot to return to their families, the center was moved to Queen Mary's Hospital in Sidcup and placed under the auspices of the Ministry of Pensions. Gillies set up private practice and, after a slow start, became widely recognized for his specialized surgical talents.

In 1920 he was made Commander of the British Empire and ten years later was given a knighthood. Summoned to treat the casulties of a chemical explosion in Copenhagen in 1924, Gillies became a hero to the Danes, who named him a commander of the Order of Daneborg.

When war broke out in 1939 Gillies was one of only four qualified plastic surgeons practicing in England. The others were his cousin Archibald McIndoe, fellow New Zealander Rainsford Mowlem, and T.P. Kilner, Gillies's former assistant at Aldershot. Anticipating an immediate influx of patients in need of reconstructive surgery, the group faced the monumental task of training sufficient numbers of surgeons. A facility was soon established at Rooksdown House near Basingstoke, which eventually became a leading center for the study and practice of plastic surgery.

Founded in 1946, the Association of Plastic Surgeons elected Gillies its first president. Two years later he was made an honorary fellow of the American College of Surgeons, and in 1955 he became the first president of the International Plastic Society based in Stockholm, Sweden.

One year after his death in 1960 the *Journal of the American Society of Plastic and Reconstructive Surgery* paid him this tribute: "He was a giant pre-eminent in his chosen field of endeavor. The ideas engendered by his fertile brain...are being spread afar, and generations of plastic surgeons will be affected by what he gave forth to the world"

Francis Glisson 1597–1677

One of the leading anatomists of the seventeenth century, Francis Glisson coined the term "irritability," thereby introducing a doctrine that would remain influential for centuries.

The notion of "irritability," or "sensibility," as the ability to respond to stimulation by contraction had existed since Galen, but it was Glisson who established it as a biological characteristic. Developing and refining his theory over a period of several years, he eventually attributed the principle to almost every part of the body. By 1677 "irritability" was defined by Glisson as the capacity to perceive an irritant and respond by attempting either to attain it or to withdraw from it. Operating independently of the nervous system, the phenomenon could occur in blood as well as muscle, Glisson argued. He suggested that conscious perception, in connection with brain function, could be superseded by a "natural perception" involving motion, appetite and irritability.

Glisson's published writings include treatises on general anatomy and advanced research methodology (*Prolegomena quaedam ad rem anatomicans universe spectantia*, 1654), the physiology of the digestive system (*Tractatus de ventriculo et intestinis hepatis*, 1662), and the structure of the liver (*Anatomica hepatis*, 1654). Describing the liver's vascular network, Glisson refers to *capsula communis*, a sac of fibrous tissue now known as "Glisson's capsule." Other notable writings discuss fermentation, embryogenesis, the nature of congenital disease and the mechanisms of nervous function and blood circulation.

English-born Francis Glisson received a degree in medical studies from Cambridge University in 1634. Maintaining a permanent position at Cambridge as regius professor of physic, Glisson conducted the greater part of his work in London at the Royal College of Physicians. Admitted as a fellow in 1635, he came to be revered as an influential member of that institution, later serving as president from 1667 until 1669.

Glisson and his London colleagues produced a series of studies on various aspects of ricketts, a bone disorder deriving its name from a corruption of the Greek *rhachitis*, an affliction of the spine. Their findings were published in *De Rachitide*, a detailed report on the clinical and anatomical aspects of the disease. Glisson was the author and major contributor to what has been considered a classic work on the subject. The book first appeared in Latin in 1650, and in response to its immediate and widespread popularity an English translation was published a year later.

In his last published work, entitled *Tractatus de natura substantiae energetica (Treatise on the Nature and Substance of Energy)* (1672), Glisson offers a philosophical argument for hylozoism, the belief that all matter is imbued with a life force. Presenting his ideas in the form of a scholastic debate, Glisson cites WILLIAM HARVEY, RENÉ DESCARTES and Francis Bacon (1561–1626) in an attempt to demonstrate the existence of a *vis plastica*—a free-floating gaslike force investing all substance with life.

Committed to the highest standards of scholarship, Glisson included in *Anatomia hepatis* a humble apology for his intellectual meanderings into unchartered fields, referring to "the allurement and sweetness of speculation."

Joseph Goldberger 1874–1929

By establishing the nutritional basis of pellagra Joseph Goldberger may have prevented millions from suffering the devastating and often fatal effects of that disease. Pellagra, meaning "rough skin" in Italian, appears initially as a debilitating malaise followed by weight loss and an agonizing burning sensation throughout the body. Then follows an eruption of symmetrical skin rashes on the hands, arms, ankles and most noticeably on the face, where victims are often branded with a butterfly-shaped rash across the cheeks and nose. Symptoms of mental disorder often accompany these signs.

As with most such fearsome diseases, pellagra has been surrounded by mythology and wild conjecture as to its source, transmission and treatment. Throughout his career in the U.S. Public Health Service Joseph Goldberger waged a crusade not only against the scourge of pellagra but against the conservative minds of the medical establishment, who resisted his findings in the face of considerable scientific evidence.

Goldberger and his family emigrated to the United States from Austria-Hungary when Joseph was six years old. As a child growing up on the Lower East Side of New York City Joseph showed early evidence of an inquiring and facile mind. At eighteen he entered Bellevue Hospital Medical School (now New York University School of Medicine), graduating with honors by the time he was 21. Four years later he entered the Public Health Service, where for the next three decades he distinguished himself as a bold and tireless campaigner for disease prevention.

As a member of a medical expedition to combat yellow fever in Mexico Goldberger contracted the disease himself. His recovery granted him immunity from the disease, allowing him to safely investigate the disease in Mexico, Puerto Rico, Mississippi, Georgia and Louisiana. In investigating pellagra he was frequently to use his own body for experimental demonstrations—what he called "filth parties"—where he would self-inject the blood of pellagra patients and ingest samples of their skin, feces and urine. Although temporarily sickening, the results of the "filth parties" contributed dramatically to Goldberger's array of evidence against the notion that pellagra was a communicable disease. Recent bacteriological revelations on the infectious properties of syphilis, diphtheria, typhoid and other diseases had inspired a number of medical researchers to search for the "Streptobacillus pellagrae," a mythical microorganism imagined to be the etiological agent of pellagra.

Based on his own field observation throughout the southern United States, Goldberger concluded that the disease could only be attributed to a fundamental deficiency in the prevailing diet among the Southern poor. In the one-crop cotton economy of the South little thought was given to raising vegetables or livestock for one's own consumption. (Pigs, requiring little space and no special feed, were an exception.)

Based on controlled dietary experiments at a number of Southern orphanages where pellagra was rampant, Goldberger observed that when meat and milk were added to the children's diet pellagra symptoms disappeared and no new outbreaks occurred. In Mississippi he conducted the famous Rankin Farm Experiment, an innovative if controversial study, using prison inmates as subjects on a "pellagra squad."

They were offered full pardons in exchange for their participation in a six-month experiment in which Goldberger would attempt to induce pellagra by controlling their diet. The results confirmed Goldberger's nutritional theory, although they did little to advance his standing in the eyes of the medical establishment or southern farmers. In 1916 the pellagra victims in the southern United States were estimated at 100,000.

During World War I Goldberger devoted several years to a statistical study of the Southern economy as it related to pellagra. His theories gradually won public acceptance, particularly in the North, but it was not until 1927 that the Southern Medical Association formally altered its position, conceding that pellagra is "intimately bound up with the economic factors influencing the character of the food supply."

The following year,in an address to the American Dietetic Association, Goldberger commented, "The problem of pellagra is in the main a problem of poverty." By that time Goldberger had already begun to trace the biochemical bases of his findings, suspecting that amino acids were a critical nutritional element. Carl Voegtlin had determined that yeast was effective in treating pellagra patients, and he and Goldberger were convinced that the pellagra-preventive factor (P-P) was to be found in vitamin B.

After Goldberger's death from cancer in 1929 work continued on the search for the P-P factor. Confirming his initial suspicions, the factor was discovered in nicotinic acid, a variant of Vitamin B. When riboflavin, another B-vitamin variant, was later included as a final component in the P-P factor, it was named vitamin G—for Goldberger.

Joseph Leonard Goldstein 1940–

While studying the process of cholesterol metabolism Joseph Goldstein and his partner MICHAEL BROWN made a discovery that provided new insight into the prevention and management of diseases related to the accumulation of cholesterol. Their cellular research revealed the existence of molecules capable of extracting cholesterol from the blood and carrying it into the cell.

Goldstein received his medical degree in 1966 from the Southwestern Medical School of the University of Texas. He conducted research in the field of biomedical genetics at the National Heart Institute from 1968 to 1970, followed by two more years of research at the University of Washington in Seattle. Returning to the University of Texas in 1972, Goldstein began his collaboration with Brown in laboratories at the Texas Health Science Center in Dallas. Investigating the genetic factors involved in high blood cholesterol levels, Goldstein and Brown compared the healthy cells to those of patients with hypercholesterolemia, an inherited tendency toward abnormally high levels of cholesterol. In exploring the physiological expression of this genetic defect they discovered the existence of cholesterol-seeking molecules known as low-density lipoprotein (LDL) receptors, which must remove cholesterol particles from the bloodstream before they can be broken down. Goldstein and Brown found that patients with this trait are lacking or deficient in these receptors and therefore unable to dispose of the cholesterol they ingest. This breakthrough gave rise to new ideas about diet and drugs in the prevention and treatment of strokes, heart attacks and other diseases caused by the clogging of arteries due to accumulated fatty cholesterol. For their significant contribution to the medical understanding of cholesterol metabolism Goldstein and Brown were awarded the Nobel Prize for Physiology or Medicine in 1985.

Robert Alan Good 1922–

Robert Alan Good was head of the pathology department and professor of pediatric medicine at the University of Minnesota Medical School. He focused his attention on pediatric immunology and demonstrated the governing role of the thymus gland in the immune system. From these studies Good developed and introduced the technique of bone-marrow transplant. This form of therapy is still considered experimental but has already been used with some success to treat a number of different forms of cancer in advanced stages. Good was chief of the Sloan-Kettering Institute for Cancer Research from 1973 to 1980.

Ernest William Goodpasture 1886–1960

Among the most significant advances in modern research methodology was Ernest Goodpasture's invention of a practical technique for growing mass quantities of sterile virus cultures.

By the 1930s bacteriologists had been steadily producing immunization vaccines for a growing number of bacterial diseases, but virologists had yet to overcome a major obstacle in the battle against viral disease. Because they will only survive and reproduce in living cells of a specific host, viruses were elusive experimental subjects. The only existing immunizing agents against viral diseases were EDWARD JENNER'S smallpox vaccine and LOUIS PASTEUR'S rabies vaccine, but these discoveries had succeeded by pure luck in circumventing the frustrating properties of viruses.

As a pathologist whose primary interest was in pathogenesis—the development of diseases—Goodpasture sought to investigate the mechanism of fowlpox, a viral disease related to human smallpox that is characterized by ulcerous nodules around the beak of the bird. In collaboration with distinguished colleagues Alice and Eugene Woodruff, Goodpasture sought to cultivate the fowlpox virus in a fertile egg. As a living host in its own bacteriologically sterile environment, the embryonic chick seemed uniquely valuable as an experimental tool. Noting that pox viruses are generally found in the skin, Goodpasture suspected that viruses were not only host-specific, but cell-specific as well. He therefore suggested that the virus be introduced in the outermost layer of the chorioallantois, the membranous sac that surrounds the chick embryo.

In 1931, after a long series of experimental refinements and innovative methods calling on all their talent, Goodpasture and Eugene and Alice Woodruff finally managed to produce a large quantity of uncontaminated fowlpox virus. A pivotal step in virology research, their discovery of a practical, inexpensive and sterile environment for the cultivation of viruses made possible enormous advances in immunological medicine.

Born on a tobacco farm in Tennessee, Goodpasture entered the recently founded medical school at Johns Hopkins in 1908, becoming a disciple of distinguished bacteriologist and pathologist WILLIAM HENRY WELCH, one of the four original faculty members who helped establish the school's international prominence. Receiving his medical degree in 1912, Goodpasture remained at Johns Hopkins to serve under Welch as an instructor and research fellow. After his marriage in 1915 Goodpasture and his wife moved to Boston, where he joined the faculty at the Peter Bent Brigham Hospital at Harvard Medical School.

Following military service in World War I he studied briefly in Vienna, where he began to develop a theory of the pathogenesis of rabies. Comparing the mechanism of the disease to that of herpes simplex, Goodpasture suggested that both diseases reach the spinal cord and the brain by traveling along a path of nerve cells.

He returned to the United States in 1922, taking over as director of the Singer Memorial Research Laboratory in Pennsylvania. Two years later he accepted the chairmanship of the pathology laboratory at Vanderbilt University School of Medicine in Nashville, Tennessee. It was in 1927, with the arrival of Eugene and Alice Woodruff, that Goodpasture embarked on the historic research that would ensure him an honored place in the history of medicine.

Goodpasture went on to investigate the wide range of applications of this new method of virus cultivation at the Louisiana State University School of Medicine, where he and Alice Woodruff were joined by enthusiastic laboratory assistant Gerritt John Buddingh, who had dropped out of medical school in order to participate in Goodpasture's research with chick embryos. Demonstrating that cowpox and cold-sore viruses could be cultured in chick embryos, Goodpasture and his colleagues created the first "chick vaccine" in 1933. Using Goodpasture's technique of mass cultivation of viruses, immunologists soon developed vaccines against a number of life-threatening diseases, including influenza, yellow fever and typhus.

Continuing to teach pathology at Vanderbilt until 1955, Goodpasture also served as dean of the medical school from 1945 to 1950. Among his distinguished colleagues and research partners was bacteriologist Katherine Anderson, with whom he performed chick embryo experiments using a number of viruses. Their collaborative research included studies on diphtheria, meningitis, shingles, rabies, plague, typhus and mumps. Anderson and Goodpasture were married in 1945, five years after the death of his first wife.

Named professor emeritus upon his retirement from the university at 69, Goodpasture served as director of the department of pathology at the Armed Forces Institute of Pathology, based at Walter Reed Army Medical Center in Washington, D.C. After four years he returned to Tennessee, spending the last year of his life living in a cottage in the hills of Montgomery County, not far from where he was born and raised.

William Crawford Gorgas 1854–1920

Wiliam Crawford Gorgas is remembered primarily for his ground-breaking work in the control of yellow fever.

In 1898 a valiant group of American doctors set sail for Cuba on a mission that would have a profound effect on both medical and political history. Yellow fever or "Yellow Jack" had been the scourage of the tropics throughout the nineteenth century. In 1882 work on the Panama Canal had to be abandoned because the disease was rampant in many of the construction areas. Evidence suggested that the disease was spread by mosquitoes, and the American Army Board, led by WALTER REED, was sent to Havana to investigate.

James Carroll was a member of the board and was the first to volunteer to be infected with this devasting disease in order to better understand its transmission. There followed many experiments, many human volunteers and a number of casualties before the board determined how the disease could be spread and, by extension, how it could be curbed.

William C. Gorgas graduated Bellevue Medical College in 1879 and immediately joined the U.S. Army Medical Corps. While stationed at Fort Brown, Texas he contracted yellow fever and recovered. He was thereafter immune to the disease and, in 1898, was sent to Havana to serve as chief sanitary officer. There he encountered Carlos J. Finlay, a local physician who had also been studying the nature of yellow fever. Finlay and Reed confirmed the role of the mosquito in spreading this disease, and Gorgas began a massive campaign to rid his territory of infection. He isolated all yellow fever patients, carefully protecting them from any contact with mosquitoes. He reasoned that if no mosquito came in contact with the disease, then none could transmit it. Within three months Havana, for the first time in history, was completely rid of the disease.

In 1904 Gorgas brought his methods to the Isthmus of Panama, where he worked on controlling both yellow fever and malaria. In spite of enormous logistical and administrative obstacles he succeeded in eliminating yellow fever from the Canal Zone, permitting construction to resume. General health conditions in the area improved tremendously, particularly in the cities of Colon and Panama, and in 1915 Gorgas completed a book on the subject called *Sanitation in Panama*.

Gorgas was called upon by disease-infested countries around the world to help with problems of sanitation and prevention. In Guayaquil, Ecuador he brought about remarkable progress in an area that had been plagued by yellow fever for many years.

Gorgas served as United States Surgeon General from 1914 to 1916 and was responsible for the organization of medical personnel during World War I. From 1916 until his death Gorgas worked in association with the International Health Board.

Norman McAlister Gregg 1892–1966

Norman Gregg discovered that rubella, or German measles, during a pregnancy could result in congenital abnormalities in the eyes, ears and heart. In 1940 he was practicing ophthalmology in Australia when he observed a group of children who had been afflicted with cataracts since birth. Gregg investigated and found that each mother had contracted rubella during her pregnancy. Armed with this remarkable clue, Gregg went on to determine the potential effects of the disease on an embryo. Until that time it had been assumed that only a defect in the genetic mechanism could cause such abnormalities.

This discovery, showing for the first time that environmental factors could cause congenital abnormalities, changed forever the prevailing attitudes toward genetic irregularities. Prevention became a possibility and a priority for the first time. Shortly after Gregg's revelations a diagnostic test for rubella and a vaccine were produced. The campaign for prenatal care took hold rapidly, particularly in Adelaide, Australia and in Boston, Massachusetts. Prevention programs directed toward young girls and pregnant women greatly reduced the incidence of rubella-induced congenital disease and improved overall health in mothers and children.

Emil Hermann Grubbe 1875–1960

American physicist and physician Emil Grubbe was among the earliest pioneers of radiology and the application of X rays for the treatment of disease. Unaware of the powerful effects of the invisible, odorless, silent ray, Grubbe exposed himself to prolonged and extensive radiation in the course of his research and practice and, like many other early investigators, suffered extensive radiation damage to his hands and face, which eventually led to several severe forms of cancer.

Born in Chicago, Grubbe obtained degrees in pharmacology, chemistry and physics from Valparaiso University in Indiana. Several months before he completed his doctorate work, in the winter of 1895, WILHELM RÖNTGEN announced his sensational discovery of a new kind of ray at the University of Würzburg. Grubbe, who was already involved in experimentation and manufacture of vacuum tubes, immediately began to produce X rays with his own tubes.

Within weeks he developed a severe form of dermatitis on his left hand and was referred to noted physician Dr. J.E. Gillman for a consultation. Gillman was intrigued by Grubbe's work in radiology, and the two discussed the possibility of a therapeutic effect from X-ray exposure. Among Gillman's patients was a woman suffering from recurring breast cancer, and in a desperate attempt to relieve her extreme pain he referred her to Grubbe for treatment. On January 29, 1896, less than a month after Röntgen's historic lecture, Grubbe gained his own place in the history of medicine as the first practitioner of radiation therapy.

Other physicians soon began to prescribe X-ray treatment, generally to reduce the severe pain of various forms of cancer. A number of patients were treated by Grubbe, who documented each case in a series of detailed reports. Focusing his attention on the medical aspects of radiology, he entered the General Medical College in Chicago in 1896 and obtained his degree two years later.

Though radiation quickly took its place as a fundamental tool of diagnostic medicine, its therapeutic application remained mainly as a palliative procedure for several decades. Elihu Thomson was the first to demonstrate conclusively the harmful effects of X-ray emissions in the early part of the twentieth century. As medical scientists came to understand the nature of radiation damage and the particular vulnerability of young, rapidly growing tissue they began to explore ways of directing X rays against malignant tissue to treat various forms of cancer. By the 1940s radiotherapy had made significant advances, most notably with the advent of radioactive isotopes—synthetic chemicals emitting radiation that can be inserted by "radium needle" directly into the cancerous tumor or injected into the bloodstream to be absorbed by the affected organ.

Grubbe's distinguished career in X-ray- and electrotherapeutics spanned more than half a century, during which time he played a significant role in the design and development of clinical radiology facilities and the establishment of hospital radiology departments. Once the dangers of X-ray exposure were recognized, he pioneered a number of protective measures, including the use of lead shields, in radiology practice and research.

A founding member of the Radiological Society, he served as president of the National Society of Physical Therapeutics and member of a great many other professional associations, including the National Academy of Sciences, the American Association of Cancer Research, and the Association of Approved Radiology. After accepting a postgraduate degree from the Chicago College of Medicine and Surgery in 1910 he joined the faculty as professor and head of the department of roentgenology and electrotherapeutics.

For his outstanding contribution to the development of radiology Grubbe received a number of honors, including the Walter Reed Society Award in 1952 and the citation scroll of the Chicago Röntgen Society in 1956. In addition to publishing numerous medical articles and monographs, he served as associate editor of the *American Electro-Therapeutic and X-Ray Era* and editor of the *Archives of Electrology and Radiology*. Other notable writings include *X-Ray Treatment—Its Origin, Birth, and Early History* (1949).

Roger Charles Louis Guillemin 1924–

For his investigation of the hormones produced by the hypothalamus Roger Guillemin was awarded the 1977 Nobel Prize for Physiology or Medicine, which he shared with ANDREW SCHALLY and ROSALYN YALOW. The Nobel Committe hailed the three researchers as having "laid the foundations of modern hypothalamic research."

The hypothalamic hormones act by regulating the secretions of the anterior pituitary gland, a small organ located at the base of the brain. Functioning as the "master gland" of the body, the pituitary gland secretes hormones that control the glands governing sexual and reproductive activity; the adrenal glands, associated with the regulation of stress and emotional response; and the thyroid gland, which is responsible for adaptation to heat and cold. Establishing the role of the brain as a master control center for the complex chemical functions of the body, Guillemin's research combined principles of neurology and endocrinology to develop a single unified discipline of neuroendocrinology.

Born in Dijon, Guillemin fought with the French Resistance during World War II. After receiving his medical degree at the University of Lyons in 1949 he emigrated to Canada to join the staff of the Institute of Medicine and Surgery at the University of Montreal as a research assistant under Hans Selye, a leading authority on endocrinology and adaptation to stress.

In 1953 Guillemin was appointed assistant professor at Baylor College of Medicine in Houston, Texas, where he and Schally launched their collaborative study of the regulatory mechanisms involved in pituitary gland secretions. These controls involved substances released by the hypothalamus, which could be studied in infinitesimal concentrations found in brain tissue. To obtain the enormous amounts of brain tissue necessary for their investigation Guillemin and Schally accumulated more than 5 million sheep brains, handling more than 45 tons of brain tissue in the course of seven years of research.

In 1960, while serving as professor of physiology and endocrinology at Baylor, Guillemin also accepted an appointment as associate director of the department of experimental endocrinology at the Collège de France in Paris. By 1968 he and other researchers in the field had isolated one of the substances released by the hypothalamus, initially identified as "thyrotropin-releasing factor" or TRF. The substance became known as TRH once it was shown to be a hormone. TRH stimulates the pituitary gland to release thyrotropin, a hormone that acts on the thyroid, which in turn releases its own hormone.

In 1970 Guillemin left Baylor University to establish the Laboratories for Neuroendocrinology at the Salk Institute in San Diego, where he continues to study the biochemical and physiological effects of hypothalamic hormones. His research team discovered and synthesized somatostatin, a substance that appears to influence several biological functions, including the production of insulin.

Allvar Gullstrand 1862–1930

An important researcher in the field of ophthalmology, Allvar Gullstrand was a professor at the University of Uppsala in his native Sweden. He applied physical mathematics to the study of optics and light refraction, an innovative approach that yielded valuable information about the process of light refraction in the eye. Gullstrand also examined the structure and mechanism of the cornea, improving a system of measuring astigmatism and determining corneal defects.

Along with his theoretical discoveries and refinements, Gullstrand's achievement extended to practical inventions in the field of clinical ophthalmology. Now considered indispensable to any ophthalmic examination, his slit-lamp and reflex-free ophthalmoscope permit the physician a detailed view of the anterior section of the eye. Gullstrand also made significant improvements in the corrective lenses used by patients after cataract surgery.

For his contribution to the advancement of practical and theoretical ophthalmology Allvar Gullstrand was awarded the Nobel Prize in Physiology and Medicine in 1911.

H

Christian Friedrich Samuel Hahnemann 1755–1843

At the turn of the nineteenth century Samuel Hahnemann formulated a medical doctrine known as homeopathy, based on the ancient principle of "The Law of Similars." The dictum *similia similibus curantur*—"let likes be cured by likes"—dates back to the teachings of HIPPOCRATES. Following this ancient teaching, Hahnemann developed his theory of medicine that he christened homeopathy (from the Greek for "like treatment of disease"). Hahnemann's doctrine was in direct opposition to established medicine, which he referred to as "allopathy"—signifying treatment of disease by "unlike" remedies.

Homeopathy takes as its premise the belief that an organism will respond to any disturbance in a way that permits the least possible damage to it. If that response is inhibited or curtailed by traditional medical treatment, the body will find the next best response under the new set of pathological circumstances. Hahnemann claimed that in removing the symptoms of a disease allopathic treatment merely diverts the expression of the disease to another, more destructive channel. The alleviation of specific symptoms is therefore considered counter-therapeutic by the homeopath, because the system as a whole is not relieved of the disease.

Hahnemann proposed a method of treatment involving the prescription of one or more of his own "non-medicines," which, he claimed sent information directly to the somatic processes, stimulating the body's "native intelligence." Based on pharmacological experimentation, Hahnemann concluded that diseases could be cured by small amounts of substances that produce the symptoms of the disease in healthy people.

Subsequent pharmacological research led Hahnemann to formulate his "Law of the Infinitesimals," which states that the smaller the dose, the more effective the medicine. Hahnemann developed the technique of "succussion," a method of mixing, diluting, and stirring his medications. He claimed that with vigorous shaking a form of dynamic contact occured within the substances, releasing their vital powers. The roots of this concept can be traced to a number of ancient and primitive cultures in which the powers of a medicine were "summoned" in rituals involving shaking, grinding and even the suffocating of birds in pharmaceutical substances. Using his own methods of preparation, Hahnemann found that the greater the dilution, the less severe the initial reaction, and the more complete the eventual healing. Amid a storm of opposition from the medical establishment, this tenet often became a prime target of derision.

Hahnemann was born in Meissen, Germany just before the start of the Seven Years' War in 1763. In 1779 he received his doctorate in medicine from the University of Erlangen, but two years after becoming a physician he gave up his practice, explaining in a letter to a friend that "My sense of duty would not easily allow me to treat the unknown pathological state of my brethren with these unknown medicines. If they are not exactly suitable (and how could the physician know that, since their specific effects had not yet been demonstrated?), they might with their strong potency easily change life into death or induce new disorders and chronic maladies, often more difficult to eradicate than the original disease."

The first intimations of homeopathic theory appear in 1790, in his translation of WILLIAM CULLEN'S celebrated work, *Treatise on Materia Medica.* At the end of a section on the use of cinchona (the source of quinine) in the treatment of malaria Hahnemann sharply criticized Cullen in a footnote while presenting his own findings on the effects.

Hahnemann developed his theory of homeopathy in the years that followed, publishing an article in 1796 entitled "Essay on a New Principle for Ascertaining the Curative Powers of Drugs, and Some Examinations of Previous Principles." In addition to his homeopathic remedies Hahnemann offered other innovative recommendations for the maintenance of good health, including exercise, proper nutrition and fresh air. Anticipating the findings of PASTEUR and JOSEPH LISTER on the mechanism of infection, Hahnemann emphasized the boiling of medical utensils and the isolation of patients with contagious diseases.

In 1810, in the face of general derision, Hahnemann published *Organon,* in which he outlined the theoretical and practical guidelines of homeopathy. He obtained a professorship at the University of Leipzig in 1812, where he taught his doctrine for nine years, until pressure from the medical establishment forced the university to dismiss him.

The most violent reaction to homeopathy came from the Council of Apothecaries, which accused Hahnemann of infringing on their medical domain. By that time Hahnemann had attracted some influential figures, including the intemperate Prince

Schwarzenberg of Austria, a cousin of the King of Saxony. The influence of the prince was short-lived, however. During what was to be his last drinking binge he lost faith in Hahnemann's remedies and allowed a team of physicians to treat him by bloodletting, a medical practice particularly loathsome to Hahnemann. The prince died five weeks later, and the responsibility was placed on Hahnemann. Soon afterward a governmental decree was issued against all unlicensed dispensation of medicines, forcing Hahnemann to leave Leipzig.

In 1821 he retreated to Kothen, where he wrote *The Chronic Diseases, Their Peculiar Nature, and Their Homeopathic Cure,* his second major work, published in 1828. More philosophical than *Organon,* the book discusses the nature of disease from an historic, cultural and spiritual perspective, in addition to its extensive clinical descriptions of symptoms and appropriate homeopathic remedies.

By 1831 a homeopathic movement had emerged, with followers throughout Europe and America. Hahnemann's behavior, however, had become erratic. Denouncing former disciples, his preaching drifted from his original principles. A widower at the age of eighty, he married a French woman of thirty-two who brought Hahnemann to Paris, where she took over his practice.

In Allentown, Pennsylvania an institution for instruction in homeopathic method was founded in 1833, and three years later the Hahnemann Medical College in Philadelphia opened its doors. Although its popularity declined with the enormous advances in pharmocology and bacteriology in the early part of the twentieth century, homeopathy continues to be practiced throughout the world.

John Burdon Sanderson Haldane 1892–1964

"Even the Pope is 70% water," John Haldane said in a characteristically unequivocal expression of egalitarianism. In addition to his important contributions to the fields of genetics and biology, this rebel son of physiologist JOHN SCOTT HALDANE stimulated scientific interest in the layman with his graphic and accessible writings on the fundamental theories and philosophical ramifications of science.

Stating that "Science is vastly more stimulating to the imagination than are the classics," Haldane threw himself into scientific research with a passion, often acting as his own experimental subject. To measure temperature fluctuations in the brain Haldane inserted a thermocouple—an electrical device for measuring such changes—through his own jugular vein and into his brain. In addition to other experimental studies of human physiology, he conducted important research in the field of enzyme kinetics (the rate at which enzymatic reactions proceed).

Applying mathematics to the biological principles of MENDELIAN genetics, Haldane was influential in the development of population genetics, a branch of biology concerned with evolution and the behaviors of populations. Haldane's work, combined with the studies of R.A. Fisher (1892–1964), Sewall Wright (b.1889) and S.S. Chetverikoff (1880–1959), gave rise to the neo-Darwinian evolutionary synthesis that emerged in the mid-1930s. Based on the relative selective values of homozygous and heterozygous genes, Haldane's mathematical demonstrations also elucidated the phenomenon of polymorphism, the occurrence of more than one form of a species in a single habitat. A leading biometrician, Haldane studied rates of mutation and evolutionary change, analyzing the statistical occurrences of hemophilia and color blindness.

Born at Oxford, Haldane received an early introduction to science from his distinguished father, John Scott Haldane. Educated at Eton and Oxford, the younger Haldane served in the Scottish "Black Watch" infantry unit during World War I. He returned to his studies in 1922, becoming a reader of biochemistry at Cambridge University. He remained there until 1933, when London University offered him a professorship in genetics and biometrics.

A committed Marxist and member of the Communist Party, Haldane served as chairman of the editorial board of the *Daily Worker* from 1940 until 1949. He left the newspaper and, a year later, resigned from the party in responses to scientific repression in the Soviet Union.

In protest over British foreign policy in Egypt Haldane left his native country in 1957 and emigrated to India, where he settled permanently and adopted citizenship. He joined the faculty of the Indian Statistical Institute in Calcutta but resigned four years later, objecting to criticism and interference from the Indian goverment. In 1962 he became director of the Orissa State Genetics and Biometry Laboratory, where he remained until his death two years later.

Despite his undisguised political views, Haldane was widely celebrated for his important contributions to science. He was elected to fellowship in the Royal Society in 1932, became a Chevalier of the Légion d'Honneur in 1937 and was awarded the Darwin medal of the Royal Society in 1953 and the Feltrinelli prize for Biology in 1961.

His enormous body of written work includes *Animal Biology,* written with J.S. HUXLEY in 1927, and *Fact and Faith,* published in 1934.

John Scott Haldane 1860–1936

John Scott Haldane conducted pioneer studies on the mechanics of respiration and pulmonary disease. In 1905 he found that the breathing process is regulated by a respiratory center in the brain that responds to the fluctuating concentration of carbon dioxide in the blood. This discovery led to extensive study of the effects of various gases on the respiratory system, particularly such poisons as carbon monoxide.

A pioneer investigator of the health problems of mine workers, Haldane contributed significantly to improving safety conditions in the mines. Analyzing the high incidence of lung disease among miners, Haldane was influential in the improvement and enforced use of safety and rescue equipment.

His studies of physiological adaptations to extreme altitudes and altitude change provided important advances in the fields of mountaineering, aviation, space exploration and deep-sea diving. Introducing the notion of a prolonged period of decompression for the safe ascent from underwater depths, he designed a chamber—now known as "Haldane's chamber"—to prevent "the bends," a painful and potentially fatal condition that occurs when a drastic drop in external pressure causes nitrogen bubbles to form in the body.

The chamber was also used in animal metabolic studies. In order to study the physiological effects of extreme barometric pressure he organized an expedition to Colorado's Pike's Peak (altitude 14,110 feet). Haldane also devised a method for measuring the amount of hemoglobin in circulation that is still used today in the diagnosis of anemia.

Born in Edinburgh, Haldane was the grand-nephew of celebrated English preacher Robert Haldane, who founded the Society for Propagating the Gospel at Home in 1797. John Scott became a fellow in physiology at New College at Oxford in 1888. He continued his research as director of a mining research laboratory in Birmingham, England and later founded the *Journal of Hygiene.*

Haldane's written works include *Organism and Environment* (1917), *New Physiology* (1919), *Respiration* (1922), *The Sciences and Philosophy* (1929), and *The Philosophy of a Biologist* (1936). His son, JOHN BURDON SANDERSON HALDANE, became a distinguished biologist, geneticist and writer.

Albrecht von Haller 1708–1777

Celebrated for his literary talents as well as for his achievements in surgery, anatomy and botany, Albrect von Haller is most widely recognized for his investigation of the nervous system, specifically the nerve fiber. He introduced the notion that a nerve was capable of firing, or sparking the irritable substance of any muscle it contacted, thereby causing a reaction.

Although Haller mistakenly portrayed "irritability" or contractility as a function of muscle fibers and "sensibility"—the conscious recognition of stimulus—as a function of nerve fibers, he served to elucidate the inherent physiological characteristics of nerves and muscles. Haller defined "sensibility" in humans as the seat of the soul, straddling the physical and the spiritual realms, but he attributed mental functions to the brain without reference to metaphysical principles. With this approach his work anticipated the modern view of the interrelationship between the brain cortex and outlying nerve fibers.

Haller also described the mechanism of breathing and elucidated the process of digestion, particularly the role of bile in the metabolism of fats.

A native of Bern, Switzerland, Haller studied medicine at the University of Leyden under the celebrated physician and teacher HERMANN BÖERHAAVE. While pursuing his wide-ranging interests in literature and the sciences Haller established a medical practice in 1729. Seven years later he was invited to join the faculty at the newly founded University of Göttingen, where he established a renowned botanical garden, an anatomical museum and a theater. While continuing to teach in the departments of anatomy, medicine and botany Haller also organized a separate school of obstetrics at Göttingen.

A prolific writer of poetry, prose and technical treatises, Haller was an influential force in the development of Göttingen's distinguished reputation as a center for scientific study. It was during his seventeen years at the university that Haller performed his intensive experimental research on the nervous system, producing his major work, *A Dissertation on the Sensible and Irritable Parts of Animals,* in 1752.

A year after the book's publication Haller returned to Bern, where he continued to experiment and write while participating in public affairs as a magistrate. His enormous body of published works includes an eight-volume treatise on human physiology entitled *Elementa physiologiae corporis humani* (1757–1766), as well as three political romance novels, four major bibliographies of surgery, anatomy, medicine and botany and a volume of lyric poetry entitled *Versuch Schweizerischer Gedichte (Swiss Poem).*

William Stewart Halsted 1852–1922

A member of the original faculty at Johns Hopkins Medical School, American surgeon William Halsted was recognized as a scholarly and meticulous surgeon who contributed important advances in surgical procedure and methodology. Trained in German and Austrian hospitals, Halsted imported the European techniques of asepsis into less-refined American operating rooms. He pioneered the use of white surgical gowns, skullcaps, gauze masks and, most notably, rubber gloves, initially introduced in 1889 to protect the hands of the operating room staff.

In particular, the gloves were meant to protect the hands of Halsted's chief nurse at Johns Hopkins Hospital, Caroline Hampton, whom he married in 1890. She had complained of skin irritation from the caustic antiseptic chemicals in use at the time. As surgical practitioners at Hopkins gradually adopted Halsted's innovation the aseptic benefits to the patient became evident.

Born in New York City, William Halsted attended exclusive private schools in New York and Massachussetts. In 1870, after graduating from Phillips Preparatory Academy in Andover, he entered Yale University as a star athlete with little enthusiasm for academics. Developing an interest in medicine in his senior year, Halsted enrolled in the Columbia College of Physicians and Surgeons. He excelled as a medical student, graduating in 1877 as one of the top ten students of his class.

After postgraduate training in surgery at Bellevue and New York hospitals Halsted spent two years in Europe, where he concentrated on advanced studies in anatomy and basic sciences. He returned to New York in 1880 to join the faculty of the College of Physicians and Surgeons. In addition to maintaining a private surgical practice he held positions as attending physician at five hospitals in the New York area.

In the early 1880s medical researchers had begun to explore the anesthetic properties of cocaine hydrochlorate. Embarking on an investigation in which they used themselves as experimental subjects, Halsted and a number of colleagues and students became addicted to the drug. Several careers were destroyed, and Halsted was hospitalized in Providence, Rhode Island at different intervals for more than fifteen months before he could exorcise the effects of cocaine. In *The Inner History of the Johns Hopkins Hospital* WILLIAM OSLER reported that Halsted was later treated for addiction to morphine in 1898.

In the midst of his battle against cocaine Halsted moved to Baltimore, where he accepted a research position in the laboratory of distinguished pathologist William H. Welch. The benevolent Welch was sympathetic and protective toward Halsted throughout his ordeal, and by 1892 the two influential physicians were appointed the first department heads of Johns Hopkins Medical School.

Once aggressive and energetic, Halsted was considerably subdued by his experience, methodically performing his duties at Hopkins at a painstakingly slow pace that infuriated some of his colleagues. Despite their annoyance, Halsted established standards of surgical precision that were widely admired, earning him a reputation as the "bloodless surgeon," a reference to his extreme gentleness in handling tissue and his tireless attention to every bleeding vessel, no matter how minute. In a letter to Harvey Cushing his brother Edward wrote of Halsted, "There is no surgeon like him in the land, his aseptic technique is perfect, and the scientific manner of his work, keeping at it from the laboratory side simultaneously with his clinical and operative work, is a revelation to man."

Although at great price to himself, Halsted derived significant findings from his experiments with cocaine in the development of neuroregional anesthetic procedures in which cocaine is injected into specific nerves. He is also known for his introduction of a radical form of mastectomy in the treatment of breast cancer, largely based on the refinement of earlier operative techniques.

Other innovations in surgical procedure include a radical treatment for the most common form of hernia, and a technique for thyroidectomy developed out of extensive experimental research on the thyroid and parathyroid glands.

After undergoing surgical removal of his gall bladder in 1919 the ailing and jaundiced Halsted died on the operating table three years later.

Alice Hamilton 1869–1970

American physician and social reformer Alice Hamilton pioneered the study of occupational medicine in the United States, establishing important principles in industrial hygiene and safety. Traveling across the country, Hamilton worked in factories, mines and ammunition plants to investigate firsthand the health hazards faced by the American work force. Tirelessly crusading for the rights of men and women in blue-collar jobs, Hamilton was a key figure in the enactment of workers' compensation laws and the reform of public health policies.

The second of five children, Hamilton was born in New York City but spent her childhood in Fort Wayne, Indiana. Encouraged by her family to pursue her interest in science, she received her medical degree from the University of Michigan in 1893. Following internships at Women's Hospitals in Minneapolis and Boston she continued her training at the universities of Leipzig and Munich, where German authorities agreed to suspend the limitations they imposed on women in higher education provided that she remain "unobtrusive."

Returning to the United States to continue studies at Johns Hopkins Medical School, she accepted an appointment as professor of pathology at the Woman's Medical School of Northwestern University in 1897. As a part of Chicago's burgeoning movement for social reform, Hamilton established that city's first health clinic for infant care in 1899. When the Women's Medical School closed three years later she joined the staff at the Memorial Institute for Infectious Diseases, serving under noted pathologist Ludwig Hektoen.

Investigating Chicago's devastating typhoid epidemic in the fall of 1902, Hamilton called attention to the importance of insects in the transmission of the disease. Her work contributed significantly to a massive reorganization of the city's health department.

Appalled at conditions she had found in factories and steel mills, Hamilton campaigned for the right to safe working conditions for all industrial workers. In 1910, when the country's first Commission for Occupational Disease was assembled in Illinois, Hamilton was elected to membership on the board. She later became its managing director. It was through the efforts of the commission that Illinois became the first state to pass a law establishing the responsibility of employers to compensate workers for injuries suffered at the workplace. Subsequently Hamilton was asked by the federal government to continue her surveys at a national level.

Her zeal for reform led her into the pacifist movement, participating, along with Jane Addams, in the peace conference of the International Congress of Women at The Hague in 1915. The U.S. government retained Hamilton's services even after the United States entered World War I, commissioning her to investigate labor conditions in the munitions industry.

In 1919 Hamilton accepted the position of assistant professor of industrial medicine at Harvard Medical School, becoming the faculty's first woman member. She remained at Harvard until 1935, when she was granted the status of professor emeritus. As the only woman appointed to the Health Committee of the League of Nations, Hamilton studied industrial hygiene in the Soviet Union and Germany. As a delegate to the International Congress on Occupational Accidents and Diseases, she returned to Germany in 1938 to investigate the impact on industrial health of the Nazi regime.

Many of Hamilton's writings are still considered classic reference works in the study of occupational medicine, most notably *Industrial Poisons in the United States* (1925), *Industrial Toxicology* (1934), and an autobiographical work entitled *Exploring the Dangerous Trades* (1943).

Gerhard Henrik Armauer Hansen 1841–1912

In 1873 Norwegian microbiologist Gerhard Hansen discovered *Mycobacterium leprae*, the leprosy bacillus. Hansen's finding was historic for reasons beyond its significance to the fight against leprosy. As the first identification of a bacteria as the causative agent of a chronic human disease, his study was a precursor to ROBERT KOCH'S conclusive demonstration of the bacterial cause of anthrax three years later. Although Hansen was unable to cultivate the leprosy bacillus in vitro as an experimental confirmation of his hypothesis, his research helped to establish fundamental principles in immunology, bacteriological medicine and public health policy.

One of fifteen children, Hansen was born and raised in Bergen, Norway, where his father worked as a cashier in a bank. Hansen worked his way through college and medical school, graduating with honors from the University of Christiania (now Oslo) in 1866. Returning home to fulfill internship requirements at the National Hospital in Christiania, he launched his medical practice in Lofoten, a string of islands off the northern coast of Norway, where he served as community physician to 6,000 fishermen.

In 1868 Hansen accepted a position in Bergen's leprosy care program, which had been organized by Daniel Cornelius Danielssen to service the city's leprosy hospitals. Bergen was recognized as the European center for leprosy research, mainly as a result of Danielssen's efforts and his distinction as a foremost authority on the pathological and clinical aspects of the disease. He mistakenly adhered to the prevailing medical theory, however, that leprosy was an inherited condition, a belief he continued to hold even after Hansen's discovery.

Based on the evidence of various epidemiological studies of leprosy, Hansen was certain that the disease was not a congenital disorder but rather the result of a specific etiological factor. In 1870 he obtained a grant to visit institutes in Germany and Austria for advanced training in histopathology, the study of diseased tissues.

During his stay in Vienna Hansen was introduced to the teachings of Charles Darwin and discovered in Darwinian doctrine a scientific ideal, particularly in its methodology of dispassionate investigation. Unfazed by accusations of blasphemy, Hansen became a leading spokesman for the dissemination of Darwinism. He delivered lectures, published articles and, in 1886, wrote the first defense of Darwin to be published in Norwegian.

On his return to Bergen in 1871 Hansen launched his search for the causative agent of leprosy, using biopsy specimens drawn from patients, and within the next two years he had observed the rod-shaped bacterial bodies now referred to as *Myobacterium leprae* or Hansen's bacilli. In an effort to remove the age-old stigma that had marked leprosy and its victims, the term "Hansen's disease" has been introduced, along with "hansenarium" to replace "leprosarium."

As Norway's leprosy medical officer, Hansen initiated a number of public health policies that drastically reduced the nationwide incidence of the disease from 1,760 known cases in 1875 to 575 twenty-five years later. The Norwegian Leprosy Act of 1877 and the amended act of 1885 empowered health authorities to impose precautionary isolation of leprosy victims to prevent the disease from infecting entire families.

Despite his unpopular advocacy of Darwinian doctrine, Hansen was widely acclaimed for his contribution to the study of leprosy, serving as honorary chairman of the International Leprosy Committee. In 1897 he was named chairman of the First International Conference on Leprosy, held in Berlin, and twelve years later was elected president of a second such conference in Bergen.

Haldan Keffer Hartline 1903–1983

Haldan Hartline isolated single nerve fibers from the eyes of frogs and horseshoe crabs and studied their individual reactions to light. Revealing the complex interaction of light receptor cells (rods and cones), his investigations led to a better understanding of how humans and animals see. Hartline demonstrated that it is the interconnection of nerve fibers and receptor cells that enables the eye to sharpen its focus and to differentiate between movement and form.

In 1931 Hartline began teaching neurophysiology at the University of Pennsylvania. He left for Johns Hopkins University in 1949, and he taught there for four years. He then joined the Rockefeller Institute (now Rockefeller University), where he continued to teach and research. His studies of the physiology of the eye were honored in 1967 with the Nobel Prize in Physiology or Medicine, which he shared with GEORGE WALD and Ragnar Granit.

William Harvey 1578–1657

"I do not profess to learn and teach Anatomy from the axioms of the Philosophers, but from Dissections and from the fabrick of Nature," declared English physician William Harvey.

Celebrated as the first modern biologist, Harvey ushered in the age of scientific medicine with his revolutionary discovery and demonstration of the circulatory system of the blood. In an innovative display of hypothesis, anatomical and experimental observations, quantitative data and deductive reasoning, Harvey established that the blood is propelled through the arteries and drawn back through the veins. He elucidated the mechanism of circulatory function by likening the beating heart to a pumping device. "The blood is driven into a round by a circular motion...and moves perpetually," he wrote. "Hence does arise the action and function of the heart, which by pulsation it performs."

As the first son of a successful businessman, William Harvey enjoyed a childhood of affluence and advantage. His life began in Folkestone, a small town on the southern coast where he was educated by tutors until the age of nine. After six years at King's School in Canterbury he entered Cambridge University, completing his undergraduate studies in 1697.

At 19 Harvey was firmly set on a career in medicine and left for Italy at once to obtain his education at the University of Padua, a world-renowned institution of the highest academic and historic distinction. Among his professors was the legendary Italian anatomist Fabricius ab Aquapendente (1537–1619), who conducted his lectures in the prefabricated dissection theater designed 50 years earlier by GABRIEL FALLOPIUS.

Despite the school's prestigious reputation, however, Harvey's diploma from Padua proved to be a liability when he returned to London in 1602. As a foreign medical student he was subject to a number of financial and practical requirements imposed by the College of Physicians. The early prosperity of his family had long since given way under the financial strain of raising nine children, and Harvey's own meager funds were barely enough to cover his living expenses in London, much less the exorbitant costs of launching a medical career.

For the next two years he struggled vainly to overcome the political and economic obstacles that stood in his professional path. His prospects improved considerably in 1604 when he married Elizabeth Browne, the daughter of one of the king's physicians. Harvey's professional standing was finally established through the efforts of his brother, John, however, whose influence at court secured William's appointment as chief physician at St. Bartholomew's Hospital in 1605.

Harvey soon attracted a devoted following among students and colleagues for the wit and originality of his lectures. His services as a physician were widely sought after, and his roster of dedicated patients included such celebrated figures as Sir Francis Bacon (1561–1626).

In 1618 he was appointed Physician Extraordinary to King James I. When King Charles I took the throne seven years later Harvey became his physician as well as personal and intellectual companion and would remain in his service until the king's death in 1649.

Harvey was 50 years old when he completed the manuscript of *De Motu Cordis et Sanguinis in Animalibus* ("On the Motion of the Heart and Blood in Animals"). Less than 80 pages long, the Latin text was originally published by a small German press in 1628. Acclaimed as a classic on its literary merits alone, Harvey's elegant description and unassailable demonstration of the circulation of the blood marked a historic achievement in the advancement of science.

Fourteen centuries of myth-laden medical dogma fell away as the ancient wisdom of Galen surrendered to the challenge of scientific evidence. Still widely accepted in the sixteenth century, Galen's theory stated that blood was produced in the liver and moved through the veins in a tidelike ebb and flow created by the rhythmic pulsations in the blood vessels. He taught that the mediation of blood, breath and body heat was a function of the heart, which acted like a furnace or refinery, transforming the blood by innate heat into a weightless but powerful substance known as "Vital Spirit." Using the metaphor of a lamp, he described how a continous supply of blood from the liver is consumed like fuel in the fire of the heart.

When Harvey embarked on his investigation of cardiovascular phenomena 1600 years after Galen the available evidence was essentially the same. Yet, with no more than a magnifying glass to enhance his powers of observation, Harvey recognized what had been overlooked by thousands of scientists before him.

Scholars attribute such "scientific blind spots" to a deficiency in technological development, claiming that hypotheses are derived from technological models. Bound to the industrial context of his own time, Galen had a limited selection of technical metaphors at his disposal, and thus far less access than Harvey to the scientific imagination. It has been suggested, in fact, that the long-awaited discovery of the circulatory system of the blood could not have occurred much before its own time, following the development of pumping mechanisms and the mechanical application of hydrostatic principles in the sixteenth century.

In his original manuscript of *De Motu* Harvey included his grim predication: "I not only fear that I may suffer from the ill will of a few, but dread lest all men turn against me...The die has now been cast, and my hope lies in the love of truth and the clear-sightedness of the trained mind."

His fears were not unwarranted. As recently as 1553 Spanish philosopher Michael Servetus had been burned at the stake as a heretic for suggesting in his theological treatise *Restitutio Christianismi* that a passage through the lungs allows blood to travel from right to left.

For Harvey's radical ideas the condemnation was professional, as criticism streamed in from the outraged scientific establishment in England and on the Continent for over twenty years. After he was forced to retire from St. Bartholomew's the only opportunity for employment was in service to the king. When Charles was beheaded in 1649 Harvey found himself, at 71 years old, an outcast facing poverty and loneliness in his last years.

Criticism of his work had subsided over the years as most of the scientific establishment had given him up for dead, but he would make his presence known once again in 1651 with the publication of *Exercitationes de Generatione Animalium* (On Animal Reproduction). Based on several decades of research, the book presented Harvey's theories on animal generation and embryology. It was quite favorably received and caused none of the uproar he anticipated, undoubtedly because his findings did not contradict traditional scientific doctrine. Handicapped by the technological deficiency of his time, he was unable to challenge such time-honored concepts as spontaneous generation.

Six years after the book was published Harvey suffered a stroke and died at the age of 79.

William Heberden 1710–1801

One of the most distinguished clinicians of his day, William Heberden was the first to describe angina pectoris, a condition characterized by severe chest pains and intense feelings of suffocation. The result of an insufficient supply of oxygen to the heart muscle, the paroxysm is also known as Heberden's asthma. Heberden is also noted for his description of a particular form of osteoarthritis in which small, hard nodules form in the bones of the fingers. Today "Heberden's disease" refers to a form of rheumatism of the smaller joints accompanied by these nodes.

In his half-century of practice Heberden made the first clinical distinction between chicken pox and smallpox. He was also the first to describe the condition known as "night blindness" (now recognized as a symptom of vitamin A deficiency).

A native of London, Heberden studied medicine at Cambridge, where he established his first medical practice. After distinguishing himself as an astute and skillful clinician he was elected to the Royal College of Surgeons in 1748 and moved his practice to London. In recognition of his significant clinical observations—many of them written in Latin, which had become obsolete even among scholars—Heberden was elected a Fellow of the Royal Society in 1749. His reputation as one of London's foremost physicians is confirmed by his celebrated list of patients, which included the legendary Dr. Samuel Johnson.

Heberden's son not only carried his father's full name as the second William Heberden (1767–1845) but became a distinguished physician as well.

Lorenz Heister 1683–1758

Lorenz Heister was an influential anatomist and medical practitioner helped to elevate the surgical standards of his time.

As a young boy, Heister spent much of his free time visiting the many fairs that toured Germany at the turn of the eighteenth century. He witnessed the usual assortment of mildly daring and lurid spectacles that have excited children for centuries. A particularly fascinating personage at these fairs was the "operator," who performed surgical feats that more established practitioners would never attempt. Irresistibly drawn to these demonstrations, Heister recorded his observations in a detailed journal. "It is usual for a number of oculists, and other operators, to resort to Frankfurt at the fair time," he wrote, "to undertake the cure of persons afflicted with ruptures, cataracts, the stone, excrescences, hare-lips, and such like disorders; there being no physician or surgeon at Frankfurt who cared to perform these operations..."

Heister also recorded the minute clinical details of many of the operations he witnessed and began to formulate his own critical view on the state of surgery and of doctor–patient relations.

Heister went on to study under the Dutch master of anatomy Frederik Ruysch. He served as surgeon in the German army and was then named professor of anatomy and surgery at Altdorf. He began the first studies on the pathology of appendicitis (1711) and introduced the word "tracheotomy" to medical terminology (1718).

As a professor as well as a physician Heister had strong ideas about surgical practice. He recommended that equipment be kept simple, "great apparatus having been invented more for the sake of pomp than real utility." As he studied the writings and practices of medical authorities in other European countries he became more and more alarmed at the poor standards in his own country. In 1718 he published *Chirurgie (Surgery)*, a profusely illustrated treatise on anatomy. This highly influential work became a standard text on the subject, and when it was translated into English in 1748 it became the first systematic reference on surgery in that language.

Hermann Ludwig Ferdinand von Helmholtz 1821–1894

Hermann von Helmholtz left his mark on a broad range of scientific study, from electrochemistry, meteorology and hydrodynamics to sensory perception and psychoanalysis. He expanded many of the evolving theories of his time while drawing on all branches of scientific knowledge to understand the most basic questions of existence and experience. Von Helmholtz's career illustrates the vital interaction of technology, knowledge and specialization. One of his inventions, the ophthalmoscope (1851), launched the study of ophthalmology, extending the range of clinical observation and opening the door for the adventurous inventions that would allow direct observation of internal processes.

Von Helmholtz was born in Potsdam, Germany. His education spanned the sciences, and he distinguished himself equally in physiology, mathematics and physics. He extended the application of the law of conservation of energy to the area of muscular action and in 1847 formulated that law mathematically. In the same year he aligned himself with three other notable scientists, CARL LUDWIG, Ernst von Brucke (1819–1992) and Emil du Bois-Reymond (1818–1896). They separated themselves from *Naturphilosophie*, a popular school of thought partly derived from "vitalism," a doctrine asserting that life processes cannot be fully explained by physical and chemical laws. (*Naturphilosophie* was originally derived from Immanuel Kant and put forth by F.W.J. Schelling [1775–1854]). Von Helmholtz and his colleagues formed a research group committed to elevating physiology to equal scientific rank with physics and proposed a physico-chemical analysis of such physiological functions as urine secretion and nerve conduction.

Although the group later recognized their goals as somewhat simplistic, much of their detailed research was invaluable, particularly von Helmholtz's measurements of the velocity of nervous impulses in terms of space and time perception. His studies of acoustics conjectured that different parts of the ear resonate at different frequencies, thus enabling us to analyze tone. To demonstrate this theory he constructed mechanical resonators that imitated the physiological process. Expanding on the research on color vision initiated by THOMAS YOUNG and J.C. Maxwell (1831–1879), von Helmholtz published *Handbuch der physiologischen Optik (Textbook on Optic Physiology)* in 1867. In this pioneer work he describes the mechanism of the eye's lens and the work that led him to the invention of the ophthalmoscope.

Von Helmholtz went on to analyze the color spectrum, the acoustics of vowel sounds, the vortex motion of fluids, the behavior of air vibrations and electric current. In 1881 he theorized that if matter is atomic, then electricity must be so, too. His research based on that idea contributed greatly to the study of electrodynamics and thermodynamics.

He was professor of physiology successively at Königsberg (1849), Bonn (1855) and Heidelberg (1858). In 1871, eight years after publication of his pioneering work *On the Sensations of Tone*, he became professor of physics at the University of Berlin. One of his assistants at the university was Heinrich Hertz (1857–1894), whose name still resounds in the study of acoustics. While von Helmholtz's reputation grew as a physician, mathematician and philosopher, he became a successful lecturer on popular science. In 1877, while continuing to teach, write and pursue his own research, he was named director at the Physiotechnical Institute at Charlottenberg.

Philip Showalter Hench 1896–1965

Affiliated with the Mayo Foundation for more than forty years, Philip Hench played an important part in the battle against rheumatoid arthritis. His pioneering work with cortisone and ACTH (adrenocorticotropic hormone) in the treatment of arthritis earned him the Nobel Prize for Physiology and Medicine in 1950 (shared with his colleague EDWARD C. KENDALL and TADEUS REICHSTEIN).

Hench obtained a medical degree from the University of Pittsburgh in 1920. Three years later he joined the

Mayo Clinic in Rochester, Minnesota, becoming head of the department of rheumatics by 1926. He taught for many years at the University of Minnesota School of Medicine and was named consultant to the Surgeon General of the United States Army in 1946.

Working with Kendall and other researchers at the Mayo Foundation, Hench recognized the important role played by the adrenal glands in rheumatoid arthritis. After Kendall had isolated the adrenal hormone, later known as cortisone, Hench became the first physician to treat arthritis patients with cortisone and ACTH.

Friedrich Gustav Jakob Henle 1809–1895

The microscope, which had been in use since the sixteenth century, became the indispensable tool of the nineteenth-century pioneers in the field of histology, the study of the cellular composition and organization of tissues. One of these early histologists was Jakob Henle.

In addition to making significant anatomical discoveries, Henle's macroscopic and microscopic observations led him to conjecture on the nature and mechanism of contagious disease. Anticipating the findings of LOUIS PASTEUR, Henle suggested that infectious diseases were caused by living microorganisms. Infectious disease must be spread by organic agents, Henle argued, because only living organisms can multiply.

Published in 1840, Henle's pioneer work, entitled *Pathologische Untersuchungen (Pathological Investigations)*, outlined the essential requirements for determining the causative agent of a particular disease. According to Henle, conclusive proof lies in the demonstration that when the disease occurs, the organism is invariably present in a pure and unadulterated form, and that the disease can be reproduced with the isolated organism. It was the celebrated ROBERT KOCH, Henle's pupil at the University of Göttingen, who several decades later confirmed and developed many of Henle's hypotheses on contagion.

Equally renowned for his anatomical studies, Henle published a number of major medical treatises. Most notable was a monumental work presented in three volumes entitled *Handbuch der systematischen Anatomie*. Produced between 1866 and 1871, Henle's influential work offered one of the first detailed and systematic discussions of the microscopic structure of tissues. It also included descriptions of a great many anatomical structures, many of which now bear the author's name. "Henle's loop" is a section of a small tube in the kidney, and "Henle's layer" refers to the outer layer of cells in the sheath of a hair follicle. Other anatomical discoveries include "Henle's elastic membrane" and "Henle's fenestrated membrane," layers of tissue found in different sections of an artery.

Born in Furth, Germany, Henle was educated at the University of Berlin, where he was a student of the great physiologist and educator Johannes Muller. Henle himself was a distinguished teacher, with professorships in anatomy at Zurich, Heidelberg and Göttingen.

Herophilus c.290 B.C.

Herophilus is acknowledged as one of the founding fathers of anatomy. As documented in later medical commentaries by CELSUS, Galen and others, Herophilus performed human dissections as a method of investigation, a practice permitted for a brief period in Alexandria in the interest of advancing medical knowledge. Celsus reports that he also practiced human vivisection using criminals and other outcasts of society as his subjects, although Galen's commentaries make no mention of this. Herophilus is noted in a number of references as the first to conduct comparative anatomical studies between humans and other animal species.

His studies included a description of the channels of venous blood in the embryo, referring to their confluence as the *torcular Herophili* (Latin for the "winepress of Herophilus"). Recognizing the brain as the seat of intelligence, sensation and the origin of motion, Herophilus described the interconnection and interaction of the brain and the nervous system, distinguishing between motor and sensory nerves.

He delineated the structures of the eyes, the liver, the genital organs, the lymphatics and the alimentary canal, and he distinguished veins from arteries.

Determining twelve finger-breadths to be the standard length of the first portion of the small intestine, he named the organ the duodenum, from the Greek *duodeni*, meaning "twelve apiece." His vascular studies led to the development of an elaborate diagnostic system based on the subtle variations in rhythm and rate of pulsation.

Along with his contemporary ERASISTRATUS, Herophilus is often cited as one of the leading figures of Alexandrian medicine. Born in Chalcedon, on what is now the Bosporus in Turkey, Herophilus studied medicine under Praxagoras of Cos and later participated in the establishment of a celebrated medical school at Alexandria.

Alfred Day Hershey 1908–

Hailed as one of the founders of modern molecular biology, Alfred Hershey conducted a landmark investigation of the genetic structure and replication mechanism of viruses, elucidating the nature of viral diseases and the hereditary process in all microorganisms.

Hershey was born in Michigan, where he completed undergraduate and graduate studies in bacteriology and chemistry at Michigan State University. After receiving a doctorate in 1934 he joined the faculty of the bacteriology department at the Washington University School of Medicine. Committed to a career in immunological research, Hershey became interested in bacterial viruses as a result of the work of bacteriologist Jacques Jacob Bronfenbrenner, a faculty colleague who had pioneered the study of bacteriophages in America.

Little was known about the functioning of viruses in the 1940s, when Hershey, along with colleagues Salvador Luria and MAX DELBRÜCK, pioneered the study of bacteriophage replication. As the first to confirm the existence of viruses, distinguished Dutch microbiologist MARTINUS BEIJERINCK wrote in 1913 that "In its primitive form life is like a fire, like a flame which appears in endless diversity and yet has specificity within it...which does not originate by spontaneous generation, but is propagated by another flame."

The term bacteriophage, introduced in 1925 by Felix d'Herelle, refers to a virus that infects bacterial cells. Comprising a core of nucleic acid coated in a protein shell, a bacteriophage lacks the necessary equipment for carrying out the genetic instructions of its own DNA. Like other types of virus, it can only reproduce by invading a living cell and commandeering its protein-making machinery. Attacked by a phage virus, the bacterial cell no longer controls its own biological mechanism, functioning instead to produce new bacteriophages.

In 1952 Hershey discovered that by the time a phage virus enters a bacterial cell it has shed its protein covering. Demonstrating that the phage DNA is responsible for altering the genetic continuity of the bacteria, the landmark finding was the result of Hershey's now-celebrated "blender experiment," so called because he used a Waring blender to rupture the cell walls of infected bacteria.

Using radioisotope markers to distinguish phage protein from phage DNA, Hershey and his assistant Martha Chase infected a bacteria culture with marked phage viruses and pulverized the material in a blender. The disintegrated bacterial cells were then placed in a centrifuge in order to separate the inner and outer portions of the cell so that Hershey could compare phage protein levels. Hershey's "blender experiment" furnished convincing evidence of the independent role of nucleic acid in heredity. In September, 1952 Hershey's findings were published in the *Journal of General Physiology*, providing a significant forerunner to the imminent discoveries of Francis Crick, ROSALIND FRANKLIN, MAURICE WILKINS and JAMES WATSON.

Recognized as the "American phage group," Hershey, Luria and Delbruck conducted subsequent studies that formed the basis for the development of the first virus vaccines, most notably against mumps, measles, polio and rubella (German measles).

Acknowledging his major contribution to "the discovery of the fundamental role of nucleic acid in the reproduction of viruses and in the transmission of inherited characteristics," the American Public Health Association presented Hershey with the Albert Lasker Award in 1958.

"In recognition of his role in the development of modern molecular genetics" he was honored again in 1965 with the Kimber Genetics Award of the National Academy of Sciences. Citing contributions that helped "to bring about an increased understanding of the mechanisms that control the development, growth, and function of tissues and organs," Hershey, Luria and Delbruck were awarded the 1969 Nobel Prize for Physiology or Medicine.

Walter Rudolf Hess 1881–1973

Known as the father of electrical brain stimulation, Walter Hess was the first person to conduct an experimental investigation of the brain using implanted electrodes. In order to study the mechanism by which the brain controls various organs, Hess inserted electrodes into the brains of cats, specifically in the diencephalon, or interbrain.

Located in the oldest, innermost layer of the forebrain, the diencephalon includes the hypothalamus, subthalamus and parts of the thalamus. When Hess activated the implanted electrodes he observed an immediate and violent reaction. His cats became enraged, wildly hissing and clawing. With further experimental study Hess concluded that the diencephalon functions as a control center for the autonomic nervous system and many of the body's other basic drives and visceral functions. In the 1930s, when Hess began these experiments, physiologists dismissed his results and his ideas. Over the next two decades, however, Hess's , theories were confirmed, and in 1949 he was awarded the Nobel Prize for Physiology and Medicine, which he shared with EGAS MONIZ.

Born in Frauenfeld, Switzerland, Hess trained to practice ophthalmology, but soon after obtaining his degree he changed his field of study to neurophysiology. Hess conducted his experimental research on the brain at the Physiological Institute at the University of Zurich, where he served as director from 1917 to 1951. His written works include *The Functional Organization of the Diencephalon* (English translation published in 1957) and *The Biology of the Mind* (English translation published in 1964).

Russell Hibbs 1869–1904

As the originator of the spine fusion operation, Russell Hibbs played a major role in the establishment of modern orthopedics. Introduced in 1911, spine fusion, or spondylosyndesis, is the fixation of an unstable area of the spinal column by immobilization.

Although he initially developed the procedure as a treatment for Pott's disease, a type of bone inflammation, Hibbs's first description was entitled "An Operation for Progressive Spinal Deformities," which suggests his notion of broader applications. In fact, spine fusion revolutionized the treatment of vertebral fractures, spinal tuberculosis, and a number of other afflictions of the lower back.

Born in Birdsville, Kentucky, Hibbs studied at Vanderbilt College and at the Medical College of the University of Louisville, where he obtained his doctorate in 1890. After several years of surgical practice in Texas he left for New York in 1894 to accept a position as resident surgeon at the New York Orthopedic Dispensary and Hospital, where he was serving as surgeon-in-chief by the time he was thirty. Widely respected for his surgical skills, Hibbs was also notable as an energetic and resourceful administrator. It was under his guidance that the dispensary grew from a modest operation in a converted boarding house to become one of New York's distinguished medical facilities. As founder of the New Jersey Orthopedic Hospital in 1903, Hibbs again displayed his aptitude for organization and management.

Despite the enormous demands of his administrative duties, Hibbs never lost sight of his commitment to medicine. Approaching the practice of orthopedics with creativity and compassion, Hibbs was highly regarded for his insight as a clinician. He served as consulting surgeon at more than a dozen hospitals in the New York area and as president of Hope Farm, a community residence for children.

In the course of his career Hibbs continued to develop the practice of spine fusion, publishing a series of reports on various applications, including scoliosis, hip fractures and joint tuberculosis. Hibbs's other notable contributions to orthopedic technique include a surgical procedure for stiffening the knee joint and a method of lengthening the tendons for use in treating muscle-bound feet.

Archibald Vivian Hill 1886–1977

Physiologist Archibald Hill helped to elucidate the biophysical and biochemical nature of muscle contraction with his experimental studies of energy production and consumption in muscular activity.

Hill, a native of Bristol, England, graduated from Cambridge University in 1907 with a degree in physiology. In 1911 he began a quantitative analysis of heat consumption in muscle contraction, discovering the series of biochemical reactions that precipitate contraction. Hill's work also revealed that oxygen is not required in that stage of muscle activity.

In 1918 Hill was elected to the Royal Society, and four years later he shared the Nobel Prize for Physiology or Medicine (along with Otto Meyerhof for their important contributions to the physiology of muscular function. In 1926 he was made Foulerton Research Professor of the Royal Society, a position he maintained until 1951.

Hill was involved in World War II politically and strategically as well as scientifically. While helping to organize air defense missions he was an Independent Conservative Member of Parliament for Cambridge from 1940 to 1945. He also served as a member of the War Cabinet Scientific Committee from 1940 until 1946.

Hill's published works include *Muscular Activity* (1926), *Muscular Movement in Man* (1927), *Trails and Trails in Physiology* (1965) and *First and Last Experiments in Muscle Mechanics* (1970).

Hippocrates 460 B.C.–377 B.C.

> To know is one thing; to believe is another. To know is science, but merely to believe one knows is ignorance.
> —from *Hippocratic Aphorisms*

It was more than two thousand years ago that historians in ancient Greece declared Hippocrates the founding father of medicine, a title he still retains. Nevertheless, very little is definitively known about his life or his work. Of the sixty medical treatises that comprise the *Hippocratic Collection*, fewer than ten are now attributed to Hippocrates himself, and he was almost certainly not the author of the renowned Hippocratic Oath.

Among the most widely known of the documents associated with Hippocrates, the Oath, in either ancient modern versions, has been invoked by graduating medical students for centuries. Though no longer formally administered, the spirit of the Physician's Oath still resonates in medical tradition. It is widely believed, however, that the Oath was the work of neither Hippocrates nor even a disciple of his.

In fact, the Oath is at variance with the rest of the *Collection* on a number of philosophic and practical issues, most notably in prohibiting abortion, contraception and surgical practices. Because of these and other inconsistencies, many historians discount the Oath as an authentic part of Hippocratic doctrine, and some suggest that it originated a century earlier with the school of PYTHAGORAS.

Hippocrates was born on the Aegean island of Cos, where his medical training may have begun at the island's celebrated temple to ASCLEPIOS. It is believed that he traveled throughout Greece and Asia Minor for several decades as an itinerant physician and then returned to Cos in his middle years to write, practice and teach. Noting that during the same period there were at least seven other physicians named Hippocrates, some writers have joked that the Hippocratic writings were not produced by Hippocrates but by someone of the same name. In fact, the *Collection* is thought to contain the work of a great many writers whose combined efforts gave rise to one of the most influential documents in history.

Calling for a separation of medicine from religion, the so-called Hippocratic doctrine introduced a rational approach to health care that relieved the gods of the responsibility for disease and the success or failure of medical treatment. By applying critical deductive reasoning and objective observation, Hippocratic physicians helped to establish medical practice as a scientific endeavor, particularly in diagnosis and prognosis.

Greek civilization was nearly at its height when the Cos approach to medicine took on the aspect of an enlightened doctrine of objective examination and analysis. Establishing the scientific principles that form the basis of modern medicine, Hippocratic teachings were presented in a collection of treatises that included *Aphorisms, Ancient Medicine, Humors, Epidemics, Diseases of Women, On the Articulations, On Airs, Waters, and Places, and On Winds,* as well as reference texts on anatomy, surgery, physiology, mental illness and general pathology.

Included in the Cos texts on surgical technique were guidelines for pre- and postoperative care, preparation of the operating table, instruments, lighting and surgical assistants. A wide variety of fractures, dislocations and other wounds were described and analyzed, along with recommendations for treatment with drugs, bandages, manipulation and surgery.

Based on the theories of EMPEDOCLES and others, Hippocratic doctrine developed the concept of disease as an imbalance of the four bodily humors—blood, phlegm, yellow bile and black bile. Rather than viewing all illness as a single abnormal condition, however, the teachings described these imbalances as the result of glandular secretions that could be affected in various ways. To determine the origins of a particular disease, physicians were taught to search for immediate internal causes as well as indirect factors in the patient's activities, diet, hygiene or physical environment.

The *Collection,* most notably in *Epidemics,* provides the first examples of comprehensive clinical studies, presenting case histories that include detailed observations on the appearance of eyes, skin, body fluids and the course and characteristics of fever. Also included are details of patients' living and working conditions. In addition, the studies note the occurrence of these symptoms within families and communities and in successive generations.

Focusing attention on the patient rather than the disease, Hippocratic method emphasized the practice of systematic investigation, logical reasoning and meticulous attention to detail in medical examination. The physician is advised to observe with all the senses and to "leave nothing to chance, overlook nothing: to combine contradictory observations and to allow enough time."

Consistent throughout the *Collection* is the underlying Hippocratic principle of nature as the highest medical authority. The function of the physician is merely to restore the body to a natural state of balance. warning against the dangers of arrogance and adherence to dogma, Hippocratic doctrine advises, "As to diseases, make a habit of two things; to help or at least not to harm."

The *Aphorisms* teach, "Life is short; and art long; the right time is an instant; the treatment precarious; and the crisis grievous. It is necessary for the physician not only to provide the needed treatment but to provide for the patient himself, and for those beside him..."

Wilhelm His 1831–1904

A dedicated student and teacher of biological sciences, Wilhelm His is remembered for advances in anatomy, histology, and embryology, and most notably for innovations in experimental methodology. In 1866 he introduced the first microtome, an instrument designed to produce extremely thin slices of tissue thus providing a continuous series of sections for microscopic study.

Striving to improve standards of accuracy in experimental observation as well as in teaching, His developed various devices and techniques for achieving exact reproductions of microscopic sections. He constructed a drawing apparatus called an embryograph that used prisms as a means of replicating the microscopic image. Pioneering the use of lantern slides in classroom lectures, His was also an early proponent of the use of photography in anatomical investigations. Students also benefited from the fine topographical detail of His's celebrated wax models, which furnished three-dimensional illustrations of anatomical development in fish, birds and humans.

Between 1880 and 1885 His wrote a developmental study of the human embryo that introduced the use of standardized charts in embryology. He also contributed to anatomical nomenclature in a work, published in 1895, entitled *Nomina anatomica* (Anatomical Classification).

Acknowledged for his contributions in theoretical embryology and cytology, His was among a number of late-nineteenth-century biologists, including H.A.E. Driesch (1867–1941) and Wilhelm Roux (1850–1924), who gave priority to mechanical principles in embryological development. Known as "causal embryology" or "development mechanics," this approach relied on an experimental analysis of individual development and heredity as a means of studying the principles of embryo formation.

With the help of mathematician Eduard Hagenbach, His developed a theory of the law of growth based largely on mechanical and mathematical interpretation of experimental observations. Credit for the establishment of a causal-analytic approach to embryology, however, is accorded to Wilhelm Roux, who substantiated his theories with experimental demonstrations.

As conflicting theories of cell structure and reproduction emerged during the mid-nineteenth century His became an important figure in the controversial areas of histology (the study of tissue) and cytology (the study of cells). Among his earliest discoveries are the nerve plexus in the outermost layer of the vessels and the existence of independent cornea cells. Other research included extensive anatomical investigations of the lymph system and the thymus.

Published in 1865, *Die Haute and Hohlen des Korpers* (*The Skin and Cavities of the Body*) was His's first major work on embryology, focusing on the development and delineating layers of the cavities of the human body. Included in the book is a discussion of tissue forms in which His distinguishes between the "true epithelia" originating from ectoderm and entoderm and "pseudo-epithelia" found most notably in blood vessels, for which he coined the term endothelia. He also asserted that the designation "bodily cavities" should be restricted to those cavities of mesodermal origin—e.g., vessels, joint cavities and connective tissue interstices.

A native of Switzerland, His studied medicine under some of the most distinguished scientists of the century. Among his celebrated mentors at the universities of Bern, Berlin, Wurzburg, Prague and Vienna were Johannes Muller, Robert Remak, RUDOLF VIRCHOW, ALBERT VON KÖLLIKER, and KARL ROKITANSKY. His doctoral dissertation on the normal and pathological histology of the cornea was presented at the University of Basel in 1855.

Later that year His left for Paris and, after additional studies in chemistry and in physiology with CLAUDE BERNARD and Charles Brown-Sequard, he returned to Basel as lecturer and later professor of anatomy and physiology. In 1863, after epidemics of typhus and cholera had devastated the city, His was appointed to Basel's parliament and placed in charge of reorganizing the city's health and sanitation systems. At the end of his term he continued to serve as municipal advisor on issues of health and hygiene as they affected schools, cemeteries and the public water supply.

Accepting the chair of anatomy at the University of Leipzig in 1872, His was asked to supervise construction of a new anatomy laboratory. Completed in April, 1875, the result was a model of modern medical laboratory facilities.

His served as university vice chancellor at both Basel (1869–1870) and Leipzig (1882–1883). A preeminent member of Germany's scientific establishment, he cofounded the German Anatomical Society, participated in the reorganization of the Society of German Scientists and Physicians, and served several terms as president for both groups. A member of the Commission for Neurological Research of the International Union of Academies, His was also named perpetual secretary of the department of mathematics and physics at the Royal Saxon Society of Sciences.

His's son Wilhelm Jr. (1863–1934), a distinguished internist who practiced in Berlin, is credited with the discovery of the heart's atrioventricular impulse-conduction system, designated as the "bundle of His." His's nephew Johann Friedrich Miescher is also recognized as the first to suggest the idea of genetically encoded hereditary information.

His's written works include *Uber die Bildung des Lachsembryos* (*On Embryones Formation in Salmon*) (1874), *Die erste Anlage des Wirbeltierleibes* (*The First Atlas of Vertebrates*) (1866–1868) and *Unsere Korperform* (*The Form of the Body*) (1874). He is also remembered for his role as presiding physician in the identification of the remains of Johann Sebastian Bach and the rediscovery of the composer's long-lost burial site.

George Herbert Hitchings 1905–

In a career spanning nearly half a century, pharmacologist George Hitchings contributed to the development of many of the most valued drugs available in modern medicine.

At the Burroughs Wellcome Laboratory in Tuckahoe, New York, Hitchings and long-time collaborator GERTRUDE B. ELION developed a pivotal principle of modern pharmacology based on inhibiting the function of nucleic acids. To understand the biochemical distinctions of normal human cells, cancer cells, bacteria and viruses, Hitchings studied the characteristics of individual components of nucleic acids, the chemical substances that control heredity and cell function. Focusing on two nucleic acid components in particular, purine and pyrimidine, Hitchings and Elion investigated the development of nucleic acid in *Lactobacillus casei,* a strain of bacteria. Discovering that the bacteria would not grow without folic acid or a combination of purines, they conceived the idea of inhibiting pathogenic cell growth by blocking the formation of nucleic acid.

Applying this principle to the development of effective forms of chemotherapy, Hitchings and Elion achieved their first success in the early 1950s with the support of the research staff at Sloan-Kettering Institute (now known as the Memorial Sloan- Kettering Cancer Center). The collaborative effort produced thioguanine and 6-mercaptopurine, the first effective drug therapy against leukemia.

In the Burroughs Wellcome Laboratories Hitchings and Elion continued to follow this line of research through the 1950s and 1960s, working with pharmacologists and biochemists at Tufts and Duke universities. During that time they produced drugs for the treatment of autoimmune disorders, malaria and other infectious diseases, herpes and gout.

By altering the chemical composition of 6-mercaptopurine Hitchings and Elion created azathioprine, which proved effective not only in preventing the rejection of donated organs but also in the treatment of severe rheumatoid arthritis. Subsequent studies have led to the discovery of trimethoprim, which is used to treat a number of respiratory and urinary tract infections as well as *Pneumocystis carinii* pneumonia, the most frequent cause of death among AIDS patients.

George Hitchings was born in the port town of Hoquiam, Washington, where his father worked as a shipbuilder. Completing undergraduate and graduate studies at the state university in Seattle, Hitchings received his doctoral degree in biochemistry from Harvard University. He taught at Harvard and at Western Reserve University in Cleveland before joining the staff of Burroughs Wellcome Laboratories in 1942.

After more than 45 years with Burroughs Wellcome Hitchings currently serves as scientist emeritus at the company's research facility in North Carolina. He remains actively involved in a number of local charitable organizations and has established an educational foundation at Research Triangle Park, North Carolina.

In 1988 Hitchings and Elion were awarded the Nobel Prize for Physiology or Medicine, which they shared with English pharmacologist James W. Black, who pioneered development of "beta blockers," a group of drugs widely used in the treatment of hypertension and heart disease that act by blocking certain receptors of the autonomic nervous system. Paying tribute to the three distinguished laureates for their innovative contributions to the advancement of pharmacological research, the Nobel committee stated that their body of work "has had a more fundamental significance than their development of individual drugs."

Hitchings's studies laid the groundwork for the development of a wide range of invaluable new drugs, including azidothymidine, or AZT, the first drug approved for the treatment of AIDS.

Admired as a "rational visionary" by many of his colleagues, Hitchings is credited with compassion as well as intellectual brilliance. He describes his approach to scientific research as "enlightened empiricism," tempering the process of trial and error with a set of rational guidelines.

Julius Eduard Hitzig 1838–1907

Eduard Hitzig is noted for his experimental contributions to the theory of cerebral localization, which asserts that different sensory and motor functions are controlled by separate and specific regions of the brain. Although it emerged as a modern neurological principle in the nineteenth century, the concept dates as far back as HIPPOCRATES, who reported the case of a soldier who had received a sword wound to one side of the head, precipitating paralysis of the other side of his body.

Hitzig rose to prominence as the result of a collaboration with German physician Theodor Fritsch on one of the earliest experimental demonstrations of cerebral localization. Lacking suitable laboratory facilities, they reportedly conducted their experiments on Frau Hitzig's dressing table, but despite the unscientific setting, their results offered conclusive evidence of separate areas of control within the brain.

Using dogs as their subjects, Hitzig and Fritsch subjected both sides of the brain to electrical stimulation at various points on the surface of the cerebral cortex. Reporting their findings in 1870, in an article entitled *"Uber die elektrische Erregbarkeit des Grosshirns"* (*On the Electrical Excitability of the Brain*), they established conclusively that electrical stimulation of certain areas of a dog's brain produces movement of the limbs on the opposite side of the body. Hitzig and Fritsch further determined that when those same cortical areas are surgically removed the corresponding limbs appear noticeably weakened. Drawing widespread attention to the electrophysiological aspects of cerebral function, the historic demonstration gave rise to the experimental study of localized cerebral functions.

Hitzig was heir to one of Berlin's most illustrious Jewish families. His grandfather, for whom he was named, was a celebrated author, publisher and criminologist; his uncle, Franz Kugler, was a distinguished art historian; and his cousin, Adolf von Baeyer, was a world-renowned chemist and Nobel laureate. Eduard's father, distinguished architect Friedrich Hitzig, was highly regarded in Berlin, where a street still bears his name.

Educated at the universities of Würzburg and Berlin, Hitzig studied under Emil du Bois-Reymond and RUDOLF VIRCHOW before gaining his degree in medicine in 1862. After practicing internal medicine in Berlin for several years he achieved instant celebrity status in 1870 with the public announcement of his experimental demonstration of cerebral localization.

In 1875 Hitzig was appointed professor of neurology at the University of Zurich and director at the nearby Bergholzli mental asylum. Universally described as arrogant, insensitive and brutish, his character was once summed up as a volatile mixture of "incorrigible conceit and vanity complicated by Prussianism." His personal and professional battles were bitterly fought, leaving him few friends willing to tolerate his personality.

Continuing his experimental investigations of specific areas of cerebral function and localization, Hitzig concentrated mainly on normal and pathological function of the visual cortex. As a fierce opponent of the "holistic" doctrine of mental processes, he attempted experimental demonstrations of the localization of all mental processes, ignoring metaphysical or philosophical considerations.

After a brief stint as director of the Nietleben asylum Hitzig was asked to head the newly established psychiatric clinic at the University of Halle, where he also served as professor of psychiatry. Suffering from gout and progressive blindness resulting from diabetes, Hitzig was forced to end his career in 1903, four years before his death at the age of 69.

An influential figure in the development of psychology and psychiatry, Hitzig contributed significantly to mental health reforms by heightening public awareness of the inefficiency of current practices in the treatment of mental patients. As a materialist, Hitzig called for a system of psychiatric care grounded in science and insisted on medical qualifications for all practicing psychiatrists.

Robert William Holley 1922–

Since 1947, American biochemist Robert Holley has been investigating the nature of amino acids, cellular proteins and the nucleic acids involved in their synthesis. Holley's ground-breaking discovery of transfer RNA enabled him to complete the first analysis of a nucleic acid and identify the particular sequence of nucleotides in the chain structure of the molecule. Distinguished for his leading role in "breaking the genetic code," Holley was awarded the 1968 Nobel Prize for Physiology or Medicine, which he shared with fellow biochemists Marshall W. Nirenberg and HAR GOBIND KHORANA.

Born in Urbana, Illinois, Holley received a bachelor's degree in chemistry from the University of Illinois in 1942. During World War II, he worked at Cornell University Medical College in New York where he was a member of the research team headed by Vincent du Vigneaud that first synthesized penicillin.

After receiving his doctorate in biochemistry from Cornell University in 1947 Holley served for a year as postdoctoral fellow of the American Chemical Society at Washington State College. Returning to Cornell, he joined the faculty at the New York Agricultural Experiment Station in Geneva, New York, where his prize-winning research originated with investigations of nitrogen metabolism, peptide synthesis and plant hormones.

In 1955 Holley accepted a Guggenheim fellowship at the California Institute of Technology, and the following year he served as a research chemist for the Department of Agriculture at the Plant, Soil, and Nutrition Laboratory at Cornell.

It was during his fellowship at the California Institute of Technology that Holley uncovered the first evidence of transfer RNA. In addition to the RNA within the ribosomes of a cell, he discovered the presence of a simpler form of RNA diffused through the cell sap. The larger, more complex molecules in the ribosomes are distinguished as messenger RNA (mRNA); the short molecules circulating outside the ribosomes are known as transfer RNA (tRNA). Holley established the function of tRNA as a sort of amino acid transport system in which each of the tRNA molecules seeks out a specific amino acid and carries it to the ribosome, where one by one the amino acid molecules are linked together to form a protein chain according to the genetic instructions of the mRNA.

In 1962 Holley obtained the first pure transfer RNA, isolating three types of tRNA specific to the amino acids alanine, tyrosine and valine, respectively. In a painstaking process of biochemical identification he broke a molecule apart into nucleotide segments and applied each of these to various enzymes known to be specific to a particular nucleotide sequence, gradually piecing together the puzzle over a period of nearly five years. The result was the complete analysis of the nucleotide structure of a 77-unit molecule of alanine tRNA.

When Holley, Khorana and Nirenberg accepted the Nobel prize in 1968 Swedish biochemist and Nobel laureate HUGO THEORELL commented on the significance of their achievement: "This means that we suddenly have come to understand the alphabet of life, as far as heredity is concerned."

In 1968 Holley was named resident fellow of the Salk Institute in La Jolla, California, where he currently serves as American Cancer Society Research Professor of Molecular Biology.

Robert Hooke 1625–1703

As mechanical philosopher, experimentalist and naturalist, Robert Hooke's sphere of influence is enormous. He recognized the phenomenon of species extinction at a time when this idea was hotly denied, contributed to the early evolution of the microscope and anticipated the invention of the steam engine. He made many improvements on the mechanical systems of clocks and watches, particularly with his invention of the spiral spring. Hooke also improved upon a number of astronomical instruments and essentially invented the Gregorian telescope. He was the first to devise a theory of planetary movement in mechanical terms, and he foresaw the gravitational theories of the next century. In 1684 he invented a practical system of telegraphy and the first mechanical calculator.

Using one of the simple microscopes newly invented by ANTONIE VAN LEEUWENHOEK, Hooke chose to examine a thin slice of cork and was astonished to observe that the cork seemed to be made up of little boxes or cavities in a honeycomb formation. He described these structural units for the first time and dubbed them "cells," from the Latin word *cella,* meaning room.

Robert Hooke was born on the Isle of Wight and educated at Westminister and Christ Church, Oxford. He had the skill and good fortune to become assistant to the brilliant chemist Robert Boyle, and to demonstrate Boyle's Law—stating that at a constant temperature the volume of a gas varies inversely with the pressure. Hooke's experiments confirmed that the elasticity of solids is dependent on the force applied to them. His work with Boyle led to a lifelong relationship with the newly chartered Royal Society of London for the Improvement of Natural Knowledge, where many of the most revolutionary ideas in science were first presented. The society's roster of fellows includes the names of some of the most distinguished and influential scientists in history.

Hooke became curator of experiments for the Royal Society in 1662 and professor of geometry in 1665 at Gresham College. In that same year he published *Micrographia,* in which he described his microscopic observations of plant tissues. He also demonstrated that an animal could be kept alive by artificial respiration and, conversely, that it would die if deprived of air. In 1667 he became secretary to the Royal Society as well as city surveyor of London. In the reconstruction that followed the Great Fire of London Hooke designed the new Bethlehem Hospital, Moorfields.

Sir Frederick Gowland Hopkins 1861–1947

With the dawn of the twentieth century came a new era in the field of biochemistry and nutrition, ushered in by the research of Sir Frederick Gowland Hopkins. In 1901 Hopkins discovered tryptophan, the first of a series of amino acids he was to identify in the course of his pioneering biochemical career. In combination, these amino acids determine the structure of the complex molecules in nearly all proteins. Referring to them as "essential amino acids," Hopkins demonstrated that although these substances were essential to the diet, they could not be produced by the body.

Born in Eastbourne, England, Hopkins studied biochemistry at Cambridge and at the University of London. He taught at Cambridge from 1914 to 1943 while continuing to expand the scope of his research.

At the time when Hopkins embarked on his studies in nutrition it was generally believed that all the elements needed to sustain life were contained in water, mineral salts, carbohydrates, proteins and fats. Demonstrating that these elements were insufficient, Hopkin's feeding experiments with animals revealed a series of small but important dietary components he called "accessory food factors." The discovery of these food factors, now known as vitamins, led to the recognition and ultimately the cure of many deficiency diseases such as pellagra, ricketts and scurvy. A new light was shed on epithelial disorders, night blindness and other deficiency-related syndromes as a result of Hopkins's studies.

In recognition of the importance of his research findings Hopkins was knighted in 1925, and in the following year he received the Copley Medal. His contribution to medicine was acknowledged again in 1929 when he shared the Nobel Prize in Physiology or Medicine with CHRISTIAAN EIJKMAN. Hopkins was elected president of the Royal Society in 1930, retaining the position until 1935, when he was given the British Order of Merit.

Hopkins's body of work also included several feeding experiments with rats, in which the addition of a small amount of milk to the diet produced a striking effect on growth. Later he made many valuable studies of muscle function and carbohydrate metabolism. Among his findings was the discovery of a connection between muscle contraction and lactic-acid formation. Through research on biochemical oxidation Hopkins isolated the tripeptide glutathione, a substance needed to maintain the biological activity of certain proteins.

Hopkins's writings include *Newer Aspects of the Nutrition Problem,* published in 1922; *The Problems of Specificity in Biochemical Catalysis,* published in 1931; and *Chemistry and Life,* published in 1933.

Sir Victor Alexander Haden Horsley 1857—1916

English surgeon and physiologist Horsley is often referred to as the "Father of Neurosurgery," and it is indeed his pioneer work as a professor, researcher and practicing surgeon that gave impetus to the great advances soon to follow in that field. Horsley specialized in surgery of the nervous system and endocrine glands and is noted for his attempt to localize brain function. His writings, based on extensive experimentation with animals, include *Functions of the Marginal Convolutions* (1884), *Alcohol and the Human Body* (1907) and, in collaboration with Edward Albert Schafer, *Record of Experiments upon the Functions of the Cerebral Cortex* (1888). Horsley performed many successful cranial operations on humans and, in 1887, was the first person to remove a tumor from the spinal cord, with an operation he devised himself. In addition he demonstrated experimentally the effects of thyroid deficiency, delineating a syndrome known as myxedema that is characterized by fatigue, weight gain, mental dullness and intolerance to cold.

Born in Kensington, in London, Horsley received his doctorate in 1881 from the Royal Institution, where a decade later he was appointed Fullerian Professor in Physiology. In 1893 he joined the faculty at University College, London as Professor of pathology. Made a fellow of the Royal Society in 1886, he was knighted in 1902. In 1911 he received the Lannelongue International Gold Medal for Surgery. Horsley died in active duty in Mesopotamia in 1916.

Godfrey Newbold Hounsfield 1919–

In 1973 British electrical engineer Godfrey Hounsfield devised and constructed the first computerized axial tomography (CAT) scanner. Now referred to as computed tomography, or CT scanning, this technique of photography relies on X-ray irradiation of an area of the body from different directions as a computer processes the varying rates of tissue absorption of the beams. From these calculations a cross-section image of the interior of the body is derived, providing far more detailed information than could be obtained by any other nonsurgical technique.

Born and raised in Newark, near Nottingham, England, Hounsfield attended City and Guild's College in London, where he received his qualification in radio communication in 1938. During World War II he served his country by lecturing on radar for the Royal Air Force. After the war he resumed his studies at Faraday House Electrical Engineering College in London and, on graduation in 1951, was immediately recruited by the research department at EMI Ltd., an international electronics and entertainment company. Heading a team of researchers, Hounsfield supervised development of the first solid-state computer built in England.

Commissioned to study X rays, the team developed a system of interpreting the signals generated by a complex object to create a two-dimensional image. Hounsfield recognized the medical application of this technology and produced the "CAT" scanner, which became a revolutionary tool for clinical diagnosis. Two years after his discovery, in 1975, he was made a fellow of the Royal Society, and, the following year, Commander of the British Empire. He was knighted in 1981.

For his contribution to the advancement of radiology Hounsfield shared with medical physicist ALLAN CORMAKk the 1979 Nobel Prize for Physiology or Medicine.

Huang Ti c. 2700–2600 B.C.

Huang Ti is glorified in legend as the founder of Chinese civilization and the first ruler of the empire who was not a god. His accomplishments are recounted in tales of epic proportion, most notably in the *Historical Records* of Ssu-ma Ch'ien, celebrated historian of the second century B.C. Referred to as the Yellow Emperor, Huang Ti was credited with the invention of music, writing and transportation by wheel. He was also said to have produced a written record of all knowledge acquired by man since the beginning of time.

Discounting the exaggerations attendant upon such exaltation, it is generally accepted that Huang Ti was among the authors of a classic medical treatise entitled the *Nei Ching Su Wen* (*The Yellow Emperor's Book of Internal Medicine*). Recognized as the oldest known written work on medicine, the *Nei Ching* presents a system of health and clinical practices in a philosophical and sacred framework, attaching particular significance to the number five.

The book teaches five basic therapeutic forms: spiritual cures, dietary control, pharmacological remedies, acupuncture techniques and treatment of the respiratory and excretory systems. Stressing the value of health education, Huang Ti emphasized the principle of preventive medicine, expressed in the maxim: "The ancients did not treat those who were already ill; they instructed those who were not ill."

The *Nei Ching* revolves around the continual interplay of yin and yang, the two elemental and opposing forces in nature, and the cosmological concept of *tao*, which describes the ebb and flow between these two extremes. As later stated by Lao- tzu in the *Tao-te-Ching*, "Return is the movement of the *tao*." A fundamental aspect of Chinese medical theory, the maintenance of a balanced and steady flow of yin and yang throughout the body is considered essential for health and well-being. As interpreted in the *Nei Ching*, any imbalance or stagnation of these forces results in disease.

The first half of the book, entitled *Su wen* (General Questions), is introduced in the form of a dialogue between Huang Ti and his minister Ch'i Po, who poses a series of wide-ranging questions, such as, "Why do people sneeze?" and "Does heaven decree that old people may no longer have children?" The emperor's answers generally involve the distribution and circulation of energy and the function of acupuncture in the maintenance of those processes. Contained within all clinical responses, however, are metaphors for Huang Ti's philosophical doctrine of man, nature and the universe. In addition to a description of the anatomy and functions of the major internal organs, this section also contains notable remarks on the causes and types of fever, including detailed clinical observations of febrile pathology.

A large portion of the *Su wen* is devoted to discussion of the theory of pulse, an outgrowth of the basic concept of yin and yang. The diagnostic interpretation of subtle variations in pulse remains an essential element in modern Chinese medical practice. In general, rapid, sharp beats of great amplitude are associated with disorders related to an excess of yang, and a slow, soft beat is a sign of excessive yin.

The discussion of pulse and pulse types is followed by a major section devoted to the fundamental notion of *ch'i*, or energy. "Essential, primordial energy gives birth to all the elements and is integrated into them," Huang Ti states. "The circulation of energy is not visible, but a great practitioner perceives it. He knows how to go with or against the flow." Coursing through all living beings, *ch'i* follows certain pathways known as *ching*, or meridians. Huang Ti's complex description of the meridian theory identifies twelve double meridian lines running symetrically along the left and right sides of the body.

In association with these paths of energy, the *Nei Ching* identifies 365 points of particular sensitivity at the skin's surface that allow access to the meridians. Forming the basis of acupuncture technique, the theory of "gatekeepers" has been recognized in Chinese and and Japanese texts throughout the centuries, with the number of points varying up to 800. In recent studies at the Medical Research Council Laboratory at Cambridge, biologists Chikashi Toyoshima and Nigel Unwin found evidence of the "gatekeeper" principle at the cellular level.

Ling shu, the second section of the *Nei Ching*, deals mainly with the principles and practice of acupuncture. Developed as a means of treating diseased organs, acupuncture functions by restoring the body's balance and flow of energy. After the nature of the disorder is determined as an excess or defiency in yin or yang, acupuncture needles are inserted at pertinent "outlet" points, effecting a cure by replenishing or diminishing the appropriate form of energy.

Huang Ti is said to have designed the nine types of needles used in classical acupuncture technique. Varying in shape and size, these earliest needles were made of flint. Later models were made of gold, silver, iron and other metals, but in modern times acupuncturists use primarily steel needles.

Acupuncture continues to play a significant role in modern Chinese medical practice and has gradually gained a limited acceptance in Europe and the United States, where some practitioners use it as an adjunct to Western medicine. Research on acupuncture dating back to the nineteenth century has suggested that the procedure works by stimulating or inhibiting the autonomic nervous system, and recent studies have demonstrated significantly lower electrical resistance at the designated "acupuncture points." In 1974 the National Institutes of Health launched a research project to study acupuncture as a treatment for chronic pain due to cancer, arthritis and other diseases.

Hua T'o c. 100–145 A.D.

Revered in Chinese historical texts as the "God of Surgery," Hua T'o is noted for the first use of anesthesia in surgical practice. As the leading surgeon of his time, Hua T'o counted among his distinguished patients General Kuan Yun, a legendary military hero. Following his death Kuan Yun was deified, with temples erected throughout China in his honor. Over the centuries the mysterious ability to stop pain became attributed to the general's exalted power, but it was Hua T'o, who prescribed the local anesthetic.

Wounded in the arm by a poisoned arrow, Kuan Yun called upon Hua T'o, who concocted a mixture of wine and hemp extract. He then applied the substance to the affected area before performing the necessary surgery. According to reports, onlookers watched in amazement as Kuan Yun calmly played chess with one hand as Hua T'o painstakingly gouged out poisoned flesh from the opposite arm.

Several years later Hua T'o received a patient named Ts'ao Ts'ao, a bitter rival of the noble general. Complaining of violent headaches, the patient relunctantly agreed to allow Hua T'o to operate on his head, but at the sight of the scalpel Ts'ao Ts'ao was suddenly seized with the conviction that his surgeon was conspiring with his rival to murder him. Powerfully connected to the regime then in power, Ts'ao Ts'ao arranged for Hua T'o's arrest. The surgeon was beheaded without a trial.

David Hunter Hubel 1926–

David Hubel and his long-time collaborator, TORSTEN WIESEL, were awarded the 1981 Nobel Prize for Medicine or Physiology, (shared with ROGER SPERRY) in recognition of their studies on the mechanism of the brain's visual cortex.

After graduating in 1951 from McGill University in his native Montreal, Hubel began research at Johns Hopkins Medical School. It was there that his collaboration with Wiesel began, a partnership that would continue when the two moved their research to Harvard Medical School in 1959. For more than two decades, Hubel and Wiesel experimented on cats and monkeys in order to study the brain's system of processing visual information by mapping specific functions of individual cells in the visual cortex.

Hubel states, "In the visual system...it is contrasts and movements that are important, and most of the first two or three steps [in visual information processing] is devoted to enhancing the effect of contrast and movement."

With the use of electrodes implanted in an animal's striate cortex (the primary visual cortex) Hubel and Wiesel monitored cell firings one by one as images were presented to the subject. The painstaking process revealed the existence of "feature detectors," cells with the specialized function of recognizing horizontal, vertical or slanting lines. Hubel and Weisel found that the six layers of the striate cortex made up an "intricate edifice of orderly columns" with an army of neurons responding to the particular orientation of lines or edges in the visual field. Hubel and Wiesel went on to chart, cell by cell, the brain's interpretation of light and color information, finally deciphering the visual code of the mind.

Charles Brenton Huggins 1901–

Surgeon and researcher Charles Huggins is best known for his ground-breaking research on the relationship between hormones and cancer. As the originator of endocrine inhibition of tumor growth in the treatment of breast and prostate cancers, Huggins was awarded the 1966 Nobel Prize for Physiology or Medicine, which he shared with distinguished pathologist PEYTON ROUS.

A native of Halifax, Nova Scotia, Huggins graduated from Harvard Medical School in 1924. Specializing in surgery, he completed four years of postgraduate training at the University of Michigan before joining the surgical faculty at the medical school of the University of Chicago. It was there that Huggins conducted the greater part of his landmark research on the endocrinological control of cancer.

In 1940, using dogs as his experimental subjects, Huggins set out to investigate the metabolism of the prostate gland. His choice of dogs was a happy accident, since dogs are the only species besides humans to develop prostatic tumors. Initially dismayed at finding these tumors in some of his subjects, Huggins shifted the focus of his research when he began observing a distinct difference between cancer cells and healthy cells in the way they each responded to hormonal changes. By modifying the hormonal environment—either by withdrawing critical hormones or by introducing large amounts of hormonal compounds—Huggins found that tumor growth could be reversed.

Huggins went on to establish that in humans, as in dogs, the administration of small doses of one type of hormone, specifically estrogen, causes a regression in prostate cancers, whereas the administration of another hormone, testosterone, stimulates cancer growth. In subsequent studies Huggins investigated hormonal influences on the biochemical mechanisms of metastatic cancer, examining alterations in acid and alkaline blood levels and the interaction between cancer cells and normal cells, particularly osteoblasts, the cells involved in bone formation.

While still a faculty member at the University of Chicago Huggins served as president of the American Association for Cancer Research in 1948 and 1949, taking over as director of the Ben May Laboratory for Cancer Research in 1951. A member of the National Academy of Sciences and the Royal Society of Medicine, he was named William B. Ogden Distinguished Service Professor in 1962.

A pioneer in the development of hormone chemotherapy in cancer treatment, Huggins received the 1963 Albert Lasker Award for Clinical Research. In 1965 he won the Passano Foundation Award, and, after receiving the Nobel Prize in 1966, he was honored yet again in 1972 with the foundation of the Laboratorio di Ricerca Cancerologia Charles Huggins, a center for cancer research in Rome, Italy.

That same year Huggins left Chicago to become chancellor at Acadia University. In addition to his contribution to cancer research, Huggins made significant advances in the study of bone formation, bone marrow function, serum enzymes and the biochemistry of proteins.

Since Huggins's introduction of endocrinologic chemotherapy for prostate cancer, a number of other forms of cancer have been found to be influenced by hormones. These include cancers of the endometrium, thyroid, kidney, breast, lymphatic system and seminal vesicle.

Commemorated in medical terminology, Huggins lends his name to a diagnostic test for cancer based on the principle that serum albumin clots more easily in healthy patients than in those with cancer. "Huggins's operation" refers to surgical castration as a treatment for prostate cancer.

John Hunter 1728–1793
William Hunter 1718–1783

The Hunter brothers, John and William, did much to introduce medical science into the eighteenth-century world of barber-surgeons, untrained midwives and venerated superstitions. While William sought to refine the art of obstetrics into a science, his younger brother John became the most celebrated surgeon of the age, devising a procedure for the treatment of aneurysms (a sac formed by the dilation of the wall of an artery, vein or the heart), writing the first scientific treatise on the teeth, defining the functions of the lymphatic system and collateral circulation, and putting together a huge menagerie to demonstrate the kinship of diverse forms of life.

Differences in the personalities of the brothers were noticeable even in their childhood on the family farm called Long Calderwood, just south of Glasgow near East Kilbride, a town of 1,000 people and 150 horses. William was personable, tractable and studious. John, ten years younger, delighted in the dissection of frogs and worms rather than in schoolwork and showed no interest in the social graces.

When William was thirteen he was awarded a scholarship of £10 a year to begin a five-year course at the University of Glasgow leading to his ordination as a Calvinist minister. He finished the course but declined to be ordained, declaring that he had lost his faith.

Instead he apprenticed himself to a young surgeon, WILLIAM CULLEN, still lacking a medical degree but already practicing in the nearby city of Hamilton. It was Cullen who introduced William Hunter to WILLIAM SMELLIE, an early pioneer in obstetrics.

To gain more experience in his chosen specialty Hunter went to London, where Smellie was running a class in obstetrics. Smellie took him along on house calls to deliver women in London's slums and sent him to attend lectures by the city's top anatomists. However, a more fashionable and prestigious sponsor, Dr. James Douglas, soon hired Hunter to help in the publication of an anatomic atlas. He was invited to live with the Douglas family and, as Douglas's protege, was admitted as a student at St. George's Hospital. He was allowed to bring down from Scotland his older brother Jamie, whom he wanted to introduce to the study of anatomy amid the extensive resources of the Douglas library. The future seemed very promising to young William Hunter. He undertook to tutor Douglas's wayward son, William George, and woo Martha Jane, the daughter of the house. In 1742, however, both his brother Jamie and his sponsor, James Douglas, died. The widow Douglas, in accordance with the will of her husband, sent her son on a tour of the Continent as a distraction from London dissipation. William Hunter, who had just published his first paper—on blood circulation in the joints—was obliged to interrupt his work in order to accompany the young Douglas as chaperon and tour guide.

When William returned to London he found that his bride-to-be had died, plunging him into a bitter grief that caused him thereafter to shun any thought of marriage as a ruinous distraction from the high pursuit of science.

He sent for another brother, John, whom he had not seen in eight years. William thought he would rescue his younger brother from the boredom of life on a Scottish farm and at the same time acquire an assistant who could do the scut work in the anatomy school he had opened in Covent Garden. John proved to be an apt dissector and very canny in assuring a supply of cadavers from the grave robbers who were unpleasant but indispensable adjuncts of any anatomy school. John learned all he could from his brother and polished his surgical skills at the Chelsea Royal Hospital under the expert instruction of WILLIAM CHESELDEN, who was widely celebrated for being able to remove a kidney stone in under a minute. John studied briefly at Oxford and acquired a richly varied clinical experience at St. George's Hospital in London, a highly prized post, though it carried no salary.

Working together or separately, the Hunter brothers were beginning to make a name for themselves. Together they demonstrated that the vas deferens (excretory duct of the testes) and epididymis (located inside the scrotum behind the testes) form a continuous duct, traced the direction of lymph flow and pointed out the clinical consequences of undescended testicles. William outlined the process of feeding and elimination in the fetus, developed a technique for draining ovarian cysts and described a retroverted virus. John charted the olfactory nerves and perfected a technique for dilating the urethra by means of flexible silver rods.

The Hunters' school in Covent Garden, which gradually expanded to include operating theaters and obstetrical clinics, attracted admiring attention from physicians all across Europe and America. While William's distinguished reputation and elegant manners were winning him a fashionable reputation and a profitable array of patients, John paid no mind whatever to the niceties of medical practice but gave himself to an idea that soon became an obsession. He wanted to establish the essential kinship of all forms of life—from insects to tigers to humans. He applied to zoos for the rights to autopsy their animals.

When his research was interrupted by military service in the Seven Years' War he utilized whatever time he could spare from the wounded to study lizards off the Brittany coast. He preserved the organs of some 200 of the rich supply of shore animals, clocked the slowdown in digestion during hibernation, and discovered that eels lay eggs. In his treatment of the wounded he was far ahead of his colleagues, who still followed the cauterizing techniques of AMBROISE PARÉ, the sixteenth-century French surgeon.

In his spare time John Hunter found geological evidence that at least part of Belle Ile, off Brittany, had once been under water and devised a system of dating fossils by the minerals in which they were found. His determination to gather evidence of the interrelatedness of all matter extended to finding points in common between the animate and the inanimate.

With the coming of peace in 1763 John was retired on half pay, allowing him to scrape by while serving in a payless post on the Board of Governors of St. George's Hospital. Meanwhile, William had risen to new heights in his career. His school had achieved considerable prestige, and he was called in as a consultant when Queen Charlotte went into labor. Marking the sharp diversion in economic and professional status between the Hunter brothers, John had to work with dentists, the lowest-ranking members in the medical hierarchy.

John utilized the rare opportunity to study teeth, advancing the novel theory that they were living tissue nourished like other body parts by the flow of blood. He studied problems of occlusion and, always seeking signs of kinship, looked for teeth in lobsters and earthworms. He put all his new-found knowledge into one of the first scientific studies on dentistry, entitled *Natu-*

ral History of the Human Teeth. It not only won him a fellowship in the Royal Society but earned him a financial return that made it possible for him to marry Anne Home, a poet, musician, composer and painter.

They honeymooned at their menagerie and farm at Earl's Court, where, in addition to lions, tigers and apes, John caged together dogs, wolves and jackals in mating experiments to demonstrate a common canine kinship. One building was a museum in which animals and plants were so arranged as to indicate similarities and differences in fetal growth, skeletons, skin and genitalia of a wide variety of creatures, including hippopotami, starfish, kangaroos and barnacles. The menagerie became a marvelous playground and school for natural history buffs and for the Hunter children, Agnes and John Jr.

The gap between the two Hunter brothers had so widened that when William died in March, 1783 John did not attend the funeral service, though privately he expressed his grief. Continuing to work, he broke new ground when he tested his theory that the collateral circulation could enable a patient to survive even a major cardiac emergency. When a patient suffered an aneurysm in a leg artery, he ligated the artery and proved that collateral circulation could pull the patient through.

He also accepted the post of surgeon general and inspector general of the army, which helped defray the enormous expenses of his animal farm. After John Hunter's death at the age of 65, the contents of his museum was bought by the government and cared for by the Royal Society of Surgeons.

Sir Andrew Fielding Huxley 1917–

British physiologist Andrew Fielding Huxley belongs to a celebrated family of scientists and literary figures that includes his grandfather, Thomas Henry, and half-brother, Julian Sorell Huxley, both noted biologists, and his father, Leonard, and half- brother, Aldous Huxley, both noted authors. Recognized in his own right for distinguished research on the electrophysiology of nerve impulse transmission and muscle contraction, Andrew Huxley received the 1963 Nobel Prize for Physiology or Medicine, which he shared with his collaborator, British biophysicist Alan Lloyd Hodgkin, and Australian neurophysiologist SIR JOHN CAREW ECCLES.

Huxley was a doctoral student at Trinity College, Cambridge, when he and Hodgkin embarked on a comprehensive physico-chemical analysis of the conduction of nerve impulses. Introducing a microelectrode into the giant axon, or nerve fiber, of the squid, they confirmed earlier findings by JOSEPH ERLANGER, HERBERT GASSER and others that the transmission of an impulse is associated with a momentary change in the permeability of the axon membrane.

In the process of their investigation of bioelectrical function, however, Huxley and Hodgkin discovered that in excitation the axon membrane does not become equally permeable to any substance, as was commonly believed. They found instead that in response to a stimulus the axon membrane suddenly becomes highly permeable to sodium ions, allowing them to flood into the interior of the fiber. The high concentration of sodium ions shifts the axon's internal electrical charge from negative to positive, and it is that sharp reversal in the internal polarity of the membrane that travels down the fiber as a nerve impulse. Within a fraction of a second the internal level becomes so highly positive that the sodium ions are electrically repelled, and the rush stops automatically. The axon membrane then returns to its normal "rest state" of low sodium- and high potassium-permeability, thereby restoring a negative charge to the interior of the nerve fiber to prepare the cell for conduction of another impulse.

Appointed a fellow of Trinity College in 1941, Huxley was later named director of research physiology at the university. In 1960 he joined the faculty at University College, London, where he served as Jodrell Professor in Physiology for twenty-three years. Huxley was knighted in 1974 and served as president of the Royal Society from 1980 until 1985.

I

Dmitri Iosifovich Ivanovsky (Iwanowski) 1864–1920)

Dmitri Ivanovsky's status in the annals of bacteriology is the subject of an irreconcilable debate between those who credit him with the discovery of the virus and those who claim the honor for MARTINUS WILLEM BEIJERINCK. While Ivanovsky's detractors do not deny that he was the first to perform the experimental demonstration, they argue that he ignored the significance of his findings, and that it was not until Beijerinck obtained the same results independently that the importance of the discovery was realized.

By the late nineteenth century microscopic bacteria had been discovered, but few scientists accepted the possible existence of organisms invisible even by microscope. The technology for detecting such microorganisms, however, was already in existence. Recently introduced by French bacteriologist Charles Édouard Chamberland (1851–1908), the "Chamberland candle" was a filter made of unglazed porcelain that allowed only clear fluid to pass through its tiny pores. Established as a bacteria-tight medium, the device was generally used as a means of ensuring the sterility of a fluid, trapping specific unicellular microbes in the pores of the filter.

As a member of the research staff at the botanical laboratory of the Russian Academy of Sciences, Ivanovsky was commissioned by the Department of Agriculture to investigate mosaic disease in the tobacco plant, an increasing problem in the plantations of the Crimea. After observing the effects of the disease firsthand he completed his study in the laboratory, presenting his report in 1892. Focused mainly on the agricultural aspects of the problem, the four-page paper mentions in passing that "The sap of leaves attacked by the mosaic disease retains its infectious qualities even after filtration through Chamberland candles." Attributing the phenomenon to a flaw in the filtration equipment, Ivanovsky dismissed the matter from further consideration.

Unaware of these findings, Beijerinck conducted similar experiments in Amsterdam in the years that followed. In 1898 he published an article reporting his own conclusion that the results were evidence of an organism smaller than any known bacteria. Christening his submicroscopic "discovery" a virus, Beijerinck caused a sensation that reached as far as Ivanovsky's laboratory in Russia.

Although he seemed to dismiss the far-reaching implications of the experimental results, Ivanovsky wrote a short article publicly demanding credit for the discovery. Beijerinck graciously acknowledged the earlier study, and the two followed their separate paths in the investigation of submicroscopic pathogens.

Despite his conviction that the causative agent of the tobacco mosaic disease was a minute form of bacteria, Ivanovsky developed a number of hypotheses that have since been confirmed. In investigations of plant pathology he discovered the existence of crystalline particles, relating their presence to the onset of tobacco mosaic disease. Studying the mechanism of the disease in 1935, Wendell Stanley demonstrated the role of crystals in the process of infection.

Maintaining that these pathogenic agents could survive only in a live environment, Ivanovsky anticipated the concept of viruses as living parasitic organisms, a theory now held by a many microbiologists.

J

John Hughlings Jackson 1835–1911

John Hughlings Jackson rose to medical eminence as the leading scientific clinician of the nineteenth century and the father of modern neurology. During a spectacular career of nearly fifty years Jackson spent most of his time observing the behavior, symptoms and particularly the speech and motor defects of epileptics and stroke victims. His comprehensive clinical investigations served to elucidate the fundamental nature of these and other neurological disorders, but Jackson's greatest contribution was in the application of his data to the understanding of normal functioning of the nervous system. He articulated the concept of cerebral localization, explored its implications, and in the process laid the foundation for the development of clinical neurology, neurophysiology and psychology in the twentieth century.

The son of a farmer, John Hughlings Jackson was born in Yorkshire, England, where he began his medical career at the age of fifteen as apprentice to a physician at York Hospital Medical School. After completing his training at St. Bartholomew's Hospital Medical School in London in 1856 he returned to York Dispensary to accept a position as resident surgeon.

After three years he abandoned the job, intending to leave the medical profession altogether. At the age of twenty-four he entered London University to devote himself to the study of philosophy, an intellectual commitment he retained throughout his life, even after returning to medicine.

Obtaining his medical degree from St. Andrews University in 1863, he joined the hospital and teaching staff at London Hospital, where he came under the influence of French physiologist Charles Brown-Sequard (1817–1894), who encouraged his interest in neurology, and English surgeon Jonathan Hutchinson (1828–1913), a professional colleague who became one of Jackson's very few close friends.

In addition to his association with London Hospital, which lasted until his death in 1911, Jackson served at the National Hospital for the Paralysed and Epileptic in Queens Square and at Moorfield's Eye Hospital. As one of the first to recognize the relationship between eye and brain disorders, he established the role of the neurologist in the diagnosis and treatment of ophthalmic diseases and pioneered the field of neuro-ophthalmology.

Although epileptic phenomena had been described earlier in the century—most notably by L.F. Bravais in his doctoral thesis on the symptoms and treatment of hemiplegic epilepsy—Jackson's comprehensive research laid the foundation for the modern understanding of the disease and its various forms. Locating the source of the disturbance in the cerebral cortex, he identified the seizure as a symptom rather than the disorder itself. His insightful description of an epileptic convulsion as "an occasional, an excessive and a disorderly discharge of nerve tissue on muscle," anticipated by nearly a hundred years the discovery of electrical activity in the brain.

Jackson's particular interest in epilepsy was the fortuitous result of his wife's affliction with a form of the disease that he distinguished as "epileptiform," confining the use of the term "epilepsy," to grand mal seizures. Her disorder is now referred to as "Jacksonian epilepsy," which was the term popularized by celebrated French neuropathologist JEAN CHARCOT. Jackson described the recurrent characteristic manifestation of the disorder as a motor seizure that begins in a small group of muscles, typically in the hand, and then spreads to other areas on the same side of the body. Although conscious throughout the attack, the affected person is unable to control these movements.

Encouraged by BROCA'S demonstration of cerebral localization in 1861, Jackson interpreted the characteristic pattern of these motor seizures as an indication of a "motor cortex"—a functional localization in the cerebral cortex. At the time it was still widely believed that the cerebral hemispheres were responsible only for thought processes, but by 1870 Fritsch and HITZIG produced experimental confirmation of Jackson's theory. Several years later Scottish physiologist and neurologist David Ferrier (1843–1928) worked out a finely detailed cortical map of motor control, and in the 1940s Canadian neurosurgeon Wilder Penfield produced a graphic illustration of the functional organization of the brain with his *motor homunculus*.

Jackson's prodigious contribution to neurology reflected the influences of various other scientific disciplines, including clinical pathology, ophthalmology and biology, but it was powerfully enhanced by his interest in philosophy. His most revolutionary neurological theory incorporated the doctrine of English philosopher Herbert Spencer (1820–1903), whose ten-volume *Synthetic Philosophy* (1862–1893) presented an interpretation of all phenomena according to the principles of evolution.

Jackson visualized the organization of the nervous system as an evolutionary hierarchy in which the levels rose from the simplest activities to the most complex and "civilized," with each level inhibiting or modulating the one beneath it. Comparing his model of the brain to an authoritarian political system, he explained that when the ruling power is besieged (by injury or disease) the "lower" levels of the system take control. Jackson referred to such an event as "dissolution"—a recapitulation or reversal of evolutionary history.

"We should be very much helped in our investigation of diseases of the nervous system by considering them as reverses of evolution," he wrote. "By evolution I mean a passage from the most simple to the most complex, a passage from the most automatic to the most voluntary. The highest centres, which are the climax of nervous evolution, are the most complex and the most voluntary...Dissolution is a process of undevelopment; it is a taking to pieces in order from the most complex and most voluntary towards the most simple and most automatic..."

As clinical evidence, Jackson pointed to the pattern of recovery after an epileptic seizure, which proceeds from the simpler nervous functions to the more complex ones.

Jackson distinguished many local manifestations of epilepsy, including, most notably, the "psychical seizure," which he described as a "dreamy state" involving hallucinations of smell or taste, déjà vu, and "reminiscences."

In the course of his exhaustive clinical investigations Jackson gained an advanced understanding of various speech and language disorders and contributed significantly to the medical literature on the subject. A prolific author, he published more than 300 articles on clinical neurology and neurophysiology. Many of these studies, along with lectures, addresses and other writings, are contained in two major collections of his work: *Selected Writings of John Hughlings Jackson* (1931) and *Neurological Fragments of John Hughlings Jackson* (1925).

Edward Jenner 1749–1823

Edward Jenner developed an effective vaccine against smallpox, an ancient, disfiguring and often fatal disease. In the eighteenth century smallpox was responsible for up to 20% of the deaths in England. As a child Jenner experienced variolation, an experimental and painful preventive procedure of the day that involved an injection of the disease itself as a means of encouraging an immunity.

As apprentice to a country doctor in Gloucestershire, England he heard a dairy maid confidently proclaim her immunity to smallpox. "I cannot take that disease," she said, "for I have had the cowpox." Cowpox is a disease common to cows and not dangerous to humans. For years Gloucestershire farmers had known about the cowpox route to smallpox immunity, but their testimony was dismissed by the medical profession as pure folklore.

Under the tutelage of the surgeon JOHN HUNTER Jenner studied the nature of pus as a response to infection and inflammation. Understanding that if pox were present in the system, it would be found in the pus, he conceived of a means of transferring cowpox from human to human through injection of pus. He tested his system on a number of children, including his own, but it was eight-year-old Jimmy Phipps who became living proof of the validity of Jenner's theory. Jenner immunized the boy with cowpox that had been passed through the body of Sarah Nelmes, a milkmaid at a nearby farm. Jenner's plan was to infect large groups of people with cowpox. They would then not only be protected from smallpox, but also provide,through their lesions from the cowpox, an ongoing supply of pus with which to continue spreading immunity through inoculation. The word vaccination comes from Jenner's Latin term *variola vaccinae*—literally, "the smallpox of cows."

Edward Jenner was a dedicated, if controversial, figure of eighteenth-century medicine. He was often at odds with the "anti-vacks," a large segment of the medical profession that remained fearful or skeptical of his ideas. He did win converts in high places, however. Thomas Jefferson had his family and slaves vaccinated and tried to encourage the practice throughout the United States. Every Indian who came to the White House had to be vaccinated before returning to his or her tribe.

Although Jenner remained convinced that his methods would wipe out smallpox within his lifetime, when he died in 1823 the disease was still claiming millions of victims. It was not until 1977 that smallpox was eradicated by a vaccine very close to Jenner's original design, though it was passed through calves rather than humans.

Niels Kai Jerne 1911–

Born in England of Danish parents, Niels Jerne is recognized for his great contribution to the advancement of immunology. His theoretical understanding of the various mechanisms of the immune system was recognized in 1984 with the awarding of the Nobel Prize for Physiology or Medicine, shared with Georges J.F. KÖHLER and Cesar Milstein.

Jerne's research elucidated the development and maturation of the immune system, describing the broader immunological process by a "network theory" that conveys the complex biological and chemical interaction necessary to protect the body from disease. Jerne also identified the mechanism with which the immune system supplies antibodies sufficient to destroy invading bacteria or viruses.

From 1943 to 1955 Jerne pursued a degree in medicine from the University of Copenhagen while also working at the Danish State Serum Institute. Already recognized as an important contributor to the field of immunology, Jerne was appointed chief medical officer of the World Health Organization in 1956. While at WHO Jerne taught at universities in Europe and the United States, continuing to develop the theories that would later help in the fight against AIDS and other immunological disorders.

In 1969 Jerne founded the Basel Institute of Immunology in Switzerland, serving as its director until 1980.

Frédéric Joliot-Curie and Irène Joliot-Curie See CURIE.

K

Howard Atwood Kelly 1858–1943

A member of the original faculty at the Johns Hopkins Medical School, Howard Kelly joined physician WILLIAM OSLER, surgeon WILLIAM S. HALSTED and pathologist William Henry Welch in establishing the institution as an internationally acclaimed center for medical education. In addition to serving for many years as an influential professor of gynecology and obstetrics, Kelly is distinguished for his achievements as a surgeon, gynecologist, teacher, researcher, author and leading authority on American medical history.

As a surgeon, he is credited with the introduction of a number of innovative techniques, including methods for aeroscopic examination of the bladder, ureter catheterization, and a surgical procedure known as "Kelly's operation" in which a displaced uterus is fixed to the wall of the abdomen. A prolific inventor, Kelly devised a variety of medical instruments, including a wax device for locating stones in the urinary tract and a rectal speculum fitted with an obturator (a natural or artificial disk or plate used to close an opening). He is perhaps most widely known as one of the earliest pioneers of radium treatment for cancer.

Kelly's first published works, entitled *Operational Gynecology* (published in 1898) and *The Vermiform Appendix and Its Diseases* (published in 1905 and co-written with Elizabeth Hurdon), were illustrated by the German medical artist Max Broedel, who had recently joined Johns Hopkins University. Broedel's clear and detailed drawings launched the field of medical illustration in the United States.

A native of Camden, New Jersey, Kelly lived most of his life along America's eastern seaboard. His mother's enthusiasm for the natural sciences was passed on to young Howard, who maintained a lifelong interest in herpetology, ichthyology and botany, as well as a great love of the wilderness.

Receiving his degree in medicine in 1882 from the University of Pennsylvania, Kelly was only 31 years old when he was invited to head the department of obstetrics and gynecology at the newly founded Johns Hopkins Medical School. At the same time he accepted the position as chief of the clinical department at the university hospital.

The author of over 500 articles on medical topics, Kelly produced an enormous body of written work, which includes *Walter Reed and Yellow Fever* (1906, 1907, 1923), *Medical Gynecology* (1908,1912), *Cyclopedia of American Medical Biography* (2 volumes, 1912), *Some American Medical Botanists* (1913), *A Scientific Man and the Bible* (1920) and *Electrosurgery* (co-written with Grant E. Ward, 1932).

The founder of Kensington Hospital in Philadelphia, Kelly later practiced as a radiologist and gynecological surgeon. Named professor emeritus at Johns Hopkins in 1919, he abandoned teaching in order to concentrate his efforts on private practice and fund-raising for medical, educational and religious causes. He died at the age of 85, several hours after the death of his wife, Laetitia Bredow Kelly.

Edward Calvin Kendall 1886–1972

By recognizing the important role played by hormones in the body's metabolism, Edward Kendall and his colleague PHILIP HENCH made a profound contribution both to biological understanding and to medical practice. By isolating a series of compounds of the adrenal gland cortex, most notably cortisone and hydrocortisone, Kendall paved the way for the synthesis and large-scale production of these hormones. Dubbed "miracle drugs" by the medical community and the public, they were used successfully to treat a wide range of diseases including rheumatoid arthritis, Addison's disease and other disorders of the eye, skin and intestines.

Born in Connecticut, Kendall obtained his doctorate in chemistry from Columbia University in 1910 and immediately began research on the thyroid gland at St. Luke's Hospital in New York City. In 1914 he left for Minnesota to head the biochemistry section of the Mayo Clinic. It was in that year that Kendall isolated the hormone thyroxin from the thyroid gland. This substance became widely used in the treatment of glandular deficiency. Soon after, Kendall established the structure of the tripeptide glutathione, which is important in maintaining the biological activity of certain proteins and in many aspects of cellular respiration.

From 1921 to 1951 Kendall taught physiological chemistry at the Mayo Foundation while continuing investigative research on hormones. Kendall and his colleagues had observed that a woman suffering from rheumatoid arthritis showed a lessening of symptoms during pregnancy. Determined to track down the biochemical substance responsible for this phenomenon, Kendall eventually isolated hormones of the steroid series in the adrenal glands in 1934. With colleagues P.S.

Hench, H.F. Polley and C.H. Slocumb, Kendall then developed a method of partially synthesizing cortisone and hydrocortisone, facilitating widespread production of these hormones. Demonstrating value of the substances in the treatment of rheumatoid arthritis, Kendall's research team also studied the effects of adrenocorticotropic hormone, or ACTH.

Kendall and his colleagues went on to discover a number of other steroid compounds, valuable not only for treating arthritis but also for control of some sexual functions, as well as mineral and carbohydrate metabolism.

In recognition of their contribution to medicine and pharmacology Kendall and Hench were awarded the 1950 Nobel Prize for Physiology and Medicine, which they shared with TADEUS REICHSTEIN. After 1952 Kendall taught chemistry at Princeton University.

Sir John Cowdery Kendrew 1917–

John Kendrew shared the 1962 Nobel Prize for Chemistry with Max Perutz for producing the first three-dimensional depiction of a protein molecule. Kendrew's detailed description of the atomic structure of myoglobin, a muscle protein found in higher mammals,was a breakthrough in the study of molecular biology. Myoglobin, found in human cardiac muscle as well as in the tissues of diving mammals such as whales and dolphins, can store oxygen by binding it to atoms of iron, an essential part of myoglobin's composition. For humans, as well as for the aquatic mammals, myoglobin permits continuous function when oxygen levels fluctuate.

Born in Oxford, England, Kendrew studied biochemistry at Clifton and Trinity College in Cambridge. He was still in his wartime Royal Air Force uniform when he began work as an assistant to Max Perutz, who was conducting crystallographic research on a modest grant from the Rockefeller Foundation. In 1946, just as their funding was running out, the Medical Research Council sponsored Perutz and Kendrew to work as a two-man team, operating out of a hut on the Cambridge campus. Called the Medical Research Unit of Molecular Biology at Cambridge, the unit attracted a distinguished roster of scientists, including Hugh Huxley, Francis Crick and JAMES WATSON. Kendrew served as deputy director under Perutz until 1975.

In 1957, using high-speed computers and X-ray diffraction photography, Kendrew produced the first three-dimensional image of myoglobin, and in the two years that followed he arrived at a thorough analysis of the molecule's atomic structure.

In 1966, four years after receiving the Nobel Prize, Kendrew published *The Thread of Life*. He was knighted in 1974,and the following year he left Cambridge to become director general of the European Molecular Biology Laboratory in Heidelberg, West Germany, where he remained until 1982.

Elizabeth Kenny 1886–1952

In 1910, while caring for victims of poliomyelitis in the bush country of her native Australia, Elizabeth Kenny developed a program of physical therapy involving applications of moist heat along with a system of passive exercise. This was in opposition to the prevailing approach to polio, in which paralyzed limbs were immobilized in casts or splints.

Born in Brisbane, she became known as "Sister" Elizabeth Kenny in the years 1914 to 1918 during her tour of duty in the Australian army as a first lieutenant nurse. Between 1933 and 1937, after many years of civilian nursing in Australia, Kenny opened several clinics where she could employ her own unconventional methods of treating polio. Although ridiculed by the medical establishment, Kenny staunchly defended her technique. She brought her findings to England, where she opened a clinic in 1937 amid vigorous opposition from the British medical establishment.

Determined to impart the value of her method of treatment, Sister Kenny left for the United States in 1940. Impressed by her demonstration, the American Medical Association was receptive and supportive. By the end of the year the Sister Kenny Foundation, where nurses and physical therapists could receive training in Kenny's techniques, was established in Minneapolis, Minnesota. As word of her success spread, clinics employing Kenny's methods opened up across America.

In 1942, with co-author John F. Pohl, Kenny wrote *The Kenny Concept of Infantile Paralysis and Its Treatment*. The following year she published an autobiography, written with Martha Ostenso, called *And They Shall Walk*. This was followed in 1955 by another autobiographical work, *My Battle and Victory*.

Har Gobind Khorana 1922–

For his outstanding investigations of the structure of DNA and its functions in protein synthesis, biochemist Har Gobind Khorana was awarded the 1968 Nobel Prize for Physiology or Medicine, which he shared with fellow biochemists MARSHALL W. NIRENBERG and ROBERT HOLLEY.

Born in Raipur, India, Khorana received a graduate degree in chemistry from the University of Punjab in 1945. After obtaining his doctorate from the University of Liverpool in 1948 Khorana served for a year as postdoctoral fellow for the Indian government at the Federal Institute of Technology in Zurich. In 1950 he was named Nuffield fellow at Cambridge University and two years later took over as director of the organic chemistry division at the British Columbia Research Council in Vancouver, Canada.

Also serving as research professor of graduate faculty studies, Khorana launched investigations that confirmed Nirenberg's discovery of the four nucleotides that constitute genetic material—adenine, cytosine, uracil, and guanine. The genetic code designates each of the 20 amino acids by a specific sequence of three of these nucleotides, using no overlapping sequences in any of the trinucleotide structures (also known as "codons"). To investigate the mechanism of protein synthesis, Khorana created synthetic molecules, each designed from one of 64 possible triplet sequences. Confirming the findings of Nirenberg and Holley, Khorana furnished new evidence that the function and chemical composition in a new cell is determined by the particular arrangement of these basic "building blocks" in a DNA molecule.

During the last two years of his tenure at the Research Council Khorana also served as visiting professor at the Rockefeller Institute. In 1960 he left both positions to join the staff at the Institute for Enzyme Research at the University of Wisconsin, where he later became co-director. Continuing his investigations of DNA structure, Khorana synthesized a complete gene, establishing a detailed picture of the "punctuation," "grammar" and "vocabulary" of the genetic code.

The author of more than 300 published papers, Khorana currently conducts research at the Massachussetts Institute of Technology, where he was named Alfred P. Sloan Professor of Biology in 1970. In addition to the Nobel Prize he has accepted a great many honors for his distinguished research, including the Merck Award of the Chemical Institute of Canada (1958), the Gold Medal of the Professional Institute of Canadian Public Service (1960), the Dannie Heineman Prize (1967), the Lasker Foundation Award (1968) and the Louisa Gross Horwitz Prize (1968).

Athanasius Kircher 1601–1680

Athanasius Kircher was the first person to observe microorganisms.

Although the existence of bacteria was not verified until the nineteenth century, the idea that tiny, invisible creatures produced and spread illness had been bandied around for centuries. In the first century B.C. Varro warned against the dangers of swampland, writing that "certain minute animals, invisible to the eye, breed there, and borne of the air reach the inside of the body by way of the mouth and cause disease."

By the middle Middle Ages people were isolating severely ill patients and frantically avoiding contact with those afflicted with leprosy or the plague. FRACOSTORO and Cardano both anticipated the idea of bacteria as live "seeds of disease," but it was Athanasius Kircher who first observed the phenomenon directly.

Kircher was a German Jesuit educated in mathematics, biology, physics, archeology and linguistics. His scientific interests ranged from the deciphering of hieroglyphics to the study of fossils and volcanic phenomena. He taught mathematics and ethics at the University of Würzburg, then left to teach physics and Oriental languages at the College of Rome. In 1643 he abandoned academia to pursue his wide-ranging interests independently. He studied music, perfected the aeolian harp and collected antiquities, but he made his mark in history with his remarkable biological discovery.

Observing sour milk and vinegar through a crude, low-power microscope, Kircher watched in amazement as "worms" wriggled around within the liquid. He proceeded to observe various blood samples and saw that victims of the plague carried minute animal organisms. These were probably red cells and not bacteria, but nonetheless he concluded that infectious disease, as well as putrefaction, must be caused by these microorganisms, and he proceeded to announce his revelation to the European medical community. There were a number of misconceptions and assumptions in Kircher's assertions and a number of technical difficulties in replicating his findings. The zeal with which his followers spread the news overrode their scientific integrity, and as reports throughout Europe grew more and more fanciful Kircher's claims were discredited and generally disregarded. The idea that disease was caused by living organisms was broached again, and more convincingly, by Agostino Bassi of Lodi (1773–1856) and others, but the theory was not widely accepted until JACOB HENLE'S reports in the mid-nineteenth century.

Shibasaburo Kitasato, (Kitazato) 1856–1931

Born in the village of Kitasato, at the foot of Mount Aso in southern Japan, Shibasaburo Kitasato gained distinction as a leading bacteriologist in his own country and throughout the world.

Although he was justifiably acclaimed for his work in tetanus and diphtheria, Kitasato was most widely celebrated for work that seems shrouded in some doubt. He and a distinguished Japanese team were dispatched in 1894 to study the epidemic of plague that was then ravaging Hong Kong. Within days of his arrival he reported the discovery of the etiologic agent of plague.

At the same time, Swiss-born bacteriologist ALEXANDRE YERSIN was in Hong Kong on a similar mission. Both announced their discovery of the agent, but Kitasato repeatedly denied that his agent (which at first he called a virus) was related to Yersin's bacillus. In fact, Kitasato's agent subsequently disappeared from the scientific scene, while Yersin's was used to prepare the vaccine that proved effective in almost completely eliminating the disease that had periodically scourged the world for millenia. While some Japanese investigators—including those on Kitasato's team—defended Yersin's title to the discovery, the Japanese government acknowledged Kitasato's claim, granting him the Third Order of the Rising Sun and later ennobling him. Many reference works in Europe and America continue to give equal credit to both Kitasato and Yersin, designating the agent as the "Kitasato-Yersin bacillus."

Educated at the newly founded medical school at Kumamoto, Kitasato completed his medical studies at Tokyo's Imperial University, where he received his degree in 1883. Two years later he left Japan to work at the University of Berlin in the laboratory of renowned bacteriologist ROBERT KOCH. A fellow member of the laboratory staff was noted German physiologist EMIL VON BEHRING, with whom Kitasato collaborated in a noted study of antitoxin immunity in tetanus and diphtheria.

In 1890 Kitasato and von Behring demonstrated that immunity to these diseases is dependent on the ability of the patient's cell-free blood serum to counteract the toxins produced by the bacillus of the disease. In recognition of his distinguished record of bacteriological research, Kitasato was made a full professor in 1892, an unusual distinction for a foreigner.

Returning to Japan later that year, he established a private facility in Tokyo, where he conducted extensive research on infectious disease. The laboratory boasted an impressive roster of students and visiting scientists, including noted German physiologist AUGUST VON WASSERMAN, who came to observe Kitasato's experimental use of dead cultures in vaccine research. Kitasato's laboratory became, in fact, an outpost of the German school of medical investigation. The Japanese bacteriologist so venerated his German teachers that he kept, as a relic, a lock of hair lifted from Robert Koch's comb.

In 1889, using anaerobic techniques, Kitasato achieved the first pure culture of tetanus bacillus. By the end of the year, however, the momentum of his work was broken by a state takeover of his laboratory, leaving the facilities under the supervision of the Imperial University. Indignant but undaunted, he handed in his resignation and proceeded to organize the Kitasato Research Institute. Established in 1904, the independent laboratory became widely recognized as an important center for the study of infectious diseases.

In 1907 Kitasato was elected to Japan's House of Peers. Appointed dean of the medical faculty at Kei University, he later served as president of the Medical Association of Japan. In 1917 he was made a member of the Upper Chamber in Tokyo, and in 1924, when he was 68, the government of Japan bestowed upon him a title of nobility.

Nathaniel Kleitman See EUGENE ASERINSKY.

Nathan Schellenberg Kline 1916–1983

Twice winner of the prestigious Albert Lasker Award, Nathan Kline was a pioneer of modern pharmacotherapy in the treatment of mental disorders. Introducing the use of tranquilizers and "psychic energizers," or antidepressants, Kline launched a revolution in psychiatric care and mental-health reform.

Born in Philadelphia, Kline grew up in Atlantic City, New Jersey, the youngest son in a family of ten children. His half-brother Benjamin is noted for developing the "Kline test" for syphilis. Nathan studied psychology and medicine at Swarthmore College, the University of Pennsylvania and Harvard University. As a doctoral candidate at New York University College of Medicine, Kline helped to finance his education by playing the horses. Granted a medical degree in 1943, he enlisted in the United States Public Health Service the following year as assistant surgeon in the merchant marine.

After his discharge in 1946 Kline pursued studies in neuropsychiatry while gaining clinical and research experience at a number of mental-health facilities in New York and New Jersey. In 1948 he joined the New York State Brain Research Project, also serving as research assistant in the department of neurology at Columbia University's College of Physicians and Surgeons.

Much of Kline's investigation was guided by his interest in the interconnection of mind and body. Approaching mental disorder as a form of physiological disease, he drew an analogy between schizophrenia and the general state of fever. Schizophrenia, like fever, is in fact a number of conditions, he argued, each requiring a different form of treatment.

In 1952 Kline became founding director of the research division of Rockland State Hospital, a position he retained until the year before his death. It was there that he launched his celebrated research on pharmacotherapy, experimenting on 700 patients with various forms of mental disturbance.

Ironically,the particular direction of the study was determined more by external circumstances than by Kline himself. In exchange for a costly piece of laboratory equipment, Kline made an agreement with a pharmaceutical firm to perform a clinical investigation of reserpine, a newly isolated compound recently introduced in the United States as a treatment for high blood pressure. Reserpine is derived from the Indian snakeroot plant (*Rauwolfia serpentina*), a small shrub of the dogbane family. The plant had been used for centuries as a cure for fevers and insanity in its native India, where it is known as *Sarpaganda*.

In clinical tests of reserpine on a variety of mental disorders Kline achieved dramatic and unprecedented results. Unlike barbiturates, commonly used to sedate patients or put them to sleep, reserpine appeared to allow subjects to retain a sense of their environment and to function within it, even in some cases of schizophrenia. Particularly effective in hypertensive patients, the substance was later found to relieve anxiety, tension and headaches while preserving the patients' sleep patterns (unlike barbiturates). Acting on the hypothalamic level of the central nervous system, reserpine reduces arterial blood pressure in a pattern of slow onset and sustained effect.

Subsequent clinical studies revealed a number of contraindications and adverse side effects of the drug, most notably in its property to induce depression. In some cases treatment was found to bring on Parkinson's disease, as well as other disturbances, including nightmares and gastrointestinal problems. Gradually replaced by phenothiazine tranquilizers, reserpine was relegated to research on psychosis.

In 1957 Kline's contribution to psychiatric medicine was honored by the American Public Health Association with the Albert Lasker Medical Research Award. By that time he had already introduced a new category of psychiatric drugs known as antidepressants. Originally used in the treatment of tuberculosis, iproniazid was found to have a stimulating effect on tubercular patients suffering from depression. When he tested the drug on patients at Rockland State Hospital Kline reported a positive response in 70% of the subjects. In granting a second Lasker award in 1964 the association noted, "Literally hundreds of thousands of people are leading productive, normal lives who—but for Dr. Kline's work—would be leading lives of fruitless despair and frustration."

After it was discovered that iproniazid produced several toxic side effects, the drug was withdrawn from use, but psychic energizers remain a significant factor in pharmacotherapy. Pursuing drug research in a wide range of areas, Kline examined the effects of antidepressants on male fertility and investigated drug intervention in the aging of the brain and deterioration of mental faculties.

Aaron Klug 1926–

Aaron Klug, the winner of the Nobel Prize for Chemistry in 1982, was cited by Sweden's Royal Academy "for his development of crystallographic electron microscopy and his elucidation of biologically important nucleic acid-protein complexes."

Twenty-nine years earlier he had left Cambridge University with a Ph.D. in solid-state physics earned at the renowned Cavendish Laboratory. From Cambridge he moved to Birkbeck College in London, where he met ROSALIND FRANKLIN, a scientist who played a vital role in the discovery of the double helix, the fundamental design of deoxyribonucleic acid (DNA), which carries the genetic code for all forms of life. Klug recalled Franklin's decisive influence on the course of his career: "She started me along the road of virus culture."

That road led him to study the structure of viruses, beginning with the tobacco mosaic virus, which had been a major preoccupation of Rosalind Franklin's before her death in 1958. Using X-ray crystallography, Klug analyzed the structure of the virus in unprecedented detail, forcing a revision of previous notions of the virus. He went on to develop an advanced technique of electron microscopy, which uses a series of two-dimensional images to create a three-dimensional representation of a submicroscopic structure. Known as "image reconstruction," Klug's innovation in research methodology enabled researchers to understand the structure of viruses, chromosomes and their subunits.

Born in Lithuania, Klug grew up in Dunbar, South Africa, attending the universities of Witwatersrand and Capetown before going to Cambridge in 1949. When he began to explore viral anatomy the tobacco mosaic virus was viewed as a "rod," with subunits twining themselves around ribonucleic acid (RNA) like steps on a spiral staircase. Klug found that the protein molecules of the virus formed not a helix, but a double-layered cylindrical disk. Analyzing the structure by X-ray crystallography, he and his team succeeded, after twelve years, in constructing a precise model that details the structure of the virus and shows how it is assembled.

Acclaimed as a leading figure in the advancement of molecular biology, Klug also pioneered the structural analysis of nucleosome core particles, thought to be the smallest subunits of a chromosome. He is noted, too, for describing the structure of transfer RNA, the short segments of ribonucleic acid involved in protein formation. Other achievements by Klug include the structural analysis of the viral agent for polio and the class of viruses to which it belongs. Klug demonstrated that these organisms, previously thought to be spherical in shape, are in fact icosahedrons—20-sided structures.

In addition to winning the Nobel Prize, Klug has received a number of other prestigious awards, including the Louisa Gross Horwitz Prize from Columbia University in 1981 and the Royal Society's Copley Medal in 1985.

Klug, who currently serves as the director of the Medical Research Council Laboratory of Molecular Biology in Cambridge—a proving ground for some of the most significant microbiological developments in this century—modestly sums up his triumphant career: "I am glad to be able to work at the beginning of structural molecular biology.

Robert Koch 1843–1910

Following immediately in the footsteps of LOUIS PASTEUR, Robert Koch was one of the leading pioneers of microbiology. Koch laid the foundation for all modern bacteriological techniques and demonstrated conclusively the germ theory of disease. Although Pasteur had attributed two diseases of the silkworm to microbes a decade earlier, it was Koch who isolated in 1876 the first known organism responsible for disease—the anthrax bacillus.

After identifying the etiological agent of anthrax, a disease of hoofed animals, Koch rose to even greater distinction with his historic discovery of the tubercle bacillus—the bacteria responsible for tuberculosis. Establishing scientific proof that the germ theory could be generalized to human diseases, Koch's findings encouraged the introduction of effective preventive measures in Europe and the United States against typhoid fever, plague, malaria and other infectious diseases.

The son of a mining administrator, Koch was born in the German village of Klausthal in the Harz. He studied under noted German anatomist and histologist JACOB HENLE at the University of Göttingen, where he received his medical degree in 1872.

Serving as a country practitioner in Wöllstein, Hanover and elsewhere, Koch gained recognition for his work on septicemia, splenic fever and the treatment of wounds. He was appointed district medical officer in 1874 and, with only modest resources, built his own laboratory, where he devoted his spare time to microscopic studies of bacteria.

To conduct his research, Koch had to devise techniques for the collection, cultivation and observation of bacteria, many of which are still in use. Establishing that microorganisms could be distinguished from one another by the way they absorbed different dyes, he developed the fundamental technique of "staining" bacteria, specifically with aniline dyes. He demonstrated the advantages of growing bacteria on solid, rather than in liquid media, and showed how to obtain a "pure culture."

To identify bacterial infection, Koch devised a procedure that remains vitally important in bacteriology and clinical medicine. As the basic principle of obtaining a "throat culture," the technique involves taking some of the presumably infected matter from a patient and smearing it on a layer of nutrient in a dish. If bacteria are present, they will grow rapidly into colonies in the nutrient to become visible under a microscope. Koch also discovered a substance in seaweed that is still widely used as a nutrient—a gelatinous material known as agar.

In addition to his technical advances and landmark discoveries, Koch's enduring contribution to the development of microbiology includes the introduction of rigorous scientific methods, most notably a formula for demonstrating that a particular disease is caused by a specific organism. Known as Koch's postulates, the formula is based on three rules: the organism must be found in all cases of the disease in question; it must be isolated in pure culture in a laboratory; and it must be capable of causing the disease when injected into an animal or human subject.

Following the discovery of the anthrax bacillus, Koch pursued his investigation of bacteria, establishing the role of microorganisms in wound infections in 1878. His clinical and experimental achievements gained him a seat on the Imperial Board of Health in Berlin in 1880, and two years later he captured worldwide attention with his discovery of the bacterial cause of tuberculosis, then one of the most dreaded diseases known to humans. A major cause of death and suffering, tuberculosis was often impossible to distinguish clinically from other diseases until Koch isolated the *Bacillus tuberculosis* in 1882.

Within the next few years, Koch discovered the microorganisms responsible for a number of other diseases, including cholera, amoebic dysentery and conjunctivitis. Joining the faculty at the University of Berlin in 1885, he served as professor until 1891, when he was named director of the newly founded Institute for Infectious Diseases.

Over the course of his association with the Institute, Koch traveled to many parts of Asia and Africa, investigating sleeping sickness, malaria, bubonic plague and other infectious diseases.

He also devoted much of his attention to the study of tuberculin, a purified derivative of the tuberculosis bacterium. Although the substance failed to provide a cure for tuberculosis, as he had hoped, it served as the basis of a test for the disease. For his contribution to the development of tuberculin as a valuable diagnostic tool, Koch was awarded the Nobel Prize for Physiology or Medicine in 1905.

Emil Theodor Kocher 1841–1917

For nearly eighty years Emil Theodor Kocher has retained his distinction as the only surgeon to receive the Nobel Prize for Physiology or Medicine. Presented to Kocher in 1909, the award acknowledged his pioneer investigation of the thyroid gland, which arose from his practice of thyroid surgery.

The risk of hemorrhage is a prime consideration in any operation, but in thyroid surgery the danger is such that, for centuries, the practice was prohibited except in cases of extreme emergency. The thyroid, an endocrine gland situated in the base of the neck, accepts far more blood than any other organ of its size, so that before Kocher, the rare attempts to remove the gland almost always proved fatal. By devising a technique for sealing off all blood vessels connecting to the thyroid, Kocher greatly reduced the chances of fatal hemorrhage during surgery, and by 1912 he had performed more than 5,000 thyroid operations at a mortality rate of only 0.5%.

A disciple of celebrated English surgeon JOSEPH LISTER, Kocher owed his success to the conscientious application of Lister's principles of antiseptic procedure and to his own technical ingenuity. He devised many appliances and tools that are still used in current surgical practice, most notably "Kocher's forceps," which were designed to compress bleeding tissue. In the advancement of operative technique his notable contributions include surgical procedures for the lungs, ovaries, cranial nerves, tongue, gall bladder, stomach, duodenum, humerus and ankle joint.

In 1876 Kocher drew widespread attention as the first surgeon to perform a thyroidectomy for the treatment of goiter. Observing a characteristic pattern of arrested physical and mental development following the total removal of the thyroid, Kocher discovered that when he did not excise the entire gland, but left some portion in place, his patients suffered only transitory signs of the disorder.

Identified as "operative" or "surgical myxoedema," the syndrome was soon recognized as a form of "cretinism" and attributed to the absence of thyroid secretion. Kocher's first findings, announced in 1883, elucidated the mechanism and function of thyroid secretions. Over the next four decades his award-winning studies explored the role of thyroid secretions in various disorders, most notably Graves' disease, a goiter or enlargement of the thyroid due to over-secretion ("thyrotoxicosis").

Born in Bern, Kocher was the son of a noted Swiss engineer. After obtaining a degree in medicine from the University of Bern Kocher sought advanced surgical training in London, Paris, Berlin and Vienna, where he studied under distinguished Austrian surgeon Christian Billroth (1829–1894). Returning to Switzerland in 1872, Kocher was appointed professor of clinical surgery and director of the surgical hospital at the University of Bern, where his distinguished forty-five-year tenure ended with his death in 1917. His notable writings include the *Textbook of Operative Surgery*, a classic reference published in 1892.

Georges J.F. Köhler 1946–

Georges Köhler, one of the pioneers in monoclonal antibody research, studied biology in his native West Germany at the University of Freiburg, receiving his doctorate in 1974. Upon graduating he was invited to join the Medical Research Council Laboratory of Molecular Biology at Cambridge as a postdoctoral fellow.

From 1974 to 1976 he worked with CESAR MILSTEIN on the development of a procedure for producing pure antibodies. Together they arrived at a system of fusing antibody-producing cells with tumor cells to produce easily reproducible "monoclonal antibodies." This technique proved an invaluable tool in biomedical research as well as in the diagnosis and treatment of cancer and other diseases. For their considerable contribution to the field of immunology Köhler and Milstein were awarded the Nobel Prize for Physiology or Medicine in 1984 (shared with NIELS K. JERNE).

In 1976 Köhler was invited to continue research at the Basel Institute of Immunology in Switzerland, where he remained until 1984. He then returned to Freiburg to take over directorship of the Max Planck Institute of Immune Biology.

Willem Johan Kolff 1911–

A leading authority on artificial organs, Dutch physician Willem Kolff is best known for developing the first practical artificial kidney in 1943, and for achieving the first effective use of dialysis for treating acute renal failure.

In kidney dialysis the blood is purified by transferring dissolved metabolic waste from an area of high concentration to an area of lower concentration through a semipermeable membrane, usually cellophane. The low-concentration dialysis fluid must be of a chemical composition closely resembling that of the blood, so that waste products are diffused through the membrane into the fluid but vital substances in the blood will not be transferred because of their presence in the dialysis fluid.

Kolff is also recognized for his design of a heart-lung machine, a membrane oxygenator (a device which allows the exchange of gases between the blood and oxygen), an early artificial heart, and preliminary designs for an artificial eye and ear. In 1982, as a member of the pioneer team that also included Robert Jarvik and William de Vries, Kolff participated in the first implantation of an artificial heart, in the body of a dying man. The patient, Dr. Barney Clark, survived 112 days with the device made of plastic and aluminum.

Kolff's father was a doctor who presided over a tuberculosis sanitarium in Holland. Having watched his father's frustration and grief over the deaths of his patients, young Willem was reluctant to follow in his father's footsteps. His interest in medicine overcame his hesitation, however, and he received his degree from the medical school at the University of Leiden in 1938. After graduation he took an unsalaried position as a teaching assistant at the University of Groningen while continuing his training at the university clinic. It was there that Kolff developed an interest in renal failure as he observed the inevitably fatal progress of the disease. He conjectured that if one could remove the toxic excretory products produced daily by the body, patients might survive renal failure.

Though not financially rewarding, his teaching job did provide Kolff the opportunity of working with two outstanding scientists at the university. Professor R. Brinkman was a biochemist who had determined the value of cellophane as a dialyzing membrane and had considered using it in the construction of an artificial kidney. Professor Polak Daniels, the director of Groningen's medical department, encouraged the innovative young scientist, whose preliminary experiments were yielding promising results. All research at Groningen ground to a halt in 1940, however, with the German invasion. Kolff accepted a position as an internist at a municipal hospital in Kampen while actively participating in the Dutch Resistance.

It was at Kampen that Kolff devised the first rotating-drum artificial kidney, a basic model for the device now used throughout the world. With assistance from H. Berk, the director of an enamel factory, and technical advice from a local car dealer, who provided the seal of a car's water pump, Kolff built the first artificial kidney out of aluminum, wood and cellophane. He is often quoted as saying, "I'll take a good technician over a mediocre doctor any day."

Having achieved successful results in Holland, Kolff donated an artificial kidney to Mt. Sinai Hospital in New York, offering to come over to demonstrate its operation. He arrived in the United States in 1947. He spoke at a number of hospitals and universities and, during his four-month stay, received the Francis Amory Award from the Academy of Arts and Sciences in Boston.

He returned to America in 1949, this time to accept a position in the research division at the Cleveland Clinic Foundation. Kolff produced significant advances at the Cleveland Clinic, including further development of the artificial kidney, the invention of a twin-coil disposable kidney, the membrane oxygenator and the heart-lung machine. He also participated in work on the intraaortic balloon pump and, with Donald Effler, introduced the technique of elective cardiac arrest in open-heart surgery, in which the temporary suspension of movement greatly facilitated the delicate job of suturing the heart.

In collaboration with Tetsuzo Akutsu, Kolff began work on developing an artificial heart in 1957. He left Cleveland ten years later to continue work on the project as director of the Institute for Biomedical Engineering at the University of Utah.

Albrecht von Kölliker 1817–1905

Albrecht von Kölliker was a pioneer in the new and revolutionary science of histology, the study of tissues and their cellular composition and organization. In the mid-nineteenth century SCHLEIDEN, SCHWANN, J. P. Müller, VIRCHOW and ROKITANSKY were all studying and expanding their theories of cellular biology, and HENLE was investigating microorganisms as a cause of disease.

Von Kölliker was born and educated in Switzerland and began teaching physiology at the University of Zurich in 1845. In 1847 he moved to Würzburg to teach microscopic and comparative anatomy at the university. It was there that he began his own research on cell theory, embryology and histology. The availability of the compound microscope and the newly emerging cell theories led von Kölliker to describe for the first time the existence of nerve cells and fibers, although the interrelationship of these two was not clarified until the 1880s (by Camillo Golgi).

As the study of cellular organization evolved the word "protoplasm" gradually lost its meaning as a structured substance and came to refer instead to the basic component of cells. Von Kölliker provided the term "cytoplasm" to refer to the material outside the cell nucleus. In light of the new cell theory von Kölliker also described the development of the embryo for the first time and contributed significantly to an understanding of the vital function of spermatozoa. His studies on embryology also led him to an analysis of spontaneous variation in evolution.

Von Kölliker wrote extensively on his findings. His most important work is the *Manual of Human Histology,* the first organized textbook for that discipline. It was written in 1852 and translated into English in 1854. Von Kölliker produced a number of other reports on his findings, including *Entwicklungsgeschichte des Menschen (The Story of Human Development)* (1861) and an autobiography entitled *Erinnerunn* (*Memoirs*) (1899).

Arthur Kornberg 1918–

In 1956 American biochemist Arthur Kornberg isolated and purified deoxyribonucleic acid polymerase—an enzyme that proved to be an essential factor in the synthesis of DNA. Kornberg discovered that the polymerase replicates genetic information by selecting the appropriate nucleotides and arranging them in proper sequence to create an exact copy of the original DNA molecule.

Polymerase, which was extracted from a common intestinal bacteria called *Escherichia coli,* permitted Kornberg to elucidate the enzymatic mechanism by which genetic material is reproduced. In 1957 he created the first artificial DNA molecule that successfully duplicated the chemical and physical characteristics of natural DNA, although, due to enzyme impurities, it was genetically inert. Kornberg's achievement was hailed as a milestone in the advancement of genetic chemistry. In his own career it marked the start of a decade of scientific breakthroughs that culminated in 1967 with his creation of biologically active DNA.

A native of Brooklyn, New York, Kornberg obtained a medical degree from the University of Rochester in 1941. The following year he joined the physiology division of the National Institutes of Health, where he conducted experimental research on nutrition.

Focusing his attention on the biochemical nature of enzymes, he took a leave of absence from the NIH in 1945 and over the next two years studied with CARL AND GERTY CORI at Washington University, H.A. Baker at the University of California at Berkeley and SEVERO OCHOA at the New York University College of Medicine.

When Kornberg returned to the NIH he was put in charge of enzyme and metabolism research in the Department of Arthritis and Metabolic Diseases. In 1952 he left for St. Louis, Missouri to accept an appointment as chairman of the department of microbiology at the Washington University School of Medicine.

Guided by the celebrated double-helix model of a DNA molecule provided by WATSON and Crick, Kornberg's research also relied on the experimental techniques of former colleague Severo Ochoa, who produced the first artificial RNA molecule in 1956. Kornberg's first major success came the following year with the first synthesis of DNA. Both achievements brought worldwide acclaim to Kornberg and Ochoa, who shared honors in 1959 as corecipients of the Nobel Prize for Physiology or Medicine.

That same year Kornberg left Washington University to join the faculty at Stanford University School of Medicine as professor and executive head of the biochemistry department. Working with colleagues Mehran Goulian and Robert Sinsheimer, Kornberg conducted pioneer research on artificial DNA throughout the 1960s, eventually producing a substance that not only had the same physical and chemical properties as naturally produced DNA but was also biologically active. The team synthesized the infectious inner core of a virus and confirmed it as fully virulent, attacking cells and reproducing with the same efficiency as the original model.

Kornberg and his colleagues announced their results at a press conference, pointing out the far-reaching implications of synthetic DNA, particularly in the battle against hereditary defects, viruses, cancer and other diseases. As he concluded the interview Kornberg conveyed his hope that the course of human evolution would not be seriously affected by his endeavors. "There is vastly more we can and must do to further human cultural evolution by political and social means," he advised. "I see the greatest rewards of genetic chemistry to human welfare in the cure of disease and ultimately in a better understanding of human behavior and understanding."

Kornberg was honored by a number of prestigious awards, including the Paul-Lewis Award of the American Chemical Society, the Max Berg Award for prolonging human life and the Scientific Achievement Award of the American Medical Association. In addition to numerous scientific papers, his published works include *Enzymatic Synthesis of DNA* (1962).

Karl Martin Leonhard Albrecht Kossel 1853–1927

An early pioneer in the development of physiological chemistry, Albrecht Kossel was awarded the 1910 Nobel Prize for Physiology or Medicine for his investigation of cell chemistry in proteins.

In 1895 Kossel embarked on a detailed analysis of nucleoproteins—organic substances made up of nucleic acids and proteins. Several decades earlier Swiss physiologist Johann Miescher Friedrich Miescher, among the first to propose the theory of a "genetic code," discovered a product of nucleoprotein breakdown he identified as a nuclein. Refining Miescher's chemical analyses, Kossel discovered adenine, thymine, cytosine, and uracil, distinguishing these nitrogenous bases as products of the decomposition of nucleic acids. With this distinction Kossel established a means of differentiating between "true nucleins" (or "cell nucleins"), defined as substances that can be broken down into protein and nucleic acid, and "pseudonucleins" (or "paranucleins"), referring to substances of similar appearance found in milk or egg yolk, now known as nucleoalbumins.

Establishing the large quantities of nuclein in embryonic tissue, Kossel's physiological studies led him to recognize the role of nuclein in the formation of new tissue. Other protein chemistry research included a biochemical investigation of fish sperm and extensive study of amino acids and peptones (the product of protein splitting). His later work foreshadowed modern findings on the fundamental significance of proteins in biological development and specificity of form and function.

Born in Rostock, Germany, Kossel was educated at the University of Strasbourg, where he studied under Felix Hoppe-Seyler, Germany's foremost exponent of physiological chemistry. Recognizing Kossel's talent and dedication, Hoppe-Seyler hired him as an assistant in 1877. Kossel's work had caught the attention of another influential figure in the German scientific establishment, electrophysiologist Emile Du Bois-Reymond, who in 1883 appointed Kossel director of the department of chemistry at Berlin's Physiological Institute.

A decade later Kossel left Berlin to take over as director of the Physiological Institute at Marburg, where he also accepted the chair of physiology. He later joined the faculty at Heidelberg, where he became influential in the careers of a number of students who would soon distinguish themselves in the field of chemistry, most notably H.D. DAKIN. After retiring from teaching in 1924

Kossel served as director of Heidelberg's newly established center for the study of proteins.

Kossel's son Walther, born in 1888, gained recognition as an important scientist in his own right in the area of atomic physics.

Hans Adolf Krebs 1900–1981

Shedding new light on the mechanism by which food is converted into energy, Hans Adolf Krebs launched a revolution in biochemical research. Although later studies were to refine and amend Krebs's biochemical analyses, his discovery of cyclical paths in cell metabolism led to the discovery of a great many other cell reaction cycles in intermediary metabolic processes.

Krebs's first landmark study, conducted in 1932 at the University of Freiburg, revealed a self-perpetuating sequence of cellular reactions in the metabolism of proteins known as the "urea cycle." Five years later he established a second cycle of biochemical events known as the citric acid cycle, or "Krebs cycle," which occurs as the second stage of the three-part process of carbohydrate metabolism.

An essential step in the biochemical conversion of glucose into physical energy, the citric acid cycle is an intermediate step in the biochemical conversion of sugars, fats and proteins into carbon dioxide and water. Krebs discovered that citric acid, the first and last product generated in a chain of chemical reactions, serves as a catalyst for oxidation, an essential event in the transformation of chemical energy, or fuel, into physical energy, or muscle power.

Descended from Jewish-Silesian ancestry, Hans Krebs was born in Hildesheim, Germany, where his father had established a successful practice as an ear, nose and throat surgeon. Intending to follow in his father's footsteps, Hans studied medicine at the Universities of Gottingen, Freiburg, Berlin and Hamburg, where he received his degree in 1925.

After graduating Krebs joined the staff of the chemistry department at the Institute of Pathology at the University of Berlin, where he was exposed to the latest developments in biochemical research. Berlin's department of chemistry became the training ground for a number of distinguished biochemists, including FRITZ LIPMANN and ERNST B. CHAIN.

Enthralled with the world of biochemical research, Krebs took a job as research assistant in the laboratory of Nobel laureate OTTO WARBURG. Though Krebs was in most ways profoundly influenced by his celebrated mentor, he pursued a career in biochemistry research despite Warburg's warnings about the shortage of jobs in the field.

Krebs left Berlin in 1930 to join the faculty at the University of Freiburg, where within the next two years he completed his study of the urea cycle. The rise of Nazism in Germany forced his emigration to England, where he was invited to join the Institute of Biochemistry at Cambridge University, under the direction of SIR FREDERICK GOWLAND HOPKINS. Krebs launched his study of the citric acid cycle at Cambridge, continuing his research at the University of Sheffield, where he began teaching in 1935. Krebs was to spend nearly twenty years on the faculty at Sheffield, during which he became recognized as a leading authority on biochemistry. During World War II he helped coordinate a government nutritional study, with particular attention to the dietary roles of vitamins A and C.

In 1953 Krebs was honored for his landmark study of metabolism with the Nobel Prize for Physiology or Medicine, which he shared with Fritz Lipmann. In the following year Krebs joined Oxford University, where he continued to study the biochemical mechanisms of cell metabolism, also examining the diseases known as "inborn errors of metabolism." In recognition of his distinguished scientific career Hans Krebs was knighted in 1958.

A frequent visitor to Israel, Krebs lent his efforts to the development of the Hebrew University in Jerusalem. In 1960 he was awarded the *Doctor honoris causa*, acknowledging his considerable contribution to the establishment of the university's biochemistry department. The Israelis expressed their respect and gratitude again in 1972, appointing Krebs an honorary fellow of the Weizmann Research Institute, their nation's highest scientific honor.

A humble and occasionally sardonic man, Krebs suggested to a meeting of the American Philosophical Society in 1970 that the way to impress upon governments the value of scientific exploration would be to do away with the vast amount of wasteful and gratuitous research he described as "occupational therapy for the university staff."

Schack August Steenberg Krogh 1874–1949

Krogh was a Danish physiologist who studied zoology at the University of Copenhagen. His chief interest was in the respiratory and circulatory systems, and he studied these processes under various conditions in humans and in other living organisms. Krogh's most important findings were in the anatomy and physiology of blood capillaries. He described the system by which the motor mechanisms in capillaries are regulated in order to provide muscle tissue with the appropriate amounts of blood. Krogh's observations expanded not only the prevalent ideas of respiration and circulation but also advanced the understanding of water balance, metabolism and related diseases.

In 1920 Krogh was awarded the Nobel Prize in Medicine for these influential studies. In the course of his research he also observed the effects of deep-sea conditions on marine life and the effect on Eskimos of their exclusive meat diet.

Krogh taught zoophysiology at the University of Copenhagen from 1916 to 1945. In 1922 he published the first edition of *The Anatomy and Physiology of Capillaries*. A revised edition came out in 1959 and included a memoir of Krogh. Other writings include *Osmotic Regulation in Aquatic Animals* (1939) and *Comparative Physiology of Respiratory Mechanisms* (1941).

Elisabeth Kübler-Ross 1926–

Swiss-born physician and psychiatrist Elisabeth Kübler-Ross pioneered theoretical and practical advances in the understanding of death. Admired for her compassion as well as the strength of her convictions, Kübler-Ross dedicated much of her life to the medical and human rights of the terminally ill and to an advanced understanding of the experience of dying. As a leading proponent of the "Death Awareness Movement," Kübler-Ross is recognized for her tireless efforts on behalf of dying patients and their families. Her best-selling book, entitled *On Death and Dying,* attempted to overcome some of society's most deeply rooted fears and taboos by encouraging a more frank and open discussion of death.

Death was no stranger to her from the start, when, as the first of a set of triplets, she weighed barely two pounds at birth. In *Death: The Final Stage of Growth* she described the last days of a child she knew in the village near Zurich where they both lived. "She was never removed from the village," Kübler-Ross wrote, "or from her home. There was no impersonal hospital where she had to die in a strange environment. Everybody close to her was near her day and night." Recalling the impact of the girl's funeral in the village, Kübler-Ross wrote: "There was a feeling of solidarity, of common tragedy shared by a whole community."

In contrast, Elisabeth's personal experience when she was hospitalized with a life-threatening illness at the age of five is described as a frightening and disorienting experience during which she was isolated from human contact for weeks in a "cage" of glass walls, without the comfort of a "familiar voice, touch, odor, not even a familiar toy."

As an adolescent during World War II she volunteered her services at Zurich's Kantonsspital, helping to care for thousands of German refugees. When peace came Elisabeth Kübler left Switzerland to observe first-hand the aftermath of the war. Working her way across Europe, she took odd jobs as a manual laborer, helped to organize medical care facilities, and even traveled with a gypsy caravan. She later commented that a pre-occupation with death and a respect for the dignity of the dying was the inevitable result of having visited concentration camps immediately after the war. Working as a hospital aide in a small, understaffed and overcrowded clinic in Poland, Kübler made the decision to pursue a career in medicine.

She returned to Switzerland to enroll in the University of Zurich, where she was granted a degree in medicine in 1957. In the beginning of the following year she married American neuropathologist Emanuel Robert Ross, who had been a fellow medical student at Zurich. Completing her internship and residency requirements in New York, she accepted a fellowship in psychiatry at the University of Colorado School of Medicine. At the Psychopathic Hospital, and later at the university's General Hospital, she achieved a significant measure of success with an unprecedented approach to the treatment of chronic schizophrenics: She allowed her patients to suggest the treatment that they thought would be most effective.

Kübler-Ross left Denver in 1965 to join the faculty at the University of Chicago Medical School, where she was appointed assistant professor of psychiatry and assistant director of psychiatric consultation. Soon after her arrival she was approached by a group of students from the Chicago Theological Seminary who requested her help in an investigation that would become the major focus of her career. Seeking to provide comfort to the terminally ill, the seminarians wanted to gain a more practical understanding of the spiritual, emotional and physical needs of the dying patient.

Kübler-Ross launched the first of a series of interviews with terminally ill patients that eventually formed the basis of a teaching seminar at Billings Hospital in Chicago. Although patients were generally eager to talk openly about the issue that governed nearly every moment of their lives, many doctors opposed the project, fearing the potentially negative effects of uninhibited discussion.

Kübler-Ross spent hundreds of hours in conversation with the dying, gradually gaining an understanding of their psychological and emotional condition. She offered counseling and support in return, eventually establishing training seminars and workshops for professionals as well as family members of the terminally ill patient.

Based on her exhaustive observations, Kübler-Ross reported a number of characteristic reactions to the prospect of imminent death. She identified five basic phases, beginning with denial, an unwillingness to accept the circumstances. This stage is often followed by anger, frequently as a result of feeling "singled out." After a period of resentment the patient may enter into "bargaining," in the hope of delaying the inevitable. A period of depression, described by Kübler-Ross as a form of grieving, is sometimes necessary to allow the patient to reach the fifth stage, in which death is finally accepted, sometimes with a growing sense of detachment.

As chief of the consultation and liaison department of LaRabida Children's Hospital and Research Center, Kübler-Ross concentrated on the particular problems of young terminally ill patients and their families. She also served as consulting psychiatrist to the Chicago Lighthouse for the Blind and medical director of the Family Services and Mental Health Center of South Cook County, Illinois.

Since 1975 Kübler-Ross has stirred widespread controversy by her research into the afterlife. For several years she had recorded the independent accounts of patients describing the experience of near-death. Struck by the many elements and motifs in these reports, she sought to establish a scientific confirmation of the phenomenon of life after life.

In the late 1970s she established Shanti Nilaya (Sanskrit for "Home of Peace"), a nonprofit center for teaching and therapy in the hills of Southern California. She also founded the American Holistic Medicine Association.

Her many published works include *On Death and Dying* (1969), *Questions and Answers on Death and Dying* (1974), *Death—The Final Stage of Growth* (1975), *To Live until We Say Goodbye* (1978) and *Living with Death and Dying* (1981).

L

René Théophile Hyacinthe Laënnec 1781–1826

Although he is celebrated for his outstanding work as a clinician and pathologist, René Théophile Laënnec is best remembered for revolutionizing diagnostic medicine with his invention of the stethoscope. As a physician, Laënnec practiced the diagnostic technique of auscultation, in which a practitioner places his ear directly on the chest of the patient in order to listen to sounds emanating from the heart and lungs. JEAN-NICOLAS CORVISART, a distinguished physician and cardiologist who would become Laënnec's mentor at the Hôpital de la Charité, had discovered the "percussion method" in he the writings of Viennese physician Leopold Auenbrugger (1722–1809).

The dignified Laënnec considered the act of listening directly to a patient's chest not only ineffective but "inconvenient, indelicate, and, in hospitals, even disgusting." He also noted that the procedure "was hardly suitable where most women were concerned, and with some the very size of their breasts was a physical obstacle." It is reported that the solution to the problem occurred to Laënnec as he watched two young boys playing with a wooden plank. The sounds created on one end of the board were clearly distinguishable at the other, inspiring Laënnec to apply the same acoustic principle to sounds emitted from the chest cavity. Rolling up several sheets of paper into a tube, he placed one end to the chest of a patient and listened at the other end. "I was as surprised as I was gratified to hear the beating of the heart much more clearly and distinctly than if I had applied my ear directly to the chest."

Dubbing the new technique "mediate auscultation," Laënnec was sufficiently encouraged by his preliminary results to futher refine the instrument. He compared the efficiency of different types and thicknesses of wood, finally determining that a foot-long cylinder of beechwood provided the best results. Further experimentation revealed that tubes of a single thickness were most efficient for listening to breathing sounds, whereas a tube of double thickness was more effective for hearing a patient's vocal wheezes and heartbeat.

Laënnec called his device a "stethoscope," although the name, meaning literally "examination of the chest," is misleading. Others referred to the device as a pectoriloquy or medical trumpet, but by any name, Laënnec's invention initially stirred great controversy in the Parisian medical community. Three years after its inception Laënnec formally introduced the stethoscope to the public in his book entitled *Traité de l'auscultation médiate* (*Concerning Mediated Auscultation*), published in 1819. Subtitled *A Study of the Diseases of the Lungs and Heart, Based Principally on the New Means of Exploration*, Laënnec's work encompassed far more than a discussion of his new invention.

Laënnec used this innovative technique to expand his study of the physiology and pathology of the chest cavity. He described the various stages of pneumonia, pulmonary tuberculosis, and pleurisy, also identifying for the first time a number of other diseases, including emphysema, bronchiectasis, pulmonary melanosis and cirrhosis of the liver, also referred to as "Laënnec's cirrhosis." His name has also been attached to the soft matter expectorated in bronchial asthma, known as "Laënnec's pearls."

Along with PHILIPPE PINEL and Pierre Louis (1787–1872), Laënnec was one of a pioneering group of French physicians in the early 19th century who greatly advanced the practice of medicine by organizing and refining the criteria for diagnosis and classification of disease. Drawing from clinical observations as well as postmortem evidence, Laënnec correlated the symptoms of a pathology with the physiological changes discovered in autopsy to describe the qualitative, structural effects of specific diseases. In cancers Laënnec emphasized the significance of the tissue of origin, recognizing the disease's tendency to spread.

From the first, the life of young René Théophile was imbued with the threat of disease and death. He grew up in the midst of the French Revolution and, to compound the mortal dangers all around him, inherited a tendency to tuberculosis, which caused the premature deaths of many members of his family before he, too, succumbed at the age of forty-five. Born in Quimper in Brittany, René was seven years old when he and his brother were sent to live with their uncle Guillaume, a physician practicing in Nantes. On July 14 of the following year the Bastille fell, but it was not until 1792 that the revolution overshadowed the lives of René and his brother, along with all those caught in the brutal battle for Nantes between revolutionary and counterrevolutionary forces. Guillaume worked tirelessly at the hospital treating war casualties, often bringing the wounded into his own home as well. The boys, barely into their teens, thus saw the casualties of revolution in their own home as well as in the streets.

Spurred on by the immediate medical emergency, the revolution gave rise to significant reforms in medical practice and education. In an effort to end a long tradition of bitter competition, physicians and surgeons were officially united in a single branch of medicine, designated "the healing art." Terminating archaic systems and antiquated methods of teaching, medical schools were reorganized to meet the needs of the time. As young doctors emerged from this revitalized system of education they established France as an international center for clinical medicine.

In 1795 Laënnec embarked on a career in medicine as an apprentice student. He pursued his profession in the midst of political turmoil, serving as a commissioned third-class surgeon, a medical officer in the army, and later resuming studies under Jean- Nicolas Corvisart at the Charité, the largest and most prestigious hospital in Paris. He also completed studies at the École Pratique, where he was influenced by noted histologist XAVIER BICHAT. Laënnec followed his term at the École with a three- year course in anatomy, surgery and dissection.

Although fighting a constant fatigue, Laënnec worked feverishly, publishing articles regularly on a wide variety of medical subjects including amenorrhea, the function of the prostate and the fibrous structures enclosing the liver, spleen and kidney. After receiving his medical degree he established a medical practice in Paris in 1804. Laënnec's list of patients expanded rapidly to include an impressive array of celebrities, and he was soon appointed personal physician to Joseph Cardinal Fesch, an uncle of the emperor Napoleon.

In the volatile political climate Laënnec's fortunes fluctuated dramatically. He worked for a time at Paris's historic hospital La Salpêtrière, treating the endless stream of wounded soldiers. In 1816 he became chief physician at the Hospital Necker, where, in addition to his clinical duties, he delivered daily lectures attended by students and colleagues from all over Paris. It was in 1816, while working at Necker, that the idea of the stethoscope first occurred to Laënnec.

By the time his book was published, Laënnec, at the age of thirty-eight, was chronically exhausted. Despite the controversy and mixed reviews, the book sold well, but Laënnec felt too weak to continue working in Paris. He left for Quimper, where he remained until economic pressures forced him to return to work. Resuming clinical practice at the Hôpital de la Charité, he also accepted the position of professor and royal lecturer at the Collège de France. On August 13, 1826, several hours before his death, Laënnec removed the rings from his fingers, saying, "Someone will soon have to render me this service. I wish to spare him this painful task."

Fernand Lamaze 1891–1957

Recognized as a leading Western authority on natural or "painless" childbirth, Fernand Lamaze developed a method of psychoprophylactic preparation for expectant mothers based on the PAVLOVIAN system of deconditioning that had become popular in the 1940s in the Soviet Union. Although Lamaze differed in both theory and practice from British gynecologist GRANTLY DICK-READ, the two leading authorities on natural childbirth shared the basic belief that the pain experienced during childbirth is of psychological origin and can be avoided by a method of physical and mental preparation.

"It is necessary to destroy prejudices based on ignorance," Lamaze declared, "to enlighten the woman by instructing her about the phenomena involved in the childbirth, the purpose being to convert delivery from the idea of pain to a series of understood processes in which uterine contraction is the leading phenomenon...Labor thereby leaves the high-lights of phantasmagoria for the quiet shadow of physiological reality."

Seeking to free his pregnant patients from the negative effects of "cultural conditioning," Lamaze devised a system of behavioral training that emphasized the woman's active participation through breathing and muscle control. "Rather than telling the patient to relax," he said, "we enable her to help herself in the various phases of labor so that she is able to relax." He described the "undramatizing" of labor as the first step in removing apprehension and allowing the expectant mother to establish a set of new and and more productive conditioned reflexes:

> Normal respiration works by inborn reflex. By modifying the rhythm of breathing, a conditioned reflex is initiated as a sort of "branch" of the normal reflex. The repeated teaching of this new respiratory style leads to the formation of a new conditioned reflex, which we may call the contraction-respiration reflex. Uterine contraction, as a sequel of this, becomes the signal for a specific respiration and not any longer for pain.

Born in Paris, Lamaze earned a degree in obstetric medicine from the University of Paris in 1922. He observed the practice of psychoprophylactic preparation during a visit to the Soviet Union, and in 1952 he introduced the "Lamaze Method" of drug- free, painless childbirth at the Maternité du Metallurgiste, a distinguished maternity hospital in Paris. Four years later he published *Qu'est-ce que l'accouchement sans douleur?*, a discussion of the underlying psychological and physiological principles of his technique, as well as a step-by-step guide.

The book appeared in English translation in 1958 under the title *Painless Childbirth,* and it was not long before the Lamaze technique was adopted, at least as an optional approach, in hospitals throughout the United

States and Great Britain. One of the most controversial features of the method was one that held an immediate appeal for many of its earliest advocates. Lamaze stressed the importance of a *monitrice*—a comforting and supportive partner during the birthing process who is trained to act as a "labor coach" during the delivery. Encouraging expectant fathers to take an active role in the procedure, he cautioned that "as long as the husband has been trained so that he knows what to expect and what his place is in the delivery room there is no problem," but to allow a husband to enter the delivery room unprepared "is the quickest way to defeat the program—it might be a very traumatic experience for the husband if he hasn't been prepared psychologically and by actual training...The husband is in there to work. His place is to provide moral support for his wife."

The virtues of psychoprophylactic preparation were celebrated by Marjorie Karmel in her popular book entitled *Thank You, Dr. Lamaze*. Published in 1959, the personal testimonial helped the Lamaze method to become the most widely accepted of all the various "natural childbirth" techniques.

Rebecca Craighill Lancefield 1895–1981

Exploring the biological and pathological characteristics of streptococci for more than six decades, American bacteriologist Rebecca Lancefield gave the world a key to the identification of these bacteria, so often implicated in disease.

Streptococci belong to a genus of sphere-shaped bacteria (cocci) that characteristically link together to form a chain. The subcategories of genus Streptococcus include the alpha-hemolytic group, which comprises parasitic forms found as normal flora of the upper resiratory and intestinal tracts; the saprophytic forms, living on dead or decaying organic matter; and the beta-hemolytic group, containing animal and human pathogens such as those found in pneumonia, tonsillitis and urinary tract infections. The Lancefield classification system of hemolytic streptococci has been adopted by physicians, immunologists, epidemiologists and biologists throughout the world.

Published in 1933, *A Serological Differentiation of Human and Other Groups of Hemolytic Streptococci* not only classified the more than 60 forms of dangerous bacteria but described techniques for producing streptococcal antigens. Lancefield noted that "the results of this study are of interest not only from the theoretical viewpoint of establishing an orderly grouping of these microorganisms but also from an epidemiological aspect in providing means of identifying the probable origin of a given strain."

Lancefield's exhaustive research also showed that a single type of streptococcal bacterium could cause a number of different conditions, such as sore throat, scarlet fever or erysipelas, an infectious skin disease. Moreover, she demonstrated that immunity to streptococcus is type-specific.

Born in Fort Wadsworth, New York, Rebecca Craighill was studying English literature at Wellesley College when she became interested in biological sciences in her junior year. Completing graduate and doctoral studies in biology at Columbia University, she received her degree in 1918, the same year in which she married biologist Donald E. Lancefield.

After graduating from Columbia University Rebecca Lancefield accepted a position at the Rockefeller Institute for Medical Research, where she served as research assistant under noted bacteriologists OSWALD T. AVERY and Alphonse R. Dochez, who later conducted extensive studies of the common cold. During World War I Lancefield investigated the role of streptococci in rheumatic fever, studying samples obtained from the victims of a series of severe epidemics of streptococcal infection.

Appointed professor of microbiology in 1922, she remained on the faculty at Rockefeller University until her death at the age of eighty-six. A member of the United States National Academy of Sciences, Lancefield is distinguished as the first woman to serve as president of the American Association of Immunologists.

Karl Landsteiner 1868–1943

Karl Landsteiner's landmark studies in immunology and serological reaction brought to light the notion of human blood types. This discovery, revealing specific and highly significant cellular differences between individuals, demonstrated the incompatibility between some blood types. Landsteiner's findings gave rise to a safe procedure for blood transfusion, contributing greatly to the eventual success of organ and tissue transplants. The revelation of blood "markers," the determinant factors in an individual's blood type, led Landsteiner and Brooklyn physician Alexander Wiener to another landmark discovery: the "Rh" marker, named for its presence in the blood cells of rhesus monkeys as well as those of humans.

Karl Landsteiner, the son of a Viennese journalist, earned his medical degree in 1891 from the University of Vienna. Landsteiner's interest in serology and biochemistry led him to study chemistry in Germany, where he worked under noted German chemist E.F. Fischer, who was later to win a Nobel Prize for his work in synthesizing sugars. Returning to Austria in 1896, Landsteiner served for ten years as a research assistant at the Vienna Pathological Institute.

Landsteiner's studies with Fischer had involved the differentiation of proteins by chemical analysis, based on observing the interaction at a molecular level between proteins and organic tissue. This process inspired Landsteiner to investigate the components in human blood by a similar procedure. Combining red blood cells drawn from two different sources, Landsteiner observed that occasionally the cells would join together. Through extensive and detailed experimentation between 1900 and 1902 Landsteiner arrived at an explanation for this phenomenon. Discerning two protein substances in red blood cells, he observed that his samples might contain one, both or neither of these substances. Using these proteins as markers, dubbed A and B, he identified his blood samples by the marker (or markers) present. Thus the four recognizable blood groups, or types, were identified as A, B, AB and O (when no marker was present).

Landsteiner saw that a serum contains antibodies against a foreign marker, so that if an individual with type A blood is injected with B or AB type blood, his antibodies will destroy the red blood cells with B markers. Type O blood will respond with antibodies against both markers but can be safely injected into all blood types.

For centuries, blood transfusions from animals to humans had been attempted with results so deadly that the process was banned in England, France and Italy. In the nineteenth century European physicians considered human blood transfusion, but only as a desperate measure, as results were at best unreliable. The record suggests that the Incan civilization introduced the procedure of human blood transfusion with considerably more success. Landsteiner explained this fact by pointing out that nearly all South American Indians have type O blood. Thus the system of blood typing served an important anthropological role, helping to chart the history of human migration and racial interrelationships.

In 1909 Landsteiner joined the faculty at the University of Vienna as professor of pathological anatomy. His remarkable findings found little public recognition or practical application until the outbreak of World War I, when millions of wounded soldiers were desperately in need of blood. Putting Landsteiner's ABO blood-typing method into effect, a large-scale blood drive was launched. Storage was made possible with the advent of sodium citrate to prevent clotting.

The war left Landsteiner's country, as well as his professional life, in ruins. He left Austria with his wife and son to continue his work in Holland. In 1922, invited to New York by the Rockefeller Institute for Medical Research, he emigrated to the United States, becoming a citizen in 1929. The following year Landsteiner's work in the classification of human blood types was honored with the award of the 1930 Nobel Prize for Physiology or Medicine.

Working at the Rockefeller Institute with Philip Levine, Landsteiner discovered two additional classifications of human blood, with markers dubbed M and N, based on studies comparing blood from a number of different species. A significant refinement of his original idea, this new direction of investigation led to Landsteiner's next medical breakthrough.

Landsteiner had begun working with Alexander Weiner on a research project involving rabbits, rhesus monkeys and human blood. Observing the behavior of the rabbits' antibodies, Landsteiner and Weiner discovered a red blood cell marker common to rhesus monkeys and a large percentage of humans. This "Rh factor" explained for the first time a generally fatal syndrome of jaundice and anemia occurring in some infants.

Landsteiner realized that this heartbreaking condition was due to a sequence of immunological events initiated when an Rh-positive child is born to an Rh-negative mother. If, during birth, fetal blood cells enter the mother's circulatory system, her body will develop antibodies against the Rh marker. If she conceives a second Rh-positive child, her antibodies will attack the red blood cells of the fetus, sometimes killing it even before it leaves the womb. This condition is now prevented by a system of antibody vaccination for Rh-negative mothers administered between the births of their first and second children.

In addition to saving the lives of countless infants, Landsteiner's work with primate blood classification had important theoretical implications. Evolutionary relationships among humans and primates can be tracked by Landsteiner's comparative studies of blood groups. Other applications of Landsteiner's research include the use of blood typing as a method of identification in legal and forensic cases.

Perhaps Landsteiner's greatest contribution, however, was to pave the way for the enormous strides taken in medicine in the decades to follow. The 1960s saw the first genetically determined markers, located in white blood cells, leading to the subsequent success of tissue and organ transplants. Immunologists continue to investigate the possibility of markers in diseases such as rheumatoid arthritis, multiple sclerosis and cancer.

At 75 Landsteiner was still conducting research when he suffered a fatal heart attack in his laboratory at Rockefeller Institute.

Landsteiner's written works include *Specificity of Serological Reactions,* published in 1933.

Mother Alphonsa Lathrop (Rose Hawthorne Lathrop)
1851–1926

In a two-room tenement apartment on the Lower East Side of New York City Rose Lathrop founded the first hospice for terminally ill cancer patients. To commemorate her death in 1926, the *New York World* printed the following tribute:

> She was a personality, one who would have been interesting whether she had ever undertaken her humanitarian work or not. To many a welfare worker it would have been enough to provide a refuge for the sick and to provide charity's indifferent hospitality. But not for her. Her guests, poor and helpness though they were, were still her guests, and treated as such; their whims were deferred to as well as their needs, and did they crave preposterous delicacies she did not chide them for being unreasonable but did her best to satisfy them, and usually succeeded. In other words she respected the eternal childishness of humanity, simply because it is childish and not amenable to reason...Such a person understands that man does not live by bread alone, that he is cursed with an imagination which sets him reaching for things a little above the necessities of life.

The youngest child of celebrated author Nathaniel Hawthorne, Rose was born in Lenox, Massachussetts, but from the time she was three she lived in Liverpool, England, where her father served as consul. The Hawthornes carefully supervised the intellectual and cultural development of their children, providing Rose and her brother and sister with the benefits of a rich and well-rounded education, supplemented by extensive travel and an erudite circle of friends.

In her early twenties she settled in London, tentatively embarking on a literary career. Within several years she published a volume of poetry, a collection of short stories and a series of articles entitled "Memories of Hawthorne" that first appeared in the *Atlantic Monthly* and were later compiled in book form. In 1873 she married George Parsons Lathrop, and together they converted to the Roman Catholic faith. A brief literary collaboration produced *A Story of Courage*, a history of the Georgetown Visitation Convent, but the Lathrops devoted the greater part of their joined efforts to philanthropic and charitable works.

In 1896 they founded the first home for victims of incurable cancer. When George Lathrop died two years later Rose became a nun of the Dominican order and dedicated her life to the welfare of the terminally ill. With four other nuns she established a small cancer hospice on Cherry Street in lower Manhattan, where patients were admitted free of charge, without regard to race or religion. Taking the name Mother Alphonsa, she founded a sisterhood known as the Servants of Relief for Incurable Cancer. In 1901 a religious community was established at Rosary Hill Home in Hawthorne, a small town in northern Westchester County, New York.

Seeking to provide for the increasing number of patients in need, Mother Alphonsa took over a five-story building in New York City to found a second and larger hospice called St. Rose's Free Home for Incurable Cancer in 1912.

Charles Louis Alphonse Laveran 1845–1922

When Alphonse Laveran received the Nobel Prize for Physiology or Medicine in 1907 the awards committee cited "his work regarding the role played by protozoa in causing diseases." As the discoverer of the malarial parasite, Laveran had attained international and historical distinction more than twenty-five years earlier.

Laveran dedicated most of his life to the study of parasitology and tropical medicine, conducting exhaustive investigations of a number of protozoan parasites in humans and animals. Defined as an animal phylum or subkingdom of single-cell, self- reproducing organisms, all protozoa, unlike bacteria, have at least one clearly defined nucleus. Protozoa (from the Greek *protos*, meaning "first," and *zoion*, meaning "animal") are subdivided into several classes, including Sporozoa, Ciliophora, and Rhizopoda. Flagellata, also known as Mastigophora, are a class of Protozoa characterized by one or more threadlike projections that provide mobility by their undulating movement caused by the surrounding waves.

Born in Paris, Alphonse Laveran was five years old when his father, an army physician, was appointed to a post in North Africa. After spending five years with his family in Algeria, Laveran was sent back to France to complete his education. In 1867 he obtained a medical degree from the University of Strasbourg, later fulfilling hospital internships in Lille and Paris. Following a tour of military duty during the Franco-Prussian War (in which he endured the siege of Metz), he was named professor of medicine at the Val-de-Grace School of Military Medicine in 1874.

Four years later Laveran was commissioned by the French Army to return to Algeria to study the cause and infective mechanism of malaria, a disease that then seriously threatened public health in Africa and many other parts of the world. Malaria was common in ancient Asian and Middle Eastern civilizations and is likely to have existed in prehistoric times. Reported in the fifth and fourth centuries B.C. by the Hippocratics, malarial epidemics had been associated with environmental conditions of heat and humidity, but it was not until Laveran's discovery—followed by the work of Camillo Golgi, Patrick Manson, RONALD ROSS, Amico Bignami (1862–1929), E. Marchiafava (1874–1935) and others—that the role of the mosquito in the transmission of the disease was clearly established. Designated at various times as "ague" or "intermittent fever," the disease derived its current name in the early eighteenth century from Italian roots meaning literally "bad air."

Malaria occurs in either chronic or acute form, generally following an episodic and recurrent pattern. Characterized by intermittent fever crises followed by symptom-free periods, the course of the disease involves fever cycles of three or four days, depending on the reproductive cycle of the parasite. If left untreated, the blood parasite causes enlargement of the spleen and liver, leading to anemia, jaundice, general debility and frequently, infection of the cerebral tissues.

Since the middle of the nineteenth century pathologists had noted the presence of black granules in the blood of malaria victims, recognizing them as products of the pathological degeneration of the blood. While in Algeria Laveran observed that these granules appeared in cysts actively moving inside the blood cells of malaria patients. Upon close examination of these cysts Laveran discovered an undulating filament extruding from the cell, providing a vital clue to the flagellate identity of the agent.

Laveran published the first announcement of his discovery in November of 1880, subsequently adding expanded papers and book- length treatises that appeared between 1884 and 1892. Despite considerable evidence based on clinical, pathological and geographic analysis, his findings were not accepted until they had been confirmed by other leading investigators. The studies of Ronald Ross and Camillo Golgi in particular furnished convincing support for Laveran's identification of the protozoan culprit, later given the name Plasmodia.

Since the army offered little opportunity to continue pathological research, Laveran left in 1896 to join the staff at the Pasteur Institute in Paris. Established as a leading authority on parasitology and protozoal agents of disease, Laveran conducted outstanding studies of other flagellata, including trypanosoma, a genus of blood parasites. Later identified as the causative agents of sleeping sickness, trypanosomes are transmitted to vertebrate animals by tsetse flies or other insect vectors. In collaboration with colleague Felix Mesnil (1868–1938) Laveran produced the first definitive treatise on trypanosomes and trypanosomiases in 1904.

Laveran published an important study of another genus of protozoa called Leishmania (see W.B. LEISHMAN) in 1917, in which he distinguished two forms of leishmaniases, identified as Indian and Mediterranean kala-azar. Other notable published works include *Traité des maladies et des épidémies des armeés (Treatise on Military Diseases and Epidemics)* (1875), *Traité des fièvres palustres (Treatise on Malarial Fevers)* (1884), *Traité d'hygiène militaire (Treatise on Military Hygiene)* (1896), *Traité du paludisme (Treatise on Malaria)* (1898).

Antoine Laurent Lavoisier 1743–1794

Considered the founder of modern chemistry, Antoine Lavoisier dedicated himself to a science based on facts, rather than on the fanciful speculations being juggled by the alchemists of his day. At the basis of his work was the principle of advancing to the unknown from the known, accepting results only from observable causes.

Lavoisier's genius lay in his ability to organize and synthesize available knowledge, editing and expanding existing scientific theory. In Lavoisier's time, medical "cures" were often conjurers' concoctions with little or no therapeutic value, and alchemy, the transmutation of metals or other substances, was an accepted part of science. Lavoisier disproved these principles and introduced the fundamental notion of chemical elements.

Born to a wealthy and distinguished Parisian family, it was assumed that Lavoisier would follow in his father's footsteps and become a lawyer. The young Antoine, who had lost his mother in childhood, had developed an early passion for science, however. Frail health provided a good excuse for him to withdraw from the world around him and devote himself to his own experiments at an early age.

At twenty-four, Lavoisier was invited to collaborate with noted geologist Jean Guettard, who had been commissioned to produce a mineralogical atlas of France. Traveling through France with Guettard for several months, Lavoisier honed his scientific skills and returned to Paris even more committed to a life of scientific study.

Although he was only twenty-five, Lavoisier was accepted as a member of France's Academy of Science. In order to earn more money for his own experimental research, Lavoisier became a *fermier*—one who bought from the government the concession of collecting indirect taxes. Although not likely to endear him to the citizenry, the job was profitable and made even more attractive by the daughter of another *fermier*. Lavoisier fell in love with Marie Anne Pierrette and they married when she turned fourteen. In addition to an impressive dowry, Lavoisier's influential new father-in-law also provided him with an additional salaried position, that of *régisseur des poudres* (director of the arsenal). Lavoisier's laboratory at the arsenal became a scientific salon entertaining such luminaries as Joseph Priestley, THOMAS YOUNG, Benjamin Franklin, and James Watt, the Scottish engineer.

Since his geologic studies with Guettard, Lavoisier had been interested in the physical characteristics of water. "Scientific demonstrations" of alchemy had been popular among scientists since the seventeenth century. People still spoke of Dutch chemist Jan Baptista van Helmont (1579–1644), who allegedly could transform water into wood. Lavoisier performed stringent and repeated experiments with water decomposition, demonstrating conclusively that any residue left after evaporation had been present in the vessel. His conclusion, that water is unalterable, signaled the downfall of alchemy.

Lavoisier followed these experiments with an investigation of the nature of air, expanding on the work of

Priestley and van Helmont. In 1777, Lavoisier publicly announced his discovery that air is made up of "two elastic fluids, one respirable, the other poisonous." He named the first "vital" fluid *oxygen*, a combination of Greek words *oxys*, meaning acid, and *gennan*, meaning to generate.

His studies of air and water led Lavoisier to postulate the chemical elements. Calling them *principes*, he defined them as substances that "chemical analysis cannot resolve into any simpler substance." Using this definition, Lavoisier created the first list of "real" substances, identifying thirty-three separate elements. In 1789 Lavoisier expounded his theories in a landmark work, entitled *Elementary Treatise of Chemistry*. Introduced in this treatise are many of the basic terms still used in the vocabulary of modern chemistry.

The scientific community responded enthusiastically to Lavoisier's work, but the political forces taking over France reacted differently. Before his days as a revolutionary, Jean Paul Marat had been a practicing physician. In 1780 he had written a paper on the physical nature of fire that was refuted by Lavoisier, among others. Whether moved by personal, political or scientific resentments—perhaps all three—Marat, in his newspaper *L'Ami du Peuple*, launched a scathing and inflammatory attack on Lavoisier, now director of the Academy of Science. Denouncing the Academy as a "defunct repository of royalist thought," the Robespierre regime conducting the Reign of Terror eventually shut it down. Lavoisier was arrested on charges of treason against the régime and extortion of taxes harking back to his days as a tax collector. Many of his fellow *fermiers* had already been sent to the guillotine.

At his trial, many of Lavoisier's supporters spoke in his defense, but when Lavoisier appealed for a reprieve to allow him to complete an experiment, he was told that "The Revolution doesn't need scientists, it needs justice."

In May of 1794, as Lavoisier was brought to the guillotine, noted French scientist Joseph Louis Lagrange is said to have remarked, "Only a moment to cut off his head, and perhaps a century before we shall have another like it."

Other works written by Lavoisier include *Physical and Chemical Essays*, and *Chemical Memoirs*, published posthumously in 1805.

Joshua Lederberg 1925–

Joshua Lederberg explored genetic mechanisms by studying the ways in which genes are recombined and transmitted in bacteria. His work provided powerful weapons in the fight organs career and other diseases.

Bacteria are the simplest and smallest of all living organisms. They are unicellular and possess no nucleus, which distinguishes then from animals and plants. In more complex organisms the nucleus is the site of genetic information. In bacteria the DNA is found throughout the cell, and the genetic code is essentially the same in all bacteria of a species. This simplicity and consistency makes the bacterium a valuable tool in genetic studies.

Lederberg confirmed that although bacteria reproduce by dividing asexually, a sexual recombination of genes also takes place. This bacterial exchange of genetic information, known as transduction, occurs with the intervention of the bacteriophage virus, which invades the bacteria and ultimately transports genetic material from one bacterial cell to another. Once Lederberg understood this process he could control and alter the genetic information inherited by bacteria. This technique became a powerful weapon in the fight against cancer and other diseases.

Lederberg was born in Montclair, New Jersey. He attended Columbia and Yale universities and received a Doctor of Science degree in 1948. Lederberg taught at the University of Wisconsin from 1947 to 1959. In 1958 his research in bacterial genetics was acknowledged with a Nobel Prize for Medicine, which he shared with George W. Beadle and Edward L. Tatum. Lederberg became a professor at Stanford University in 1959 and remained there until 1978. Since then he has served as president of Rockefeller University in New York.

Antonie van Leeuwenhoek 1632–1723

An amateur biologist with minimal formal education, Antonie van Leeuwenhoek won a pioneer's distinction in the history of science for his studies of microorganisms at a time when such forms of life were scarcely imagined. Although he cannot be credited with inventing the microscope, van Leeuwenhoek is acknowledged as the first to effectively use the instrument in scientific observation. Applying his own advanced techniques for lens grinding, lighting and focus, he produced instruments with a magnification of up to 270X, a tremendous improvement over the microscopes available in his day.

Despite his lack of training, van Leeuwenhoek possessed a highly motivating sense of scientific curiosity, and it is this intellectual adventurousness that led him to use the microscope to explore the invisible. As the first person in history to observe protozoa, bacteria and other single-celled organisms, Leeuwenhoek showed that within a raindrop, a tear, a drop of sweat or even a single animal hair exists a teeming population of living beings, or "animalcules," as he called them.

Observing the frenzied activity in a drop of semen, van Leeuwenhoek became the first to describe spermatozoa, asserting that these animalcules must enter the ovum for the creation of a fetus. Along with Nicolaas

Hartsoeker (1656–1725), who published drawings of tiny homunculi, or preformed men, inside the "spermatic animalcules," Leeuwenhoek maintained that each spermatozoon contained a preformed embryo, relying on the ovum merely as a safe location for prenatal development.

Known as the "animalculist view of preformation," Leeuwenhoek's mistaken theory challenged the prevailing and equally misguided "ovist" concept, which maintained that a preformed embryo is encapsulated in the egg. It was not until the end of the eighteenth century that both theories were abandoned.

Leeuwenhoek's remarkable observations are documented in the form of a lengthy correspondence with Henry Oldenburg, first secretary of the prestigious Royal Society in England. Admitted to the society in 1673, following the intervention of fellow Dutch scientist Rejnier de Graaf, van Leeuwenhoek was to recount his observations in 190 letters written over a period of fifty years. In these descriptions of a microscopic world he emphasized the similarities in all living creatures as evidenced in the common functions of reproduction, ingestion and digestion of nutrients and elimination of waste. He attributed variety in nature to varying degrees of anatomical complexity.

Leeuwenhoek described a universal network of biological conduits, indicating separate tubes for the transport of blood, air and nerve impulse; and, unaware of earlier findings by Italian microscopist Marcello Malpighi, he independently discovered the capillary system, responsible for transporting nutrients to the tissues.

Van Leeuwenhoek took great pains to conceal his methods, remaining courteous to visitors but notoriously secretive about his techniques. Although the scientific community has long celebrated his monumental contribution to microbiology and microscopy, many of Leeuwenhoek's observations continue to baffle historians. Of the 247 microscopes he constructed, only a precious few remain, and the power of these instruments cannot account for the extraordinary precision of his work. A leading authority on Leeuwenhoek, British microbiologist Clifford Dobell, suggests that the secret lies in a system of dark-ground lighting, possibly using a field of black taffeta silk illuminated by candlelight to highlight the subject by contrast.

Born in Delft, Antonie left school at the age fourteen and was sent to live with an uncle who provided him with a foundation in mathematics and basic physics. With little interest in any other form of intellectual pursuit, Leeuwenhoek left for Amsterdam at sixteen to learn a trade, opting for an apprenticeship in the Cloth Workers' Guild. A successful textile merchant by the age of 22, he purchased a house and an adjoining shop in Delft, where he was to spend the rest of his life.

His personal life was devastated by deaths, first of his three infant sons, then, in rapid succession, of his mother and his wife. Leeuwenhoek set out to rebuild his life on a new foundation. By the time he was named Chamberlain of the Council Chamber of the Worshipful Sheriffs of Delft in 1666 he had already begun to broaden his scientific horizons, studying navigation, astronomy, mathematics and natural sciences. A family inheritance provided sufficient resources to launch his exploration of uncharted microscopic worlds.

As one of Delft's distinguished citizens, van Leeuwenhoek was appointed to a variety of honorary and active municipal positions, serving as the city's "wine and liquor gauger" as well as the trustee of the property of the celebrated Dutch artist Jan Vermeer.

Initiated in 1673, his correspondence with the Royal Society appeared regularly in *Philosophical Transactions*, the society's journal, and was later collected and published separately, shortly before his death. Unanimously elected a fellow of the Royal Society in 1680, Leeuwenhoek was by then widely recognized as a scientific celebrity, receiving a steady flow of distinguished callers. Among the notables who visited Leeuwenhoek at his former dry-goods shop were Peter the Great of Russia, Queen Mary II of England, James II of England and Frederick the Great of Prussia.

Van Leeuwenhoek dictated two final letters to the Royal Society 36 hours before his death at the age of 90.

William Boog Leishman 1865–1926

Scottish bacteriologist William Boog Leishman is remembered for his discovery of the parasite, now known as the Leishman-Donovan body (*Leishmania donovani*), responsible for the fatal disease known as kala-azar. Also referred to as visceral leishmaniasis, febrile tropical splenomegaly and Assam, Hindu, black or Dum-Dum fever, the condition is characterized by fever, dropsy, progressive anemia and atrophy. Transmitted to humans by the sandfly, kala-azar is endemic to the warm regions of Asia, Africa, South America and parts of the Mediterranean basin.

In 1903 British protozoologist RONALD ROSS introduced the term Leishmania to refer to a genus of flagellate protozoan parasites responsible for a range of infectious diseases in humans and animals, including canine leishmaniasis, infantile leishmaniasis, nasopharyngeal leishmaniasis and cutaneous or dermal leishmaniasis. This last form, caused by *Leishmania tropica*, is a chronic condition characterized by the development of nodules, known as leishmanids that pass through a characteristic sequence of ulcerative stages.

Born in Glasgow, Leishman attended that city's university, where his father, William Leishman (1833–1894), was regius professor of midwifery. After receiving a masters degree in chemistry Leishman enlisted in the Army Medical Service, serving in India for ten years as staff surgeon under Sir George Wolseley. Promoted to the rank of major in the Royal Army Medical Corps, Leishman was recalled to England in 1899 to take charge of the clinical department at the military hospital and medical school in Netley.

Although he had conducted some experimental work in India, Leishman's position at Netley allowed him the first opportunity for extensive independent research, and it was there that he developed a stain for microscopic observation of blood samples. Using "Leishman's stain," he identified the kala-azar parasite in 1900, although the discovery was not published until it had been confirmed three years later by Irish physician Charles Donovan (1863–1951) of the Indian Medical Service.

Leishman went with the Royal Army Medical College when it was relocated to London in 1903, and in the decade that followed he served as professor of pathology while continuing to study kala-azar, tick fever and typhoid fever. During that time he perfected ALMROTH WRIGHT'S vaccine against typhoid, directing that a large supply be produced and held on reserve at the Army Medical School. The precaution paid off in August, 1914 at the beginning of World War I, when the vaccine was distributed to the Allied troops, saving many hundreds of thousands from the debilitating and sometimes fatal effects of the disease. Although typhoid fever, an infection of the bacteria *Salmonella typhi,* is now treated successfully with various antibacterial drugs, the vaccine is still recommended as a method of short-term prevention for military personnel and travelers to areas with poor sanitary conditions.

A leading authority on tropical diseases, Leishman served as a member of the Army Medical Advisory Board as well as chairman of committees on "trench fever" and "trench nephritis." In 1909 he was awarded a knighthood, and in the following year he was elected to the Royal Society and named president of the Society of Tropical Medicine and Hygiene. Internationally acknowledged for his contribution to medicine, Leishman received the Distinguished Service Medal of the United States of America and the title of Grand Officer of France's Legion of Honor. In 1923 he rose to the highest rank in the medical branch of the military when he was named lieutenant-general director of Army Medical Services in 1923.

Rita Levi-Montalcini 1909–

For distinguished research on the biochemistry of cell growth, microbiologist Rita Levi-Montalcini, along with American biochemist STANLEY COHEN, was awarded the 1986 Nobel Prize for Physiology or Medicine. The Nobel committee cited Levi-Montalcini in particular for her role in the discovery of "nerve growth factor," hailing her work as "a fascinating example of how a skilled observer can create a concept out of apparent chaos."

Levi-Montalcini was born to a Jewish family in Turin, Italy, where she grew up in the atmosphere of turn-of-the-century Europe, in which most young girls were educated, as she noted, "...not for self-development but for self-renunciation," and destined for "a future divided between family obligations and receptions." In *My Life and Work,* an autobiography published in 1987, she recalled her determination to avoid these constraints: "My experience in childhood and adolescence of the subordinate role played by the female in a society run entirely by men had convinced me that I was not cut out to be a wife...Babies did not attract me, and I was altogether without the maternal sense so highly developed in small and adolescent girls."

The University of Turin, in an unusual concession to women's rights, admitted her as a medical student and in 1936 awarded her a doctorate. As Levi-Montalcini embarked on her career in biological research, however, World War II broke, forcing her and her family to flee south to the relative safety of Florence. In addition to serving as a volunteer physician for Allied troops when they invaded Italy, she continued her experimental studies in a makeshift laboratory set up in her bedroom.

In 1947 Levi-Montalcini emigrated to the United States to join the research team at Washington University in St. Louis, led by noted zoologist Viktor Hamburger. It was on a trip to Rio de Janeiro in 1952 that she began the work leading to the discovery of a soluble protein substance that stimulates the growth of nerve fibers. Corresponding with Hamburger at Washington University, Levi-Montalcini described her experience in the cell-culture laboratory of a colleague in Rio as "one of the most intense periods of my life in which moments of enthusiasm and despair alternated with the regularity of a biological cycle."

Until that time, little was known about the process by which embryonic nerve cells develop into a network of nerve fibers extending to all parts of the body. Levi-Montalcini and her colleagues in Rio and in St. Louis established the existence of a protein compound found in mammals, birds, reptiles, amphibians and fish that stimulates the growth of embryonic nerve cells. Attracted by the substance, known as "nerve growth factor," the axon of an immature nerve cell grows toward the appropriate "target cell" and makes contact.

In addition to identifying the growth factor as a key to the orderly development of the nervous system, Levi-Montalcini also suggested that other soluble growth factors might be responsible for regulating the growth and development of other cell types.

Her hypothesis was later confirmed, notably with the discovery of "epidermal growth factor" by fellow

Nobel laureate Stanley Cohen. Working both independently and in collaboration, Cohen and Levi-Montalcini offered vital clues to the mechanism of cancer formation, as well as to that of other degenerative and development diseases.

Naturalized as a citizen of the United States in 1956, Levi-Montalcini served as professor of biology at Washington University until 1977, when she was granted the status of professor emeritus. At the age of 78 she continues to conduct biochemical research in her current position as senior scientist at the Institute of Cell Biology in Rome.

Li Shih-chen 1518–1593

Since the first appearance of Chinese medical treatises (see HUANG TI), countless reference texts have appeared on pharmacological prescriptions and formulas. The *Pen-tsao Kang-mu (General Compendium of Remedies),* Li Shih-chen's encyclopedia, is acknowledged as the definitive compilation of medications derived from plants, animals and minerals.

Presented in fifty volumes, the *Pen-tsao Kang-mu* contains the basis of the modern Chinese pharmacopoeia, including over 12,000 recipes for drugs, balms, salves, teas and other forms of therapeutic compounds. The source of every substance is examined as biological entities, as well as the physical and chemical qualities of the materials used. Also described are methods of extracting any desired substance as well as techniques for preparing and preserving pharmacological compounds.

Profusely illustrated, the *Pen-tsao Kang-mu* is not only a schematic listing of all pharmacological products, but a systematic analysis of the elements of pharmacotherapy. In an effort to establish a scientific basis for his discipline, Li Shih-chen countered many of the superstitions and misguided practices that had prevailed for centuries. He repudiated the belief, commonly held in Europe as well as China, that the presence of parasites such as body lice or intestinal organisms was a sign of health and normal function. In bold opposition to the conventional wisdom of the day, he denounced the alchemists' magic potions and elixirs, suggesting that the content of arsenic, cinnabar and other caustic elements was more dangerous than therapeutic.

Encouraged by his father to pursue a career in medicine, Li Shih-chen, at the age of 20, failed his final examinations for medical qualification. Undaunted, he embarked on several decades of exhaustive independent research, accumulating knowledge of medical and pharmacological history and theory. At the Imperial Academy of Medicine at Peking he gained advanced training in the principles and techniques of acupuncture, which he compiled in *The Network of Nerves and Vessels,* his first publication.

Li Shih-chen devoted the remainder of his life to creating the *Pen-tsao Kang-mu,* producing three completed drafts before the final version of 56 chapters, which did not appear until after his death. Recognized as a leading pioneer in the development of modern Chinese medicine, he was acknowledged by the People's Republic of China in 1956 with a postage stamp bearing his likeness.

Clarence Walton Lillehei 1918–

Recognized as a pioneer surgeon and inventor and one of the leaders of modern cardiology, C. Walton Lillehei was among those who blazed a trail for the successful heart transplant operations in the 1960s.

Born and raised in Minneapolis, Minnesota, Lillehei entered the state university at the age of seventeen, receiving a degree in medicine before he was twenty-four. In the summer of 1942 he was commissioned a first lieutenant in the Army Medical Corps. After four years of distinguished service, during which he served as director of the field hospital at Anzio, Lillehei received a Bronze Star and was discharged as a lieutenant colonel.

Returning to the University of Minnesota to complete his surgical residency, Lillehei was awarded a number of fellowships and grants, including a sponsorship from the Rockefeller Foundation. Under the direction of noted surgeon OWEN WANGENSTEEN he developed advanced skills in research as well as in surgical practice, and by 1950 Lillehei's professional success seemed assured.

The bright prospects seemed suddenly to vanish, however, when Lillehei was diagnosed as suffering from a virulent form of lymph cancer. After extensive surgery and a grueling postoperative period he gradually recovered, and by 1951 he had resumed his busy career and normal, healthy life.

At that time heart surgery was still in a primitive stage, performed mainly on infants born with a congenital defect. With only a partial view of the patient's heart the surgeon was forced to operate at a terrible disadvantage. Seeking to reduce the risk of cardiac surgery, Lillehei and a staff of research associates developed a method of open-heart surgery in which a patient's life could be sustained without relying on his own heart to perform its vital functions.

Lillehei's team conceived of a procedure in which a controlled cross-circulation of blood is effected between the patient and a matched donor. Two sets of plastic tubes passing through a mechanical pump transport the patient's venous, oxygen-poor blood to a donor as the donor's clean, oxygenated blood is recirculated back to the patient. Lillehei supervised the first operation of this kind in March, 1954, and by the end of that year the technique had been used in the repair of various form of heart damage that would otherwise have been inoperable.

Forming the basis of heart-lung bypass techniques, Lillehei's system of cross-circulation gave rise to a number of other technical innovations that brought about a revolution in cardiac medicine. With colleague Richard A. DeWall he introduced a series of artificial heart-lung machines, most notably the helix reservoir bubble machine, a device in which venous blood is mechanically oxygenated outside the body. Hailed as a milestone in the advancement of heart surgery, the machine allowed surgeons sufficient time to perform effectively.

In 1957 Lillehei reached yet another milestone, becoming the first to replace an entire aortic valve with a plastic prosthesis. In the years that followed he performed numerous replacement operations as he set the stage for the first successful heart transplant in 1967. The historic operation was in large part due to the efforts of Lillehei's two distinguished students, Norman Shumway, who devised the heart transplant procedure, and CHRISTIAAN BARNARD, who performed the operation.

Tirelessly pursuing all aspects of cardiac surgery, Lillehei co-wrote a report published in 1960 discussing the use of artificial pacemakers in cases of heart block. He left Minnesota in 1967 to become surgeon-in-chief at New York Hospital. He also took on the duties of professor of surgery as well chairman of the department at Cornell University Medical College.

Thomas Linacre (Lynaker) 1460–1524

Linacre was a pioneer in clinical medicine, especially in the early regulation and licensing of physicians. One way to gauge the prestige of Thomas Linacre's medical practice is to consider his rather impressive list of patients, who included Henry VII and Henry VIII, Cardinal Wolsey, Desiderius Erasmus and Sir Thomas More.

Linacre was a graduate of both Oxford and Padua, from which he received an all-encompassing Renaissance education as well as the finest medical training available. He learned Greek during the Italian phase of his education and later translated works of Aristotle and Galen from Greek to Latin. When Linacre returned to England he tutored Erasmus and More in Greek, and in 1501 Henry VII requested that he teach the language to Prince Arthur, his son. Linacre also wrote a Latin grammar for the young princess Mary. His scholarship endeared him to the entire family, and he was soon made physician to the king. When the reign of Henry VIII began he retained the position.

Although Linacre's London practice was flourishing, he was concerned, along with other London physicians, about the informality of their profession. In the absence of rules and standards of practice for medical practitioners, Linacre felt it important to protect the status of responsible physicians, and at the same time to prevent unreliable ones from practicing. He enlisted the support of Henry VII, who in 1518 granted establishment of the College of Physicians of London, with Linacre as its president. The goal of the college was to act as a licensing and examining board, a regulatory system that lasted for many centuries. Although the medical school at Salerno had begun this endeavor several centuries before, it was the London College that launched the tradition of licensing and regulating medical practice, protecting patients from unscrupulous practitioners and later enforcing and improving standards of medical care.

Linacre was a champion of Renaissance humanism, a philosophical movement that emphasized a cultivation of the classics, a respect for scientific scholarship and an abiding concern for human values and the capabilities of man. In 1520, four years before his death, Linacre was ordained as a Roman Catholic priest. Perhaps Linacre's greatest contribution was his translation of a number of ancient Greek medical works into Latin.

Overall, it may be stated that Linacre's life of scholarship, service and faith has been of interest to artists and scientists over the centuries and was the subject of biographies written by Samuel Johnson (published in 1835) and WILLIAM OSLER (published in 1908).

James Lind 1716–1794

In 1747 Scottish physician James Lind became the first to associate a disease with dietary deficiency when he prescribed lemons and oranges as a remedy for scurvy. The author of a classic work entitled *A Treatise on Scurvy*, Lind is hailed as the "father of naval surgery" for his dedication to the health and welfare of sailors. It is largely due to Lind's landmark discovery, along with the subsequent efforts of Sir Gilbert Blane (1749–1834), that the British Admiralty eventually recognized the economic wisdom of preventive medicine in 1795, making citrus fruit a requirement in naval rations.

A condition characterized by weakening of the capillaries, which causes bleeding into the tissues, scurvy became prevalent in the fifteenth century with the advent of long sea voyages. Without the nutritional benefits of fresh fruits and vegetables, sailors often fell victim to the disease, which induces irritability. Scurvy took the lives of more than half of the crew accompanying Vasco da Gama on his first journey around the Cape of Good Hope between 1497 and 1499. Shipboard mortality rates had not improved 150 years later when George Anson, first Lord of the Admiralty, reported that four fifths of his crew were lost to the disease during a trip around the world. Lind's *Two Papers on Fevers and Infections* (1763), which furnishes the only medical history of the Seven Years' War—known in American history as the French and Indian War—reports that the "number of seamen in time of war who died by shipwreck, capture, famine, fire, or sword" was greatly exceeded by those who died from "ship diseases and the usual maladies of intemperate climates."

Lind entered the British navy as a surgeon's mate in 1739 after completing his apprenticeship to a physician in Edinburgh. Promoted to the rank of surgeon in 1747, Lind set sail with the crew of H.M.S. Salisbury in May of that year on what was to be a brief but historic cruise.

Suspecting a relationship between scurvy and diet, Lind conducted a clinical experiment using twelve scurvy-ridden sailors as his subjects. He paired them off into six groups, providing them all with the same basic diet but adding a different food supplement for each of the six pairs. Within one week the results were dramatic proof of the antiscorbutic effect of the lemons and oranges. The ten sailors who were fed vinegar, cider or any of the other test foods showed no marked change in their condition, but the two given citrus fruit were soon cured and pronounced fit for service.

Appearing in 1753, Lind's *Treatise on Scurvy* was dedicated to Lord Anson, who returned the tribute by appointing Lind chief physician at the Royal Naval Hospital at Haslar in 1758. As administrator and medical director for twenty-five years, Lind conducted exhaustive clinical research on the treatment of scurvy, as well as other aspects of shipboard hygiene and preventive medicine.

Among other contributions to the improvement of living conditions for sailors was Lind's invention of a method for obtaining healthful drinking water by nonchemical distillation of seawater. In 1768 he published his last written work, entitled *An Essay on Diseases Incidental to Europeans in Hot Climates,* which served for more than fifty years as a definitive reference text on tropical medicine.

In the mid-1800s British navy rations replaced lemons with less expensive and more readily available West Indian limes, giving rise to the slang word "limeys" for Englishmen. It was not until 1917, however, that preserved lime juice was found to have far less value than lemon juice as an antiscorbutic agent, thereby accounting for the mysterious resurgence of scurvy in the late nineteenth century.

The cause of scurvy was eventually established as a deficiency in vitamin C (first isolated by ALBERT SZENT-GYORGYI in 1928). Increased understanding of nutritional requirements has contributed to a significant decrease in the incidence of scurvy.

Fritz Albert Lipmann 1899–1986

In 1953 distinguished biochemist Fritz Lipmann was awarded the Nobel Prize for Physiology or Medicine in recognition of his discovery of "coenzyme A," an essential element in the metabolism of sugars, fats and proteins. Lipmann shared the honor with British biochemist HANS ADOLPH KREBS, who established a metabolic cycle now known as the "Kerbs cycle."

Lipmann was born in Königsberg, Germany, where, in 1917, he embarked on a decade of scientific study that took him to the Universities of Munich, Konigsberg, and Berlin, which in 1927 awarded him doctoral degrees in medicine and biochemistry.

Joining the research staff at Berlin's celebrated Kaiser-Wilhelm Institut, Lipmann served as laboratory assistant to Nobel Prize-winner, OTTO MEYERHOF, a leading authority on physiological chemistry.

In 1931 Lipmann came to New York on a fellowship grant from the Rockefeller Institute for Medical Research. Returning to Europe the following year, he accepted a position at the Biological Institute of the Carlsberg Foundation in Copenhagen, where for seven years he worked with the noted biochemist Albert Fischer.

In 1939, as World War II threatened even neutral Denmark, Lipmann emigrated to the United States. After two years as a fellow at Cornell University Medical College he joined the research department at Massachussetts General Hospital as senior biochemist. By 1946 Lipmann was a naturalized American citizen and a faculty member of the Harvard Medical School.

Focusing on the chemistry of metabolism, with particular attention to the role of phosphates in animal tissue, Lipmann developed the "metabolic dynamo" in 1941. Four years later he isolated "coenzyme A," an organic substance not produced in the body that activates the catalytic process of converting chemical energy into physical energy. In the process of determining the critical role of coenzyme A in the metabolism of fatty acids, amino acids, steroids and hemoglobins Lipmann elucidated the biochemical activity involved in growth, regeneration and the release of energy in the cells of the body. His wide-ranging investigation of the biochemistry of metabolism included notable studies on the process of carbohydrate conversion, the structure of cancer cells, and the function of pantothenic acid, one of the B-complex vitamins involved in the formation of coenzymes.

In 1948 Lipmann's outstanding research achievements were honored with the Carl Neuberg Medal of the American Society of European Chemists and Pharmacists and the Mead Johnson and Company Award for pioneer studies on vitamin B-complex. Appointed professor of biological chemistry at Harvard Medical School the following year, Lipmann established the molecular structure of coenzyme A in 1953.

After receiving the Nobel Prize Lipmann turned from the study of coenzymes to endocrinology, particularly the energy-regulating thyroid hormone. From 1957 until 1970 he served on the faculty of Rockfeller University, from which he retired as professor emeritus in biological chemistry. In a research laboratory he maintained at the university Lipmann conducted research up until his death at the age of 87.

A distinguished member of the New York Academy of Sciences, the Danish Academy of Sciences, the National Academy of Sciences, and the Harvey Society, Lipmann added to his list of scientific publications an autobiography, *Wanderings of a Biochemist*, published in 1971.

Joseph Lister, First Baron Lister of Lyme Regis 1827–1912

Joseph Lister revolutionized the practice of surgery when he introduced the notion of antisepsis. Basing his work on LOUIS PASTEUR'S landmark discovery that organic decomposition was caused by invisible, self-multiplying organisms transported through the air, Joseph Lister reasoned that he could greatly improve the survival rate of his surgical patients if he could keep their open wounds free of these harmful microorganisms.

Pasteur formally announced his findings in 1861, launching Lister on a long and often bitter battle to convince the medical establishment of the importance of antiseptic procedures. Long the target of scorn and opposition, Lister lived to see his victory confirmed in 1884, when a German physician was sued for malpractice because he had not followed antiseptic precautions.

Having recognized the need for protecting his patients from an invisible but dangerous threat, Lister recommended that carbolic acid be used to destroy the microorganisms. The substance, also known as "phenol," was a liquid developed by a Manchester chemist as a deodorizer for the Carlisle sewage works. Lister experimented with various strengths and methods of dispersal. Convinced that spraying would be the most effective use of the substance, Lister devised a large atomizer that was operated by a treadle. For many years surgeons operated on their patients cloaked in a yellow mist, giving rise to the playful presurgical admonition "Let us spray."

In addition to antiseptic procedure, Lister made other notable contributions to the advancement of surgery. These include significant observations on the processes of inflammation and blood coagulation. He also developed the drainage tube and absorbable stitches, both of which became widely used in the management of wounds and incisions. Among other surgical inventions he devised a silver-wire suture needle, an aortic tourniquet, and a hook for removing foreign objects from the ear.

Joseph Lister was born at Upton Park, the family estate on the outskirts of London. His father, a successful wine merchant, was a student of science. Fascinated by the properties of glass and microscopic lenses, Joseph Jackson Lister developed an achromatic lens that permitted the passage of white light without the iridescence that diminished the clarity of earlier lenses. His paper describing the achromatic lens was published in the *Philosophical Transactions of the Royal Society;* in spite of his amateur status, Joseph Jackson Lister was eventually granted membership in the Royal Society in 1832.

In 1845 young Joseph entered the arts college of the University of London, settling into a rooming house on Ampthill Square. It was there that he met Edward Palmer, a medical student who would have an important influence on Lister's career. The two friends together witnessed a historic event on December 21, 1846 when they observed the landmark operation performed by Scottish surgeon Robert Liston at University College Hospital, in which anesthesia was demonstrated for the first time in England.

Stricken by a protracted depression, Lister abandoned his college studies for several years. In 1849 he returned as a committed student of surgery, a discipline he described as the "bloody and butcherly department of the healing art." After receiving his bachelor of medicine degree in 1852, Lister served as house surgeon at the University of Edinburgh under the legendary James Syme. Lister's teacher became his father-in-law in 1856, when Lister married Syme's eldest daughter, Agnes.

Lister became an assistant surgeon at the Royal Infirmary and at the Edinburgh Lock Hospital, delivering medical lectures to supplement his income. Greatly influenced by the studies of celebrated surgeon JOHN HUNTER, Lister had already begun research on coagulation and inflammation. In 1860 he accepted the position of regius professor of surgery at Glasgow University, and he was elected to the Royal Society in the same year.

In 1867 *The Lancet* published Lister's paper expounding the values of antiseptic practice. Unfortunately, the ensuing controversy focused more on the use of carbolic acid than on the more basic medical principle. The British Medical Association referred to "the latest toy of medical science so-called...the carbolic mania."

In 1869 Lister took over Syme's position as chair of clinical surgery at the University of Edinburgh, and in the years that followed he crusaded passionately for the cause of antisepsis. In 1876 he came to the United States to preside over the surgical section at the International Medical Congress in Philadelphia.

He also traveled throughout Europe expounding his theories, which soon won international acclaim. Chosen by Queen Elizabeth as her surgeon-in-ordinary in Scotland, Lister was knighted in 1883.

By the mid-1880s resistance to the practice of antisepsis had diminished, though more slowly in England than in other parts of Europe. Lister changed his technique from employment of a spray to the use of a gauze impregnated with carbolic acid, and later he devised a more sophisticated formula employing mercury and zinc cyanides.

In the last decade of the nineteenth century Lister's efforts were widely honored. He was named president of the Royal Society in 1895 and president of the British Association the following year. In 1897 Queen Victoria made him a baron, permitting him to call himself Lord Lister of Lyme. In 1902 he was awarded the Royal Order of Merit, which had been instituted to mark the coronation of Queen Victoria's son, King Edward VII.

Distinguished fellow surgeon HARVEY CUSHING memorialized Lister by describing him as "the liberator of surgery from the shackles of sepsis." A more lighthearted tribute came from a disciple of Lister's, noted orthopedic surgeon George F.L. Stromeyer:

> Mankind looks grateful now on thee
> For what thou did'st in Surgery,
> And Death must often go amiss,
> By smelling antiseptic bliss.

Robert Liston 1794–1847

Although Robert Liston's renown as a surgeon was already well established, he took his place in medical history in December, 1846, when he performed the first public operation in Great Britain using general anesthesia. As early as 1799 HUMPHRY DAVY suggested using nitrous oxide to dull the pain of the surgeon's knife, and CRAWFORD LONG, among other doctors and dentists in America, had already begun to use ether for minor surgery. Still, the only relief offered to English patients undergoing surgery was mesmerism, an early form of hypnosis. Its effectiveness was questionable, though hotly debated.

Liston had developed a reputation for remarkable surgical skill and dexterity and was often called upon to remove tumors considered inoperable by other practitioners. When he finished his first operation using general anesthesia, he is said to have commented, "This Yankee dodge beats mesmerism hollow."

Robert Liston, the son of a parish minister, was born at Ecclesmachen Manse in Linlithgow, Scotland. He studied in London, attending JOHN ABERNETHY'S lectures on surgery at St. Bartholomew's Hospital. Liston completed his medical studies in Edinburgh, where he settled in 1818 to lecture on surgery and anatomy at the university. Developing both his surgical skill and his reputation, he was named operating surgeon at the Royal Infirmary in 1828. In 1931 he published his first book, *Elements of Surgery*. Assuming that he was next in line for the chair of clinical surgery at Edinburgh, Liston was indignant and humiliated when, in 1835, the position was given to James Syme, a former colleague and longtime rival.

Relying on his ever-widening reputation, Liston left for England, where he was immediately offered the Chair of Clinical Surgery at the University of London. In 1837 Liston published a second manual entitled *Practical Surgery*.

Liston's legendary operation using general anesthesia was performed on December 21, 1846 at the Hospital of University College on Gower Street in London. Administering the anesthesia was Peter Squire, a doctor affiliated with the hospital. The patient, a butler named Frederick Churchill, was to have his leg amputated at the thigh. Among those who observed Liston's successful completion of the difficult surgery was the young JOSEPH LISTER, dutifully impressed by the innovation that would revolutionize the practice of surgery.

Robert Liston introduced a number of surgical innovations that still carry his name. These include Liston's forceps, used for cutting through bone; Liston's knives, long-bladed instruments used in amputation; and Liston's operation, a surgical technique for the excision of the upper jaw.

Jacques Loeb 1859–1924

As physiology developed into an experimental, biochemical discipline in the late nineteenth century a mechanistic view of man became more and more popular. This materialism, as expanded by T.H. Huxley and others, appealed to Jacques Loeb, who regarded science as a philosophically liberating force. It described the human being as a machine operating according to understandable physical and chemical laws.

Loeb was born in Germany and studied physiology and biology in Berlin and in Munich. He received a medical degree from the University of Strasbourg in 1884, and seven years later he emigrated to the United States, where he became a naturalized citizen. He taught at a number of prestigious American schools, including Bryn Mawr and the University of Chicago. In 1910 he was asked to join the Rockefeller Institute for Medical Research (now Rockefeller University), where he remained as head of the physiology department until 1924. In that time he also founded and edited the *Journal of General Physiology*.

Loeb's mechanistic philosophy included the view that human ethics were merely an outgrowth of man's inherited physiological responses to external stimuli. Loeb used the word "tropism" to refer to any directed movement of an animal in response to a stimulus and interpreted all of behavior in physiochemical terms (e.g., heliotropism as a directed movement toward light). Loeb's "tropism" theory of animal conduct" has since been discredited, particularly by H.S. Jennings (1868–1947), who saw the actions of animals as efforts of trial and error rather than as direct reaction to external conditions. "Tropism" has been replaced by "taxis" as the term for the orientation responses of animals, but

Loeb's research in comparative morphology, physiology and psychology is still studied today.

Loeb also conducted well-known experiments inducing parthenogenesis (a process of reproduction without fertilization) and regeneration of organs or tissue by chemical stimulus. Loeb, who was a pioneer in this field, maintained that to fully understand fertilization, science had to go beyond the study of genetics and investigate the physiological and chemical aspects of the process. His written works include *Dynamics of Living Matter* (1906), *The Mechanistic Conception of Life* (1912), *Artificial Parthenogenesis and Fertilization* (1913) and *The Organism as a Whole* (1916).

Otto Loewi 1873–1961

Pharmacologist Otto Loewi shared the 1936 Nobel Prize for Physiology or Medicine with HENRY DALE for their discovery of the chemical mediation of nerve impulse transmission. Bringing together the disciplines of physiology, pharmacology and biochemistry, Loewi's experimental research demonstrated the role of a chemical—later identified as acetylcholine—in the transmission of impulses at the point of synapse between nerve cells.

Born in Frankfurt of Jewish parents, Loewi was educated in Strasbourg and Munich. Settling in Austria, he became a professor of pharmacology at the University of Graz in 1909. Physiological research led him to his now-famous experiments with an isolated heart, conducted in 1921. As Loewi slowed the heartbeat by stimulating the organ with its attached vagus nerve he noticed the release of a chemical substance. Suffusing a second isolated heart with this substance, Loewi observed a similar slowing of the heartbeat. These studies were the first conclusive evidence of the chemical nature of nerve impulse transmission.

In 1938 the Nazi purge of professors forced Loewi into a two-year exile. He escaped to the United States and resumed teaching and research at New York University College of Medicine, where he remained until 1955. Continuing experimental work with the heart, kidneys and nervous system, Loewi investigated the pharmacology and physiology of metabolism, also studying adrenaline and the nature of diabetes.

Loewi's invention of a diagnostic test for diabetes, hyperthyroidism and pancreatic insufficiency still bears his name. In 1954 he was invited to join the Royal Society of London.

Friedrich August Johannes Löffler 1852–1915

Pioneer microbiologist Friedrich Löffler was a key figure in the early development of bacteriological theory. Along with fellow German microbiologists Max Oertel and EDWIN KREBS, he discovered the bacterial agent of diphtheria, establishing the characteristics of the bacillus as well as the mechanism of the disease.

Löffler is also recognized as the first to establish a virus as the causative agent of any disease. A pivotal step in the development of bacteriological medicine, loffler's 1897 investigation of aphthous fever, or foot-and-mouth disease, preceded by four years WALTER REED'S Cuban campaign against the viral disease yellow fever.

The son of a physician and general in the Prussian army, Friedrich Löffler was born in Berlin, where he received his education at the French Gymnasium. While still a medical student at the University of Wurzburg loffler joined the army to serve as a medical assistant in the Franco-Prussian War. After receiving his degree in 1874 he served at the Charité Hospital in Berlin, and later as public health officer and military surgeon in Hanover and Potsdam.

In 1880 Löffler was selected by celebrated bacteriologist ROBERT KOCH to assist in setting up a bacteriological laboratory in Berlin. In the four years that followed loffler absorbed Koch's innovative and demanding definition of scientific method, which guided him in all his subsequent bacteriological studies. Reminiscing about his days as a member of Koch's laboratory staff, he fondly recalled: "Almost daily new wonders in bacteriology arose before our astounded vision, and we, following the brilliant example of our chief, worked from morning to evening…Then it was that we learnt what it means to observe and work accurately and with energy to pursue the problem laid before us."

In 1884, adhering to Koch's experimental postulates, Löffler embarked on his study of the bacterial agent of diphtheria. After isolating the bacillus he intended to culture it, reinject it into experimental animal subjects, then repeat these steps again to observe the symptoms of the second set of experimental subjects. To overcome the difficulties of culturing the diphtheria bacilli on the standard gelatin plates, Löffler developed a new culture medium using heated blood serum rather than gelatin. Increasing the incubation temperature to 37°, Löffler successfully cultured the bacilli. He then recreated the disease in successive sets of subjects, thereby satisfying Koch's requirements for conclusively establishing the causative agent of a disease.

Löffler's study of diphtheria is additionally significant for its elucidation of the toxic action of the disease Anticipating the findings of Émile Roux, ALEXANDRE YERSIN and EMIL VON BEHRING, Löffler suggested that although the diphtheria bacillus is found only in the throat membrane, the bacteria produce a poisonous substance that is transported through the bloodstream to other parts of the body.

In related investigations of the diphtheria bacillus Löffler made another significant discovery when he isolated the bacillus from a subject who showed no sign of the disease. Introducing the notion of a "healthy-carrier state," Löffler's study led to important advances in modern theories of public health and preventive medicine.

After publication of his findings on the diphtheria bacillus Löffler was named director of the Hygiene Laboratory at the First Garrison Hospital in Berlin. Though he lectured regularly on bacteriological principles in public sanitation and hygiene, Löffler nevertheless managed to continue a productive career as a research scientist. During his two years at the Hygiene Laboratory he discovered the microorganisms responsible for swine erysipelas and swine plague.

Recognized as a leading figure in the development of bacteriological science, Löffler founded the *Centralblatt für Bakteriologie und Parasitenkunde* (*Journal of Bacteriology and Parasitology*). First appearing in 1887, the journal soon distinguished itself as one of the most influential publications in its field.

In 1888, after a brief stint at the University of Berlin, he accepted the chair in hygiene at the University of Greifswald, serving as professor and later as rector of the university until 1907. At Greifswald, in the course of investigating the bacteriological cause of mouse typhoid, Löffler first introduced the notion of using bacteria as a means of controlling the growth of an animal population. In Greece, where the spread of rodents was a serious threat to crop production, the government agreed to try Löffler's theory. Dispersing bacteria through the fields, the system did effectively cut down the field mouse population, but the plan was discontinued when it appeared that the bacteria might present some risk to humans.

In 1897 Löffler was commissioned by the German government to investigate the problem of foot-and-mouth disease, a highly contagious condition that continually threatened the livestock industry. Five years earlier Russian microbiologist DMITRY IVANOWSKI had demonstrated the existence of a disease-causing organism that was too small to be observed even under a microscope. Demonstrating that apthous fever in cattle was caused by just such a microorganism, Löffler and his assistant Paul Frosch concluded that these "invisible" viruses spread disease by multiplying within the living cells of the host.

In addition to his findings Löffler contributed significantly to the advancement of bacteriological research technique. Refining laboratory methods of isolating and identifying bacteria, he developed various stains, most notably the alkaline methylene blue stain.

Also recognized for his contribution to the advancement of public health, Löffler lectured and wrote on techniques of disinfection and sewage disposal and the maintenance of hygiene in milk and water. At the outbreak of World War I he was requested to participate in the organization of an army hygiene program.

Pierre Charles Alexandre Louis 1787–1872

> There is something rarer than the spirit of discernment; it is the need of truth; that state of the soul which does not allow us to stop in any scientific labors at what is only probable, but compels us to continue our researches until we have arrived at evidence.
>
> —P. C. A. Louis

Physician and pathologist Pierre Charles Louis was one of the most widely acclaimed clinicians of the nineteenth century. Maintaining detailed records of the development of disease in his patients, the effects of his treatment and his postmortem observations, Louis accumulated an enormous store of data for pathological analysis. Such statistical reports contributed significantly to diagnostics and disease classification.

The son of a vineyard keeper, Pierre Charles Louis grew up in the region of Champagne, near Paris. After several years of law school he shifted his interest to medicine, pursuing studies at Rheims and Paris. Obtaining his medical degree in 1813, Louis accepted an invitation to accompany an official mission to Russia. He served as an itinerant doctor in that country for more than three years before setting up practice in Odessa.

Seeking additional training, Louis returned to Paris, where he joined the staff of the celebrated hospital La Charité. It was there that he began his intensive investigation of disease, maintaining detailed and systematic accounts of all clinical observations. Accumulating enormous files of data for comparative analysis, Louis retired from practice for a year to organize his findings.

Among his most influential works was a study on tuberculosis entitled *Researches on Phthisis*. Published in 1825, the report introduces "Louis's law," which states that tuberculosis usually originates in the left lung, and that tuberculous lesions found anywhere on the body accompany a primary localization of the disease in the lungs. Louis also discussed the epidemiological aspects of tuberculosis, including the issues of public health and education.

When his only son died of tuberculosis in 1828 Louis left Europe, joining an expedition to Gibraltar to investigate the yellow fever epidemic. His detailed report, first published in English, appeared in 1839 under the title *Anatomical, Pathological and Therapeutic Researches on the Yellow Fever of Gibraltar of 1828*.

Returning from Gibraltar in 1829, Louis resumed a statistical analysis of his clinical observations, presenting his findings in a landmark work entitled *Anatomical, Pathological and Therapeutic Researches upon the Disease Known under the Name of Gastro-Enterite, Putrid, Adynamic, Ataxic or Typhoid Fever*. Covering all bases, Louis presented a detailed clinical and pathological description of this group of conditions, which was still seen as a single pathology. His report outlined various physiological changes at each stage of the disease, as well as complete descriptions of postmortem findings. It was one of Louis's many notable students, American physician W.W. Gerhard (1809–1872), who later distinguished separate entities in this cluster of diseases, differentiating between typhus and typhoid.

As a distinguished clinician, pathologist and medical statistician, Pierre-Charles Louis significantly influenced the development of medicine in the United States. A surprising number of leading American physicians came to Paris to study under Louis. Oliver Wendell Holmes was among his many distinguished students.

Richard Lower 1631–1691

On January 18, 1661 British physician and physiologist Richard Lower sent a letter to Robert Boyle, noted scientist and cofounder of the Royal Society, in which he announced his first transfusion experiment. Seeking to learn "how long a dog may live without meat, by syringing into a vein a due quantity of good broth," Lower described his methodology: "I shall try it in a dog, and I shall get a tin pipe made, about two inches long, and about the usual bigness of a jugular vein, and hollow, which I may put into the vein."

Three years later Lower sent another report to Boyle describing his plan for a more advanced experiment in which he intended to "get two dogs of equal bigness [and] let both bleed into the other's vein..."

Though he is best known for being the first to perform a direct transfusion of blood, Lower also explored the circulatory system and pioneered the use of modern iatromathematics–the application of mathematical and physical principles to medical research. He also determined on the basis of animal experiments that the difference in color between venous blood and arterial blood resulted from exposure to air in the lungs. Collaborating with ROBERT HOOKE, Lower experimented with air-blocked lungs, confirming his hypothesis that the scarlet color of arterial blood is "due to the penetration of particles of air into the blood."

Since WILLIAM HARVEY'S studies of the respiratory and circulatory systems, a number of other physiologists had begun to investigate the function and mechanism of the lungs, but Lower was the first to refer to a "nitrous pabulum" of the air that was "impregnated" by the lungs into the blood.

Born to a prominent family in the village of Tremeer, near Cornwall, Lower rose quickly in his chosen profession. In 1675 he was elected to the Royal College of Physicians, and it was not long before he established a reputation as one of London's most eminent physicians. He became a fellow of the Royal Society in 1667 and served as financial auditor for several years, but he resigned when the strained finances of the society made his official position too demanding.

Replicating the experiments of English architect, astronomer and mathematician Christopher Wren (1632–1723), who had tried to inject therapeutic fluids into the blood by using quills and other instruments, Lower noted the ease with which fluids combined with the test blood of animals. He then ventured to "try if the blood of different animals would not be much more suitable and would mix together without danger or conflict" (see KARL LANDSTEINER).

The first successful transfusion of blood "from an artery of one animal into a vein of a second" was performed at Oxford in 1665. It was replicated the following year in the presence of the Royal Society and published in the *Philosophical Transactions* of December, 1666.

Lower's other submissions to the Society's *Philosophical Transactions* include such memorable titles as *An Observation Concerning a Blemish in a Horse's Eye* and *On Making a Dog Draw His Breath Like a Broken-winded Horse* (both 1667). His more noted written works include *Diatribae Thomas Willisii...de febribus vindicatio adversus Edmundum DeMeara* (1665) (*In support of Thomas Willis against the criticism of Edmund DeMeaver*), a defense of a treatise written by his friend and colleague John Willis on cardiopulmonary function. Within several years of its publication, however, he had come to doubt many of Willis's basic assertions and published his revised conclusions four years later in a definitive treatise entitled *Tractatus de corde (Treatise on the Heart)*. Describing the functions of the heart and blood, the book also includes a section on the history of transfusion leading up to Lower's own experimental results.

Carl Friedrich Wilhelm Ludwig 1816–1895

Carl Ludwig belonged to a small group of biologists and physicians of the mid-nineteenth century who pioneered the establishment of physiology as an autonomous scientific discipline. Long considered a subdivision of anatomy, the field of physiology became established as a separate and significant area of concentration largely as a result of the efforts of Carl Ludwig, along with Emil Du Bois-Reymond, William Sharpey, Johannes Muller and CLAUDE BERNARD. Investigating the phenomena of vital processes, the founders of modern physiology sought to define the functions of living organisms as mechanical operations following the laws of physics and chemistry.

By the 1840s Ludwig had already begun to consider biological principles in physiochemical terms, applying the methodology of these sciences to the study of physiology. The development of this approach was facilitated by Ludwig's numerous methodological inventions. In 1846 he introduced the kymograph, an instrument designed to produce a continuous recording of variations or modulations for use in evaluating muscle contraction, arterial activity, pulse etc. Intrigued by the nature of circulatory function, Ludwig devised a mercurial blood pump in 1859, enabling him to evaluate and isolate various substances found in a specified quantity of blood taken directly in vivo.

In the year Carl was born his father returned from service as a cavalry officer in the Napoleonic wars, resuming family life as a civil servant in Witzenhausen, Germany. In 1834 Carl enrolled as a medical student at the University of Marburg, but his strong political views, compounded by a volatile and combative nature, led to his expulsion. After several years of study at Erlangen and Bamberg he was readmitted to Marburg, receiving his medical degree in 1840.

Two years later, on the basis of his dissertation on the mechanism of renal function, Ludwig was offered a position on Marburg's medical faculty, and in 1846 he was appointed associate "professor extraordinarius." It was at Marburg that he began an investigation of the physiology of secretion that would later yield significant findings on the role of nerve stimulation in the activity of the salivary glands.

Arriving in Switzerland in 1849, he joined the faculty at the University of Zurich as professor of physiology and anatomy. Attracted by Ludwig's energetic and innovative spirit, students flocked to his laboratory to assist in his experimental studies. In 1852, with the enthusiastic collaboration of his students, he produced the first half of a two-volume reference entitled *Lehrbuch der Physiologie (Textbook of Physiology)*. Completed four years later with the publication of the second volume, Ludwig's landmark work presented the first modern treatment of physiology.

Ludwig left Zurich in 1855 to teach at the University of Vienna, devoting the next decade to an exhaustive study of the physical and chemical aspects of respiration, particularly lung mechanism, gas exchange and tissue respiration. He was convinced to leave his established position in Vienna by the offer of the newly instituted chair of physiology at the University of Leipzig. Supervising design and construction of the first physiological institute, Ludwig created a facility that would accommodate the broad scope of the discipline as he saw it. His plan included physical, chemical and anatomical laboratories interconnected in an E-shaped structure.

Under Ludwig's direction the institute established itself as a prominent center for physiological training and research. He continued to teach and conduct research until his death, producing a number of important studies, including a quantitative and histological (the study of tissues), analysis of the lymphatic system, an investigation of the structure of the kidneys, and an influential treatise on heart mechanisms. In extensive research on the physiology of circulation Ludwig examined the interrelationship of blood pressure, muscle action and cardiac function.

André Lwoff 1902–

In 1965 André Lwoff shared the Nobel Prize in Physiology or Medicine with Francois Jacob and JACQUES MONOD for his study of the genetic mechanism of a bacteriophage, or bacteria-killing virus.

Born in central France of Russian-Polish extraction, André Lwoff became associated with the Louis Pasteur Institute in Paris in 1921. Lwoff's earliest studies investigated the structural development of protozoa, unicellular animals with at least one well- defined nucleus. This research gave rise to the discovery of extranuclear genetic material in these organisms.

During World War II Lwoff was an active participant in the French Resistance. His pioneer work, *L'Evolution Physiologique (Physiological Evolution)*, introducing the thesis of biochemical evolution, appeared in 1941. Lwoff's Nobel Prize-winning research revealed the phenomenon known as bacterial lysogeny—the destruction of bacteria by integrating the genetic information of a bacteriophage into the bacterial chromosome, thereby replicating the destructive element along with the bacteria's original DNA.

Since 1959 Lwoff has been a professor of microbiology at the Sorbonne.

Feodor Lynen 1911–1979

Feodor Lynen was the first to isolate "active acetate," an element critical to the formation of cholesterol and fatty acids. His work, which revealed important pieces of the puzzle of coronary and respiratory disease, was recognized in 1964 with the Nobel Prize for Physiology and Medicine, which Lynen shared with KONRAD BLOCH. Lynen was studying biotin, a B-complex vitamin formerly called vitamin H. He came to understand the role of biotin in the cellular processing of carbon dioxide and its function in aiding body growth.

Born in Augsburg, Germany, Lynen received his doctorate in 1937 from the University of Munich and taught biochemistry there until he joined the faculty at the Max Planck Institute for Cell Chemistry Research ten years later. By then he had already begun the research that would lead him to the Nobel Prize. Lynen took over directorship of the Cell Chemistry Department of the Max Planck Institute in 1954. In 1972 he moved to the Institute's Biochemistry Division, where he remained director until his death seven years later.

M

Elmer Verner McCollum 1879–1967

A pioneer in experimental research on nutrition, Elmer McCollum isolated vitamins A and B, instituting the use of letters in vitamin nomenclature. Vitamins are a group of naturally occurring substances that are essential to the growth, reproduction or continued health of an organism. As they are not synthesized in the body, these factors must be obtained from diet.

The notion of essential nutritional substances was established in 1906 by English biochemist F.G HOPKINS, who originally called them "accessory factors." The term "vitamine" ("vital amine") was first coined by noted biochemist Casimir Funk (1884–1967) to identify his discovery of a substance that reduces inflaurientation of the nerves, antineuritic substance, later found to be thiamine. As the term is currently used, however, there is no substantive chemical property common to all vitamins.

In independent studies McCollum and fellow American biochemists T.B. Osborne (1859–1929) and L.B. Mendel demonstrated the existence of more than one vitamin, but it was McCollum who first isolated two different nutritional requirements for normal development in rats.

Born in Fort Scott, Kansas, McCollum studied organic chemistry at the University of Kansas and at Yale University, where he received his doctorate in 1906. While working at the state agricultural research centers in Connecticut and Wisconsin he became interested in what was then known as agricultural chemistry. Commissioned to investigate the effects of various foods on the health and reproductive capacity of cattle, he decided to expand his investigation by choosing smaller, more manageable experimental subjects.

In a small laboratory at Wisconsin's College of Agriculture McCollum assembled the first colony of white rats to be used for experimental research on nutrition, and in 1913 he identified a fat-soluble substance (A) and a water-soluble substance (B), both essential to normal health in rats and obtainable only from food.

Later research studies by J. GOLDBERGER revealed two subcomponents of water-soluble vitamin B, distinguishing separate factors against pellagra (a disease caused by deficiency of niacin or tryptophan) and beriberi (caused by a deficiency of thiamine B_1). While serving as head of biochemistry research at Johns Hopkins School of Hygiene and Public Health McCollum contributed to the discovery of two distinct subcomponents of vitamin A. One of these, found to be the factor against rickets, was renamed vitamin D.

In affiliation with the World Health Organization and the Nutrition Board of the National Research Council McCollum continued to conduct experimental research on nutrition until his retirement in 1943. His book *A History of Nutrition*, published in 1957, was considered a classic reference on the subject for many years.

Warren Sturgis McCulloch 1898–1969

Recognized for his significant contribution to the understanding of the organization of the nervous system and the mechanism of the brain, Warren McCulloch is also regarded as one of the founders of the science of cybernetics and information theory. Combining the disciplines of neurophysiology, mathematics and electrical engineering, *cybernetics*, from the Greek *kubernan*, meaning "to steer," refers to the study of control and communication in animals and machines. The discipline was introduced in 1948 with the publication of *Cybernetics*, written by McCulloch's friend and colleague Norbert Weiner, the noted mathematician and engineer.

A fundamental element in control and communication theory is the principle of feedback, which is the regulation of performance by the consequences of the work performed. To function adequately the brain must receive and manage the flow of information so that the individual can effectively interact with a continually changing environment. Feedback control is a basic functional attribute universally found in any biological and computer systems that must interact adaptively with a complex environment.

Born in Orange, New Jersey, McCulloch studied neurology, psychiatry and physics at Columbia University, where he received a degree in medicine in 1927. After serving at Rockland State and Bellevue Hospitals he joined the faculty at Yale University, where he taught and conducted research for more than eighteen years. In collaboration with Walter H. Pitts he developed a theory of the human brain as a computerlike machine relying on an electrical network for the manipulation and management of information. Published in 1943, *A Logical Calculus of the Ideas Immanent in Nervous Activity* introduced the "McCulloch-Pitts theory," now a widely accepted model of brain mechanism.

In 1952 McCulloch accepted a research position in the electronics laboratory at the Massachusetts Institute of Technology, where he pursued his investigation of the nervous system and the circuitry of the brain until his death at the age of seventy. A prolific writer, his notable technical articles include "Finality and Form" and "Where Was Fancy Bred?" A partial collection of his papers entitled *Embodiments of Mind* was published in 1965.

François Magendie 1783–1855

By demonstrating the separation of motor and sensory impulses in the nervous system Francois Magendie laid the cornerstone in the structure of modern experimental physiology. SIR CHARLES BELL independently arrived at similar results, so credit for the discovery is shared in the "Bell-Magendie Law," which states that the anterior roots of the spinal nerves transport impulses to the muscles, and the posterior roots receive sensory impulses, transmitting them to the spinal cord. The Bell- Magendie Law was an important step in the scientific understanding of nervous activity and the advancement of physiology as a separate and significant branch of medical study.

Magendie is also remembered for his pioneering studies of pharmacology. Through extensive investigation of the active elements of specific foods and drugs Magendie isolated and systematically examined the physiological effects of a number of substances, particularly such alkaloids as strychnine, emetine and morphine. A solution containing morphine sulfate is now referred to as "Magendie's solution."

In a tradition of "polypharmacy" dating back to Galen, therapeutic medicines were often complicated mixtures of several active substances (sometimes known as "Galenicals"). Magendie systematically discredited these prescriptions in his *Formulary*, a treatise on the effects and medicinal uses of various pure substances published in 1821.

A native of Bordeaux, France, Magendie practiced medicine at the Hôtel-Dieu in Paris. In 1831 he joined the faculty at the Collège de France, where he taught anatomy while continuing to conduct experimental research on animals. In the early nineteenth century, as experimental physiology and medicine gained importance, vivisection became an important part of research procedure. Magendie experimented extensively on live animals, documenting his findings in his *Journal de la physiologie expérimentale*. (*Journal of Experimental Physiology*).

Aside from his nerve studies, Magendie's interests included the effects of air in the arteries, the functions of veins and the mechanics of vomiting. In 1813 Magendie published a monograph with the unsavory title *Mémoire sur le vomissement*, (*Report on Vomiting*) in which he demonstrated that the activity of vomiting is not a function of the stomach, but rather a concerted effort of the abdominal wall and the voluntary muscles of the diaphragm.

Marcello Malpighi 1628–1694

A controversial figure in the scientific community of the seventeenth century, Marcello Malpighi was a pioneer of microscopic exploration at a time when the intellectual calcification of absolutists had begun to crack under the pressure of modern thinkers such as WILLIAM HARVEY, Galileo and German astronomer Johannes Kepler (1571–1630).

Malpighi was among the precursors to the age of reason, significantly advancing scientific understanding of the anatomy of the skin, the liver, the kidneys, the spleen, the nervous system, the lungs, the blood and, most notably, the capillary system. Expanding on William Harvey's study of blood circulation, Malpighi traced for the first time the "fantastic red network." His many other observations include the sensory function of the papillae of the tongue, indicating the mechanism for the sense of taste. Observing a relationship between the spinal cord and the brain, Malpighi also suggested a connection between nerve fibers and cortical cells.

His description of glandular diseases, particularly those involving the lymphatic glands, anticipated the findings of Thomas Hodgkin by nearly two centuries. Malpighi's embryological studies revealed for the first time the optic vesicles (small liquid- filled sacs in the eye) and the aortic arches—the series of arterial folds in the neck region of the embryo.

Malpighi's investigations were not limited to the study of human anatomy and physiology. His scientific curiosity led him to explore the natural world in colorful and often poetic terms. In glowing prose he described the spiral intestinal valves of sharks, the bladders of sea bass, the optical nerves of swordfish, the anatomy of fallen eagles and the life history of the silkworm. In a microscopic study of the abdominal membranes of a hedgehog he noted a "rosary of red corals," referring to red corpuscles.

Malpighi was born in the small farming town of Crevalcore, Italy, not far from the cosmopolitan city of Bologna. His family were minor landowners with sufficient means to send Marcello, one of ten children, to the distinguished medical college at Bologna. It was there that Malpighi joined the ranks of the medical avant-garde, becoming a member of the Coro Anatomico, a group of forward-thinking medical students who convened at the home of a sympathetic teacher, Bartolomeo Massari. Dedicated to the modernization of medical education and practice, the Coro directly opposed the equally fervent conservative faction at the

University of Bologna, launching a bitter feud that would forever haunt Malpighi.

After receiving his degree in 1656 Malpighi joined the Accademia del Cimento (The Adventurous Academy), a scientific society more formal than the Coro but also guided by the modernist views held by its founders, Ferdinand II, Grand Duke of Tuscany, and his brother, Prince Leopold. The duke arranged for Malpighi's appointment to the chair of theoretical medicine at the University of Pisa, also providing him with free access to the latest microscope. Probably designed by Eustachio Divini, the finely crafted instrument had a device for focusing and four different powers of magnification, ranging from 41 to 143X.

At Pisa Malpighi formed what was to be a long and influential relationship with mathematician and physicist Alfonso Borelli. A supportive friend and confidant, it was Borelli who first suggested to Malpighi the use of mercury instead of ink as a staining method.

Malpighi returned to Bologna in 1658, accepting the position of "lecturer extraordinary" on theoretical medicine. In 1661 he published *De Pulmonibus (On the Lungs)*, in which he introduced the principle of a closed circuit of internal blood flow. Based on examinations of vivisected animals, Malpighi observed, "It was clear to the senses that the blood flowed always along tortuous vessels and was not poured into spaces, but was always within tubules, and that its dispersion is due to the multiple winding of the vessels."

Studying the vessels of the kidney and spleen, he also noted "grapelike clusters," now known as "malpighian bodies" or "Malpighi's corpuscles." Other eponymously named anatomical structures include Malpighi's vesicles in the lungs, the pyramids of Malpighi in the kidney, and the malpighian layer, referring to the germinal, or deepest, layer of the epidermis, which Malpighi recognized as the site of skin pigmentation.

The political climate in Bologna grew increasingly inhospitable to Malpighi, who was quickly becoming a hero among radicals. Borelli persuaded him to retreat to Messina, where Malpighi was offered a faculty chair at the university. His time at Messina was well spent, and in 1665, his final year in Sicily, he published three significant monographs describing his findings on the tongue, the skin and the brain.

After returning to Bologna Malpighi's physical and emotional health was eroded by chronic kidney disease and recurrent fits of depression. Although personal relationships grew increasingly difficult, the 39-year-old Malpighi decided to marry. His bride, 19 years his senior, was Francesca Massari, the sister of his former instructor.

The aging and cantankerous Malpighi gradually gained official acceptance, and in 1690 he reluctantly accepted an offer to serve as physician to the newly elected Pope Innocent XII. Former enemies continued to denounce his work, however, and several days after the publication of one such blast against anatomists and modernists Malpighi died during an apoplectic fit.

Patrick Manson 1844–1922

Recognized as one of the founding fathers of tropical medicine, parasitologist Patrick Manson spent more than twenty-four years in China conducting pioneer studies of malaria, tinea and elephantiasis. His experimental research established the link between the filarial worm and elephantoid disease, a condition in which various parts of the body develop lesions and fibrous tumors leading to impaired blood circulation and a hardening of the tissues. The result of obstructed lymphatic channels, these grotesque symptoms are often extremely difficult to manage, as the patient must carry around masses of hardened, distended tissue.

Having established that the tiny, threadlike worms or filariae found in the blood of elephantiasis patients were a causative factor in the disease, Manson discovered that these worms were transported by several species of mosquito. In addition, Manson made the puzzling observation that the embryo parasites appeared in the blood only after sundown, increasing in numbers until midnight and declining thereafter. By morning all embryonic filariae had disappeared. After many months of pondering these curious findings Manson arrived at the conclusion that the parasite was developing partly in a human or animal host and partly in the tissues of the mosquito. When a mosquito bites an infected animal or human, filariae embryos are introduced into the insect's bloodstream. The filariae pass the larval stage of development in the body of their insect host and are reintroduced into a larger animal host for their growth to maturity. Perpetuating the cycle, the female worms produce more embryos to be extracted by the next biting mosquito. This was perhaps Manson's most significant discovery, with far-reaching implications in the study of tropical diseases.

Born and raised in Scotland, Manson initially intended to become an engineer. He apprenticed himself to a local firm in Aberdeen but soon lost the job due to a protracted illness. During his convalescence he became intrigued with the study of natural history and biology, and quickly gave up any thoughts of becoming an engineer. He entered the school of medicine at the University of Aberdeen, receiving his doctorate in 1866.

Through the influence of his older brother, who had settled in the Far East, Manson was appointed medical officer of Formosa by the Chinese Imperial Maritime Customs. He held the position for nearly five years, until political unrest forced his departure. Manson retreated to Amoy, where he took over as head of a missionary hospital and dispensary while establishing a private practice.

In Amoy Manson began to investigate the mechanism of elephantoid disease, building his hypothesis based on clinical observations as well as on findings from earlier elephantiasis studies conducted by Timothy Richards Lewis in Calcutta.

Manson arrived in Hong Kong in 1883, reestablishing a private practice while continuing to study the nature of various parasitic diseases. He also devoted much of his time to the founding of a medical school specializing in the study of tropical diseases. Formally established in 1886, the school became a department of the University of Hong Kong.

Manson returned to Europe in 1889, taking up medical practice in London. Appointed chief physician to the Seamen's Hospital Society in 1892, Manson seized the opportunity to resume research on the causes and mechanisms of tropical diseases, particularly malaria. Seventeenth-century Peruvian Jesuits had discovered that quinine was effective in treating the symptoms of malaria, but little was known about its mechanism. In 1884 ALPHONSE LAVERAN had published his *Treatise on the Marshy Fevers with a Description of the "Malaria microbe,"* identifying the protozoan Plasmodium as the causative agent. Applying Laveran's theories along with his own findings on elephantiasis, Manson intensified his investigation of malaria. In the course of his research he encountered RONALD ROSS, a young physician who was to become Manson's protege. With the combined efforts of Ross, Manson, Camillo Golgi, Italian physician Amico Bignami (1862–1929) and other researchers around the world, the life cycle of the malaria parasite was described, and the role of the mosquito in the transmission of the disease was finally determined.

Manson left his position at the Seamen's Hospital to join in the founding of a second medical school specializing in the study of tropical disease: The London School of Tropical Medicine, which was formally established in 1898.

Rudolph Matas 1860–1957

The modern practice of vascular surgery was launched in 1888, when New Orleans physician Rudolph Matas performed the first operation on an arterial aneurysm. The term "aneurysm" (from the Greek *aneurysma*, an opening or broadening), refers to a saclike widening of an artery or vein that may rupture, causing hemorrhage, or may lead to the blockage of an important blood vessel. When occurring in the arteries—generally as a result of hypertension, hardening of the arteries, trauma or infection—the condition is characterized by pain, paralysis from nerve pressure and the development of a pulsating tumor emitting a strange rumbling sound, referred to as "aneurysmal bruit."

One of the earliest treatments for arterial aneurysm was a technique devised by pioneer surgeon JOHN HUNTER in which he ligated, or tied off, the artery at either side of the dilated section. Unsatisfied with Hunter's method, Matas introduced the practice of endo-aneurysmorrhaphy, later known as "Matas's operation," in which the sac is opened by surgical incision, deflated and sutured. Among other important advances in vascular surgery and medicine Matas developed a procedure using an aluminum strip, now known as "Matas's band," designed to block off the larger blood vessels as a means of evaluating the efficiency of secondary circulatory passages.

Matas was born in New Orleans of Catalonian ancestry. Orginally emigrating to America to pursue a career in pharmacy and medicine, Matas's father was distracted by the rich business opportunities amid the chaos of the Civil War. Rejecting his father's way of life, Rudolph worked his way through medical school, earning his degree from the University of Louisiana (later known as Tulane University) at the age of nineteen.

A year before graduating he took part in a research expedition to Cuba arranged by the U.S. National Health Service. An investigation of the pathology and etiology of yellow fever, the study was analyzed by Carlos Finlay, who later reported the role of the female Culex mosquito in the transmission of the disease. Matas, who was fluent in Spanish as well as French and Catalonian, translated Finlay's landmark studies in 1882 while serving as editor of the *New Orleans Medical and Surgical Journal*.

During his tenure as editor Matas also treated victims of the terrible yellow fever epidemics that continued to ravage the southern United States. Among his patients in Brownsville, Texas was the celebrated WILLIAM GORGAS, who, after gaining immunity from the disease, would eventually conquer yellow fever in Cuba and Panama.

After his initial success in the treatment of arterial aneurysm by vascular surgery Matas did not perform the operation again until twelve years later. During that time he was appointed professor of surgery at Tulane. Despite the loss of vision in one eye, incurred during the surgical laceration of a gonorrheal abscess, he continued to write extensively on clinical and medical subjects. Obtaining honorary doctoral degrees in law and science from five universities, Matas maintained a lifelong association with Tulane, eventually endowing the teaching library with a gift of one million dollars.

William James Mayo 1861–1939
Charles Horace Mayo 1865–1939
William Worrall Mayo 1819–1911

One of the world's most distinguished facilities for medical treatment and teaching, the Mayo Clinic in

Rochester, Minnesota is the culminating triumph of a family of physicians loyal to one another and to a tradition of medical service.

That tradition goes back to seventeenth-century England, when members of the Mayo family figured prominently as chemists. It undoubtedly influenced William Worrall Mayo, who was born in Manchester, England and worked in hospitals before he emigrated at the age of 26 to the United States. After a stint of work in the pharmacy at Bellevue Hospital in New York City he followed the pioneering tide westward as far as Lafayette, Indiana. There in 1848 he set himself up in a tailor shop, but he had been in the business less than a year when a cholera epidemic broke out.

Called on to help one of the few doctors in town, he subsequently attended one session of a medical school that functioned only between harvest time and the spring sowing season. Upon completion of the semester and payment of $100 he received a license to practice. He set up an office in a drug store on a salary of $75 a month. On the strength of that income he married Louise Abigail Wright, who opened a notions store to make ends meet.

William worked for half a year at the University of Missouri as assistant to a professor of anatomy, which won for him a second medical degree considerably more respectable than his first. Throughout his career as doctor in the little town of Le Sueur, Minnesota he had to augment his earnings by prospecting for copper, farming, piloting a river boat, acting as justice of the peace and publishing a newspaper. He tended the wounded in Indian wars and served during the Civil War as a medical officer and recruiter.

By the end of the Civil War he and Louise had three daughters (one of whom died in infancy); a son, William James, born in Le Sueur on July 29, 1861; and another son, Charles Horace, who was born in Rochester, Minnesota on July 19, 1865.

Both boys grew up in a total preoccupation with medicine. Their father occasionally went to New York to polish his surgical technique, and when he returned his sons would learn from him. When he became the county coroner the two boys learned their anatomy from autopsies.

William graduated from Niles Academy in Rochester and from the University of Michigan in Ann Arbor, where he received his medical degree in 1883. He went directly into practice with his father in Rochester, where the family then lived. That year Rochester was hit by a devastating tornado, and the Mayo family pitched in to care for the hundreds of injured who had to be sheltered in private homes, dance halls, or whatever facilty could be improvised, for there were neither hospital nor nurses in Rochester. The elder Mayo supervised all medical care in the emergency, his sons at his side. It was in the aftermath of that storm that the Franciscan nuns of a Rochester convent determined to raise money for a hospital in town if Dr. Mayo would head the medical team.

In 1888, when Charles came out of Chicago Medical College, he joined the Mayo medical partnership, and a year later the new hospital, with funding by the nuns and medical planning by the Mayos, opened its doors. Named St. Mary's, it had 40 beds in three wards, a nursing staff of six Franciscan nuns and a medical staff of three doctors, all named Mayo. In the first year some 300 patients were admitted, of whom only two percent died, a phenomenal achievement for that year in a hospital with relatively primitive equipment.

The Mayos established the practice of giving the same care to all patients but charging only those who could afford to pay. The system of setting fees to suit the patient's means has been continued ever since at the Mayo clinic.

Gradually the younger Mayos took their father's place in the operating room, seeking his advice but introducing sterilization techniques and equipment that seemed strange to the old doctor. Occasionally the father would act as the anesthetist while one of his sons performed the surgery. As his sons relieved him from medical responsibilities he turned to politics and served as alderman and mayor of Rochester and later as state senator. William, who had learned from his father the techniques of gynecological care, expanded his interest to include all abdominal problems. Among the first to perform appendectomies, he also perfected a technique for removing gallstones and applying skin grafts. Charles specialized in surgery of the eye, ear, nose, throat, brain and nerves, frequently using instruments of his own invention. He gained his greatest fame for his thyroid operations.

In 1884 the Mayos hired their first intern, Dr. Joseph Graham, whose sister Edith married Charles Mayo. William had married Hattie May Damon, daughter of a Rochester jeweler, some ten years earlier.

Despite the services performed without fees, the joint bank account in which the two brothers kept their savings grew. They agreed to put half of their earnings into a fund to be used for the advancement of medicine. They thought of lowering their fees but feared that this would antagonize their colleagues. Instead, they followed the practice of treating without fees not only all doctors and nurses but ministers, teachers and those of lower incomes in the state civil service.

Still the hospital prospered. As the surgical reputation of the Mayo brothers grew in the early years of the twentieth century patients were attracted to Rochester from all parts of the world. They established a clinic composed of a variety of specialists who could consult one another freely and plan together for the patient's welfare—an early form of group practice. The elder Mayo took a hand in planning that clinic, traveling the world for ideas even in his eighties. In 1911, however, when he was 92, his arm was hurt in an accident with farm machinery. When he died, after three operations, the city of Rochester put up a monument to William Mayo in what had already become known as Mayo Park.

In 1915, when the fund they had established with half their earnings—which had been profitably invested—totaled $1,500,000, the brothers organized the Mayo Foundation for Medical Education and Research, which has become a prime resource in medical education for fellowships and scholarships. Both brothers were honored for their contributions to medicine, education and public service, particularly during World War I, after which both attained the rank of brigadier general in the army reserves.

The brothers had collaborated all their lives in total harmony. The death of Charles Mayo from pneumonia at the age of 74 on May 26, 1939 was therefore a bitter blow to William. He died on July 28 of the same year.

The clinic, the foundation and the tradition survive as later generations of Mayos continue to serve medicine and the institutions launched by William Worrall Mayo and sons.

Sir Peter Brian Medawar 1915–1987

Peter Brian Medawar was first to demonstrate that it was possible to transplant tissue from one animal to another having a different genetic inheritance. Monozygotic twins (i.e., those who develop from a single ovum) had been known to tolerate grafts from each other, but twins born from the same pregnancy but different ova (dizygotic or fraternal twins) completely rejected each other's tissue.

The genetic barrier seemed insurmountable because, as Sir Peter himself noted, "the rejection of genetically foreign grafts has a history of more than a hundred million years, being already present in force at the time bony fish evolved."

For his work, which not only proved the feasibility of transplantation but disclosed the underlying immunological nature of the rejection process, Medawar shared the 1960 Nobel Prize for Physiology or Medicine with Australian virologist and physician FRANK MACFARLANE BURNET.

Peter Medawar was born in Rio de Janeiro on February 28, 1915. His Lebanese father and English mother had met in England, where the senior Medawar was hired to represent a manufacturer of dental supplies in Brazil. As a boy Peter played and swam at Copacabana Beach, but he, along with his older brother Philip, was sent to a series of prep schools in England, most of them depressingly mediocre, as he was to note in his memoirs.

In 1932, at the age of seventeen, he entered Magdalen College, Oxford, where his tutor, John Zachary Young, instilled in him a passion for science, hard work and logical thought. After completing his studies, Madawar received scholarships that enabled him to do postgraduate work and tutoring at Magdalen. One of his students was Jean Shinglewood Taylor. The two married in February 1937, despite the serious disapproval of Jean's family, who thought that Peter was not only un-English but seemed to lack the social graces of the English upper middle class. After he won the Nobel Prize and was subsequently knighted, and after the marriage produced two sons and two daughters, the family was reconciled.

Peter and his bride both went to work in the tissue culture laboratory at the William Dunn School of Pathology in Oxford under Professor Howard Florey, who was later to develop the therapeutic values of penicillin. When World War II broke out, Peter, his application for military service rejected because of his height (6'5") and flat feet, became interested in the problems of treating badly burned air-raid victims who desperately needed skin grafts they could tolerate.

The incident that set him on the course he was to follow for the rest of his life occurred on a Sunday afternoon early in the war when a plane roaring over the Oxford street on which he lived crashed into a neighbor's garden and exploded. The flier, who turned out to be British, suffered from burns on over 60 percent of his body. Frustrated at his inability to devise an acceptable graft, Medawar became preoccupied with the biology of rejection. A paper he wrote for the *Bulletin of War Medicine* secured him a grant to study at the Burns Unit of the Glasgow Royal Infirmary. There he found convincing evidence that the grafting process was essentially immunological, akin to that by which the body defends itself against invasions of foreign agents such as bacteria.

This was confirmed by meticulous and laborious experimentation on rabbits when Medawar returned to Oxford. While serving as professor of zoology at the University of Birmingham, Medawar found that cattle could tolerate grafts taken from identical or fraternal twins. Furthermore, in a book by Frank Macfarlane Burnet and Frank Fenner, he came across a reference to the work of American geneticist Frank Owen, who disclosed that cattle twins, even dizygotic ones, always had the same blood group. This was apparently due to the fact that cattle twins are fed through the same placenta and therefore are constantly being transfused with each other's blood at the fetal stage.

While Macfarlane Burnet developed the theory behind the body's ability to differentiate between "self and nonself" Medawar proceeded to demonstrate, by meticulous and arduous experimentation on mice, the mechanism involved in the phenomenon.

Propounding the thesis he had set out to prove, he wrote: "A brown mouse of strain CBA, which before birth received an inoculation of living cells from white mice of a strain A, would, when adult, accept a skin graft from mice of strain A." When he succeeded by fetal inoculation to make his animals tolerant of each other's grafts and to identify the process as essentially immunologic, he called the resulting condition "acquired immunogical tolerance."

In 1953 he and his team published their findings in *Nature*, and in 1960 he and MacFarlane Burnet were awarded the Nobel Prize for Physiology or Medicine. Two years later Medawar took over the directorship of the National Institute for Medical Research at Mill Hill, the foremost investigative enterprise in the British Commonwealth.

While leading that organization into new areas of ethology and neurophysiology, he changed Mill Hill's atmosphere, making it more human—some said more "civilized." His directors' lunches became celebrated for their wit and flow of ideas. He dispatched his administrative duties in two hours and spent most of the rest of his day at his laboratory bench. At least two days a week he cut himself even from the telephone, whose ring he regarded as an unpardonable intrusion.

He elicited from his staff an extraordinary devotion and admiration not only for his scientific leadership but for his charm. Knighted in 1965, and his reputation as a witty speaker and writer grew. His honors included not only degrees from innumerable universities but the Copley Medal and a ceremonial appointment as Commander of the British Empire.

In 1969 he was to accept the presidency of the British Association for the Advancement of Science, read the traditional "lesson" at Exeter Cathedral (a traditional duty of the association's president) and deliver some twenty other talks in one week. It was while reading the "lesson" at Exeter Cathedral that he was felled by a massive stroke that paralyzed his left arm and left leg and severely impaired the vision on the left side of both his eyes.

Nevertheless he was back in his lab in 1970, though he and his personal laboratory staff were moved out of Mill Hill to the Clinical Research Center in North London. His courage in the face of monumental handicaps won the admiration of all who knew him. People with whom he worked recall the time when, having lost an eye, he ordered its replacement to be "beer-bottle brown with just a hint of sparkle."

As subsequent strokes made lab work almost impossible despite the efforts of his loyal staff, Medawar took to dictating essays into a cassette recorder. His books, a blend of science and philosophy, seasoned with rumor and anecdote, include *The Uniqueness of the Individual, The Future of Man, Advice to a Young Scientist, Pluto's Republic, The Limits of Science*, two collaborations with his wife—*The Life Science and Aristotle to Zoo*—and his autobiographical *Memoir of a Thinking Radish.*

After his death on October 2, 1987, obituaries in scholarly journals and in the general press spoke not only of Medawar's contributions to science but of his gallantry and high spirits.

Father Gregor Johann Mendel 1822–1884

The mathematical laws of heredity were first discerned in a monastery garden by a nineteenth-century Augustinian monk named Gregor Johann Mendel. It was Father Mendel who first outlined the patterns by which certain "factors," whether dominant or recessive, were transmitted from generation to generation of *Pisum sativum*, the ordiary edible pea.

Later Mendels' "factors" would be called "genes," and the science fathered by the botanist/monk would be known as genetics.

Johann, as he was called in his childhood, was born in 1822 to a peasant family living in the Moravian village of Heizendorf in what is now Czechoslovakia. His father, Anton, however, had traveled widely as a soldier in Napoleon's army and had learned to read, a rare accomplishment in rural Moravia in those years. Johann proved to be an apt student in the little school of Heizendorf, and so eager to learn that, instead of sending him to work in the fields, his father permitted him to go on to the gymnasium in the nearby town of Troppau. However, the family could not afford to pay for more than half-rations for the boy.

Poverty continued to dog Johann throughout his higher education at the Philosophical Institute of Olmutz, and his attempts to earn a living while at school left him prey to recurrent illnesses. The stress of failure or the fear of it tended to send young Johann into a state of nervous collapse.

His scholarly talents and chronic poverty suggested the church as a means of achieving security along with the time to study. He had not shown any interest in religion as a calling but accepted the church as a safe port in a stormy sea. A former physics professor of his recommended the Augustinian monastery at St. Thomas. On entering the monastery at the age of 21 Johann took the name of Gregor and began his life of study.

The abbot of St. Thomas sent Gregor to Brunn Theological College, where he took not only the required courses in theology doctrine but also the elements of pedagogy, Greek and Hebrew. At the age of 25 he was ordained a priest and sent out to serve the sick and dying in a local parish. The high-strung priest found the duty too painful, and he was assigned to teach in a local school, where he excelled. He did not do well, however, in the tests for a license required by the authorities of the Austro- Hungarian Empire. His abbot nevertheless arranged for him to take a two-year course at the renowned University of Vienna, where he encountered men and ideas that were then breaking new ground in the sciences. It was there that he was introduced into the mysteries and significance of the cell and to the wonders of plant biology, particularly hybridization as discussed by the early writers on Darwinian evolution.

When his course was completed he resumed teaching school in Brunn as an unlicensed "temporary." In the monastery gardens, however, he explored the transmissability of traits in hybrids. Choosing as his experimental model the edible pea, of which there are 34 distinct varieties, he bred and cross-bred until he formulated what has since become known as a "Mendelian law," which declares that if you cross a plant having a dominant characteristic, A, with one possessing a recessive factor, a, the resulting progeny will include an A, exhibiting the dominant trait; an a, indicating the recessive element; and two hyrids, seemingly identical with the dominant A but actually including the elements of A and a.

By meticulous breeding and note-taking he accumulated convincing data, which he refined into a series of "laws" of heredity. He incorporated his findings into a lengthy paper that he read at a meeting of the Brunn Society for the Study of Natural Science in February, 1865.

Though Mendel's paper was published in the society's *Transactions* the following year, it caused scarcely a ripple. His work might have been buried for all time if, 35 years later, in 1900, it was not rediscovered and independently confirmed by three scientists—Hugo de Vries (1848–1935), a Dutch biologist; Erich Tsermak von Seysenegg (1871–1962), an Austrian botanist who stumbled on the Mendelian laws when he was working on peas; and Karl Erich Correns (1864–1933), a German botanist who traced Father Gregor's patterns in maize as well as peas.

By that time Mendel had been dead for 16 years. He had been promoted to abbot of the monastery, where he was known as a genial, humorous man who smoked some 20 cigars a day as he puttered in the garden, apparently unaware of the enormous influence his "laws" would have. He died in January, 1884 from uremia and dropsy. He had left instructions that an autopsy be performed, not out of any scientific considerations but to make absolutely sure that he was dead. One of his nightmarish fears had been that he might be buried alive.

Karl Augustus Menninger, 1893–

The Menninger Clinic was established in 1920 by Karl Menninger and his father, Dr. Charles Frederick Menninger, as a center for psychiatric therapy and research. Located in Topeka, Kansas, the clinic gathered together specialists from all areas of mental health in order to provide patients with the broadest scope of possibilities for effective treatment.

Committed to the advancement of mental health care, Karl and his brother William Menninger (1899–1966) sought to promote public awareness and understanding of psychiatric therapy. They founded the Menninger Foundation as a center for psychiatric research, professional training and public education. One of the world's largest and most respected centers for psychiatric care, the Menninger Foundation played an important role in the American public's acceptance of psychiatry.

Born and raised in Topeka, Karl Menninger left Kansas to attend Harvard University Medical School, where he was trained as a psychiatrist. After graduation he returned to Topeka to join forces with his father in the creation of the Menninger Clinic. William Menninger, also a psychiatrist, joined the clinic five years later.

After establishing the Menninger Foundation in 1941 Karl Menninger continued to work toward the advancement and accessibility of mental health care. As World War II was ending he was influential in the development of an institute for psychiatric training in association with the Winter Veterans Administration Hospital in Topeka. In addition to its distinguished mental health care facilities, the institute offers one of the largest and most comprehensive psychiatric training programs in existence.

Karl Menninger wrote extensively on human psychology, producing in 1930 the first best-selling book on psychiatry, *The Human Mind*. Continuing to publish letters, articles and books on psychiatric subjects, Karl Menninger was also professor of psychiatry at the University of Kansas from 1946 until 1962. Other written works include *Man against Himself* (1938); *Theory of Psychoanalytic Technique* (1959); *The Vital Balance* (1963); *The Crime of Punishment* (1968); and *Whatever Became of Sin?* (1973).

Franz Anton Mesmer 1734–1815

The sensational career of Franz Anton Mesmer developed in the mysterious realm that still exists today, hovering somewhere in between medical science and charlatanism. Mesmer's therapeutic system was based on the concept of a universal, life-enhancing force that he called "animal magnetism." Claiming to manipulate the vital force, he practiced what became known as "mesmerism"—a hypnotic procedure for the treatment of a variety of symptoms. The healing power of "mesmerism" was particularly effective against headaches, hysteria, arthritis, eczema and other conditions that are now recognized as having a significant psychological component.

Mesmer was born at Itznang, a small village in Germany near Lake Constance. After completing undergraduate studies in medicine and theology at the University of Ingolstadt, he left for Austria to pursue his medical training at the University of Vienna. By the time he received his medical degree in 1766, he was deeply involved in his exploration of the occult.

Convinced that human health was influenced by the stars and planets, Mesmer presented his daring views in a doctoral thesis that sought to reconcile the arcane traditions of the Renaissance with the scientific principles of the Age of Reason, in particular the doctrine of Isaac Newton. It was Newton who had suggested the notion of an invisible "fluid" flowing through space and animating the universe as a possible explanation for such phenomena as gravity, magnetism, and the transmission of light.

While investigating the effects of magnets on the human body, Mesmer developed the idea that he himself could exert a power comparable to the force of magnetism or the influence of the stars—a therapeutic energy that could be used to heal. Identifying the transmission of such power from one human being to another as "animal magnetism," he launched his mission of healing in Vienna in 1775.

He established "hypnotic séances" as an effective therapeutic procedure, particularly for relieving symptoms of hysteria or other emotional disturbances, but despite his impressive results, the practices were denounced as quackery by the medical establishment in Austria. In 1778 a commission was ordered by Maria Christina to investigate Mesmer's claims and within 24 hours he was forced to leave the country.

After a brief stop in Belgium, Mesmer headed for Paris, where he immediately captivated the public with his charismatic powers. He soon established a successful salon on the Place Vendôme where his mystical services were sought after by a long line of wealthy and fashionable clients. Conducting the seance as a theatrical event, he wore a lavender robe embroidered with astrological symbols, played entrancing music, waved a "magnetic wand," fixed his patients with a penetrating stare and led them into "conducting tubs" to receive treatment. Fitted into the the tubs were strips of iron that presumably served to collect the demonstrator's "animal magnetism."

Though he was offered vast sums of money to reveal his methods, Mesmer kept the key to his practice a fiercely guarded secret. He did expound his theory of therapeutic energy and human transmission in a book entitled, *Mémoire sur la découverte du Magnétisme Animal*, published in Paris and Geneva in 1779.

The French mania for mesmerism brought him fame and fortune within the first few years but it was not long before his opponents in the medical establishment launched accusations of professional fakery. In 1784 Mesmer came under investigation once again, this time by a Royal Commission that included such distinguished scientists as Benjamin Franklin and Antoine Lavoisier. The decision of the committee was unanimous—Mesmer had managed to cure a certain number of patients, they acknowledged, but his success was purely a result of the power of suggestion rather than that of "animal magnetism."

At the age of 50, Mesmer was barred from practice and driven into exile for the second time. He retired to Switzerland to spend the last 30 years of his life in obscurity.

Although Mesmer's career ended in 1784, the magnetic craze would persist until the middle of the next century. It was not until long after his death that hypnosis emerged as a valuable tool in clinical practice. The conclusions drawn by the French Commission reflected a growing awareness of the powerful effects of the mind on the body, however. Examining their findings nearly 60 years later, noted British surgeon JAMES BRAID explored the nature of "psychological suggestion" in *Neurypnology*, an influential text in which he renamed the phenomenon, coining the term "hypnotism," or "nervous sleep."

Elie Metchnikoff 1845–1916

Russian microbiologist Elie Metchnikoff investigated cellular responses to injury and infection and defined the meaning and mechanism of inflammation as a defense of multicellular animals against disease. "The organism digests the food substances outside the gastrointestinal canal by means of an inflammatory recation," he announced in 1884. Though Metchnikoff was not the first to suggest that wandering cells might ingest and destroy bacteria, he discovered the central role of these scavengers of foreign substances in the process of inflammation and named them "phagocytes." Derived from the Greek words *kutos* and *phagos*, the term means literally "a cell that devours."

"Besides a tactile sense, the phagocytes possess a kind of sense of taste or chemotaxis," wrote Metchnikoff, "which enables them to distinguish the chemical composition of the substances with which they come in contact." He described the ways in which these white blood cells surround, engulf and digest microorganisms and cellular debris, discerning their effects not only on bacteria but on the body's own red cells. A century later Dr. Alex Comfort would develop a theory of aging based on his observation of a proliferation of phagocytes in aging cells.

In his own lifetime the impassioned Metchnikoff was hailed as a brilliant prophet by many of the leading lights of his profession, including LOUIS PASTEUR, RU-

DOLF VIRCHOW, and JOSEPH LISTER. Celebrated bacteriologist Émile Roux, with whom he collaborated at the Pasteur Institute in Paris, dubbed Metchnikoff the "Daemon of Science."

The more traditional scientific establishment, particularly in Germany, was less sympathetic to Metchnikoff, whose phagocyte theory seemed to contradict the accepted doctrine of the day. Belonging to the "humoral school" were such distinguished bacteriologists as Hans Buchner (1850–1902) and EMIL VON BEHRING, who believed that the body's system of defense against disease relied on the ability of blood serum to lyse, or destroy, bacteria. As Robert Koch and others avidly sought to discredit Metchnikoff's radical theories the feud became more and more divisive, so that it was not until many years later that it became clear that both sides were in fact partially correct.

The imagination of the public was captured by Metchnikoff's fierce combatativeness as well as his feverish and prophetic genius. As early as 1906 the notion of phagocytes found its way to the stage in George Bernard Shaw's *The Doctor's Dilemma*, in which the idea serves as an example of the latest advance in medical theory. Metchnikoff's legendary status was further enhanced by Leo Tolstoy, who described him as an "Old Testament prophet." "He believes in his science as in Holy Scripture," wrote Tolstoy. "He is a sweet and simple man but as some weak men get drunk on alcohol, so he gets drunk on science."

Born in the village of Ivanovka in the Ukraine, Metchnikoff attended secondary school, then the nearby University of Kharkov, where he obtained his doctorate in microbiology before he was twenty years old. Plagued throughout his career by headaches, nervous exhaustion and depression, Metchnikoff was nursed through one of his breakdowns by a young woman named Ludmilla, whom he subsequently married. The couple had little hope for a bright future, however, since the bride was a chronic consumptive who had to be carried to her wedding in a chair. When she died several years later Metchnikoff took a dose of morphia in the first of several suicide attempts over the course of his life.

Appointed lecturer at the University of Odessa in 1870, Metchnikoff met and married his second wife, Olga, and settled into the quiet life of an academic. Though he had been impatient with the unscientific aspect of revolutionary theory, he remained relatively apolitical until the wave of right-wing repression that followed the assassination of Czar Alexander II in 1881. Metchnikoff's outspoken views cost him his position at the university, and,in a dramatic demonstration of despair, he again resorted to suicide.

After his second failed attempt he went with Olga and her brothers and sisters to recuperate at Messina, a resort on the northern coast of Sicily. Finding himself alone for an afternoon, he amused himself by watching the mobile cells of transparent starfish larvae under his microscope. In a burst of inspired intuition he wondered whether "...similar cells might serve in the defense of the organism against intruders..." and proceeded to conduct a series of experimental demonstrations that confirmed his hypothesis.

Over the next twenty-five years Metchnikoff continued to explore the nature and mechanism of inflammation as he developed his phagocyte theory. He returned to Russia, where he was put in charge of a newly established bacteriologic station at the University of Odessa.

In 1881 he left on a tour of Europe to defend and disseminate his radical ideas and was warmly received by much of the scientific community in France. He left a strong first impression on the celebrated Louis Pasteur, who later described his first meeting with Metchnikoff: "I saw an old man, rather undersized, with a left hemiplegia (paralysis affecting only one side of the body), very piercing grey eyes, a short beard and moustache and slightly grey hair, covered by a black skull cap. His pale and sickly complexion and tired look betokened a man who was not likely to live many more years...'I at once placed myself on your side,' he told me...'I believe you are on the right road.'"

Pasteur invited him to join the research staff at the new Pasteur Institute,which was then being built, and in 1881 Metchnikoff and his wife settled in a small hotel in the Latin Quarter of Paris. While Germany remained unreceptive to his ideas, England showed its respect with the award of an honorary degree at Cambridge in 1891. After accepting the honor Metchnikoff remained at Cambridge to deliver a series of lectures on phagocytosis and inflammatory response, which were complied as *Leçons sur la Pathologie Comparée de l'Inflammation (Studies on Comparative Pathology of Inflamation).*

In 1901 he published *L'Immunité dans les Maladies Infectieuses* (*Immunity in Infectious Diseases*), a discussion of the phenomenon of aging in which he presented a great deal of wild conjecture along with incisive speculation. He also introduced with in the book the notion of autoimmunity and suggested the role of pernicious intestinal flora in the aging process.

Noting that bacteria respond to changes in pH, or acid-base balance of its environment, Metchnikoff asserted that sour milk, which contains acid-producing lactobacilli, could be used to curb the baneful flora and thus retard the deterioration of the body. His doctrine of sour milk was given support by the reports of record-breaking longevity in certain regions of Bulgaria where the consumption of sour milk was particularly high. The romantic pessimism of Metchnikoff's youth gave way to a new enthusiasm for finding ways to sustain the "life wish" so that humans might live out their "natural span," and he described his mortal battle against intestinal flora in a collection of writings entitled *Essais Optimistes* (*Optimistic Essays*).

In 1908, at the age of 63, Metchnikoff was awarded the Nobel Prize for Physiology or Medicine, which he shared with another pioneer immunologist, PAUL EHRLICH. Despite rapidly declining health, Metchnikoff continued to work at his laboratory, and after a series of episodes of tachycardia (attacks of excessively rapid heart rate), he moved into the apartment at the Institute where Pasteur has lived until his death in 1895. Twenty-one years later, as Metchnikoff lay dying, he requested that his corpse be cremated in the same furnace that had incinerated his laboratory animals and that his ashes remain at the institute.

César Milstein 1927–

Argentine-born César Milstein, a leader in the development of monoclonal antibodies, received his education at the University of Buenos Aires, completing his doctoral work on enzymes at Cambridge in 1960. Milstein continued enzyme studies at the Medical Research Council Laboratory of Molecular Biology at Cambridge for several years, eventually turning his attention to the field of immunology.

In what proved to be a highly successful collaboration, Milstein and GEORGES J.F. KÖHLER, a visiting post-doctoral fellow in immunology, embarked on a revolutionary study of antibodies. Together they developed a method of producing an unlimited number of pure and uniform antibodies by fusing tumor cells with antibody-producing cells. The unlimited production of these easily reproducible "monoclonal antibodies" greatly expanded the scope of biomedical research and provided a valuable diagnostic and therapeutic tool in the management of cancer and other diseases.

In 1984 Milstein and Köhler were recognized for their contribution to the advancement of immunological medicine with the Nobel Prize for Physiology or Medicine (shared with NIELS K. JERNE).

George Richards Minot 1885–1950

Through tireless investigation of the nature of pernicious anemia George Minot discovered a nutritional method of controlling the disease by means of a diet rich in liver. This particular form of anemia, first described by Thomas Addison in 1855, was dubbed "pernicious" because of its subtle onset and eventually fatal outcome. Minot, in conjunction with WILLIAM MURPHY, GEORGE WHIPPLE and William Castle, studied the clinical aspects of pernicious anemia for many years before recognizing and eventually understanding the therapeutic factor in liver.

George Minot was born to a distinguished Massachussets family with a long tradition in the medical profession. Minot's father, grandfather and great-uncle were all noted physicians, and his uncle, Charles Sedgwick Minot, a respected biologist, was the author of a philosophical treatise entitled *Age, Growth, and Death*. Minot, a sickly child, dedicated himself to medicine, concentrating early in his career on diseases of the blood.

After graduating from Harvard Medical School in 1912 Minot interned at Massachussetts General Hospital, where he began a lifelong discipline of recording detailed observations of many of his patients, particularly those suffering from various forms of anemia. Pernicious anemia, a result of a stomach defect, prevents young blood cells, or reticulocytes, from becoming fully developed red blood corpuscles. With the help of newly introduced experimental stains Minot could recognize these reticulocytes in blood samples taken from pernicious anemia patients and monitor their levels at various stages of the disease. Working with pathologist James Homer Wright, Minot became convinced that the disease was related to ill-functioning bone marrow, but various attempts at treatment were unsuccessful.

In 1921 Minot's fragile health worsened dramatically. He diagnosed diabetes and followed the drastic diet recommended by a diabetes expert, but it was the recent and revolutionary discovery of insulin by FREDERICK BANTING that saved Minot's life.

With a heightened awareness of diet as a therapeutic agent, Minot came across a number of studies documenting the restorative, therapeutic values of liver. In particular, George Whipple's work at the University of Rochester indicated a therapeutic factor in liver, although his animal experimentation was performed in cases of induced or secondary anemia, which had pathology quite different from that of pernicious anemia. As the cure for both disorders was only coincidentally to be found in the same food, it is fortunate that Minot did not recognize that Whipple's subjects were suffering from iron deficiency.

Minot began recommending an increased amount of liver to patients in various stages of pernicious anemia. In addition to his growing private practice Minot served as an associate in medicine at Peter Bent Brigham Hospital, as a consultant on blood diseases at Massachussets General and as head of a division of Huntington Memorial Hospital specializing in cancer.

His experimental high-liver diet was proving highly successful, corroborating the results achieved by Murphy with a similar diet. In 1926 Minot and Murphy reported their findings to the medical community, giving rise to a concerted effort to isolate the factor in liver that was proving consistently effective in treating pernicious anemia. Two years later Minot joined the Harvard faculty as professor of medicine, also taking over directorship of the Thorndike Memorial Hospital, affiliated with Boston City Hospital.

In 1929 William Castle, a junior member at Thorndike Laboratory, contributed important findings in the search for what he called the "extrinsic factor" in liver—the dietary element that allows pernicious anemia patients to produce sufficient amounts of red blood corpuscles. Eventually this factor was identified in 1948 as vitamin B_{12}, or cyanocobalamin, by Berk and his colleagues. In pernicious anemia gastric secretion is severely deficient, preventing the absorption of vitamin B_{12}, a necessary factor in normal red blood cell production. Iron was discovered to be the other therapeutic substance in liver, of critical value to patients with secondary anemia.

Daily ingestion of liver as treatment for pernicious anemia soon gave way to injections of liver extract, and eventually of isolated B12. In recognition of their great contribution to the conquering of this devastating disease, Minot, Murphy, and Whipple shared the Nobel Prize for Physiology or Medicine in 1934. At the award presentation, it was estimated that their dedication had already saved the lives of 15,000 to 20,000 patients in the United States alone.

Silas Weir Mitchell 1829–1914

American author and physician Silas Weir Mitchell contributed important studies on the physiology of the brain, the distribution of nerves in the skin, the principle of sensory reinforcement and the description and treatment of hysteria.

As a practicing physician during the Civil War, Mitchell served at Turner's Lane Hospital in Philadelphia, where he treated thousands of patients debilitated by neurological injuries and disorders, including post-traumatic epilepsy, traumatic neuralgia, hysteria and neurasthenia. In 1864 he published the first definitive report on post-traumatic neurological pathology, entitled *Gunshot Wounds and Other Injuries of Nerves*. Later expanded to a broader study entitled *Injuries of Nerves and Their Consequences* (1872), Mitchell's observations established him as a preeminent authority in clinical neurology. His illustrious circle of friends and colleagues included physician WILLIAM OSLER and pathologist and medical historian William Henry Welch. Born in Philadelphia, Mitchell was the son of a respected professor of medicine at Jefferson Medical College, where he received his medical degree in 1850. After pursuing postgraduate studies in France with noted physiologist CLAUDE BERNARD and biologist and microscopist Charles Philippe Robin (1821–1855) Mitchell returned to join his father's clinical practice in Philadelphia.

His earliest investigations were in the area of toxicology and pharmacology, with a particular emphasis on the effects and mechanism of snake venom. His extensive writings on the subject include a detailed study entitled *Researches upon the Venoms of Poisonous Snakes*. In 1886 Mitchell and American physiologist E.T. Reichert (1855–1931) collaborated to demonstrate the protein composition of snake venom.

Widely sought after by patients with a broad range of neurological problems, Mitchell established a system of therapy for nervous exhaustion, hysteria and other related conditions now referred to as "Weir Mitchell treatment." The therapeutic method, advanced in his articles "Rest in Nervous Disease: Its Use and Abuse" (1875), "Fat and Blood" (1877), "The Evolution of the Rest Treatment" (1904) and "Rest Treatment and Psychic Medicine" (1908), consists of an enforced period of bed rest accompanied by abundant feeding and techniques of electrical stimulation and massage.

Mitchell's numerous published monographs include the first clinical observations of post-paralytic chorea (a condition characterized by involuntary spastic body jerks) and the effects of weather on pain, particularly in amputees. In an influential work entitled *Headaches from Heat Stroke, from Fevers, after Meningitis, from Over Use of the Brain, from Eye Strain* (1874) he makes the first association between headache and astigmatism. Mitchell is also distinguished for the identification of a syndrome he called erythromelalgia, also known as "Mitchell's disease," which he described as a "rare vaso-motor neurosis of the extremities" characterized by sudden and intense vascular dilatation causing redness and burning pain, particularly in the feet.

Mitchell's other general reference works in neurology include *Wear and Tear* (1871), *Lectures on Diseases of the Nervous System—Especially in Women* (1881) and *Clinical Lessons on Nervous Diseases* (1897).

As a popular and well-respected author of fiction and poetry, Mitchell also published a number of novels, including *Hugh Wynne, Free Quaker*, an historical romance appearing in 1896, and *Constance Trescot*, a psychological study written in 1905.

Jacques Monod 1910–1976

Recognized for his philosophical perspective as well as his scientific contribution to the study of biology and medicine, Jacques Monod shared the 1965 Nobel Prize in Physiology or Medicine with Francois Jacob and ANDRE LWOFF for their valuable research on the genetic mechanism at the cellular level.

Born in France, Monod earned his doctorate in biochemistry from the University of Paris in 1941. Decorated for valor in World War II, Monod was an important figure in the French Resistance. In 1945 he became affiliated with the Louis Pasteur Institute in Paris, eventually assuming the directorship of the department of cellular biochemistry in 1954. It was at the

Pasteur Institute that Monod and Jacob embarked on a ten-year collaboration that had an enormous impact on scientific understanding of the genetic process, and ultimately on the progress of cancer research.

Genetic information is encoded in the form of a chain of various small molecules whose sequence corresponds to that of amino acids in a given protein. The assembly of protein molecules is the mechanism by which this information is expressed. For this process to occur, the information must be carried to the site of protein synthesis in the cell. Monod and Jacob introduced the notion of the "operon"—the part of a chromosome containing the "structural genes" that control protein synthesis and those that determine whether or not those structural genes will function.

They also identified and described the concept of "messenger RNA"—the ribonucleic acid molecule that conveys from the DNA the information used to determine the structure of a particular polypeptide molecule. It is the sequence of nucleotides in the messenger RNA or mRNA, that dictates the sequence of amino acids in the polypeptide.

In 1967 Monod left the Pasteur Institute to teach molecular biology at the Collège de France. His published writings include *Of Microbes and Life*, edited with Ernest Borek and published in 1971. In the same year Monod published *Chance and Necessity*, a treatise offering a philosophical and ethical perspective on the study of genetics. Presented as "An Essay on the Natural Philosophy of Modern Biology," it discusses the vast implications of what Monod calls a "universe without causality."

Giovanni Battista Morgagni 1682–1771

Giovanni Morgagni is generally considered one of the champions of eighteenth-century medicine and one of the founders of the discipline of anatomy and pathology.

Morgagni's teaching career at the renowned University of Padua spanned 56 years and was crowned by the publication in 1761 of his masterpiece, *De Sedibus et Causis Morborum* (*On the Sites and Causes of Disease*). The book was a beautifully designed presentation of Morgagni's observations of over 500 autopsies, accompanied by his own correlations between each patient's clinical symptoms and the postmortem findings. Morgagni was careful to pay tribute to Théophile Bonet (1629–1689), who had previously published *Sepulcretum* (Graves), a poorly organized and inconclusive description of autopsy findings, but it is Morgagni's work that established principles and methods of clinical medicine still practiced today. Morgagni drew more inspiration from HIPPOCRATES, whose methods of observation and reasoning he revived and expanded.

While Hippocrates had systematically differentiated diseases by their external, symptomatic appearances, Morgagni described and classified the internal conditions of the body in relation to their external expression. Hippocrates could only know and differentiate diseases by their symptoms, but for the first time Morgagni examined the nature of the internal damage to the body that had given rise to those symptoms. Morgagni would carefully record his patients' symptoms during illness, and in postmortem examinations he would try to trace those responses to an organic or pathological cause. Through extensive research Morgagni was able to predict or visualize the nature and extent of internal derangement from his observation of external evidence.

With this new perspective Morgagni also debunked a long-standing medical assumption: the ancient humoral theory of one cause for all disease. In his book he clearly identifies a number of individual pathologies, notably hepatic cirrhosis, renal tuberculosis, pneumonic solidification of the lungs and syphilitic lesions of the brain. A number of the anatomical parts identified by Morgagni have since been given his name. XAVIER BICHAT was an admirer of Morgagni's and studied hundreds of cadavers in his attempt to classify the body's different tissues.

Morgagni's half century of work as a professor at Padua is greatly responsible for the university's powerful influence during that period.

William Thomas Green Morton 1819–1868

At Mt. Auburn Cemetery in Massachussetts a gravestone bears the following inscription:

> William T.G. Morton, inventor and revealer of anaesthetic inhalation, by whom pain in surgery was averted and annulled; before whom, in all time, surgery was agony; since whom science has control of pain.

The epitaph honors the first medical practitioner to use ether as a surgical anesthetic. Inaugurating the technique at Massachussetts General Hospital on October 16, 1846, Morton administered the drug to a young and frightened patient named Gilbert Abbott, who was to have a vascular tumor surgically removed from his jaw. The excision was performed by distinguished Boston surgeon John Collins Warren (1778–1856) before an audience of influential physicians and surgeons who watched in amazement as Abbott endured the procedure with no sign of pain.

After successfully completing the operation Warren hailed the advent of "painless surgery" by announcing, "Gentlemen, this is no humbug!" His endorsement deliberately echoed the words spoken 47 years earlier by a Boston physician in praise of the newly introduced smallpox vaccination.

Born in Charlton, Massachussetts, Morton studied at the Baltimore School of Dental Surgery and became a member of the American Society of Dental Surgeons. He practiced dentistry in Boston for several years, during which time he shared a brief partnership with Horace Wells (1815–1848), who preceded Morton as a pioneer in the advancement of anesthesia in surgery (see HUMPHREY DAVY).

Dentistry was still a primitive craft in the early 1800s, requiring a certain pioneer spirit of its practitioners. In the course of his practice Morton developed a number of innovations, including a new solder for attaching false teeth to the gums. Though clearly an improvement over earlier methods, his procedure, requiring root extractions, was brutally painful. To make the technique more practical, Morton sought a chemical substance to reduce the pain. Exploring the value of sulphuric ether as a localized numbing agent, Morton developed a method of inducing a more general desensitization by applying the drug to the system as a whole through the respiratory system. (The words "anesthesia" and "anesthetics," derived from the Greek meaning "lack of feeling," are attributed to celebrated American physician and scholar Oliver Wendell Holmes, who coined the terms shortly after he learned of Morton's discovery.)

Within weeks of its historic introduction Morton's technique for "painless surgery" was recognized for its wide range of applications. Intoxicated by the prospect of unlimited financial dividend, Morton sought to monopolize distribution by adding inactive ingredients to color and disguise the ether. Before the end of the year he presented the mixture as a mysterious new compound called "Letheon" and applied for a patent. Morton's scheme was soon discovered, however, and ether anesthesia entered the public domain, untrammeled by private greed.

Despite the disclosure of Morton's lapse of ethics he was internationally acclaimed for his contribution. The innovation caused a sensation in London, where noted English physician JOHN SNOW soon became established as the city's unofficial master of "ether practice."

Morton pursued studies in medicine and surgery at Harvard Medical School and at Washington University of Medicine (now the College of Physicians and Surgeons in Baltimore). Although he did not complete the curriculum, he was granted a degree in medicine *honoris causa* from Washington University in 1852.

While visiting New York City with his wife in 1868 Morton suffered an apoplectic fit during a carriage ride through Central Park, and he died later that afternoon at the age of 49. Massachussetts General Hospital memorialized the advent of "painless surgery" with the construction of an "Ether Dome" inscribed with Morton's name on a listing of fifty-three Massachussetts-born heroes of surgery. Morton is also among the five hundred illustrious men whose names are engraved on the facade of the Boston Public Library.

Paul Hermann Müller 1899–1965

Swiss chemist Paul Müller is credited with the discovery of dichloridiphenyltrichloroethane, a toxic insecticide more familiarly known as DDT. Educated at the University of Basel, Müller joined the staff at J.R. Geigy Co. in 1925, where he remained as a chemical researcher until his death in 1965.

Müller was assigned by his employer to develop an effective and economical substance that would kill insects on contact. Intended for the protection of crops as well as for prevention of insect-transmitted diseases, the pesticide was produced in 1939 and was soon widely distributed. During World War II DDT was successfully used to arrest a typhus epidemic in Naples, Italy.

For his discovery Müller was awarded the Nobel Prize for Physiology or Medicine in 1948. After twenty years of use on crops throughout the world, however, DDT was found to be acutely toxic not only to insects, but to plants, animals and humans. Inhalation or other means of ingestion can cause vomiting, convulsions, tremors and abnormalities of the heart, lungs and nervous system, ultimately leading to coma and death. Treatment may be achieved by irrigating the stomach, a procedure known as gastric lavage. DDT has been replaced with safer chemicals in many parts of the world, although not all countries have discontinued its use.

N

Daniel Nathans 1928–

In one of the earliest applications of biotechnology, American microbiologist Daniel Nathans identified the DNA structure of a virus by using endonucleases, the Type II "restriction enzymes" discovered by Nathans's colleague and fellow Nobel laureate HAMILTON SMITH.

Endonucleases are protein molecules that seek a particular sequence of nucleotides on a strand of DNA and break it apart at that point. Nathans followed this unique guide to the genetic code to derive a map of the DNA in simian virus 40—a virus known to produce cancerous tumors.

Using the endonuclease as a chemical scalpel, Nathans and Smith pioneered the techniques of "gene splicing" as they discovered ways to extract any given gene from a chromosome, splice it to another, and shuttle genetic material back and forth in various combinations. Nathans applied these principles in experiments on simian virus 40 in an effort to establish a molecular basis for cancer and a means of carving out the cancer-causing DNA molecules.

In 1978 Nathans, Smith and Swiss geneticist WERNER ARBER shared the Nobel Prize for Physiology or Medicine in recognition of their trail-blazing exploration of recombinant DNA technology.

Nathans was born and raised in Wilmington, Delaware, where he completed undergraduate studies in 1954 at the state university. After receiving his medical degree from Washington University in St. Louis, Missouri he embarked on his prize-winning genetic investigations at Johns Hopkins University in Baltimore. Appointed professor of microbiology in 1962, Nathans took over direction of the department ten years later and continues to investigate the genetic aspects of cancer and the various ways in which experimental science can exploit the remarkable properties of endonucleases.

Charles Jules Henri Nicolle 1866–1936

Charles Nicolle, a French physician and microbiologist, is best known for his discovery that typhus—an infection characterized by headache, chills, high fever and skin rashes—is transmitted by body lice. Historically the disease has been particularly threatening during wartime, when conditions are generally overcrowded and unsanitary. As a result of Nicolle's discovery in 1909, all army units in World War I included delousing as a regular part of military routine.

After studying under the great LOUIS PASTEUR Nicolle worked in Paris with another of Pasteur's protegés, bacteriologist P.P.E. Roux. In 1903 Nicolle left for North Africa to take charge of the Pasteur Institute in Tunis. In addition to his research on typhus Nicolle studied a number of other diseases, including trachoma, whooping cough and influenza. His work on measles produced the first immune sera for that disease.

Through experimental research on a wide variety of illnesses Nicolle demonstrated for the first time that individuals could carry and transmit diseases without exhibiting any symptoms. Under Nicolle's influence the Pasteur Institute in Tunis developed an international reputation as an important center for bacteriological research.

In 1928 Nicolle was awarded the Nobel Prize for Physiology or Medicine in recognition of his work on typhus. He remained in Tunis until 1932, returning to Paris to teach at the College de France for the last four years of his life.

Florence Nightingale 1820–1910

So dedicated was Florence Nightingale to the establishment of nursing as a dignified and respected profession that her name has become forever associated with her occupation. A legendary and heroic figure of her time, Florence Nightingale was dubbed "the Lady with the Lamp," referring to her tireless efforts to provide nursing care whenever and wherever it was needed.

When Florence Nightingale informed her family of her intention to become a nurse their reaction was one of horror and dismay. In the mid-nineteenth century nursing was considered a lowly profession, and the reputation of its practitioners was assumed to be at best dubious. In 1854 Florence Nightingale recorded in her diary the remarks of a head nurse at a London hospital who said "she had never known a nurse who was not drunken, and there was immoral conduct practiced in the very wards, of which she gave me some awful examples." With an almost fanatical dedication Florence Nightingale brought about widespread changes in nursing practices and training, establishing the modern standards of her profession.

Born in Florence, Italy to British parents, Nightingale and her family returned to England, where young Florence grew up in an atmosphere of luxury, with family homes in Derbyshire and New Forest and rooms in London's Mayfair for the social season. At an early age, however, Florence expressed her discomfort in this privileged environment. Later she wrote, "The thoughts and feelings that I have now...I can remember since I was six years old. A profession, a trade, a necessary occupation, something to fill and employ all my faculties, I have always felt essential to me, I have always longed for. The first thought I can remember, and the last, was nursing work..."

Florence's restlessness grew, and her desire to minister to the sick attained almost obsessive proportions. She secretly collected hospital reports, health pamphlets, medical treatises and any information available on hospitals in England and abroad. At seventeen her fervor took a different form when she began to hear the voice of God instructing her to devote her life to "divine" service.

Her commitment was strong enough to override her feelings of love for a young man who had asked her to marry him. "I have an intellectual nature which requires satisfaction," she wrote in her journal, "and that would find it in him. I have a passional nature which requires satisfaction, and that would find it in him. I have a moral, an active nature which requires satisfaction, and that would not find it in his life." She felt that marriage would force her "to be nailed to a continuation and exaggeration of my present life...to put it out of my power ever to be able to seize the chance of forming for myself a true and rich life."

Already concerned about their daughter's "unnatural" behavior, her parents were horrified at her decision to join the "vulgar" profession of nursing and tried in every way to prevent her from acting on it.

Florence Nightingale ultimately prevailed. After observing patient care practices in various hospitals in England and France, she spent three months at a nursing institution in Kaiserwerth, Germany, where she gained the foundation of her nursing training. She returned to London in 1853 to take over the supervision of a run-down and poorly managed nursing home on Harley Street. Under her tough-minded administration the institution was soon functioning smoothly.

In the fall of 1854, at the outbreak of the Crimean War, Nightingale began reading reports on the horrifying conditions in British military hospitals, where wounded soldiers lay on dirt floors, with cholera spreading through the wards like wildfire. Quickly organizing a unit of thirty-eight female nurses, Florence Nightingale set out for Scutari, a suburb of Constantinople, on the eastern banks of the Bosphorus. Arriving on November 4, 1854 with money and provisions, they were unprepared for the misery, confusion and neglect that awaited them. There were 10,000 soldiers in desperate need of medical care, living in filthy, unventilated, vermin-infested wards without food, water, clothing or beds. Florence Nightingale tackled the awesome task with characteristic devotion, seeing to it that these men were cared for as well as possible while raising money so that the hospital could function effectively.

A significant, if less concrete contribution to the wounded at Scutari was Florence Nightingale's profound sympathy for the suffering, combined with almost superhuman energy and courage. By the time she left for England in 1856 her heroism and devotion had become legendary. Upon her return she was met with public adulation and an expression of gratitude from Queen Victoria, who sent her a diamond brooch with the inscription "Blessed are the Merciful."

Florence Nightingale's work in Scutari served to elevate public opinion of both soldiers and nurses. She continued her crusade to reform and reorganize army medical services, producing a document of more than 1,000 pages entitled *Notes on Matters Affecting the Health, Efficiency and Hospital Administration of the British Army*.

A royal commission was established to investigate the problems described in her notes, and between 1859 and 1861 many of her recommended reforms were put into effect. These included remodeling many army hospitals to provide proper heat, lighting and ventilation. Hospital cooking facilities were overhauled, and for the first time attention was given to the personal and spiritual needs of the soldiers. An army medical school was created, and a military medical department was organized to formally acknowledge the army's responsibilities to its personnel.

In 1859 Nightingale published *Notes on Hospitals*, an authoritative study of hospital management and construction. The following year, with money raised by public subscription as a tribute to her achievement during the war, she opened the Nightingale Training School for Nurses at St. Thomas's Hospital. Recognized as a leading expert on nursing care, Florence Nightingale attracted scores of applicants, and soon other nursing schools were established in Britain and throughout the world.

Florence Nightingale's feverish intensity took its toll in her later life. Acknowledged internationally as the founder of modern nursing, she lived her last years in seclusion, gradually succumbing to senility. In 1907, three years before her death at the age of 90, she was awarded the Order of Merit. When the insignia was brought to her at her small London house on South Street, it is reported that she could only murmur, "Too kind...too kind."

Hideyo Noguchi 1876–1928

The bacteriologist Hideyo Noguchi, who died a martyr to science, had to his credit a long list of significant contributions to the study of infectious diseases.

He isolated the spirochete that causes syphilis and developed a reliable test for that disease. Noguchi also demonstrated that two deadly diseases ravaging Latin America, Oroya fever and *verruga peruana*, were different phases of a single fatal condition known as Carrion's disease. He identified both the organism that caused the multileveled disease and the agent of transmission, a female bloodsucking sandfly.

Investigating another bacteriological scourge known as kala-azar, or the "black fever," Noguchi tracked down the flagellate organism responsible. His studies also revealed the existence of a new genus of microorganisms, now called *Noguchia*. His technique for culturing a variety of pathogenic organisms provided a valuable tool for clinical and experimental research.

The heights attained by Noguchi were all the more extraordinary given the unfortunate circumstances of his childhood. He was born Seisaku Noguchi in the town of Oyajima in Northern Japan, where he grew up with his mother and older sister. (As a young man he changed his surname to Hideyo, meaning "great man of the world.") His father abandoned the family after Noguchi's birth, and the infant was left in his sister's care while their mother, Shika, worked in the rice paddies to support her family. At the age of three Hideyo was badly burned in an accident that permanently maimed his left hand.

At an early age Noguchi's intellectual gifts were apparent, and through his mother's perseverance and his own he managed to find benefactors to sponsor his education. In 1894 Noguchi was accepted by the Tokyo Medical College, and Shika had enrolled in a course in rural midwifery. Determined to leave the rice paddies, she became a competent practitioner.

In 1897, at the age of twenty-one, Noguchi received his doctorate in medicine. While working at Juntendo General Hospital he was introduced to SHIBASABURO KITASATO, the distinguished bacteriologist. Noguchi became his assistant at the Institute for Infectious Diseases, where he had the opportunity to meet an American medical luminary on a visit to Japan—the celebrated American microbiologist SIMON FLEXNER. Convinced that to achieve the success he desired he would have to leave Japan, he took a well-paid job at the quarantine office to improve his financial situation. Several months later he volunteered to join a Japanese medical expedition to China, where an outbreak of plague had been reported. Noguchi stayed there for several months, practicing as a physician until the xenophobic Boxer Rebellion forced his return to Japan.

In December of 1900 Noguchi arrived at the Philadelphia home of Simon Flexner, presuming on the basis of scant acquaintance and minimal encouragement to ask for a job. Somewhat taken aback, Flexner introduced Noguchi to Dr. SILAS WEIR MITCHELL, who needed assistance in his work on snake venom. Noguchi's tireless commitment and creative experimental skills won Mitchell's admiration. Within two years Noguchi published his first papers on the immunologic properties of snake venom. His scientific career finally launched, Noguchi began receiving offers for various research projects, including a Carnegie fellowship awarded in 1903 to study at Copenhagen's Staatens Serum Institute.

Returning to the States in 1904, Noguchi joined Flexner's staff at the newly established Rockefeller Institute for Medical Research in New York. After German microbiologist Fritz Schaudinn reported his discovery of the spirochete *Treponema pallidum* in 1905 Noguchi and Flexner demonstrated that this was the organism responsible for syphilis. Noguchi was to become a leading authority on the disease, publishing a great number of articles on the subject, as well as a book on the serology and diagnosis of syphilis. Noguchi's studies in this area led him to devise methods of culturing spirochetes so that experimental research need not rely on specimens in their wild state. From *Treponema pallidum* Noguchi drew a substance called luetin, which forms the basis of a diagnostic skin test for latent or congenital syphilis. He also succeeded in culturing the etiological agents of yaws and relapsing fever.

Noguchi's reputation in the scientific and medical community grew steadily at institutes and universities throughout the world. His crowning victory, he hoped, would be the discovery of the cause of yellow fever, which on seemingly good evidence, he thought to be a spiral-shaped bacterium known as a spirochete. (It was later shown to be a filterable virus.) While seeking to test his theory in Africa he became infected with yellow fever and died in Accra, Ghana, at the age of fifty-two.

O

Sir William Osler 1849–1919

Although born and educated in Canada, Sir William Osler is celebrated as one of the founding fathers of American medicine. Distinguished as a brilliant and highly principled physician, he contributed significant findings in clinical medicine but his greatest influence was in the development of medical education both in Europe and the United States. In 1893 he was recruited as head of the department of medicine at the newly founded Johns Hopkins Medical School in Baltimore, Maryland, joining with noted colleagues WILLIAM S. HALSTED, HOWARD A. KELLY and William H. Welch (1850–1934) to establish the institution as one of international reputation and authority.

Of the "Big Four," Osler was probably the most widely renowned, a larger-than-life medical hero who inspired countless careers through his innovative teaching methods and influential writings, including, most notably, *The Principles and Practice of Medicine*. Published in 1892, the text was to become a classic of modern medical literature. In addition to his extraordinary command of physiology, pathology, bacteriology, chemistry and pharmacology, Osler was also a leading authority on the history of medicine. He played a key role in focusing interest on the subject in the United States and wrote a number of important works, including *A Concise History of Medicine,* which was published in the last year of his life.

After graduating from McGill Medical School in 1872, Osler left Montreal to spend the next two years in Europe, observing clinics and hospitals in England, France and Germany. He returned to Canada to establish private practice but was soon invited by one of his former professors at McGill to join the faculty as lecturer in physiology and pathology.

Continuing to pursue clinical practice while developing his skills as an educator, he launched his techniques of bedside teaching in 1879 when he was appointed physician at Montreal General Hospital in 1879. Five years later he accepted the chair of clinical medicine at the University of Pennsylvania and in 1889 he moved to Baltimore to become chief of medicine at the new Johns Hopkins Hospital.

Osler was 44 years old when he greeted the first class at Hopkins Medical School in 1893. Rejecting what he called "that base and most pernicious system of educating them with a view to examinations," he launched a practical method of "learning by doing," in which students were taught to apply scientific knowledge to the care of living patients. The underlying principle of Osler's approach was summed up in the title of his address to the New York Academy of Medicine in 1903: "The Hospital as a College." Outlining the basic steps in the curriculum, he declared that "even the dullest learn how to examine patients, and get familiar with the changing aspects of important acute diseases. The pupil handles a sufficient number of cases to get a certain measure of technical skill, and there is ever kept before him the idea that he is not in the hospital to learn everything that is known, but to learn how to study disease and how to treat it, or rather how to treat patients."

More than a thousand students were trained at Hopkins during Osler's 12-year tenure but his influence among American physicians extended far beyond those "first-generation Oslerians" as they proudly called themselves. His revolutionary methods were adopted by institutions across the country to become a fundamental part of American medical education.

In 1905, at the age of 56, Osler left Johns Hopkins to become Regius Professor of Medicine at Oxford University in England. He was awarded a baronetcy at the coronation of George V in 1910 and resigned from teaching following the death of his son on the western front. Osler died in England in 1919.

P

George Emil Palade 1912–

For his landmark investigation of the structure of living cells George Emil Palade was awarded the 1974 Nobel Prize for Physiology or Medicine, which he shared with collaborators ALBERT CLAUDE and CHRISTIAN DE DUVE. Using the electron microscope Albert Claude had recently adapted for biological research, Palade significantly advanced scientific understanding of the structure and inner workings of a cell. He charted this tiny universe by first locating an organelle (an organized, membrane-bound substance present in all cukaryotic cells) with the microscope and then examining the centrifuged sediment to determine its chemical constituents.

Discovering a tiny organelle in the cell's cytoplasm, Palade identified the structure as a ribosome, establishing its function as "interpreter" of the chemical message encoded in the messenger RNA. As the cell's "protein factory," ribosomes play a major role in the most fundamental biological processes, assembling the appropriate protein molecule based on the DNA's genetic instructions. Elucidating the mechanism of protein synthesis, Palade took an important step toward understanding and treating degenerative disease.

Joining Claude at the Rockefeller Institute in 1946, Palade devised a number of techniques for specimen preparation, further developing Claude's application of the high-speed centrifuge in electron microscopy. Making possible a detailed biochemical analysis, these refinements were key to the discovery of many of the major cellular components.

A native of Jassi, Rumania, Palade received his medical degree in 1940 from the University of Bucharest. Inducted into the army immediately after graduation, he continued to conduct research at the university while on active military duty.

Palade was invited to serve as visiting professor and medical researcher at the Rockefeller Institute, where he worked for two years before returning to Rumania. After the communist takeover Palade emigrated to the United States, becoming a citizen in 1952. In 1946, at a New York University symposium, Palade introduced himself to Albert Claude, who was speaking on his innovations in the application of electron microscopy. Palade joined Claude's laboratory at Rockefeller University and, with Christian de Duve, launched a distinguished collaboration. Trained as physicians, all three scientists were dedicated to the medical application of their experimental findings.

In addition to the Nobel Prize Palade has been honored with numerous awards, most notably the prestigious Albert Lasker Basic Research Award in 1966 and the 1970 Louisa Gross Horowitz Prize of Columbia University, which he shared with Albert Claude and Keith A. Porter.

In 1972 Palade left Rockefeller University to serve as director of the Department of Cell Biology at Yale University's School of Medicine. He continues to conduct cellular research in partnership with his wife, cell biologist Marilyn Farquhar.

Daniel David Palmer 1845–1913

As founder of the Palmer School of Chiropractic, Daniel David Palmer introduced a new therapeutic discipline based on the theory that disease is caused by a disruption of the nervous system.

Born at Lake Scugog in Ontario, Canada, Palmer left home at the age of 16 to try his luck in the United States. While teaching school in Illinois and Iowa he became interested in "magnetic healing," a practice based on the belief in a "psychic energy" presumed to flow through the nervous system from the brain to all parts of the body. Seeking to formulate a general principle of disease, he investigated various methods of establishing a smooth and uninterrupted flow of energy as a means of restoring health.

Palmer established the fundamentals of chiropractic theory in 1895 following his experience in treating a case of deafness, for which he reportedly effected an instantaneous cure by repositioning one of the patient's vertebrae. Recalling the incident, Palmer wrote,

> I made inquiry as to the cause of his deafness and was informed that when he was exerting himself in a cramped, stooping position, he felt something give way in his back and immediately became deaf. An examination showed the vertebra racked from its normal position. I reasoned that if that vertebra were replaced the man's hearing should be restored.

Palmer developed a general theory and set of therapeutic procedures establishing the "science and art of Chiropractic." He derived the term (from the Greek words *kheir,* meaning "hand" or "manual care," and *praxis,* meaning "practice") to define a "system of manipulations which aims to cure diseases by mechanical restoration of displaced or sub-luxated bones, especially the vertebrae, to their normal relation" (see ANDREW TAYLOR STILL).

Palmer's lack of academic credentials, along with his seemingly outlandish techniques of spinal adjustment, gave rise to strong opposition from conventional medical practioners. Widely denounced by the establishment despite a growing number of followers, Palmer was arrested and imprisoned in Davenport, Iowa in 1914 for practicing medicine without a license. By then he had opened a school to spread his theory and technique. His teachings continued to gain adherents despite his jail sentence, and in the last years of his life Palmer lectured on chiropractic principles throughout the Midwest, eventually establishing the College of Chiropractic in Portland, Oregon in 1898. The original school in Davenport was taken over by his son Bartholomew, the offspring of Palmer's fifth and final marriage.

After his father's death Bartholomew Joshua Palmer became a leading exponent of chiropractic treatment, publishing *Textbook on the Technique of Palmer Chiropractic* in 1920. Through his efforts, along with subsequent refinements in the discipline, chiropractic gradually gained acceptance in many parts of the world. Although it remains a source of controversy in the medical establishment, the practice is now legally sanctioned in the United States and elsewhere, along with certified training programs. Modern chiropractors continue to perform hand manipulation and message to adjust the alignment of the spine and relieve nerve pressure, in addition to using more recent innovations such as therapy by heat, cold, light and electricity.

George Nicholas Papanicolaou 1883–1962

George Papanicolaou invented an invaluable tool in cancer detection known as the Pap smear.

When George Papanicolaou arrived in the United States from his native Greece he had already received an M.D. from the University of Athens and a Ph.D. from the University of Munich, and he had served as a medical officer in the Greek army; but he had to begin life over again in America as a salesman. He soon changed jobs to become an anatomical assistant at Cornell Medical College in 1924, where he worked his way up to a full professorship.

At Cornell Papanicolaou began studying the menstrual cycle in animals and incorporated into his research the science of exfoliative cytology (the study of cast-off cells). In 1927, while investigating the reproductive cycle by using vaginal smears obtained from human and animal subjects, he recognized the presence of cancer cells. This discovery led Papanicolaou to develop his famous test. A scraping, or smear, is taken from a woman's cervix or vagina and examined under a microscope. Cells may appear as normal, cancerous or suspicious, indicating either malignancy or some other abnormal condition or infection. This technique is also used to detect cancer of other tissues, most commonly in the bladder. Due in part to Papanicolaou's significant findings, exfoliative cytology came into use as a valuable tool in the study of all hollow organs and secreted fluids.

Papanicolaou devoted much of the remainder of his life to campaigning for widespread use of the Pap smear as a simple, painless and effective means of early cancer detection. The procedure is now fully accepted by the medical community, although much attention has lately been given to improving techniques of interpretation.

Paracelsus (Theophrastus Bombastus von Hohenheim) 1493–1541

Paracelsus was an alchemist and medical practitioner of the Renaissance whose legendary career was one of frenzied passion and garrulous exploits. Challenging two thousand years of medical orthodoxy, he gave himself the name Paracelsus as a permanent advertisement of his claim to medical wisdom "beyond CELSUS," the celebrated Roman physician of the first century. Though he fiercely condemned the dogma of others, Paracelsus declared with equal fervor the infallibility of his own teachings and vaunted himself as a second HIPPOCRATES.

Rejecting the long-accepted precepts of herbalism, astrology, superstition and the doctrine of humours, he argued that disease was not a punishment for sin but rather the result of natural causes. "Study nature, not books," Paracelsus advised his students at the University of Basel, where his first act as a member of the faculty was to wage a ceremonial book-burning of the works of GALEN and AVICENNA.

He spent most of his life roaming around Europe in search of knowledge and claimed to have learned more from "old wives, gypsies, sorcerers, and wandering tribes" than from the "high asses at the high colleges." "In order to understand the wonders of nature," he wrote, "I went not only to the doctors, but also to the barbers, bathkeepers, executioners, learned physicians, women, and magicians who pursue the art of healing; I went to alchemists, to monasteries, to nobles and common folk, to the experts and the simple."

Born as Philippus Aureolus Theophrastus Bombast von Hohenheim, he grew up in Einsiedein, a village in what was then Germany but is now central Switzerland. Though his original name was abandoned, a family tie remains in the eponym bombastic, an etymological allusion to one of his more notable characteristics.

It is unlikely that Paracelsus inherited his rambunctions spirit from his father, a modest country physician and chemist who also traveled throughout southern Austria and Germany to teach alchemy to the miners and farmers of that area. Father and son were opposites in temperament, but they shared a passion for knowledge, and it was from his father that Paracelsus gained his introduction to science and medicine.

Restless for new experiences, Paracelsus left home at fourteen and set off on a lusty survey of life that would lead him from the towers of erudition and scholarship to seedy beer halls and back-street haunts all across the continent. He studied at universities of world renown, consulted with alchemists, physicians and pharmacologists, practiced as an army surgeon in Italy, escaped from prison in Russia and spent countless nights in drunken revelry as he crisscrossed the map from Dublin to Vienna to Constantinople and back for more than twenty years.

He accepted a teaching position at the University of Basel in 1527, and it was not long before the faculty and the administration were scandalized. Not only did he conduct his lectures in German, rather than the customary Latin, but he dared to invite the public to attend. Far more disturbing, however, were the teachings themselves, which promptly brought charges of heresy.

The world is composed essentially of mercury, sulphur and salt, claimed Paracelsus, and ruled by a single divine order. As elements of a fully spiritual universe, the movements of the stars, the properties of metals, the action of fire and the functions of the human body all follow an inner harmonic progression and are thus replications of the cosmos.

In accordance with the notion of microcosms and macrocosms, Paracelsus claimed that for every disease there was a specific remedy. As a further elaboration of the "theory of specifics" he developed the "doctrine of signatures," which states that the remedy for a particular condition is found in a plant that imitates the "look" of the disease (e.g., yellow flowers for jaundice).

Paracelsus explored natural correspondences and diversity in a wide range of environments and biological phenomena, with particular attention to the properties of various plants and minerals. Merging ancient principles of folk medicine with a modern experimental approach, he introduced into his practice and pharmacopoeia a number of organic and inorganic substances, including sulphur, iron, lead, arsenic, laudanum (from opium) and antimony (under the name stibium).

Paracelsus's most notable contributions to medicine include the first clinical investigation of syphilis, in which he presented not only a description of the symptoms and progressive stages of the disease and its transmission to infants, but his prescription of mercury as a treatment, in a sequence of graduated dosages. Other distinguished studies include his identification of silicosis and tuberculosis as occupational diseases of miners resulting from the inhalation of toxic substances. He also sought to establish a medical basis for various neurological and psychological disorders and associated the conditions of cretinism and goiter.

As a dedicated iconoclast and outspoken adversary of dogma, Paracelsus was not destined for success in an academic career. His relentless campaign against the establishment enraged his colleagues and caused even greater indignation among the physicians and apothecaries of Basel. As the public began to challenge the absolute authority of practitioners Paracelsus became the target of death threats from the medical community. After less than a year he made his escape in the dead of night and fled the country.

Resuming a peripatetic life, Paracelsus concentrated his efforts on writing while he roved around Europe for the next eight years. In 1536 he published *Die Grosse Wunderarztney (The Wonders of Medicine)*, a treatise on surgery that includes a notable passage on unnecessary surgical intervention. A wound will heal itself, he advised, provided that the practitioner limits his activities to the prevention of infection.

The critical success of his book brought Paracelsus back into public life, and in the next five years he amassed a considerable fortune as one of the leading physicians of his day. At the age of 48 Paracelsus was found dead in a Salzburg tavern under mysterious circumstances.

Ambroise Paré c. 1510–1590

> Five things are proper to the duty of a surgeon: to take away that which is superfluous; to restore to their places such things as are displaced; to separate those things which are joined together; to join those things which are separated; and to supply the defects of nature. Thou shalt far more easily and happily attain to the knowledge of these things by long use and much exercise, than by much reading of books or daily hearing of teachers.

So asserted Ambroise Paré in stating the code of the barber-surgeon. Although Paré was the foremost surgeon of sixteenth-century France, he was accepted and licensed by the elite community of academic surgeons only after he had been practicing for almost thirty years.

However, formal titles, as well as religious or political loyalties, meant little to Paré, who was dedicated to the refinement and improvement of surgical practice. Throughout his influential and innovative career Paré emphasized humanity in the practice of his art, with particular attention to sensible pre- and postoperative care. He recognized the physical toll of surgery on the patient, recommending rest and proper nourishment, and always emphasizing the importance of hygiene. During wartime Paré was said to have convinced the prostitutes who followed the soldiers to the battlefields to help wash linen and bandages for the wounded.

Among Paré's most significant contributions to the advancement of surgical method was his repudiation of the practice of pouring boiling oil on an open wound as a means of cauterizing it. In place of this ineffective and agonizing procedure he reintroduced the use of stitches; combined with salves of his own concoction, to aid in healing.

His patients benefited from a number of curious techniques or appliances either devised by Paré himself or rediscovered in his reading of ancient medical texts. He constructed trusses for his hernia patients and used ingenious prostheses, including artificial hands and noses. He created a sling designed to support a particularly unwieldy pregnancy and demonstrated the technique of inducing labor as a means of stopping the profuse bleeding of a woman in childbirth.

Born and raised on the outskirts of Laval, in northern France, Paré got his introduction to the field of surgery as an apprentice to a barber, a position held by his father and two of his brothers. In Paré's time a barber was considered the lowest form of medical practitioner, responsible for pulling teeth, applying poultices and dressing wounds in addition to the nonmedical chores of shaving whiskers, cutting hair and curling wigs. To attain the status of master barber-surgeon several years of apprenticeship were required, followed by the completion of a difficult examination.

At 23 Paré left Laval to complete his apprenticeship at the Hôtel-Dieu, a historic hospital in the heart of Paris. As a *compagnon chirurgien*—the equivalent of a modern-day surgical resident—Paré worked under the guidance of Jacques Dubois, the distinguished anatomist known by the pseudonym Sylvius. During his residency Paré encountered daily a vast array of medical conditions and procedures, which he later described as the foundation of his education.

His education was enhanced in 1537, when he was appointed a military surgeon during the French army's campaign to take Turin. Paré's horrifying introduction to battlefield medicine inspired him to develop techniques and tools to better attend to the terrible requirements of the wounded.

Discrediting the application of boiling oil as a method of cauterizing open wounds, Paré developed soothing *digestives*, or balms, used to quell swellings and infections. He learned to stop a hemmorhage by stitching blood vessels and discovered that the best technique for removing projectiles from the body was to place the patient in the position he was in when he was shot, which limited further damage by allowing the surgeon to retrace the path of entry.

He also developed a technique of amputation that sacrificed as little as possible of healthy tissue while providing for a proper course of healing, stressing, as always, the maintenance of sanitary conditions before, during and after the operation. Not only was Paré well paid for his wartime service, but he also gained a distinguished reputation for his skillful and innovative surgical technique.

Licensed as a master barber-surgeon, Paré settled in an apartment on the Left Bank of Paris, established a successful practice and married Jehanne Mazelin, who bore his first son in 1845. Paré was to serve as surgeon on a number of military campaigns, and between battles he published his first book, entitled *The Method of Treating Lesions Made by Arquebuses and Other Firearms: as Well as Those Which Are Made by Arrows, Darts and the Like: also Burns Caused Especially by Cannon Powder*. His second publication, *A Brief Compilation Concerning Anatomic Management with the Technique of Joining Bones*, further enhanced Paré's growing prestige at home and on the battlefield.

While officially still no more than a master barber-surgeon, Paré, at the age of 44, was formally appointed surgeon-in-ordinary to King Henry II. Influenced by the sign of royal favor for Paré, the confraternity of academic surgeons grudgingly granted him certification as a licensed surgeon. Henry II was the first of five kings to retain Paré's medical services, although his service in the court of Charles IX was short-lived due to the king's premature death at 24. "Dead from too hard blowing of his horn out hunting" was Paré's wry comment after completing the autopsy.

After his death of his wife, Paré, at 64, was left with Catherine, the couple's only surving child. Within several months he married Jacqueline Rousselet, who was to bear him six more children. Having previously produced a number of respected written works, including his *Ten Bookes of Surgery with a Collection of Necessary Instruments* and *Essay on Plague*, Paré, in 1575, published a 945-page edition of collected writings including discussions on obstetrics, the removal of cataracts, the use and fitting of prosthetic devices and surgical practice on and off the battlefield.

Paré's work questioned the value of a number of nostrums frequently prescribed by physicians of the day. On the subject of treating bruises with scrapings taken from Egyptian mummies Paré declared that "the ancient Jews, Egyptians, and Chaldees never dreamed of embalming their dead to be eaten by Christians."

Although sanctioned by the king, Paré's edition of collected works, written in "vulgar French" instead of Latin, enraged the academic medical establishment, who tried in vain to stop publication. Paré put together a second edition in 1578 and held off publication for more than a year before finally receiving the reluctant approval of the Council of the Faculty of Physicians. When it was finally published, Paré's work was an enormous success. It was translated into Latin, and later into Dutch, German and English.

Although Paré has often been called the father of modern surgery, he modestly summed up his own career in the words *"Je le pansait; Dieu le guarit"* (I treated him; God healed him).

William Hallock Park 1863–1939

William Park and his colleague Dr. Anna Williams developed a serum derived from horse antitoxin that provided the first effective treatment for diphtheria.

Diphtheria is an acute contagious infection caused by *Corynebacterium diphtheriae*, which produce a toxin that passes into the bloodstream and affects the heart and nervous system. Most commonly found in children, the disease was once epidemic in many parts of the world, and in 1895 the mortality rate was higher than 50%. Within five years Park's antitoxin serum reduced the figure to 12%, and subsequent advances in methods of treatment and prevention have virtually eliminated the disease as a major threat.

Born in New York City, Park graduated from City College in 1883, receiving his degree in medicine three years later from the Columbia College of Physicians and Surgeons. After pursuing advanced training in bacteriology at the University of Vienna he returned to New York in 1890 to establish a general practice. Appointed director of the Bureau of Laboratories at the New York Health Department in 1893, Park earned the respect of his medical colleagues, the general public and government officials. He organized the first municipal health laboratory and directed extensive research on the control and prevention of tuberculosis, typhoid, influenza, scarlet fever, measles, pneumonia and polio. In 1911 Park introduced a system of milk purification that dramatically reduced the incidence of tuberculosis.

When he was due for retirement from public service New York's five country medical societies sent a petition to Mayor O'Brien urging that Park be allowed to retain his office. The mayor obliged, and a *New York Times* editorial enthusiastically supported the his decision, declaring that

> Dr. Osler himself would not doubt have urged that Dr. William Park be kept in the service of the Health Department despite his 70 years. There must be thousands upon thousands in this city and in other parts of America who are, many of them unconsciously, in his debt for being themselves alive. It is authoritatively stated that he has contributed more than any other living man to the development of bacteriological diagnosis and serum treatment which has made possible the conquest of diphtheria.

In addition to his duties at the Bureau of Laboratories Park taught bacteriology, hygiene and preventive medicine at New York University and Bellevue Hospital Medical College for more than forty years. In 1914 he was appointed consulting bacteriologist for the state department of health, and he later served as medical examiner in bacteriology and consulting bacteriologist for the United States Quarantine Service. Internationally acclaimed for his contribution to the advancement of public health, Park was granted honorary degrees from institutions throughout the world and was admitted as a member of the French Academy of Medicine in 1924. New York University paid him tribute in 1928 as "defender alike of the homes of the rich and the poor, a happy warrior against the battle lines of disease."

Considered one of the century's leading authorities on public health, Park served as vice president of the New York Academy of Medicine and president of both the Society of Experimental Pathologists and the American Public Health Association.

On the fiftieth anniversary of his graduation the College of the City of New York awarded Park the Townsend Harris Medal on November 18, 1933. Park's notable published writings include *Public Health and Hygiene* (2nd edition 1927) and *Who's Who among the Microbes* (1929).

Louis Pasteur 1822–1895

Universally acclaimed in his own time and ever since as one of the truly monumental figures in chemistry and microbiology, Louis Pasteur was a master of scientific theory and its application to down-to-earth problems concerning the health of people, animals and industries.

In brilliantly devised experiments he showed that microorganisms were responsible for fermentation and for many diseases. He developed a vaccine against rabies, which had been considered inevitably fatal, and for animals he offered similar protection from anthrax and chicken cholera.

He also saved the wine and silk industries of France and made it possible for British brewers to send their beer around Africa to the outposts of empire in India. He developed the process of using heat to kill pathenogenic bacteria in milk or other substances, a technique known the world over as "pasteurization."

His earliest crystallographic research, however, dealt in fundamental molecular physics. The first controversy in his career came in response to his decisive refutation of the ancient but persistent notion of "spontaneous generation," according to which bacteria and other microorganisms were thought to originate in inorganic life. Life, Pasteur demonstrated, can only arise from life.

Tanning was the family profession of the Pasteurs. Louis, born in Dôle in the Jura Mountains of eastern France, was the only son of Jean Joseph Pasteur, a sergeant in Napoleon's army who went back to tanning after his emperor was exiled. Though Louis's great-grandfather had been an indentured laborer, the family had risen to a moderate prosperity by the time Louis was born. Accordingly, he was sent to a succession of adequate but not aristocratic schools. As the only son among three daughters he was much favored. One sister, who was diagnosed as suffering from "cerebral fever" at the age of three, was raised in a convent. The other two joined their parents in lifelong adoring support of their brother.

Louis was an average student in his early days when he attended primary school in Arbois, not far from Dôle, where the family had moved. A career in art was his primary ambition between the ages of 13 and 18. He painted portraits of his family and the people of Arbois not only with enthusiasm but with considerable skill. His interest in science became apparent in his secondary school days at the Royal College of Besançon, where he was given the equivalent of a modern degree of bachelor of science in 1842.

In that year he qualified for admission to the science section of the École Normale Supérieure in Paris but ranked sixteenth in the freshman class, which he regarded as so humiliating that he postponed entry until the following year, by which time he had achieved a more respectable standing of fifth in the class. Two years later, in 1845, he was awarded a master's degree, and he was graduated in 1847 with a doctorate. "Will make an excellent professor" was the curt prediction noted on his records.

On May 22, 1848, at the age of 26, Pasteur presented a paper to the Paris Academy of Sciences outlining the results of his crystallographic research revealing that certain substances may divide into two components—their atomic arrangements being reverse images of each other, as in a mirror. Though otherwise identical, he revealed, they have very different properties. The contribution won the first accolades for the young scientist, but his celebration that year was muted by the death of his mother.

His career as an educator was launched with an appointment as physics professor at a lycee in Dijon, where he taught for barely a year before being appointed chemistry professor at the University of Strasbourg. An intense and somewhat humorless young man, Pasteur announced to his father that he would like one of his sisters to come and preside over his household, since he had no plans to marry for a very long time. Those plans changed abruptly when, several weeks after he met Marie Laurent, daughter of the rector of the university, he asked her to marry him.

In love as in science he was ardent. To Marie he wrote: "I have not cried so much since the death of my dear mother. I woke up suddenly with the thought that you did not love me and immediately started to cry."

The marriage—which was to be also a collaboration, since Marie took an active interest in Louis's scientific projects—was to be lifelong and produce five children, of whom three died before the age of 12. A daughter and a son survived.

Though Pasteur's greatest accomplishments were not as an educator, he nevertheless showed himself remarkably innovative when he served as dean of the newly created science faculty at the University of Lille. It was then that he saw clearly the close links between academia and industry. He made his classes tour factories to investigate the applications of science and, conversely, organized evening classes for young working men in the city.

His fermentation studies, which he began at Strasbourg when an industrialist queried him about the production of alcohol from grain and beet sugar, were continued when in 1857 he accepted the post of Director of Scientific Studies at the École Normale Supérieure in Paris. Establishing the fact that yeast is an organism capable of reproducing itself even in vitro, he went on to demonstrate that fermentation is the work of microorganisms. In his experiments he showed that sweet milk could be soured by the injection of organisms but kept in its pristine state if sealed against such contamination.

His swift rise to celebrity status brought his election to the Paris Academy of Sciences in 1862, and in the following year an offer to chair a newly created department at the École des Beaux Arts designed to teach the applicability of science to the fine arts. Administrative chores connected with that post diverted him too much from his experimental studies, however, and with the backing of Emperor Napoleon III a special laboratory was devised for him at the Beaux Arts, and he was relieved from school business to follow his predilections.

In a remarkable series of experiments he proved conclusively that bacteria are not generated spontaneously but derive from other bacteria. He then proceeded to develop the technique of destroying these contaminants by heat—the essence of "pasteurization," which he applied to the preservation of vinegar, wine and, some years later, beer. The last was in response to a request from British breweries that had desparied of supplying their product to Englishmen holding down the far- flung imperial frontier.

He saved another industry from desolation when silk production was threatened by a baffling epidemic that was wiping out silkworms. In 1865 he was asked by the government to investigate. For four years he worked, with only occasional breaks, until in 1869 he announced to an increasingly worried nation that he had isolated the bacilli responsible for the two diseases that were plaguing the worms, and that he had discovered how to detect the maladies and halt their spread.

He had worked on the silkworm under exhausting pressure compounded by the deaths of two of his daughters and of his father. During the final stages he himself suffered a devastating form of paralysis that deprived him forever of the use of his left hand.

His management of the silkworm epidemic had set him on the path of inquiry into infectious diseases, which led ultimately to his development of an attenuated vaccine against anthrax in cattle, chicken cholera and finally rabies. He had demonstrated that rabies was an acute viral infection of the cerebrospinal system and had immunized dogs by an injection of an attenuated preparation of the crushed spinal cords of rabid rabbits, but he hesitated to try it on humans until July 6, 1885, when a nine-year-old boy was brought to his door, apparently doomed because he had been bitten by a rabid dog two days before. Daily inoculations of Pasteur's preparation saved the boy, and the world rejoiced.

Louis Pasteur had been honored by universities, industrialists, royalty and republics. He had been made a member of the Académie Française and was appointed to the faculty of the Sorbonne. His last triumph brought not only fresh honors but the promise of an institute, funds for which were to be raised by popular subscription. It would be devoted to the treatment of rabies and the study of other microbiological diseases.

When the Pasteur Institute was opened by the president of the French republic in November 1888, Pasteur was so moved that his son had to read his speech. He and his wife moved into an apartment in the institute, where Pasteur lived for another seven years until his death on September 28, 1895. He is buried in a chapel in the Paris Institute, but his actual monument is considered to be the 60 Pasteur Institutes around the world, which constitute one of the world's great scientific resources.

Linus Pauling 1901–

The American physical chemist Linus Pauling has delineated ways in which molecules and atoms bond together, a momentous contribution which, in 1954, won him the first of his two nobel Prizes. The second—a Peace Prize—was awarded in 1963 for his work in bringing about an international ban on the atmospheric testing of nuclear weapons. In neither instance did he have to acknowledge a partner in his prize-winning accomplishment, a rarity among Nobel Laureates, though he frequently credited as a collaborator his wife, Ava Helen Miller Pauling.

Pauling threw new light on the mystery of protein structure, determined the effects on hemoglobin wrought by the gene for sickle cell anemia and modified the prevailing theory of anesthesia. His work is regarded as a milestone on the way to the discovery of the double helix of DNA (deoxyribonucleic acid), the sequence within the cell nucleus that determies an individual's heredity.

Pauling's early preoccupation with chemistry was evident in some of his favorite reading matter found in his father's drug store in Portland, Oregon. After he absorbed, at the age of nine, the *United States Pharmacopeia* and the *Dispensatory of the United States of America*, his father wrote an anguished letter to the editor of the *Portland Oregonian:* "My son has read all the books in sight and is demanding more. Would you please suggest some appropriate titles that would be best for him?"

His father died shortly after writing that letter at the age of 33, leaving his widow to raise Linus and two younger sisters. Before he was 16 he had graduated from high school and entered Oregon State Agricultural College (since renamed Oregon State University.) He earned his way by chopping wood, working in the school's kitchen and, in the summer, assuming the job of paving inspector for the state's roads. In addition to a precocious familiarity with the sciences, Pauling had in his high school years acquired a working knowledge of Latin, Greek and, according to some biographers, Chinese.

When World War I drained the college faculty Pauling, as the school's star student, was asked to serve as a chemistry teacher, even though he had just entered his junior year. Most of his students, sophomores, were older than he was. Free to take whatever course he wished, and to use the college laboratories and library, Pauling educated himself far beyond the confines of the curriculum.

It was then that he began to explore the chemical means by which atoms are joined to other atoms. Years later he wrote, "I was simply entranced by chemical phenomena, by the reactions in which substances disappear, and other substances, often with strikingly different properties, appear: and I hoped to learn more and more about this aspect of the world. It has turned out in fact, that I have worked on this problem year after year."

In his senior year he taught second-year chemistry to a class of women, among whom was Ava Helen Miller, the woman he was to later marry. He subsequently recalled that their courtship began with a discussion on ammonium hydroxide. After being graduated from the college in 1922 at the age of 21 Pauling undertook two years of doctoral studies at the California Institute of Technology in Pasadena. During that time he published five papers on the molecular structure of crystals, continued to spend his summers inspecting roads and entered a 58-year marriage with Ava that ended only with her death in 1982.

After winning his doctorate *cum laude* he continued his research at the university until, in 1925—a year already made memorable by the birth of his first child—he was granted a Guggenheim fellowship to learn what European laboratories were doing in the field of molecular structure. When he returned a little over two years later he became the youngest member of the Cal Tech faculty. As a 26-year-old he relied on a beard to lend him the dignity befitting an assistant professor.

When physicist J. Robert Oppenheimer gave Pauling his collection of rock speimens the gift might have turned him toward a career in mineralogy, but the Geological Society of America rejected his request for $4,800 to buy equipment. The Rockefeller Foundation offered more inviting prospects in biochemistry.

In December 1930 the long years of thinking about the nature of the atomic bond culminated in what seemed a flash of inspiration. "I worked at my desk nearly all that night. I was so full of excitement I could hardly write," he told Horace Freeland Judson, author of *The Eighth Day of Creation*. Essentially his theory ascribed the chemical bond to the spread of an electron's charge around the atom allowing the electron to function in two atoms simultaneously—a phenomenon Pauling labeled "resonance." As developed in a series of papers—later combined into a celebrated text, *The Nature of the Chemical Bond and Structure of Molecules and Crystals*—the concept has profoundly affected subsequent work in molecular reactions, whether by biologists, physicists or mineralogists.

In the thirties, while the arrival of three more children made for a satisfying but apparently not distracting family life, Pauling explored molecular structures in living organisms, particularly proteins, amino acids and peptides. After the outbreak of World War II, while serving as head of Cal Tech's Division of Chemistry and Chemical Engineering, he supervised some 20 projects for the military, ranging from efforts to devise blood substitutes for battlefield use to the development of new explosives. He was so busy, in fact, that he had to turn down an invitation from J. Robert Oppenheimer to join the team at Los Alamos that was developing the atomic bomb.

He did not oppose the bomb's development until the full extent of its power was revealed at Hiroshima and Nagasaki in 145. 1945. The prospect of nuclear annihilation preoccupied Ava and Linus Pauling in the postwar years, driving them to oppose any course that threatened war or attempted to mute the efforts of peace groups. As a member of the board of trustees of the Emergency Committee of Atomic Scientists, he was a target of congressional committees seeking to identify peace activists as communists. The award of the Presidential Medal of Merit conferred no immunity on Pauling. In refuting charges that he followed a sinister political path, he told investigators, "Nobody tells me what to think—except Mrs. Pauling."

Despite his tireless campaigns for peace, his scientific work did not slacken in the tempestuous postwar period. He and his team demonstrated conclusively that patients whose chromosomes carried the gene for sickle cell anemia could not make normal hemoglobin. He also clarified the phenomenon of anesthesia, refuting the notion that it was due to the interaction of an anesthetic with lipids. He described the effects of anesthesia on protein molecules and crystalline structures as well.

Those were the years when the world stood on the brink of breaking the genetic code. Efforts were underway in England, and Pauling himself had embarked on a road that might have led him to the double helix of DNA if the politics of the fifties had not intervened. A series of lectures he delivered at Cal Tech in 1951 on the helical structure of polypeptides reportedly influenced many investigators, notably JAMES DEWEY WATSON, one of those who finally described the famous double helix.

In 1952 Pauling was denied a passport when he was invited by the Royal Society of London to attend a conference on proteins structure. In response Pauling summoned his own conference on protein, which was attended by some of the world's most prominent scientists as a tribute to him and a tacit rebuke to those who sought to isolate him. In 1953 he was allowed to go to Israel to ceremonially lay the cornerstone of the Weizmann Institute, but all other invitations, including one from Prime Minister Nehru of India, had to be declined.

Pauling and an associate, Robert Corey, published a paper outlining a theoretical structure for DNA, but, based to some extent on the limited and often faulty data available in the United States, their findings were fatally flawed. The travel ban held until 1954, when Pauling was called to Stockholm to receive the Nobel Prize for Physiology or Medicine in recognition of his work on the chemical bond.

Pauling and his wife continued to campaign for an end to nuclear testing above ground, but the political atmosphere in the country had changed dramatically. On at least one occasion he picketed the White House in the afternoon and was welcomed to the executive mansion that evening by President John F. Kennedy. Though he continued to serve as professor, Pauling gave up his post as department chairman at Cal Tech to devote more time to his peace efforts. He wrote *No More War*, a plea for an end to the nuclear arms race.

On October 10, 1963, the day chosen for the signing of a treaty by the United States, the Soviet Union and Great Britain banning all nuclear tests above ground, the Nobel Committee announced the award of its Peace Prize to Linus Pauling for his efforts to bring about such a ban.

Awards, honorary degrees and medals were showered on Pauling, most of them for his scientific achievements, but many also for his peace efforts. In 1964 he relinquished his faculty post at Cal Tech to assume a research professorship at the Center for the Study of Democratic Institutions at Santa Barbara. Later accepted faculty positions at the University of California in San Diego and at Standford Stanford University.

In 1969 he established the Linus Pauling Institute of Science and Medicine in Palo Alto,primarily to explore the possibilities of ascorbic acid—vitamin C—as therapy not only for the common cold, but for cancer and mental illness as well. Although many scientists are as yet unconvinced by the evidence for such therapies, they tend to hedge all comments on what may yet be achieved by their maverick colleague as he and the century enter their nineties.

Ivan Petrovich Pavlov 1849–1936

The name of Ivan Petrovich Pavlov is inevitably associated with the image of dogs salivating in response to the tinkling of a bell—that dramatic example of the "conditioned reflex" by which a bell, or any other contrived stimulus, may be so associated with a natural one that it produces the same biological effects. However, the great Russian physiologist had been awarded the Nobel Prize long before he so memorably demonstrated the conditioned reflex.

It was his discovery of the highly specific and subtle responses of the digestive system that in 1904 made him the first physiologist to become a Nobel laureate at the age of 55.

Even before his work on the mechanism of digestion Pavlov had won fame—within Russia, at least—for determining the role of the vagus nerve in controlling blood pressure and heart rate. (That accomplishment might have been given worldwide acclaim if an English team had not reported similar findings a few years earlier, though the news had not yet reached Russia.) Pavlov went on to demonstrate other important vascular effects produced by nerves.

Ivan Pavlov was the firstborn child of a priest in the village of Ryazan, about 100 miles southeast of Moscow. When he was not officiating in church Ivan's father worked in the fields like his parishioners. His uncle was also a priest (though he was demoted to sexton after he acquired local fame as a prizefighter). Ivan, too, would undergo training at a seminary, but science came to outshine theology in his eyes. Ten children followed Ivan in the Pavlov family, but only five survived into adulthood. Ivan and the brother closest to him in age, Dmitri, became close friends and classmates.

They were in the same class because Ivan, at the age of nine, had fallen off a wall onto a tile floor, landing on his head. He was nursed back to health at a monastery in which his godfather was the abbot, but his two-year convalescence set back his schooling. Together he and his younger brother went from the seminary to the University of St. Petersburg, where they shared a cold and squalid flat.

In his third year at the university Pavlov was much impressed by his physiology professor, the distinguished Elie Tsyon, who was the first to interest him in the problems of digestive innervation. The faculty of the Military Medical Academy elected Tsyon a professor of physiology, and Tyson promptly appointed Pavlov as his assistant; but the bright prospects of teacher-student collaboration were dashed when politicians insisted on the dismissal of Tsyon from a post considered too lofty for a Jew.

Tsyon's successor offered to keep Pavlov on as an assistant, but the indignant young man refused to work for anyone who would profit from such an outrage. Pavlov's resignation, accomplished with a flourish that gave it considerable notoriety, reduced Ivan and Dmitri to a very skimpy standard of living for their three remaining years at the academy.

In 1870 Pavlov passed the examinations that qualified him as a physician, but, since medical practice had never figured in his ambitions, he accepted a fellowship offering two years of graduate study. His doctoral thesis, which used as a starting point Elie Tsyon's work on neural control of cardiac rythms, demonstrated other effects of nerves on the heart, and particularly the influence of the vagus nerve on blood pressure.

The thesis won him a grant to undertake two years of study abroad. He had in the meantime married Serafima Vasilievna Karchevskaya, a bright and attractive student of pedagogy. Romantic, impractical and impecunious, Ivan Pavlov seemed temperamentally unsuited to a serene marriage. Serafima, exhausted by the strains of life on the edge of poverty, endured first a miscarriage and then the death in infancy of their first child. A son, Vsevelod, did grow to maturity, but he died of cancer.

On his return from strenuous research, mainly in Leipzig, Pavlov joyfully accepted a job that offered a very small salary but—more important to him—an excellent laboratory. It was there that he devised his ingenious experiments that, in effect, gave a dog two stomachs, one in which the animal would digest food in the normal way, the other in which no food would enter but where gastric juices flowing normally in response to smell and taste could be observed in minute detail.

The same type of biological redesign opened the gullet to in vivo study. Pavlov, noting that his laboratory animals cooperated "with real gusto," summed up his work: "Thanks to our present surgical methods in physiology, we can demonstrate at any time almost all phenomena of digestion without the loss of a single drop of blood, without a single scream from the animal undergoing the experiment."

Pavlov disproved the older concepts of digestion, which described the process as purely mechanical—resembling the opening of a trap door through which food is dropped to be acted upon by automatically released digestive agents. Instead, according to Pavlov, "Food excites the gustatory apparatus; the excitation is transmitted by the gustatory nerves to the medulla from which it is conducted by the vagus nerves to the gastric glands; in other words, a reflex is produced which travels from the oral cavity to the gastric glands."

The acclaim of scientists around the world for this revision of conventional thinking finally brought some security to the Pavlov family. In 1888 the Military Medical Academy granted Ivan Pavlov a full professorship, albeit in pharmacology rather than physiology, and he was subsequently appointed director of a newly founded, well-equipped animal hospital. In 1890 he published a work that summed up 15 years of experimentation. Under the title *Lectures on the Work of the Digestive Gland,* it soon became a classic of medical literature and assured Pavlov's position in Russian academia. In 1904 his efforts were crowned with the Nobel Prize for Physiology or Medicine.

His next objective followed naturally from his achievement in demonstrating that stomach reflexes responded to taste and smell. He proposed to explore the connections between digestive processes and brain activity. The connection at first seemed obvious. The smell of meat made dogs slaver, the mouths of humans watered at the suggestion of pickles and the French physiologist CLAUDE BERNARD had noted that even the sight of a bale of hay stirred a horse's gastric secretions.

Pavlov established his dogs in soundproof chambers and showed that by associating mouth-watering stimuli with specific sounds or sights, his subjects could be conditioned to respond to the substitute as to the original stimulus. He noted the precision with which his dogs could distinguish among the stimuli to which they could be conditioned. For example, dogs would salivate at a sound of 1000 cycles per second but not at 1010 cycles. They could be conditioned to respond to a circle but not to an ellipse even when the ratio of the vertical to horizontal axes was greater than nine to eight.

Working in an environment as free as possible from extraneous stimuli, he established the existence of the conditioned reflex in all animals and located the center of such reactions in the cortex. After the Russian Revolution the Bolshevik government supported Pavlov's work and might have made life personally comfortable, but the rigorously principled Pavlov refused to accept political favors while his colleagues went hungry. He shared his family's meager wartime rations with his dogs and often brought them into his house to give them warmth and affection.

Later the Soviet government was to grant Pavlov far more money than had the Czarist regime, but this did not affect the scientist's critical views. Though he was put at the head of three medical research facilities with a staff of 50 scientists under him, he referred to the government's political practices as "foolery, autocracy, and savagery." On one occasion, however, he did express the "passionate desire" of "an experimenter from head to foot" to see "the victorious conclusion" of his government's "historic social experiment."

When in the 1920s he lectured in the United States under the auspices of the Rockefeller Foundation he talked freely of the difficulties in the Soviet Union but never considered exchanging his native land for the temptations of the West.

In a "Tower of Silence"—insulated from uncontrolled stimuli—that the Soviet government built for him in the 1920s he continued to work on the conditioned reflex, but also on experimentally inflicted neuroses and on the phenomenon of sleep characterized by an inhibition of reflexes. Described by associates as a pink-cheeked, diminutive George Bernard Shaw, Pavlov continued to work until 1936, when, at the age of 87, he died of pneumonia.

"It was cold and he was an old man and he thought he could go about like a young man," said Serafima on the occasion of her husband's death. Many of his colleagues agreed that Ivan Pavlov had rarely accepted limits, whether on himself, his colleagues or his science.

Louise Pearce 1885–1959

Louise Pearce's work in the laboratory and the field led to methods of preventing and curing trypanosomiasis, or African sleeping sickness.

Trypanosomiasis is an infectious disease with an agonizing series of symptoms usually ending in death. These include heart damage, personality change, headaches, tremor, drowsiness, emaciation and a prolonged comatose state. Variations of this disease were ravaging Africa at the turn of the century when Louisy Louise Pearce and her partner Wade Hampton Brown began searching for a cure.

Pearce studied physiology at Stanford University and obtained a medical degree from Johns Hopkins University in 1909. She was one of the first women to pursue a career as a medical researcher, and she jumped at the chance to participate in a project sponsored by the Rockefeller Institute. A team including Pearce and Brown, was organized to find a cure for sleeping sickness and set about investigating various organic compounds that might be effective. Researchers had already determined that the disease was caused by a protozoan (of the genus *Trypanosoma*) and transmitted to humans by the tsetse fly. In the blood the *trypanosomae* become parasites, inducing the lethal symptoms of the disease.

Pearce and Brown ultimately arrived at a successful series of experimental trials using a compound later called "tryparsamide." Pearce wanted to confirm the effectiveness of the serum on humans, and in 1919 she traveled alone to Leopoldville, in what was then the Belgian Congo. She established a scientific procedure for distribution of the drug, and within weeks she observed positive results.

Her work in the laboratory and in the field yielded a preventive measure as well as a cure for African sleeping sickness, earning Louise Pearce the deepest gratitude from the Belgian government. In 1920 she was awarded the Order of the Crown of Belgium, and in 1953 she was again honored with the Prize of King Leopold II.

Wilder Graves Penfield 1891–1975

> Immediately the old grey house upon the street...rose up like a stage set to attach itself to the little pavilion opening on to the garden...and with the house the town, from morning to night and in all weathers, the square where I used to run errands, the country roads we took when it was fine...so in that moment all the flowers in our garden and in M. Swann's park, and the water-lilies on the Vivonne and the good folk of the village...taking shape and solidity, sprang into being, town and gardens alike, from my cup of tea.
>
> —from *Swann's Way*
> by Marcel Proust

> The brain is messenger to consciousness.
>
> —Hippocrates

In the original "Proustian experience," the narrator is transported to a place and time in the back reaches of his memory by the evocative taste of tea and madeleines. Neurologist Wilder Penfield inadvertently triggered a similar response in his patients, without the aid of cookies, when he touched an electronic probe to certain areas of brain. That phenomenon, however, appeared as a by-product in the course of an effort to chart the brain's functions.

Working at Montreal's Neurological Institute in the early 1940s, Penfield pioneered the technique of systematic electrical stimulation at various points of the cerebral cortex in the surgical treatment of focal epilepsy. The procedure required that the patients remain conscious, receiving only local anesthesia, so that their responses to Penfield's gentle applications of current would help him to pinpoint the damaged region. In addition to advancing their own treatment these patients guided Penfield through the uncharted geography of the cerebral cortex, enabling him to create his celebrated *motor homunculus* (a Latin phrase meaning "the little man of movement"). In cartoonlike drawings Penfield showed the surface of the brain and a proportional representation of the external parts of the body, not according to their actual size, but rather to the degree of subtlety in their movements. By indicating the relatively large proportion of the brain involved in sensitive and complex movement, particularly of the face and hands, Penfield's *homunculus* helped to illustrate a fundamental principle of brain organization.

Born in Spokane, Washington, Penfield obtained a degree in medicine at Johns Hopkins University in 1918. Later that year he left for Europe to complete postgraduate studies in neurology. He studied neurophysiology and nerve-cell cytology in the Oxford laboratory of celebrated English neurologist CHARLES SHERRINGTON, and at the University of Breslau he studied under Otfried Foerster, a leading authority on epilepsy. Returning to the United States in 1921, Penfield was appointed neurosurgeon at Columbia Presbyterian Hospital in New York City.

He joined the faculty at McGill University in Montreal in 1928, also accepting appointments in neurosurgery at Royal Victoria and Montreal General Hospitals. Six years later he was appointed director of the Montreal Neurological Institute as well as chairman of McGill's newly established department of neurology and neurosurgery.

Confirming the hypothesis of his distinguished predecessor, neurologist JOHN HUGHLINGS JACKSON, Penfield's "sensory and motor maps of the brain" represent a landmark contribution to the advancement of neurophysiology and neurosurgery. However, his cautious probing of the temporal lobes revealed a far more extraordinary phenomenon. In *The Mystery of the Mind*, published in 1975, he recounted his first observations of the Proustian "flashback" effects of temporal cortex stimulation: "When one of these flashbacks was reported to me by a conscious patient, I was incredulous...for example, when a mother told me she was suddenly aware, as my electrode touched the cortex, of being in the kitchen listening to the voice of her little boy who was playing outside in the yard."

In countless experimental demonstrations Penfield activated these "*tableaux vivants*" in which a patient would suddenly become aware of the sensations, emotions and interpretations of a past experience as it unfolded in vivid detail. Penfield further noted that the flashback would end as soon as the stimulus was withdrawn. "It was evident that these were not dreams," he wrote in *The Mystery of the Mind*. "They were electrical activations of the sequential record of consciousness, a record that had been laid down during the patient's earlier experience."

Based on the characteristic consistency of these observations, Penfield concluded that all experience must be permanently stored in the brain in its original form. He argued, "Since the electrode may activate a random sample of this strip from the distant past...and since the most unimportant and completely forgotten periods of time may appear in this sampling, it seems reasonable to suppose that the record is complete and that it does include all periods of each individual's waking conscious life."

Penfield also pointed out that in this state the patient does not lose awareness of his physical surroundings, nor does he imagine that the experience is actually occurring. Applying these remarkable findings to the ancient question of dual consciousness—the relationship between mind and brain—Penfield eventually came to believe that knowledge of the mind could not be drawn from an understanding of the brain. Convinced of the existence of two parallel "streams of consciousness," he wrote that "the consciousness of man, the mind, is something not to be reduced to brain mechanisms."

Penfield's distinguished writings on neurological subjects include *Cerebral Cortex of Man* (with Theodore Rasmussen, 1950), *Epilepsy and the Functional Anatomy of the Human Brain* (with Herbert Jasper, 1954), *Excitable Cortex in Conscious Man* (1958) and *The Second Career* (1963). He is also the author of two novels, entitled *No Other Gods* (1954) and *The Torch* (1960), and a biography of noted American physician Alan Gregg (1890–1957) entitled *The Difficult Art of Giving* (1966).

Lionel Sharples Penrose 1898–1972

A pioneer investigator of human genetics, Lionel Sharples Penrose explored the biological aspects of abnormal Psychology and mental disorders. His discovery of the genetic basis for Down's syndrome led to important advances in the field of psychiatric medicine and the study of hereditary disease, thereby promoting a positive application of what FRANCIS GALTON termed "eugenics"—the practice of genetic intervention.

In 1866 English physician John Langdon Down (1828–1926) described a developmental disorder characterized by mental retardation and general vulnerability as well as a series of observable physical defects, including a flattening of the skull and facial features. Associating this facial features with those of the Mongols, a group native to a region of northern China, Down referred to the affliction as "mongolism" and presented it as an example of the phenomenon of atavism—the reversion to a more primitive human condition. Because of the racial connotations as well as the theoretical misinterpretation inherent in the original name, the disease is now widely known as Down's syndrome.

Research in the 1950s had revealed that every cell nucleus of the human body normally contains 46 chromosomes arranged in 23 pairs (with each parent contributing one chromosome to every pair). As Galton Professor of Eugenics at University College in London, Penrose was among the first to correlate a numerical aberration of chromosomes with a particular pathological condition, attributing the occurence of Down's syndrome to the presence of an extra chromosome with the twenty-first pair. Referred to as trismony-21, a triple number 21 chromosome is the most common of all chromosomal abnormalities, the likelihood increasing with the age of the mother, particularly after 35. A rarer form of Down's syndrome results from the translocation of material from another chromosome to the twenty-first pair; unlike trisomy-21, the defect is an inherited trait unrelated to the maternal age.

Born in London, Penrose and his four brothers were raised in accordance with the rigorous teachings of the Quakers, following several centuries of family tradition. At 18 Lionel left school to serve in France on the Friends' Ambulance Train of the British Red Cross, and at the end of World War I he entered St. John's College at Cambridge. In addition to attending classes in logic with celebrated English philosopher and mathematician Bertrand Russell, Penrose studied psychology and philosophy, receiving his bachelor's degree in 1921. Pursuing an exhaustive course of graduate study, he spent next four years in Austria and Germany, where he studied psychiatry with such luminaries as J. WAGNER-JUAREGG, and Sigmund Freud. Returning to Cambridge in 1925, Penrose completed his graduate studies in medicine, fulfilling clinical requirements at St. Thomas's Hospital in London in 1928.

In 1931, after completing postdoctorate studies at the City Mental Hospital in Cardiff, Penrose was appointed research medical officer at the Royal Eastern Counties Institution in Colchester. It was there that the launched the pioneer studies of genetics and mental retardation that would form the basis of his distinguished research career.

Penrose moved to Canada in 1939 to accept an appointment as director of psychiatric research for Ontario. Returning to England six years later, he joined the faculty at University College in London, where he held the Galton Chair until 1965. During that time the served as president of the Genetical Society of Great Britain from 1955 until 1958. For seven years following his retirement from University College he directed the Kennedy-Galton Centre at Harperbury Hospital near St. Albans, presiding over the Third International Congress of Human Genetics in Chicago in 1966.

Hailed as an influential figure in the development of human genetics, he is remembered not only for his own outstanding research contributions but also for the significant achievements of his many distinguished students. Penrose received many honors and awards throughout his distinguished career, including the Weldon Medal for Biometrics from the University of Oxford in 1950 and the Albert Lasker Award in 1960.

Candace B. Pert 1947–

In his firsthand account of a lion attack the celebrated explorer David Livingstone (1813–1917) described the brain's "merciful" response to pain:

> I heard a shout. Starting and looking half-around, I saw the lion just in the act of springing upon me. I was upon a little height; he caught my shoulder as he sprang, and we both came to the ground below together. Growling horribly close to my ear, he shook me as a terrier does a rat. The shock produced a stupor similar to that which seems to be felt by a mouse after the first shake of a cat. It caused a sort of dreaminess in which there was no sense of pain nor feeling of terror, though quite conscious of all that was happening. It was like what patients partially under the influence of chloroform describe, who see all the operation, but feel not the knife.

More recently that anecdote has been validated in modern terms by neuroscientist Candace Pert. "People are just very complicated electronic mechanism," she said. "Our emotions of love, hate, anger, and fear are wired into our brains."

In 1973 Candace Pert was a 26-year-old graduate student in pharmacology when she made a revolutionary discovery that launched neuroscience into the "Age of the Receptor." Working under Solomon H. Snyder at Johns Hopkins University, Pert identified the opiate "receptor" in the brain, a site on the surface of the cell demonstrating a particular affinity for heroin, morphine and other opium derivatives. The molecules of these drugs bind to opiate receptors, interacting in a relationship that is often compared to a lock and key.

In addition to Pert and Solomon, Swedish pharmacologist Lars Terenius and American neuroscientist Eric Simon were also on the hunt for opiate receptors, and, in independent investigations, the three teams devised similar research procedures. Pert used mouse brains for the experiment, blending them in a homogenized mixture and then separating out different tissues with a high-speed centrifuge. By means of a radioactive tagging system she tracked the activity of various opiates and nonopiates and was the first to determine the cellular brain component specifically designed for opiates.

Pert's breakthrough discovery posed an important question: Why does the brain have a specific affinity for the derivatives of the poppy plant? She and other investigators suspected that the body produces its own opiates, a hypothesis confirmed two years later when Aberdeen researchers Hans Kosterlitz and John Hughes identified the first natural opiate, which they named *enkaphalin* (from the Greek, meaning "in the head"). It was not long before investigators throughout the world began to discover a wide variety of other such naturally occurring substances, referred to collectively as endorphins. Produced in the brain, endorphins are proteins with opiate like properties, such as the ability to eliminate pain and enhance pleasure. Larry Stein, chairman of the pharmacology department at the University of California, defined the function of natural opiates as the brain's internal reward system, endowing various human activities with pleasurable associations.

Pert describes thc system of endorphins as a subjective filtering system for all incoming sensory information: "I've stopped seeing the brain as the end of the line," she explains. "It's a receiver, an amplifier, a little wet, mini-receiver for collective reality...Our brain defines how much reality is let in...Each organism has evolved so as to be able to detect the electromagnetic energy that will be most useful for its survival." Because that selective process is always in effect, claims Pert, "nobody really knows what the world looks like."

Born in New York, Pert graduated from Bryn Mawr College in 1970. She was married by then to psychologist Agu Pert and had given birth to the first of their two children. Obtaining her doctorate in pharmacology from Johns Hopkins University in 1974, Pert stayed on for a year as postgraduate fellow at Johns Hopkins and then joined the staff at the National Institute for Mental Health.

In 1978 Solomon Snyder, Hans Kosterlitz and John Hughes were given the Albert Lasker Award for their contributions to the study of opiate receptors. Conspicuously absent from the list of honorees, Pert became the center of a storm of controversy when news of the omission leaked to scientific press and then to the public. Although some observers attributed the decision to the influence of academic tenure, the fact that Pert was equal in seniority to Hughes convinced many others that she had been discriminated against on the basis of gender. Declining an invitation to attend the awards luncheon, Pert sent a letter of protest to the Lasker Foundation despite the admonitions of her superiors at the National Institute for Mental Health.

Since Pert's discovery of opiate receptors more than forty other brain receptors have been identified by similar methods. As senior researcher at NIMH Pert applied the procedure in her investigations of receptors for diazepam (Valium), a tranquilizer and muscle relaxant, and phencyclidine hydrochloride, or PCP, a hallucinogenic drug also known as "angel dust."

In 1981 Pert was appointed director of a neuroscience research division at the Institute, where she joined in collaboration with neuroanatomist Miles Herkenham to create a map—or, more precisely, a wiring diagram—of the brain. "What we're working on now," she explains, "is connecting up neurochemical facts—the brain's juices—with circuit diagrams of the brain...the actual connections between the neurons, the wiring of the brain." Pert believes that she and her colleagues will soon be within reach of their goal: to describe the brain "in mathematical, physical, neurochemical, and electrical terms."

In summing up her vision of a more unified field of science, Pert wrote: "There used to be two systems of knowledge—chemistry, physics, biophysics on the one hand, and, on the other, a system of knowledge that included ethology, psychology, and psychiatry. And now it's as if a lightning bolt had connected the two. It's all one system—neuroscience...The brain obeys all the physical laws of the universe. It's not anything special. And yet it's the most special thing in the universe."

Jean-Louis Petit 1674–1750

Early in the eighteenth century Jean-Louis Petit led a campaign to elevate the standards and status of his fellow surgeons. During eight years of service on the battlefield Petit developed the surgical skill that would later win for him a glittering reputation throughout Europe. His many notable inventins include the "screw-type tourniquet," also known as "Petit's tourniquet," in which a strap controlling the circulation at a particular area of the arm or leg is tightened by means of a wooden screw.

Born and raised in Paris, Petit expressed an interest in medicine, and particularly anatomy, at a very young age. He was appointed *chirurgien militaire* (military surgeon) by the time he was 22, having already completed clinical training and an apprenticeship in surgery at the Hopital de Charite.

Attaining the status of *maitre de chirurgie* (master surgeon) in 1700, Petit was widely admired as a teacher ad clinician, attracting a retinue of followers. Noted for his amputation techniques, Petit is thought to have performed the first ganglionectomy for the treatment of breast cancer. In 1736 he became the first to surgically remove a mastoid abscess.

A distinguished anatomist, Petit identified a structure in the lumber region, now known as "Petit's triangle," and described a hernial condition specific to that area, now referred to as "Petit's hernia." He also furnished the first description of osteomalacia, a degenerative condition characterized by weight loss, muscular weakness and a softening of the bones (now recognized as a result of a vitamin D deficiency).

A member of the Academie des Sciences as well as London's Royal Society, Petit was co-founder of the Academie des chirurgiens (France's Academy of Surgeons), becoming that organization's first director in 1731. His notable written works include *L'art de guerir les maladies des os (Treatments for Bone Disease)*, published in two volumes in 1732, and an unfunished reference entitled *Traité de Chirurgie (Treatise on Surgery)*.

Philip Syng Physick 1768–1837

Known as the father of American surgery, Philadelphia-born physician Philip Syng Physick is credited with the establishment and development of surgical practice in the United States at the end of the eighteenth century. One of JOHN HUNTER'S many notable pupils, Physick received a degree in medicine from the University of Edinburgh in 1792. Although Hunter invited him to remain in London as his assistant, Physick returned to America, bringing with him the Hunterian principles of surgery as well as the firm foundation of an Edinburgh medical education.

As a physician and surgeon in Philadelphia, Physick introduced many of the innovative ideas and practices he had learned in Europe, refining and developing them in the course of his own practice. Questioning the advantages of mechanical traction, Physick introduced manipulation as a method of adjusting dislocations. He also advocated the surgical use of animal ligatures, such as catgut, pointing out that they could be left in the body to be gradually absorbed. His inventions include a needle forceps, several new types of catheters, and a snare for use in tonsillectomies. Physick is also credited with the invention of the guillotine tonsillotome, a knife designed specifically for tonsillotomies.

Like Hunter, Physick was reluctant to perform surgery unless no other method of treatment seemed appropriate. Although Physick was a conservative surgeon, he significantly advanced surgical technique in bladder-stone and urinary tract operations. He also pioneered the use of the stomach tube, a device used for feeding or washing out the stomach.

Familiar with cataract surgery procedure, Physick developed a technique for surgical removal of a portion of the iris, now referred to as "Physick's operation." His name is also applied to a rectal condition of inflammation known as "Physick's pouches."

Almost immediately upon his return to Philadelphia a major epidemic of yellow fever broke out, providing Physick with a grueling initiation into medical practice. He himself caught the fever, which very nearly killed him and permanently sapped much of his original energy and strength. He resumed his work, however, practicing and teaching surgery at Pennsylvania Hospital from 1794 until 1816. At the turn of the century he joined the faculty at the University of Pennsylvania, also becoming house surgeon at the Almshouse Infirmary.

A distinguished and influential member of the American medical establishment, Physick was professor of surgery at the University of Pennsylvania from 1805 until 1819. Elected to numerous European medical societies, he was named the first president of the American Academy of Medicine.

Gregory Goodwin Pincus 1903–1967

Recognized as a leading authority in endocrinology and reproductive physiology, Gregory Pincus is best known for his major contribution to the development of oral contraception.

Working with M.C. CHANG at the Worcester Foundation for Experimental Biology, Pincus conducted extensive studies on the effects of various hormones on reproductive function in laboratory animals. They discovered that progesteronelike substances, administered orally, would effectively prevent pregnancy by inhibiting ovulation. In collaboration with gynecologists JOHN ROCK and C.R. Garcia, Pincus and Chang tested the synthetic hormones on human subjects to create the cyclic estrogen- progestin regimen that is still used by millions of women throughout the world.

Born in Woodbine, New Jersey, Pincus completed his doctorate in biology at Harvard in 1927. He pursued advanced training in reproductive biology at Cambridge University under F.H.A Marshall and John Hammond and worked with noted German geneticist R.B. Goldschmidt at the Kaiser Wilhelm Institute.

Returning to the United States in 1930, Pincus accepted a position at Harvard as assistant professor of general physiology. The central focus of his early research was on the genetic transfer of physiological traits and the mechanisms involved in mammalian reproduction. His pioneer study on the nature of fertilization, entitled *The Eggs of Mammals,* was published in 1936.

Pincus taught for a year at Cambridge University and then at Clark University in Worcester, Massachussetts, where he was named professor of experimental zoology. In 1944 he joined with Hudson Hoagland to found the Worcester Foundation for Experimental Biology, which soon gained international recognition as a center for the study of endocrinology and reproductive physiology.

As director of the institute's laboratory, Pincus concentrated much of his research on the newly synthesized steroid hormones and the role of these substances in reproductive function. In 1946 he organized the annual Laurentian Hormone Conference, and he edited the record of its proceedings, *Recent Progress in Hormone Research,* for more than twenty years.

While social reformer Margaret Sanger and others were voicing the need for an oral contraceptive in the early 1950s, a number of powerful, orally active, hormonelike substances were being produced, including a synthetic form of progesterone called progestin. Although proven virtually 100% effective in preventing pregnancy, the compound developed by Pincus and his colleagues was federally licensed only for the treatment of various reproductive disorders when it was first put on the market in 1957.

In addition to the moral controversy surrounding birth control, the medical safety of "the Pill" was challenged by some members of the medical community, who expressed concern over its long-term side effects. More than thirty years later the safety of the Pill, particularly when taken for prolonged periods, is still in question. Despite the controversies, more than 4,000,000 women in America were on the Pill by 1964, and over the next two decades the social and demographic impact of oral contraception was profound.

Pincus pursued research at the Worcester Foundation on hormone biogenesis and metabolism, particularly with regard to cancer, diabetes, schizophrenia, aging and stress. In the 1960s he produced a landmark study of ovum implantation in animals with collaborators J. Jacques and U.K. Banik.

A member of the American Academy of Arts and Sciences and the National Academy of Arts and Sciences, Pincus was honored for his outstanding work in reproductive biology with the Albert D. Lasker Award and the Cameron Prize in Practical Therapeutics. With K.V. Thimann he edited a five-volume reference work entitled *Hormones: Physiology, Chemistry, and Applications* (1948–1964). In addition to more than 350 published articles, his notable writings include *The Control of Fertility* (1965).

Philippe Pinel 1745–1826

In a Paris madhouse known as the *ménagerie,* medical history was made on August 26, 1793, when French physician Philippe Pinel unchained the inmates and released them from their cells. By recognizing them as patients rather than savage beasts, Pinel's dramatic and unprecedented action restored human dignity to the mentally ill.

When he brought the enlightenment of the eighteenth century to the treatment of mental illness Pinel had served only one day as director of the notorious Hôpital Bicêtre. In a sprawling complex of in ancient and decrepit buildings along the banks of the Seine, the Bicêtre housed not only an insane asylum for men but also a workhouse, a prison, an orphanage and a home for the aged. Referring to the hospital's reputation as a repository for the human refuse of society, a journalist commented, "The name of Bicêtre is a word no one can pronounce without inexplicable feelings of repugnance, of horror and contempt."

The city's prevailing standards of taste did not preclude the Bicêtre's popular appeal as an entertainment attraction. On Sundays the public was admitted onto the hospital grounds , where, for the price of a ticket, Parisians could gawk at the chained inmates. On a sunny day as many as 2,000 visitors might spend an afternoon at the "human zoo," watching the continuous show with great amusement, and rooting for an appearance by one of the "stars" of the *ménagerie*—the transvestite "Mme. Houbigan," for example.

Born in Languedoc, Pinel was given a medical direction by his father and grandfather, both of whom were surgeons, and an early education in the classics by his mother, who also instilled in him a pious and humane spirit that endured throughout his life. After her death in 1760 he studied privately with a local abbé until he was 18 and then enrolled in the Collège des Doctrinaires in Lavaur.

In 1773, after graduating from the Medical Faculty in Toulouse, Pinel went to Montpellier to acquire clinical experience in hospital and private practice. Five years later he left for Paris, where he met many of the country's leading philosophers and scientists, including the distinguished chemist ANTOINE LAVOISIER, the mathematician Antoine de Condorcet, and Pierre-Jean-Georges Cabanis (1757–1808). A French physician and outspoken social scientist, Cabanis contributed significantly to Pinel's investigation of mental hygiene and the possibilities for diagnostic, prognostic and prophylactic techniques. Also prompting Pinel's increasing interest in mental illness was the affliction of a friend of his, who had been committed to one of the less barbaric and more expensive private mental institutions in Paris. Pinel kept a detailed record of his observations during his almost daily visits to the clinic, noting the varying responses of his friend as well as the efforts and effectiveness of the staff. In one of a series of articles published in the *Gazette de Santé* Pinel commented on the "marked indifference of the director to the possible recovery of his wealthy boarders, or actually his unambiguous desire to see the failure of any remedy."

After becoming editor-in-chief of the *Gazette* he was admitted as a member of the Academy of Sciences in 1785. It was eight years later that Pinel became director of the Bicêtre and at once unchained the inmates. At a time of revolution, any unauthorized reform presented a risk, but because both the old and the new regimes used mental institutions as prisons for "political undesirables," there was the possibility that medical innovation might expose political diagnoses.

As a herald of the Age of Reason, Pinel declared that the disturbance of reason is a disease rather than the result of divine or demonic possession. Convinced that a patient's mental condition can improve significantly under improved living conditions, he stressed the therapeutic values of fresh air, exercise and social interaction. Among the first to recognize the potential dangers of overinstitutionalization, Pinel also introduced the notion of support groups as a way in which patients might find some of the emotional rewards of a family unit.

After the *ménagerie* was shut down, Pinel took charge of another of the most scandalous institutions in Paris—the Salpêtrière, where more than 6,000 female inmates lived under barbaric conditions of filth and degradation. Accused of crimes or madness or both, women were held for months and even years. On Sundays they were displayed for public titillation, drawing even larger crowds than those that flocked to the Bicêtre during its heyday.

Pinel transformed the hospitals from wretched prisons to medical facilities emphasizing health and humanitarian principles. Although generally conservative in his practice, he was an early advocate of LAËNNEC'S stethoscope and CORVISART's percussive technique for diagnosis. Pinel is also distinguished as the first physician in Paris to have administered a vaccination against smallpox.

In 1801 he published *Traité médico-philosophique sur l'aliénation mentale (A Medico-philosophic Treatise on Mental Disturbance)*, a summation of his professional experiences and observations on mental illness. Defining his "moral" approach to mental hygiene, Pinel also discussed the emotional, environmental and inherited factors contributing to mental disturbance and distinguished several categories of patient, including manic, melancholic, demented and idiotic.

Pinel's distinction as a pioneer in mental health care rests not only on his humanitarian reforms but also on his determination to establish mental illness as a concern of medicine. It was more than century before some of his innovations were rediscovered and adopted, but by the beginning of the 1800s Pinel was recognized as a leading authority in mental hygiene. He was made a Chevalier of the Légion d'Honneur and was consulted by Napoleon on the nature of madness.

For 27 years Pinel served as professor of internal pathology at one of the new medical colleges in Paris, until it was closed down by student riots against clerical influence in the reign of Louis XVIII. When the school reopened in 1822 all the "liberal" professors had been purged from the faculty, and Pinel was not rehired.

Four years later, at the age of 81, he suffered a stroke. Among those who walked in the funeral procession were a number of elderly ladies given a day's leave from the Salpêtrière to honor their "liberator."

Clemens von Pirquet 1879–1925

The scratch test used to screen children for tuberculosis is perhaps the best-known monument to the career of Baron Clemens von Pirquet. In the first few decades of the twentieth century, however, the baron was widely celebrated as a pioneer in pediatrics, immunology, nutrition, biostatistics and as a developer of the concept of allergy. His experimental studies in immunology paved the way for a modern understanding of many immune-complex diseases, such as lupus erythematosus, a chronic and sometimes fatal inflammatory disease characterized by weakness and disfiguring skin lesions.

The baron's choice of profession had upset his family, who scorned his medical career as "ungentlemanly."

Von Pirquet entered the University of Vienna Medical School, then attended the University of Konigsberg and the University of Graz. The newly emerging field of psychiatry fascinated him, but he chose to devote his academic attention to pediatrics. During his residency at the Vienna University Kinderklinik in 1903 he met two people who were to profoundly effect his life. The first was Maria Christine van Husen, who became his wife, and the second was BELA SCHICK, a Hungarian doctor who became his close friend and professional collaborator.

Von Pirquet's collaboration with Schick advanced the theory that the symptoms of a disease do not appear until the host's antibodies react to an antigen. Incubation time is the period in which the immune system produces antibodies and acquired immunity is the body's capacity to speed up the production of antibodies to cause earlier onset of clinical symptoms, while simultaneously defeating the toxic effects of the antigen. Von Pirquet suggested the word allergy—from the Greek *allos*, meaning "other"—to describe all immunologic response. More recently the term has been limited to hypersensitivity reactions.

Von Pirquet developed a test for tuberculosis based on his discovery that a subcutaneous injection of tuberculin causes a local inflammatory reaction in tuberculosis subjects. In 1907 the test was presented to the Medical Society of Berlin, and it soon became an invaluable tool throughout Europe and the United States. In 1909 von Pirquet and his wife spent a year in Baltimore, where he taught at Johns Hopkins University and worked as chief physician at the pediatric hospital there. In 1910 they returned to Vienna, where von Pirquet, barely 31 years old, was by then an international celebrity at the Kinderklinik. His young patients were still his first priority, however, and this concern led to a number of innovations in the hospital, such as isolation cribs and open-air wards for tubercular children. Even more revolutionary were his ideas on the connection between psychological and clinical symptoms in children. He examined both the physiological and emotional conditions of a patient and often drew conclusions about one from the other.

This approach met with tremendous opposition from colleagues and from the parents of his patients, who particularly resisted the idea that physiological symptoms in their children might be echoing an emotional condition. He also gave consideration to climatic conditions, nutrition and diet as factors in the diagnosis, treatment and prevention of disease, and he proposed a system of nutritional requirements for children based on body volume, rather than height or weight. Instead of counting calories this system measured "NEMs"—Nutritional Equivalents in Milk. During the American effort to feed the European hungry after World War I President Hoover named him commissioner general for Austria, and von Pirquet put his NEM system to use in the distribution of U.S. relief supplies.

Although von Pirquet had achieved great professional prominence at a relatively young age, his private and internal life was mysteriously troubled. By the last years of their lives, Maria Christine's mental and physical health had deteriorated rapidly, and they both began to display more and more bizarre behavior. On the morning of February 28, 1925, with their two adopted children away at school, Clement and Maria Christine were found in their bedroom, dead from cyanide poisoning in a mysterious double suicide.

Hans Popper 1903–1988

Hans Popper gained worldwide recognition as a pioneer in hepatology, the study of the liver. Popper's early biochemical research laid the groundwork for this discipline, establishing diagnostic guidelines for a number of major liver diseases. A leading authority on liver diseases for more than four decades, Popper contributed significantly to the understanding of hepatitis viruses. By offering experimental proof that the liver does not deteriorate with age, Popper paved the way for the eventual success of liver transplantation.

Popper also played an important role in the establishment and development of the Mount Sinai School of Medicine of the City University of New York. As one of the founders of the school, Popper remained actively involved in its administration and academic direction until his death at the age of 84.

Born and educated in Austria, Popper received his medical degree from the University of Vienna. He began biochemical research during his first years as a practicing physician, but the Nazi invasion of Austria forced him to flee to the United States, where in 1938 he accepted a research fellowship at Cook County Hospital in Chicago. While earning a doctorate in pathology at the University of Illinois Popper rose in the the ranks at Cook County Hospital, where he eventually became director of pathology.

In 1957 Popper was offered the position of chief pathologist at Mount Sinai Hospital in New York City, where he helped to found Mount Sinai's medical school in 1968. As the school's first dean, Popper was influential in the institution's academic policies and philosophy. He resigned as chairman of the school's pathology department in 1973 but continued to teach and conduct research until his death in 1988.

Rodney Robert Porter 1917–1985

Rodney Robert Porter participated in the precise determination of the sequence and configuration of an antibody molecule. Working independently, Porter and American biochemist GERALD EDELMAN obtained results that led each other closer and closer to a detailed model until their complementary findings combined to form an exact description of the molecular structure of an antibody.

Produced in vertebrate animals, antibodies circulate throughout the body, serving as a critical element in the body's ability to resist bacteria and viruses. Antibodies belong to a group of protein molecules known as gamma globulins, with a distinctive keylike structure that allows them to lock onto specific foreign protein molecules, or antigens. Once an antibody chemically recognizes a particular antigen, it binds to the invading microbe, temporarily disabling it until the antigen can be destroyed by white blood cells. The body mobilizes a force of antibodies at the first infection of a particular antigen, retaining a reserve supply for several years to guard against reinfection.

Seeking to establish the structural components of an antibody, Porter used papain, an enzyme produced by the pawpaw fruit, as a means of breaking down the gamma globulin molecule into functionally different fragments. The first results of his structural analysis, appearing in the late 1950s, suggested a single chain of amino acids, and it was several years before Edelman and others had established that the antibody was made up of several chains of varying molecular weight. Porter and Edelman led the way as increasing numbers of biochemists and immunologists joined the investigation of immunoglobulins, and by 1969 a complete model had emerged, comprising over 1200 amino acids. In 1972 Porter and Edelman were honored for their contribution to this landmark achievement with the joint award of the Nobel Prize for Physiology or Medicine.

Porter was born in the town of Newton-le-Willows in Lancashire, England. The son of a clerk with British Railways, Porter, reflecting on his early fascination with chemistry and biological science, once said, "I don't know why I became interested in this work. It didn't run in my family." Educated at Liverpool and Cambridge universities, he worked at the National Institute for Medical Research at Mill Hill from 1949 until 1960, when he accepted a position as professor of immunology at St. Mary's Hospital Medical School in London. It was there that he conducted a large portion of his ground-breaking research on antibodies. He joined the faculty at Oxford University in 1967, continuing to teach there until his death in 1985.

Percival Pott 1714–1788

One of the most successful and influential surgeons of the eighteenth century, Percival Pott was the first to describe a great number of medical conditions, including two that still bear his name: "Pott's disease," a rare condition of the spine caused by tuberculosis, eventually leading to bone disintegration and skeletal deformity; and "Pott's fracture," a particular type of compound fracture of the ankle.

After an apprenticeship under surgeon Edward Nourse London-born Pott joined the staff at St. Bartholomew's Hospital, first as an assistant, then as a senior surgeon and professor. His reputation as a compelling speaker spread beyond the student body, drawing frequent visitors to his regular lectures at St. Bartholomew's. Among the many students inspired by Pott's teachings was renowned surgeon JOHN HUNTER, who carried on Pott's legacy in the field of surgery.

Pott's writings were extensive, documenting the wide scope of his clinical observations. In *Fractures and Dislocations*, published in 1765, he identified the two conditions bearing his name, as well as many other diseases and complications related to bone structure. Other works included discussions of various head injuries, hernia, *fistula-in-ano* (an abnormal channel between the lower bowel and the skin of the perineum) and hydrocele, a swelling of the scrotum. Pott also recognized a form of cancer located in the skin of the scrotum as an occupational hazard common to chimney sweeps. The long list of Pott's contributions to medical knowledge is particularly impressive in view of the limited scope of surgery in his day. Before the advent of anesthesia, surgeons were largely restricted to the surface of the body, rarely delving into the head, neck, chest or abdomen.

Pott was elected to the Royal Society in 1764. Other published works include *That Kind of Palsy of the Lower Limbs which is Frequently Found to Accompany a Curvature of the Spine*, published in 1779.

Vincenz Priessnitz 1799–

Vincent Priessnitz was known to thousands of devoted patients as "the Genius of Cold Water." His faithful followers were so grateful for his ministrations that they built a fountain dedicated to him. Essentially, Priessnitz had seized on a method of "cure" already gaining popularity, known as hydropathy. The medicinal value of water had been recognized for centuries, but it was not until the eighteenth century that hydrotherapy was used as a systematic method of treatment for a wide variety of disorders. In 1697 English physician Sir John Floyer published *The Ancient Psychrolusia*, a treatise extolling the wisdom of immersing oneself in icy water. When an admirer of Floyer's, Dr. Thomas Browne, subsequently published *An Account of the Wonderful Cures Performed by the Cold Baths*, England was on its way to the hydropathy craze. In 1790 Horace Walpole wrote, "One would think the English were ducks; they are for ever waddling in the waters."

Ten years after Walpole's disdainful comment Vincent Priessnitz was born into a family of farmers living in the tiny village of Grafenberg, two thousand feet above sea level in the mountains of Silesia. (The town is now known as Jesenik and is located in Czechoslovakia.) The waters of Grafenberg had no remarkable qualities, and there was never an attempt by Priessnitz to promote the place as a fashionable spa. Instead, he established a therapeutic community where people from miles around gathered to benefit from elaborate water treatments that Priessnitz himself had devised. Despite the sparse accommodations, royalty flocked to Grafenberg and competed with hundreds of other eager patients for the attention of "the Genius." In his book *Taking the Cure,* E.S. Turner counted 22 princes and princesses, a duke, a duchess, 88 barons and baronesses, 14 generals, 53 staff officers, 196 captains and subalterns, 104 civil servants, 65 divines, 46 artists and 87 physicians and apothecaries, all appearing for the "cure" in the year 1839. Ailments included apoplexy, melancholia, epilepsy, impotence, syphilis, scrofula, rheumatism, cancer, gangrene and gout.

Priessnitz would examine each new patient, paying close attention to the quality of his or her skin. Many visitors were struck by his intensity, exclaiming that they felt he could see inside them. Based on his observations, Priessnitz would prescribe a system of treatments, all relying on the use of water. He is credited with the invention of the sponge bath, the douche, and the wet sheet pack, a treatment that involved wrapping the patient tightly in a soaking wet linen sheet, then covering him, still wrapped, with layers of dry blankets and quilts. After an initial discomfort the patient would become warm and perspire profusely. Duration would vary, depending on the illness being treated, and occasionally the patient would be vigorously rubbed with the wet sheets in order to stimulate and heat the skin.

Initially Priessnitz relied on such treatments, but by 1840 his methods had grown more extreme. Along with "sweating blankets," "sitz baths" and "ascending douches" a trusting visitor might expect to experience the "cold douche" procedure created by Priessnitz, in which columns of water would cascade down from heights of eighteen feet, battering the patient for up to an hour at a time. Many of the treatments were outlandish, and most of the medical community scoffed, but Priessnitz's methods allegedly achieved remarkable results. His cure rate, or at least his survival rate, was quite high. According to one source, Priessnitz treated 7200 patients between 1831 and 1841, and of those only 38 people died.

Priessnitz claimed that his methods drove out all the poisonous and degenerative elements in the body, but it should be mentioned that as part of the program Priessnitz maintained strict controls on all forms of physical indulgence and enforced an almost ascetic way of life on his patients. Their grateful and enthusiastic response encouraged others to establish water-based health centers throughout Europe. Priessnitz is thus credited with contributing to the rise of the European health spa movement.

Sir John Pringle 1707–1782

Recognized by many historians as the founder of modern military medicine, British Army surgeon John Pringle established a set of guidelines for protecting the health of army personnel and campaigned to improve conditions for prisoners of war.

Pringle's influential work, entitled *Observations on Disease of the Army*, was recognized as a classic reference on the subject of military hygiene and contagious diseases, going through six editions within twenty-five years. Published in 1752, *Observations* introduced fundamental principles of sanitation and housing, most notably the necessity of latrines and ventilated barracks.

Based on extensive clinical studies conducted during his tenure as director of the British Army hospital in the Flanders, Pringle's book investigated many of the infectious diseases associated with military life, including typhus, malaria, epidemic meningitis and dysentery. In considerable detail it described the stage-by-stage development of these diseases, adding clinical evidence in support of the theory of contagion by the spread of "animalcules."

Born in Roxburgh, Scotland, John Pringle was sent at an early age to receive a classical education at the University of St. Andrews, where he studied under his uncle Francis Pringle. In 1727 John entered the University of Edindburgh but, intending to pursue a career in business, he left after a year to work in Amsterdam in order to gain practical experience in commerce. It was during a casual visit to the University of Leyden that he happened to attend a lecture given by HERMANN BÖERHAAVE. Inspired by the powerful presence of this distinguished Dutch physician, Pringle made the decision to pursue a career in medicine. Studying anatomy and surgery at Leyden under Boerhaave and Bernhard Siegfried Albinus (1697–1770), Pringle received his degree in 1730 and completed postgraduate medical training in Paris. He returned to Scotland in 1734 to establish private practice while serving as professor of metaphysics and moral philosophy at the University of Edinburgh.

In 1741 he accepted an appointment as attending physician at the British Army hospital in Flanders during the war of the Austrian succession, and within a year he underwent a baptism of fire in the bloody battle of Dettingen. Recognizing the overwhelming obstacle faced by medical personnel in times of war, Pringle proposed an international convention protecting all medical facilities from attack. It was more than a century later, with the establishment of the Red Cross, that military hospitals and medical personnel were officially granted neutrality status (see JEAN HENRI DUNANT)

With the return of peace in 1748 Pringle settled in London to practice medicine as a civilian, although he retained his position as military physician and surgeon. In recognition of his distinguished service the royal family honored him with medical appointments to the Duke of Cumberland, Queen Charlotte and King George III, as well as the award of a baronetcy in 1766. A distinguished member of the Royal Society, Pringle served as president from 1772 until 1778, at which time he succeeded noted Swedish botanist Carl Linnaeus as one of the eight foreign members of the Academie des Sciences in Paris.

Pythagoras c. 582–507 B.C.

Pythagoras and his disciples followed a way of life based on philosophical, moral and religious principles partially influenced by the earlier cult of Orphic mysticism. Directing attention toward the spiritual universe, Pythagorean doctrine was predicated on the notion of a transmigration of souls. While the body inevitably decays, the soul is continuously reborn, in human or animal form, until eventually liberated from the "wheel of birth." It is said that Pythagoras once came to the rescue of a dog in pain because he recognized in its howl the voice of a friend he had known in an earlier incarnation. Dedicated to self-purification, believers followed rules of moral and physical asceticism with an abiding respect for the sanctity of life.

Although he was elevated to the status of a demigod by his disciples, little is known of Pythagoras's life or his writings, and one must conjecture as to what proportion of the Pythagorean doctrine represents his own teachings, rather than those of his followers. Pythagoras was born on the island of Samos, off the coast of Asia Minor. In his native land he became acquainted with the doctrines of the early Ionic philosophers, and through his travels he broadened his education with Egyptian and other teachings. In 530 B.C. Pythagoras emigrated to Crotona, a burgeoning center of philosophy in Magna Graecia (now southern Italy).

Drawing on many of the tenets of a sect venerating the legendary Greek hero Orpheus, Pythagoras founded a school of morality and religion. As in the teachings of the cult of Orpheus, Pythagoras prescribed a rigorous program of physical exercise, meditation, music and celibacy. Pythagoreanism required a vegeterian diet, further dictated by other food restrictions and recommendations. Beans were forbidden, but cabbage, anise and squill were considered of great therapeutic value both for maintaining health and for the treatment of disease. Pythagoras is said to have produced a book detailing the medicinal properties of plants, with a guide to internal and external application. Because of the potential threat of the integrity of the soul, surgery was strictly prohibited.

According to Pythagoran teachings, the highest form of self-purification was philosophy, a term Pythagoras himself is said to have introduced. Pythagoras is credited as well with the first use of the term *psyche,* or soul. A student of acoustics, Pythagaros was the first to recognize that the relationship between notes on the musical scale could be expressed by numerical ratio. Believing that the fundamentals of knowledge were to be found in mathematics and music, Pythagaros devised a far-reaching philosophical theory based entirely on numbers. Each number held meaning beyond its mathematical properties, representing the essences of all things in the universe. In an attempt to give a form to abstract concepts, Pythagoran teaching expressed concepts such as justice or marriage in numerical terms. Applying the lore of numbers to medicine, Pythagoras introduced the concept of "critical days," referring to a predictable pattern in the progress of a disease based on the numbering of days, counted from the onset of symptoms. This numerical principle, and others applied to medical science, were further developed by HIPPOCRATES and Galen.

After the defeat of the Sybarites by the Crotonians in 510 B.C. the elitist school of Pythagaros came under public attack. Their rejection of traditional religious beliefs and practices enraged the local citizens and led to violent persecution of Pythagoras's followers. Many were killed before the last remaining disciples fled from Magna Graecia. One legend has it that Pythagoras was captured and killed because in his flight he stopped at bean field, refusing to dash across it out off respect for plant life.

R

Bernardo Ramazzini 1633–1714

In 1700 Bernardo Ramazzini published the first treatise on occupational medicine, entitled *De Morbis Aritificium Diatriba (On Artificially Caused Diseases)* In his pioneer work Ramazzini systematically identified the potential health hazards in more than forty different occupations, including mining, midwifery, pharmacy, painting, printing and gilding. Recognizing a relationship between certain metals and the symptoms of poisoning exhibited by the artisans who used them, Ramazzini launched the science of industrial medicine.

His investigation included a study of poisonous elements in some pigments used by painters, the dangers of lung disease for miners and the eye disorders associated with the precision work of printers. In conjunction with his discussion of occupational disease Ramazzini also examined the possibilities for preventive measures.

Born in Modena, Ramazzini studied medicine and taught at the University there until the beginning of the eighteenth century. He left to join the faculty at the University of Padua, where he taught pathology until three years before his death.

As a physician Ramazzini made important epidemiological observations, describing and differentiating a number of disorders according to the region of the country in which each was endemic. He also disputed the prevalent use of cinchona bark (the source of quinine) as a nonspecific treatment for disease, recognizing that the drug should only be used in cases of malaria.

Santiago Ramon y Cajal 1852–1934

Spanish artist and neuroscientist Santiago Ramon y Cajal described the nerve cell as "the aristocrat among the structures of the body, with its giant arms stretched out like the tentacles of an octopus to the provinces on the frontier of the outside world, to watch for the constant ambushes of physical and chemical forces."

Establishing the fundamental principle of the neurone theory, Cajal demonstrated the anatomical structure and function of the nerve cell as a discrete and well-defined unit of the nervous system. Along with distinguished investigators WILHELM HIS Edward Sharpey-Shafer (1850–1935), August Forel (1848–1931), George Romanes (1848–1894) and others, Cajal helped to create a histologic approach to the study of the nervous system that led to the modern understanding of cerebral cortex and the cerebellum.

Reproducing his microscopic observations in meticulous detail, Cajal depicted the anatomical structure of the neuron and charted the course of a nerve impulse from the cell body and dendrites out along the neuron's axon toward the tendrites of another neuron. These elegant sketches were the first neural road maps, not only indicating the existence of functional pathways of impulse transmission, but suggesting the concept of gaps, or synapses, between nerve cells as well.

Cajal's demonstration of the cellular structure of the nervous system laid to rest the more widely accepted "reticular" theory of an impenetrable network of inextricably intertwined nerve fibers. Italian histologist Camillo Golgi was among the many zealous supporters of the network theory who maintained that, rather than following any particular track, an impulse is conducted through the continuous contact of masses of undifferentiated nerve cells. Ironically, it was Golgi who developed the potassium dichromate-silver nitrate stain that enabled Cajal to reveal the entire histologic structure of the gray matter and eventually to disprove the reticular theory.

For their independent contributions to the establishment of the individual neuron theory, Cajal and Golgi shared the Nobel Prize for Physiology or Medicine in 1906, an experience which in no way mitigated the adversarial relationship of the two men.

Born in the Spanish farming village of Navarre, Santiago Ramon y Cajal was a romantic and artistic boy, thereby disappointing his father, a noted surgeon and professor of medicine who nevertheless convinced his son to pursue a career in that field. At seventeen Santiago entered the University of Saragossa, where, for the next four years, he concentrated mainly on physiology and anatomy and achieved barely passing grades in the rest of his courses.

Almost immediately after receiving his medical degree Cajal was drafted into military service and appointed assistant physician in the Spanish Republican army. He was dispatched to Cuba, where he volunteered to serve at a jungle outpost and promptly contracted an acute case of malaria. Declared unfit for duty, Cajal received his discharge and was sent back to Spain.

Resuming his studies at Saragossa, he obtained the necessary qualifications for an academic career but found that professorships were hard to come by. He accepted a position as director of the local anatomy museum and began to train himself as a medical investigator.

In 1884 he was appointed professor of anatomy at the University of Valencia and, after several years, accepted the same position at the more prestigious University of Barcelona. It was at Barcelona that Cajal seized on the idea of studying the gray matter in animal embryos as an area in which to examine nerve fibers before they became encased in myelin, a sheath of fatty substance. By using Golgi's stain he was able to observe neurons as separate and well-defined structures, communicating with one another at interneuronal articulations, or synapses. After establishing the nerve cell as an anatomically and physiologically autonomous unit of the nervous system, Cajal went on to distinguish among subgroups of motor, reticular, funicular and tract cells.

Influential Swiss anatomist RUDOLF VON KÖLLIKER recognized the enormous significance of Cajal's achievement and helped to bring it to the attention of the scientific establishment. Rapidly gaining distinction as an international celebrity, Cajal was celebrated in his own country as a national treasure—Spain's only scientist of world renown.

In 1892 he joined the faculty at the University of Madrid, where he served for thirty years as professor of histology and became founding director of the university's Laboratory of Biological Research (later renamed the Instituto Cajal).

In addition to hundreds of articles and monographs, Cajal produced a monumental treatise entitled *The Nature of the Nervous System in Man and the Vertbrates.* Originally published in Spanish in 1904, the classic text is still considered the most important single work in neurobiology. Other notable writings include *Degeneration and Regeneration of the Nervous System* (1913–14) and the autobiographical *Recollection of My Life* (1907).

Walter Reed 1851–1902

In 1900 American army surgeon Walter Reed was sent to Havana as head of a commission to investigate a serious outbreak of yellow fever. Based on the suggestion of Cuban physician Carlos Finlay that the disease might be transmitted by mosquito rather than through human contact, Reed launched a series of experiments in which members of the research team volunteered as subjects for the study. His findings, announced in 1901, not only confirmed Finlay's theory of a mosquito vector but demonstrated that yellow fever was caused by a virus.

As part of Reed's investigation, seven members of his mission agreed to wear clothing that belonged to patients suffering from the disease, but without being bitten by mosquito, none of them came down with yellow fever. The results seemed to indicate that the disease could not be communicated from one human being to another except by some form of inoculation. When he found that it could, in fact, be transmitted by the injection of blood that had been taken from afflicted patients and carefully filtered, Reed had conclusive proof that the disease was caused by a virus of some kind.

Three years earlier FRIEDRICH LOFFLER (1852–1915) and P. Frosch (1860–1928) had recognized a virus as the causative agent of hoof-and-mouth disease, but yellow fever was the first human disease proved to be caused by a filterable virus. Reed and his colleagues determined that the virus was borne by the *Stegomyia fasciata* mosquito (later designated as *Aedes aegypti*).

Born in Belroi, Virginia, Reed completed his training at the Army Medical College in Washington in 1875. He remained in the medical corps throughout his career, serving as professor of bacteriology from 1893 until his death in 1902.

Tadeus Reichstein 1897–

Tadeus Reichstein is recognized for his enormous contribution to the field of pharmacology. The first to synthesize ascorbic acid (vitamin C), in 1933, Reichstein went on to conduct Nobel Prize-winning research on the hormones of the adrenal gland.

Born in Poland, Reichstein was educated in Switzerland, where he earned a doctoral degree in organic chemistry from the Technical School of Zurich in 1922. He taught chemistry there until 1938, when he was made head of the Pharmacological Institute at the University of Basel. As director and later as professor of organic chemistry at Basel, Reichstein continued experimental study of the hormones of the adrenal cortex, eventually synthesizing 29 hormones, including cortisone.

Reichstein was awarded the Nobel Prize for Physiology and Medicine in 1950, which he shared with PHILIP HENCH and EDWARD KENDALL.

Rhazes (Al-Razi) 854–925

> All that is written in books is worth much less than the experience of a wise doctor.

The influential author of more than 200 medical treatises, physician-philosopher Rhazes gained distinction as a leading figure in the history of Islamic thought for his outspoken and antiauthoritarian views on religion and politics as well as science. At a time when medical care was a luxury reserved mainly for the rich and noble, Rhazes was widely admired for his willingness to treat poor patients at no charge and for his compassion and dedication to clinical practice.

Rhazes was born at Rayy, in Persia, where he obtained his medical education and later served as director of the city's largest hospital. Although little is known of his life, it is said that Rhazes was often persecuted for his open-minded and egalitarian attitudes. He rejected any form of dogma as fanaticism and argued that religious fanaticism inevitably engendered hatred and war. In contrast to the Aristotelian belief in a "point of intellectual perfection," Rhazes viewed science as a continual and unlimited progression based on an accumulation of past knowledge and an advancement into the unknown.

Dedicating much of his life to the systematic compilation and organization of all available knowledge, Rhazes produced a monumental compendium of medical and surgical knowledge entitled *al-Hawi*. The 25-volume encyclopedia, his most celebrated work, contains information on a great many diseases, including the first accurate descriptions of smallpox and measles.

For each of the disease entries Rhazes listed theories from Greek, Syrian, Indian, Persian and Arabic medicine, followed by a comparative discussion of past and current ideas and finally a presentation of his own observations and opinions. In this section Rhazes furnished case histories in the HIPPOCRATES tradition, as well as pragmatic suggestions for treatment. Recommending dietary supplementation as preferable to the use of drugs in therapy, Rhazes advocated simple remedies and cautioned against the potential dangers of complex chemical preparations.

An essential requirement of scientific study, he maintained, was intellectual receptivity, so that any observed phenomenon, however peculiar or inexplicable, can be given proper consideration.

Because of his controversial views as well as the continually shifting political situation, Rhazes was forced to leave his native city on several occasions. At various times he taught and practiced in Baghdad and also served as director and chief physician of that city's hospital.

When he was in his seventies Rhazes was beaten and blinded by order of a caliph who found his candor offensive. Although he had gained distinction, honor and a considerable amount of money over the course of his life, Rhazes died in poverty, having given all his earnings to those less fortunate.

Dickinson Woodruff Richards Jr. 1895–1973

> He was a humanist; he was a Hellenist; he was a scientist; he was a superb clinician; and he was an outstanding gentleman. I have never met another man as remarkable as he.

This description of Dickinson Richards came from his friend and collaborator of more than forty years, ANDRÉ COURNAND. The two were pioneers in the study of heart disease and operational techniques, and their substantial contributions were honored in 1956 by a Nobel Prize in Physiology or Medicine (shared with WERNER FORSSMANN).

Richards was born in Orange, New Jersey and attended Yale and Columbia University Medical School. In 1928 he became associated with the College of Physicians and Surgeons at Columbia, where he taught medicine—in particular, cardiac surgery—from 1945 to 1961. His research focused on the heart and lungs, and his fruitful partnership with Cournand began in 1931. Based on the work of Werner Forssmann presented ten years earlier, they developed an improved method of cardiac catheterization that could reliably measure blood pressure within the heart. With the catheter tube inserted in the heart (by way of a vein), it permitted an immediate assessment of cardiac condition. The technique also presented a way to observe the effects of drugs, facilitated diagnosis of disease and laid the groundwork for open-heart surgery.

Scipione Riva-Rocci 1863–1937

In 1896 Italian physician and surgeon Scipione Riva-Rocci introduced the mercury sphygmomanometer, a practical and reliable instrument for measuring blood pressure that became the prototype for the device used today. A blood pressure reading indicates the force of blood against the arterial walls at the height of a heart's contraction of the left ventricle (maximum or systolic pressure) and during the "smooth flow" as the heart chambers relax and expand (minimum or diastolic pressure).

With an inflatable arm band connected to a graduated tube containing mercury (the manometer), Riva-Rocci sought to constrict the arm by inflating the cuff until it had completely blocked the artery. Since the level of mercury in the tube is proportional to the pressure in the cuff, systolic and diastolic pressure can each be assigned a numerical value based on the height of the mercury in millimeters. A blood pressure reading is generally expressed as the maximum reading over the minimum reading, preceded by the letters RR (for Riva-Rocci).

Although he did not create the first sphygmomanometer, Riva-Rocci's ingeniously simple solution for achieving a uniform distribution of pressure and subsequent release offered medical practitioners an efficient method for obtaining relatively accurate readings.

The earliest technique for measuring blood pressure was a dangerous and elaborate process requiring the insertion of a hollow tube in the artery of the neck. Introduced in 1733 by Stephen Hales as a veterinary procedure, the system was not practical for standard medical examinations. It was more than a century later that the first sphygmomanometer (from the Greek word *sphygmos*, meaning "pulse") was invented by Ritter von Basch. Although it required no surgical incision, the device was inefficient and unwieldy.

In the second half of the nineteenth century, as emphasis gradually shifted from qualitative observation to quantitative measurement, a demand sprang up in European medicine for accurate mechanical gauges of biological events.

Born in Almese, in Piedmont Italy, Riva-Rocci received his medical degree from the University of Turin in 1888. He then served for more than twelve years as lecturer in special pathology at the Propaedeutic Medical Clinic, where he introduced his refined sphygmomanometer in 1896. In addition to serving on the faculty at Pavia University, he was appointed director and physician-in-chief of the Ospedale di Varese, retaining that position until 1928. It was at Pavia that Riva-Rocci demonstrated his invention to the distinguished American neurosurgeon HARVEY CUSHING who helped bring the mercury sphygmomanometer to the attention of the medical world.

Frederick Chapman Robbins 1916–

For his contribution to the isolation and cultivation of the poliomyelitis virus Frederick Robbins was awarded the 1954 Nobel Prize for Physiology or Medicine, which he shared with his collaborators JOHN F. ENDERS and THOMAS H. WELLER. In facilitating the supply of poliovirus these three distinguished scientists paved the way for the production of the polio vaccine, developed by JONAS SALK in 1954.

Born in Missouri, Frederick Robbins was the son of Jacob Robbins, a noted plant physiologist and professor of botany. In 1932 Frederick enrolled as a chemistry engineering student at the University of Missouri. Two years later he transferred to Harvard, where he found himself rooming with two medical students, Donald Sweeny and future collaborator Thomas Weller. It was through Weller that Robbins initially became intrigued with virology, with particular attention to pediatrics.

After receiving his medical degree from Harvard in 1940 Robbins served in World War II as head of a viral and rickettsial laboratory in Naples, Italy. Troops were being decimated by epidemics of what appeared to be viral pneumonia, but by isolating the rickettsial agent Robbins determined that the disease was in fact Q fever (Q for query). Previously misdiagnosed as a variety of other diseases, Q fever had never been identified in Italy until Robbins proved it to be endemic there.

Returning to civilian life, Robbins completed his residency requirements and was invited to join Enders and Weller at the new Infectious Disease Laboratory at Boston's Children's Hospital. A fellowship award from the National Foundation for Infantile Paralysis provided for one year of work with Enders, after which he performed a two-year stint in Australia in the laboratory of noted virologist MACFARLANE BURNET.

Working at Boston's Children's Hospital with Enders and Weller was Alice Northrop, a lab technician specializing in microbiology. Six months after Robbins joined the team he and Northrop were married.

The successful cultivation of the poliovirus occurred in 1948, the result of an accidental, or at least spontaneous, act. Having successfully cultured the mumps virus, Enders, Weller and Robbins set out to perform the same operation on the chicken pox, or varicella, virus. As the laboratory also stocked a quantity of the Lansing strain of poliovirus, the team impulsively decided to attempt to grow a culture from that virus as well. The varicella virus culture failed, but the poliovirus was a historic success.

The ability to produce unlimited amounts of the poliovirus enabled development and mass production of the polio vaccine, introduced by Salk in 1954. The laboratory cultures also facilitated diagnosis of the disease, even permitting identification of the particular strain of the virus.

Robbins went into the hospital wards to collect samples of the poliovirus from patient after patient. Back in the laboratory the team eventually isolated and cultured thirteen different strains of the virus.

After a year's deferment Robbins resigned from his National Foundation fellowship, which would have required a move to Australia, so that he could continue working with the poliovirus. As word of their work spread Enders, Weller and Robbins were all courted by the scientific establishment. After turning down an offer to work with Jonas Salk, Robbins finally left his partners in 1952, accepting a position at Case Western University in Cleveland. Remembering the events surrounding the Nobel Prize award as "a trying experience," Robbins said, "I figured a very great mistake had been made. A Nobel laureate should not be someone like me."

Robbins served as professor of pediatrics at Case Western as well as director of pediatrics and contagious diseases at Cleveland's Metropolitan Hospital. In 1966 he was named dean of the school of medicine, retaining the post until 1980, when he became president of the National Academy of Sciences.

John Rock 1890–1984

Boston gynecologist and obstetrician John Rock pioneered the development and advancement of oral contraception.

A leading authority on embryology and reproductive physiology, Rock's initial area of concentration was the study of infertility and reproductive dysfunctions. He served for thirty years as founding director of the Fertility and Endocrine Clinic at the Free Hospital for

Women in Brookline, Massachussetts, one of the first American institutions dedicated to reproductive research. Among Rock's many outstanding accomplishments was the first in vitro fertilization of a human ovum, achieved in collaboration with Harvard biologist Miriam F. Menkin in 1944. He also pioneered long-term preservation of sperm cells, successfully maintaining potency in frozen sperm for over a year.

Seeking alternate methods of conception for infertile couples, Rock investigated therapeutic use of the female hormone progesterone. Associated with the onset of ovulation, progesterone is secreted in the body by the corpus luteum in the ovary to prepare and strengthen the womb and fallopian tubes in the event of fertilization. Unsatisfied with results obtained by supplements of natural progesterone, Rock experimented with synthetically produced hormones in order to better regulate progesterone levels.

In the early 1950s progesterone research was launched in an entirely different direction by physician and endocrinologist GREGORY PINCUS, a colleague of Rock's at the Worcester Foundation for Experimental Biology. Pincus and research associate M.C. CHANG hoped to use progestins—synthetic compounds simulating progesterone—as a means of inhibiting fertility, based on the fact that the hormone acts to prevent overlapping pregnancies by inhibiting ovulation once fertilization has taken place. By 1954 Pincus and Chang had developed three steroid compounds derived from the root of the wild Mexican yam, and within two years the substances were industrially produced in pill form.

Testing progestins on his patients in Brookline and later in experimental studies in Puerto Rico, Haiti and elsewhere, Rock determined that the steroids prevented pregnancy with apparently few side effects. In 1957 the drugs were federally licensed for the treatment of various reproductive disorders. While some doctors refrained from prescribing oral birth control until they had further evidence of its safety, by 1964 some 4,000,000 women in America were on "the Pill."

Rock, a devout Roman Catholic, had been an outspoken advocate of birth control since 1931, when he campaigned for the repeal of a Massachussetts law against the sale of any birth control device. Staunchly defending the right of individual choice in a pluralistic society, Rock led the crusade for Catholic reform on the issue of birth control in the 1960s.

Traditionally, the Church has opposed as "unnatural interference," all forms of contraception with the exception of the "rhythm method," which consists of abstinence from sex during ovulation. Arguing that the mechanism of the birth control pill is the same as that of the body's endocrine system, Rock maintained that the use of oral contraception falls within the bounds of "natural" sexual activity.

In 1963 he presented his case in a scholarly and impassioned work entitled *The Time Has Come: A Catholic Doctor's Proposal to End the Battle for Birth Control.* Rock's book sought to rally the international scientific and religious community in a united effort to establish practical and ethical systems for population control throughout the world.

A graduate of Harvard Medical School, Rock was appointed clinical professor of gynecology there in 1947. In 1956 he gave up his faculty position at Harvard, along with his post at the Fertility and Endocrine Clinic, to establish his own foundation, known as the Rock Reproductive Clinic, in Brookline, Massachussetts.

Karl Rokitansky 1804–1878

Karla Rokitansky was recognized as one of the great pathologists of his period, devoting nearly half a century to the study of disease and anatomy, and, with his staff, performing over 50,000 autopsies.

Rokitansky was born in Königgratz, in Bohemia, and went to Austria to study medicine. From 1834 until 1875 he taught pathological anatomy at the Vienna Institute of Pathology and gained worldwide recognition for his painstaking work in that field. Using extensive postmortem studies, Rokitansky strove to classify the organic effects of disease. His important treatises dealt with heart defects and the effects of disease on the arteries. Between 1842 and 1846 he published a widely acclaimed three-volume work, *Handbuch der pathologischen Anatomie (Handbook of Anatomic Pathology)* (Eng. trans. in four volumes, 1849–1854), in which he described and classified hundreds of specific conditions such as acute yellow atrophy of the liver and gastric ulcer. As important as his conclusions were the standards he established for autopsy methods and protocol, still widely respected.

In his attempt to reconcile traditional medical theories with modern anatomical knowledge he drew criticism from some of the up-and-coming medical theorists, most notably young RUDOLF VIRCHOW, who took exception to Rokitansky's reliance on "humoralism." Gabriel Andral, a contemporary of Rokitansky's, had revived an interest in this ancient theory (see HIPPOCRATES), which identified four essential fluids in the body, assigning particular properties to each one and to their interaction. Possibly under Andral's influence, Rokitansky developed a theory maintaining that all disease was a result of dyscrases, or imbalances, in the blood. In light of Virchow's radical new theories of cellular pathology, he was forced to retract his assertions.

Wilhelm Konrad von Röntgen (Wilhelm Conrad Roentgen) 1845–1923

By 1895 Wilhelm Röntgen was already recognized as a distinguished physicist, having conducted important research in the fields of mechanics, electricity and heat conductivity. His other scientific contributions came to be overshadowed, however, by his discovery of the X ray, a physical phenomenon that has radically altered the evolution of science and technology. Although he did not fully understand the principles at work, Röntgen was the first to recognize the ability of these rays to pass through low-density substances and to apply this phenomenon to photography.

X rays are electromagnetic waves similar to light waves, but much shorter in length. Although, like visible light waves, X rays register on photographic plates, they pass through materials of low density and low atomic weight more easily and completely than through materials of high density and high atomic weight. This characteristics of low absorption in low-density substances is a result of the X-ray wave's extremely short length, which reduces its ability to interact with atoms. Because bones are of a more opaque material than flesh, they will appear lighter than the areas of flesh in an X-ray photograph.

Wilhelm Röntgen was born in the town of Lennep in the Ruhr valley of what is now West Germany. At the age of three he traveled with his family to Apeldoorn in Holland, where he was raised and educated. Röntgen entered the Technical School at Utrecht in 1862 but transferred to the mechanical technical department of Zurich Polytechnic Institute.

The decision to enroll at the Polytechnic proved fortunate, for it was there that Röntgen encountered August Kundt, who had taken over the chair of physics in 1868 and who became his mentor. After receiving his degree in engineering Röntgen stayed on at the institute to continue studies in mathematics and physics under Kundt's guidance. While working in Kundt's laboratory Röntgen conducted important studies on the specific heat of gases, for which he was awarded a doctorate in physics on 1869.

Kundt was to hold the chair of physics at a number of distinguished universities, always inviting Röntgen to accompany him as his assistant. The inspiring, although occasionally tempestuous, relationship lasted for six years. In 1875 Röntgen left his mentor to accept a professorship at the Agricultural Academy in Hohenheim, Wurttemberg. He continued the experimental research he had begun with Kundt on electromagnetism and thermography in crystals and gases. In the course of chairing the physics departments at universities in Hohenheim, Strasbourg and Giessen, Röntgen established an international reputation for innovative research.

In 1888 Röntgen joined the University of Wurzburg, where he served as professor of physics and headed the university's new Institute of Physics. It was at Wurzburg that Röntgen became aware of the studies being done with cathode rays by William Crookes in England and by Johann Hittorf and Philipp Eduard Anton Lenard in Germany.

Reproducing Lenard's experiments with cathode-ray tubes, black paper covers and tin-foil shields, Röntgen observed a fluorescent effect a short distance away from the apparatus. Through extensive experimentation Röntgen determined that these rays could pass through solid, light-proof materials, leading him to test their effect on a photographic plate. Röntgen had his wife hold her hand over a photosensitive plate, and the resulting photograph still appears in medical history books, showing the skeleton of Frau Röntgen's hand, complete with the shadowy images of her rings. Aware of the enormous impact of his findings but unable to fully explain them, Röntgen dubbed his discovery the X ray.

In the last week of December, 1895 Röntgen sent a paper to the Wurzburg Physical Medical Society entitled *On a New Kind of Ray, a Preliminary Communication*. Enclosing X-ray images of his wife's hand, along with prints of other subjects that he felt would indicate the scope of his remarkable discovery, Röntgen asked that the society committee bypass the customary requirements and publish his article as soon as possible. By New Year's Day of 1896 the article was on its way to many of Europe's most distinguished scientists. The medical establishment soon recognized the enormous diagnostic value of Röntgen's discovery, and his findings were generally met with accolades from all parts of the scientific community. However, a few scientists and a small segment of the public felt that Röntgen had released insidious rays capable of destroying the world.

In 1896, after demonstrating his discovery at the imperial court of Kaiser Wilhelm II, Röntgen was decorated by the emperor with the Prussian Order of the Crown, Second Class. In that same year he was awarded the distinguished Rumford medal, which he shared with Philipp Lenard. Three years later Röntgen left his position at the University of Wurzburg to become professor of physics at the University of Munich, where he remained until 1920. In 1901 Röntgen's great contribution to science and medicine was again recognized with the first Nobel Prize for Physics, awarded in 1901.

Initially seized upon as a major diagnostic tool in the area of orthopedics, X rays were soon used to reveal other abnormalities, particularly in the chest and gastrointestinal tract. They permitted early detection of tuberculosis and various forms of cancer and were eventually recognized as a form of cancer therapy as well. As a memorial to him X rays are also known as "Röntgen rays," and the unit of measurement for radiation emission is the "Röntgen."

Nils Rosen von Rosenstein (Nils Rosenstein) 1706–1773

A leading authority on pediatric medicine, Swedish physician and anatomist Nils Rosen von Rosenstein is best known for his classic reference work entitled *Diseases of Children and Their Remedies*. Originally published in Stockholm in 1753, von Rosenstein's influential treatise was reissued in a series of Swedish editions as well as in Dutch, Danish, English, French, German, Italian and Hungarian translations.

Based on exhaustive laboratory and field research, the book reports significant insights, particularly in discussions of smallpox, scarlet fever, whooping cough and ascarides, a genus of intestinal parasites commonly found in children throughout western Europe in the eighteenth century. Considered one of the earliest pioneers of bacteriology, von Rosenstein described the phenomenon of bacterial infection in discussing the nature and mechanism of whooping cough. Anticipating the findings of LOUIS PASTEUR by more than a century, he wrote,

> The hooping-cough [sic] always appears as an epidemical disease...I have many times plainly perceived it to be contagious, and that it infects only such children who have not yet had it. Therefore it infects in the same manner as the measles or small-pox. I knew the hooping-cough conveyed from a patient to two other children in a different house by means of an emissary. I myself have even carried it from one house to another undesignedly...The true cause of this disease must be some heterogenous matter or seed which has a multiplicative power, as is the case with small-pox. Whether this multiplicative miasma be a kind of insect I cannot affirm with any certainty.

Von Rosenstein's remarks on scarlet fever were based on direct clinical observations during the Swedish epidemic of 1741. Of particular note is a reference associating the symptom of bloody urine with anasarca, a generalized swelling of the body due to an excessive accumulation of fluid.

In the section devoted to parasitic worms von Rosenstein distinguishes five different types of ascaris, along with detailed recommendations for the practice of "worming" a child. Presenting recipes for a variety of relatively gentle laxatives and "clysters," or enemas, von Rosenstein particularly emphasized the purgative values of raw carrots and tobacco smoke.

The son of an army chaplain, Nils studied theology at Lund before embarking on a professional course in medicine at the University of Uppsala. His doctoral thesis, entitled *The Description of the History of Disease*, was delivered at Harderwijk, Holland, where he received his medical degree in 1731.

After practicing in hospitals throughout western Europe von Rosenstein was appointed professor of practical medicine and anatomy at Uppsala, later joining Swedish botanist and taxonomist Carl Linnaeus as a professor of natural history. An articulate and engaging speaker, von Rosenstein was greatly sought after by students and faculty alike for his open manner as well as his medical expertise.

His first published work, entitled *Compendium Anatomicum*, appeared in 1738, attracting considerable attention within Sweden's medical community. This was followed by a number of important monographs, including a case study of poisoning from ingestion of the *Hyoscyamus* plant (henbane). His report of the mydriatic or pupil-dilating effect of the plant was confirmed more than a hundred years later when parts of *Hyoscyamus niger* were established as mydriatic as well as narcotic and analgesic. A tincture made from dried leaves of the plant is now used to block the action of the parasympathetic nervous system.

In 1745 von Rosenstein accepted the position of Archiater, or physician-in-chief, at Uppsala's teaching hospital. When he was ennobled in 1762 he changed his name to Rosenblad, following the example of his brother Eberhard.

Widely acknowledged for his distinguished contribution to medicine, he was awarded the Royal Order of the North Star in 1757 and was honored posthumously by the Swedish Academy of Sciences.

Ronald Ross 1857–1932

After fifteen years of uninspired and undistinguished service in public health it seemed unlikely that Ronald Ross would leave any lasting mark on the history of medicine. Nevertheless, Ross provided the key to controlling one of the most devastating diseases in the world: malaria.

Ross was born in Almora, India, where his father, General Campbell Claye Grant Ross, was a member of the Indian Army. Young Ronald was sent to England to be educated, and although he yearned for the life of an artist, his father persuaded him to enroll in St. Bartholomew's Hospital Medical School when he came of age.

He endured the experience but did not meet the qualifications to become a practicing physician. However, he did manage to pass the exams qualifying him for the position of ship's surgeon. He took several voyages in this capacity, spending most of his time writing poetry, plays and one novel.

In order to return to India Ross decided to enter the Indian Medical Service. He took a course in elementary bacteriology, passed the necessary examinations and was given a public health diploma. He held various posts in Indian station hospitals, enjoying a pleasant and relaxed atmosphere that allowed him much time for his artistic and literary pursuits. Ross took a short leave from these duties to visit England, where he met

PATRICK MANSON a physician specializing in tropical diseases. This encounter had a profound effect on Ross, who returned to India with new drive and purpose.

Manson had communicated his own commitment to finding the cause of malaria, and Ross decided to join in the search. Manson's studies of the malaria parasite steered Ross to the gastrointestinal tract of the mosquito, but this still left a vast field to investigate. In 1898, after two years of studying 250 different species of mosquitoes, Ross made a striking discovery. In the stomach of a larval mosquito of the *Anopheles* species he found the malaria parasites that he (and Manson) were looking for. It had already been established that most female mosquitoes must ingest blood before their eggs can mature and hatch. Ross's discovery, along with his further parasite studies, cleared up a widespread misconception. Malaria was not contractable through the air or water but was an infectious disease spread from human to human by mosquitoes. W.G. MacCallum clarified the physiology of the malaria parasite, further confirming this theory.

Ross was heaped with honors for his work and was offered a post at the School of Tropical Medicine in Liverpool. He arrived there in 1899 and gained a professorship in 1902. That same year he was awarded the Nobel Prize for Physiology or Medicine for his contribution to the battle against malaria.

After he had made a name for himself, Ross's inauspicious beginnings returned to haunt him. It seemed that Italian medical scientist, Battista Grassi had also been studying malaria and was furious that Ross had gotten all the acclaim. In fact, Grassi had established a more detailed picture of the complex physiological process of development of the malaria parasite and its passage through the gastrointestinal tract of the mosquito. He impugned Ross's scientific background and launched a feud that lasted many months. It was Manson's influential support that finally ended the controversy over who had been the first to achieve these findings.

Ross devoted the remainder of his life to the elimination of malaria. Although this has not yet been fully achieved, his recommendations have been followed throughout the world and have done much to help reach this goal. In recognition of his work, the Ross Institute and Hospital for Tropical Diseases was founded in 1926, and he was invited to serve as director-in-chief.

In addition to poetry and several plays, Ross's writings include *The Prevention of Malaria,* written in 1910, and *Memoirs,* written in 1923. A biography of Ross written in 1958 by John Rowland was entitled *The Mosquito Man.*

Francis Peyton Rous 1879–1970

Peyton Rous had to wait decades for the scientific establishment to catch up to his ideas. He studied the physiology of the blood and liver and was a significant force in the movement to establish blood banks, but he is best known for cancer research that was initially dismissed by the medical community as ridiculous.

Rous received his medical degree from Johns Hopkins University in 1905. He taught pathology at the University of Michigan until he joined the Rockefeller Institute in 1909. It was there that he began experimenting with cancerous tissue removed from chickens with sarcoma (tumor). He placed the diseased tissue in a salt solution and filtered out all cellular material, then injected the tissue into healthy chickens and found consistently that they developed malignant tumors.

The idea of cancer-producing viruses contradicted all current assumptions about the disease's mechanisms. Rous reported his findings in 1910, but it was not until his ideas were confirmed by later research that their impact was felt in the medical community. In 1962 Rous received the U.N. prize for cancer research, and in 1966 he was awarded the Nobel Prize for Physiology or Medicine (shared with CHARLES B. HUGGINS). Rous conducted a lifetime of research at the Rockefeller Institute from 1910 until his death in 1970.

Benjamin Rush 1746–1843

Benjamin Rush, one of four physicians to sign the Declaration of Independence, was a vocal and influential figure in revolutionary America. His innovative ideas and opinions in politics and medicine were influenced by legendary giants of his era, including Benjamin Franklin, WILLIAM CULLEN, WILLIAM AND JOHN HUNTER, Oliver Goldsmith and Samuel Johnson. Nevertheless, he was also a victim of the illusions of his era, such as the misguided practice of bloodletting.

With the inadequate medical background of his time, Rush bravely offered his services in the care of yellow fever victims during a severe epidemic in Philadelphia in 1793. Despite the unsound epidemiological theories then available, Rush anticipated bacteriological studies of the next century by suggesting that mosquitoes might be involved in the spread of yellow fever.

A strong supporter of the revolutionary movement, Rush also fought against slavery, establishing the first abolitionist society in America. Championing the cause of the mentally ill, he instituted reforms in the conditions of mental asylums. His ideas on treating mental illness foreshadowed the psychiatric breakthroughs of the next century.

Believing in the social responsibilities of a community, Rush helped to establish a city agency in Philadelphia to provide free medical care for the poor. He was also intrumental in the establishment of Dickinson College in 1783.

Born in the rural village of Byberry, north of the Delaware River, Rush grew up in Philadelphia, embarking on a career in medicine at the age of sixteen. He apprenticed himself to Dr. John Redman, a graduate of the University of Leyden and founder of Philadelphia's College of Physicians. Rush attended medical lectures given by William Shippen and John Morgan at the College of Philadelphia and then set out to compete his education at the internationally acclaimed University of Edinburgh.

There Rush studied with the noted physician and educator William Cullen, who became an important influence on the eager American student. Cullen's ideas on pathology, nervous energy and mental illness helped to form Rush's advanced views on the care and treatment of mental disorders. Based on an experimental study of gastric processes, Rush's doctoral thesis showed remarkable insight into the chemical and physiological aspects of digestion, predating the work of William Beaumont, the recognized pioneer of gastric physiology.

Rush returned to Philadelphia in 1769 to establish a practice among the city's poor. Apart from his espousal of bloodletting, Rush generally followed the sensible teachings of his mentor William Cullen, prescribing fresh air, exercise in the form of dancing, swimming, golf or at the least a brisk daily walk. At the age of 24 Rush became the youngest member of the faculty at the College of Philadelphia, where he also gained distinction as the first chemistry teacher in the colonies. In addition to his responsibilities as a faculty member and private practitioner, Rush took on duties as a physician at the county poorhouse, otherwise known as the House of Employment.

A member of the Continental Congress of 1774, Rush was responsible for inoculating John Hancock against smallpox. Intensely involved in the volatile political atmosphere of the time, Rush read the final draft of Tom Paine's pamphlet on the cause of independence with great enthusiasm, suggesting only that he change the title from "Plain Truth" to "Common Sense."

From 1797 until his death Rush served as treasurer of the United States Mint. His published writings include a five-volume work entitled *Medical Inquiries and Observations* (1794–1798), *Essays, Literary, Moral, and Philosophical* (1798) and *Medical Inquiries and Observation upon the Diseases of the Mind* (1812).

Howard Archibald Rusk 1901–1989

American physician Howard Rusk developed a system of physical reconditioning, educational retraining and psychological readjustment that offered a disabled patient the opportunity for a self-sufficient and productive way of life.

Rusk maintained that rehabilitation is as much a medical responsibility as diagnosis and treatment, not only for amputees, paraplegics and the blind, but also for victims of cardiac and pulmonary disease, stroke, cancer and mental illness. By inviting patients to participate in the design and progress of their own therapy he encouraged the development of existing capabilities as a means of regaining independence. Rusk's notion of constructive rehabilitation also included a massive reeducation of society in order to eliminate the prejudices and misconceptions that further handicap a disabled person.

Born in Brookfield, Missouri, Rusk planned to become a doctor from the time he was a child. He worked his way through medical school as a hospital orderly and laboratory aide and received his degree at the University of Pennsylvania by the time he was 24. After completing his residency at St. Luke's Hospital in St. Louis he established a successful private practice as an internist.

In 1942 Rusk was called to active duty in the Army Air Forces Medical Corps and served nine months as director of medical services at a Missouri military hospital. Appointed chief of the convalescent training division, Rusk introduced a comprehensive program that included counseling as well as various types of physical therapy tailored to the needs of each patient.

After his discharge Rusk established the first faculty of rehabilitation and physical medicine at New York University medical school. In 1948 he was commissioned to organize and direct a center for inpatients—the Institute for Physical Medicine and Rehabilitation.

Rusk designed the center to function as a training facility rather than a hospital, employing social workers, vocational counselors, psychologists, psychiatrists, prosthetics technicians and physical and occupational therapists in order to meet the wide- ranging needs of disabled children, adults and elderly. Internationally acclaimed for forty years of distinguished service, the center was renamed the Institute of Rehabilitation Medicine in 1966, but since its founding day the facility has been popularly known as the Rusk Institute.

S

Albert Bruce Sabin 1906–

Albert Sabin is known worldwide for his invention of a safe, orally administered vaccine against poliomyelitis. Polio, also known as infantile paralysis, is a devastating, often fatal disease, highly contagious and endemic to all parts of the world.

The incidence of the disease dropped dramatically with the advent of the first polio vaccine, developed by JONAS SALK and introduced in the United States in 1955. Salk's vaccine, administered in a series of four injections, was a noninfectious or "killed" vaccine in which the immunizing agent, or antigen, was treated with formaldehyde to render it harmless. Sabin's system of immunization, relying on a live though attenuated antigen, promised a number of important advantages. Easily administered, Sabin's vaccine offers a stronger and longer-lasting immunity. In addition, Sabin's partisans claim that his vaccine protects against both infection and paralysis whereas the Salk vaccine can protect only against paralysis.

Born in Bialystock in Russian Poland, Sabin and his family emigrated to the United States when he was fifteen. At nineteen he entered New York University, receiving a bachelor's degree in science in 1928. He became a naturalized American citizen in 1930 and a year later was granted a degree in medicine. After serving as a medical researcher at Rockefeller Institute Sabin joined the faculty at the University of Cincinnati Medical School in 1939, continuing research in microbiology and immunology. Having devoted much of his career to the study of childhood viral diseases, Sabin was named professor of research pediatrics at Cincinnati in 1946.

After participating in the development of vaccines against dengue fever and Japanese B encephalitis Sabin became interested in the possibility of a live vaccine against polio. Developed and tested in the 1950s, Sabin's vaccine came into widespread use in the early 1960s.

Sabin accepted a professorship at the University of South Carolina Medical School in 1974, where he continued medical research until 1982.

Florence Rena Sabin 1871–1953

As author of *An Atlas of the Medulla and Midbrain*, Florence Sabin produced a landmark study of the anatomy of the brain of a newborn infant. Her three-dimensional reconstruction, known as the "Sabin model," was duplicated and manufactured, becoming a standard teaching aid for medical students.

Sabin also conducted pioneering studies of the lymphatic system, discrediting a number of long-standing misconceptions. Her innovative investigation of the lymphatic system was made possible in part by a vital staining technique of her own invention.

Sabin's work on tissues in vivo led her to the identification of small and large lymphocytes and neutrophils—specific types of white blood cells—and to an understanding of the activities of target cells—those cells with specific receptions for other substances—in relation to immunity and in inflamation.

Florence Sabin's career as a scientist is all the more impressive in light of the many obstacles she faced as a woman. Among the first women students to earn a medical degree from a major institution, she graduated third in her class from Johns Hopkins University, where she later became the first woman to obtain a full professorship at a medical school. In 1925 she became the first woman to be elected to the United States National Academy of Sciences.

Florence Sabin was born in the gold mine region of Colorado, where her father struggled to earn a living from mine holdings. With the death of their mother in 1879 Florence and her sister Mary were sent to their grandparents in New England. In 1889 Florence entered Smith College, where she first became interested in science and medicine.

When she graduated four years later she learned that the newly established Johns Hopkins Medical School was to accept female applicants, following the proviso of its main benefactor, the Women's Fund Committee. Sabin worked for three years as a teacher to save enough money for tuition at Johns Hopkins. She was admitted in 1896, and four years later she received her degree in medicine, along with Dorothy Reed and nine other women. Sabin had already completed her painstaking study of the cell grouping and nerve fibers of the brain, completing the text for publication shortly after graduation. Amid much controversy Sabin and Reed were granted two of the four internships available in the department of medicine.

Supported by a fellowship from Johns Hopkins, Sabin embarked on a systematic investigation of the lymph system. In 1902 she was invited to join the Department of Anatomy as an assistant, becoming the school's first female faculty member. After fifteen years she was made a full professor of histology.

She had earned the position of chairman in the Department of Anatomy but had been passed over by the school's board of trustees. She accepted the professorship but resigned from Johns Hopkins without regret to join SIMON FLEXNER'S staff at the Rockefeller Institute for Medical Research. She left Baltimore in 1925, accepting Flexner's invitation to organize a department of cellular studies at the prestigious institute. Working in conjunction with other departments and with outside institutions, Sabin conducted important research on immunity and tuberculosis.

Following the institute's mandatory retirement policy, Sabin left the Institute in 1938. She returned to Colorado, where she was active in the crusade for preventive medicine and for public health service reforms.

Bernard Sachs 1858–1944

A pioneer in the field of organic neurology, Bernard Sachs presented the first comprehensive description of a congenital disease of cerebral development appearing in very young children. Originally identified as "amaurotic family idiocy," the condition is now referred to as Tay-Sachs disease in acknowledgment not only of Sachs, but also of the work of British ophthalmalogist WARREN TAY, who independently reported some features of the disease. The disease, generally associated with blindness, is characterized by a rapid degeneration of physical and mental abilities leading to spasms, dementia and death, usually before the age of four.

Born in Baltimore, Maryland, Sachs was one of six children whose German-Jewish parents had immigrated to the United States in 1847. Although he decided to pursue a medical career early in his schooling, Sachs concentrated on literature and the classics throughout his premed years, graduating with honors from Harvard University in 1878. Noted psychologist and philosopher WILLIAM JAMES, a member of the Harvard faculty at the time, interested Sachs in the study of mental disorders.

In 1879 Sachs went abroad for a European gloss to his medical studies. As a student in the universities of Strasbourg, Vienna and Berlin, Sachs met many of the world's leading authorities in medical and psychiatric science. He studied pathology under RUDOLF VIRCHOW and Friedrich von Recklinghausen (1833–1910), physiology and medicine under noted German physicians Friedrich Leopold Goltz (1834–1902) and Adolf Kussmaul (1822–1902) and neuropsychiatry under Carl Westphal (1833–1890). After receiving his degree from the University of Vienna in 1882 Sachs, along with fellow student Sigmund Freud, remained to continue postgraduate studies in cerebral anatomy and neuropsychiatry with Theodor Meynert (1833–1892). Sachs later wrote an English translation of Meynert's classic treatise *Der Psychiatrie* (1885).

To round off his education in medicine and neurological science Sachs spent a year with JEAN CHARCOT in Paris and JOHN HUGHLINGS JACKSON in London before returning to the United States in 1884. After spending three years in New York as an assistant to Issac Adler, Sachs established a private practice for the treatment of mental and nervous diseases based on a synthesis of psychiatric and neurological medicine. He viewed the principles of neuropathology, neurophysiology and clinical medicine as inextricable elements of a single unified discipline.

Gaining prominence as one of America's leading clinical neurologists, he served as professor at New York Polyclinic Hospital, and later at the College of Physicians and Surgeons at Columbia University. In 1893 he was appointed consulting neurologist at Mount Sinai Hospital and helped arrange for the provision of a neurological bed service, the first separate division of its kind in a New York health care facility. He later served as president of Mt. Sinai's medical board between 1920 and 1923 and president of the New York Academy of Medicine from 1933 until 1935.

A leading spokesman for international cooperation and collaboration in neurological research, Sachs participated in the establishment of the first International Neurological Congress, held in Bern, Switzerland in 1931.

For more than 35 years Sachs served as editor of the *Journal of Nervous and Mental Disease*. Among his more than two hundred published works, most notable is a classic reference text entitled *Nervous Diseases of Childhood* (1895).

Jonas Salk 1914–

American microbiologist Jonas Salk, who developed the first successful vaccine against poliomyelitis and founded one of the world's most distinguished scientific communities, has declared that in his early struggle and ultimate triumph he "was concerned with a principle, not a product." That principle, he says, established he fact that "it is possible to immunize with a noninfectious agent as effectively as with an infectious one."

On the other side of that argument was ALBERT SABIN, who campaigned for his oral live-virus vaccine. Sabin's vaccine is currently in wider use, though the Salk vaccine continues to have its ardent defenders. Salk maintains that in many parts of the developing world, where polio remains a formidable threat complicated by intestinal ailments, "inhibitors in the intestinal tract" may negate the results of the oral vaccine.

Whatever the subsequent challenges, in 1955 Salk stood alone in his triumph as the savior who first freed vast numbers of the world's population from a deadly scourge. In that year he was awarded a Congressional medal for "great achievement in the field of medicine."

He grew up in what is now known as East Harlem in New York City, the firstborn child of Daniel and Dora

Salk. His father was a designer of lace collars and cuffs whose spare time was devoted to sketching. Jonas's mother was fiercely ambitious and saw in her small, frail son the person who would fulfill her grandest hopes. Those dreams were well founded in her son's keen intelligence and intellectual drive, which became evident at an early age.

At 13 Jonas passed the rigorous examinations required for entry into Townsend Harris Hall High School, a three-year prep school that charged no tuition but demanded high intellectual performance. At sixteen he entered the College of the City of New York and was soon so enamored of the scientific approach that he resolved to seek a career in medicine.

At New York University Medical School he made it clear to his teachers as well as his parents that he would not practice medicine but would devote himself to research. Years later, when asked why he chose research over practice, Salk replied: "Why did Mozart compose music?"

At the end of his first year Salk was given a fellowship for research in protein chemistry. It was the first of a long series of grants and awards that relieved his parents from paying for the rest of his education. In his senior year he went to work on a vaccine utilizing killed influenza virus under the guidance of Thomas Francis, a distinguished researcher on influenza who had been appointed to the chair in bacteriology at New York University.

On June 8, 1939, the day after he graduated from medical school, Salk married Donna Lindsay, a Phi Beta Kappa psychology major. During his internship at Mount Sinai Hospital in New York he worked mainly for board, lodging and the honor of his selection.

When a residency at Mt. Sinai seemed impossible to a young doctor without influential connections, Salk applied for and was granted a fellowship from the National Research Council that gave him $2,100 a year and a chance to work with Francis at the University of Michigan School of Public Health. The involvement of the United States in World War II focused attention on the threat of influenza, spurring Francis and Salk to develop a vaccine against both A and B types of the disease, which had played havoc in World War I.

In 1947, when the National Foundation for Infantile Paralysis was seeking research facilities to sort out the various forms of poliomyelitis, Salk, then at the University of Pittsburgh, received a grant to share in the laborious spadework. At that time JOHN ENDERS, THOMAS WELLER and FREDERICK ROBBINS had succeeded in cultivating the poliovirus in non-neural tissue, a development that made polio research possible without the complicating involvement of nerve cells and eased the financial burden by freeing researchers fom a dependence on expensive experimental monkeys. As Salk later described the situation, "The Enders team had thrown a long forward pass." He was one of those in the race to catch it.

Selecting three of the most common types of polio as his targets, he developed a trivalent (uniting with or replacing three hydrogen atoms) vaccine using viruses killed by formalin. When animal tests produced a gratifying increase in antibodies he proceeded to human tests in a home for crippled children near Pittsburgh. Danger was minimized because all of the subjects had had polio and therefore possessed a certain number of protective antibodies. The results were promising and were confirmed by tests on children who had never suffered from the disease.

In 1953 the National Foundation for Infantile Paralysis organized elaborate and extensive field tests to validate the vaccine. The period of testing was marked by wild rumors. The widely syndicated columnist Walter Winchell, citing Paul de Kruif as his source, reported that the Salk vaccine could be a "killer." Some monkeys tested with the vaccine had died, he insisted, despite denials by the foundation.

When, on April 12, 1955, Francis announced that, in some areas, the immunity provided by the Salk vaccine had proved 90% successful, the nation and the world hailed Jonas Salk. He declined an invitation to a ticker-tape parade up Broadway (sending his parents as stand-ins) but addressed the American public from the White House rose garden after receiving a citation from President Eisenhower.

The celebrations of April were cooled in May following the revelation that six children who had been given the Salk vaccine had died. All of the vaccine implicated in the disaster had been made by one laboratory, which, investigation showed, had not followed Salk's prescribed manufacturing procedure. The vaccination program was suspended for two weeks, alarming the country and heartening the proponents of the live-but-attenuated-virus vaccine.

Governmental support for the program was renewed before the end of May, but it took time to regain public confidence. Nevertheless, within three years half the nation's population under 40 had reveived the Salk shots, and the polio incidence had declined by 86%.

Gradually Sabin's oral live-virus vaccine was adopted in the Soviet Union, most of the United States and many parts of Europe, though Scandinavia and parts of the Third World remained faithful to the Salk vaccine. In time Jonas Salk left the battle of polio vaccines and devoted himself to gathering a glittering array of scientists to work at the Salk Institute for Biological Studies, which was established in La Jolla, California in 1963. The institute had been subsidized to the extent of $1 million a year by the March of Dimes, which sought new outlets for its generosity as the the threat of polio diminished. With an annual budget of $22 million the institute currently has a staff of 500, including 160 celebrated scientists from around the world.

Though Salk maintains a laboratory at the institute, he retired from the directorship in 1975 to concentrate quietly on problems in cancer, multiple sclerosis, demography and philosophy. He stepped into the limelight again when he separated from his first wife in 1967 and three years later married Francoise Gilot, a distinguished painter, companion of Pablo Picasso and mother of two of the artist's children.

In his writings, which include *Man Unfolding, The Survival of the Wisest, World Population and Human Values* (cowritten with his son Jonathan) and *Anatomy of Reality*, Salk examines the social consequences of science and technology and discusses what he calls "metabiological evolution"—"the evolution of human consciousness and creativity." "In order to survive the dangers created by the evolution of the human brain, we've got to understand evolution in the metabiological realm," Salk explains. "The human mind may be seen as a form of matter that has become conscious of itself, conscious of evolution, and conscious of its capacity to participate in evolution. We are a product of evolution, and the embodiment of the process as well." He states that "the threat that we are to ourselves manifests itself in the form of nuclear weapons, the economic crisis, problems associated with the development of the Third World, problems associated with resources, with the pollution of the planet—with all of those things which are threatening to the life of the organism of humankind and therefore to the individual members of the organism...I look upon each one of us as I would an individual cell in the organism...For me, the critical determinant of human evolution is the realm of human values—and that is a matter of education and choice."

Daniel Elmer Salmon 1850–1914

A leading authority on veterinary sciences, Daniel Salmon contributed greatly to the control of contagious diseases in humans as well as in animals. Salmon is associated with a number of important developments in infectious disease pathology, most notably with his demonstration of the transmissibility to humans of tuberculosis in cattle, thereby confirming the role of animal vectors in the spread of disease.

Commemorated in medical terminology, his name forms the basis of the designation of a tribe and genus of microorganisms known respectively as *Salmonelleae* and *Salmonella*, which includes the typhoid-paratyphoid bacilli and bacteria. Salmonellosis refers to an infection of these microorganisms, generally resulting from exposure to animals or food containing the bacteria. Among the common types of human infections, in addition to typhoid and paratyphoid fever, is a form of gastroenteritis characterized by violent diarrhea, cramps, nausea, vomiting and fever. This condition is often due to inadequate cooking of mass-prepared food, which fails to kill the pathogenic bacteria.

Born in Mount Olive, New Jersey, Daniel Salmon was granted a doctoral degree in veterinary medicine from Cornell University in 1876. Distinguished as a key participant in the New York State campaign to wipe out pleuro-pneumonia in cattle, he was selected by the Department of Agriculture to study the widespread problem of livestock disease in the South. In 1883 he became founding director of the Veterinary Division of the Bureau of Agriculture, later recognized as the Bureau of Animal Industry. Salmon became a leader in the field of public health administration, gaining federal support for intensive research investigation of contagious pleuro-pneumonia and Texas fever in cattle. It was due in large part to his efforts, as well as those of noted pathologist THEOBALD SMITH, that these two major threats to health and industry were eventually controlled.

During his tenure as bureau chief Salmon inaugurated a number of significant public health policies, including a nationwide system for meat inspection and a quarantine requirement for imported livestock. While serving as an influential administrator he retained his commitment to research science, collaborating with Theobald Smith on the development of killed microorganisms for use in vaccines.

Embroiled in a dispute with the head of the Department of Agriculture, Salmon was forced to resign from the bureau in 1905. He left the United States for South America, where, at the invitation of the Uruguayan government, he supervised the establishment of the Department of Veterinary Medicine at the University of Montevideo.

Returning in 1910, Salmon became head of a private pharmaceutical concern in Butte, Montana, where, four years later, he died of pneumonia.

Bengt Ingemar Samuelsson 1934–

For his research in the chemical study of prostaglandins Bengt Samuelsson was awarded the 1982 Nobel Prize for Physiology or Medicine along with fellow chemists SUNE K. BERGSTROM and JOHN VANE. Prostaglandins are a group of more than ten different compounds derived from arachidonic acid, an unsaturated fatty acid. Produced in small amounts throughout the body as they are needed, prostaglandins have far-reaching effects in many of the body's critical functions, acting on the endocrine and nervous systems, regulating blood pressure, stress, pain, smooth muscle contraction etc. Samuelsson's research revealed the chemical processes involved in the body's use of prostaglandins.

Investigating other metabolites of arachidonic acid, Samuelsson discovered thromboxanes and leukotrienes. These subtypes of prostaglandins may contribute significant advances in the prevention and treatment of strokes, heart attacks and asthma. Samuelsson continues to study other relatives of the prostaglandins, in particular lipoxin, another oxidation product of arachidonic acid.

A native of Sweden, Samuelsson attended the internationally celebrated Karolinska Institute, where he studied under Sune Bergstrom. In 1960 Samuelsson earned a doctorate in biochemistry from Karolinska, receiving a degree in medicine the following year. He returned to Karolinska as a professor, later becoming dean of the medical faculty. Currently serving as president of the institute, Samuelsson remains actively involved in scientific research, devoting a large portion of his time to laboratory studies.

Santorio Sanctorius 1561–1636

Clinical observation and experimental medicine entered the domain of the physician in the late sixteenth century. It was Santorio Sanctorius in Italy and WILLIAM HARVEY in England who were largely responsible for bringing scientific procedure to the doctor's examining table.

Sanctorius was a physiologist who introduced the use of physical sciences into the field of medical study. He observed the process of metabolism by keeping detailed records of his own weight fluctuations in the course of a day and during various metabolic events such as digestion. For these and other investigations he used a specially constructed balance scale and designed a number of other measuring systems, including a pulsilogium, or pulse monitor, a hygrometer used to measure the moisture content in gas and a steelyard chair designed to measure what he called "insensible perspiration."

Sanctorius is best known, however, for his invention of one of the first thermometers. At approximately the same time Cornelius Drebbel (1572–1633), Robert Fludd (1574–1637), Galileo and Sanctorius all devised variations of an "air thermoscope." These devices consisted of an enclosed vessel containing air that would expand or contract with the temperature, forcing water to move up or down a tube with arbitrary calibrations.

Sanctorius was professor of physiology at the prestigious University of Padua from 1611 to 1624. In 1614 he wrote *De statica medicina (On Statistical Medicine)*, an important reference that reached its fifth edition in 1737.

Frederick Sanger 1918–

Honored with two Nobel Prizes for his work in the field of biochemistry, Frederick Sanger is noted for his studies for the molecular structure of insulin and nucleic acids, which laid the groundwork for the eventual laboratory synthesis of these substances.

Sanger earned his Ph.D. in molecular biology at Cambridge University in 1943, and he remained at Cambridge for his entire career. In an investigation of the nature and biological function of enzymes, hormones and antibodies Sanger began work at the molecular level, studying the configuration of amino acids in protein molecules. In 1955 he identified the arrangement of amino acids in a molecule of insulin, a protein isolated 34 years earlier by F.G. BANTING and C.H. BEST. Sanger's findings were a breakthrough in biochemical research, enabling the eventual synthesis of insulin (in 1964) and paving the way for important advances in complex protein research, such as the work of J. KENDREW and M.F. Perutz.

Sanger's first Nobel Prize for Chemistry was awarded in 1958 for his molecular study of insulin. His second award, shared with WALTER GILBERT and Paul Berg, was in recognition of his biochemical description of the structure of nucleic acids. Sanger's description of the base sequences in these molecules made possible the laboratory synthesis of genetic material.

Margaret Sanger (Margaret Higgins) 1883–1966

As the founder of the birth control movement in the United States Margaret Sanger faced threats, harassment and legal prosecution, but her fervent belief in the need for family planning fueled her determination to integrate the practice of contraception into American life.

Born in New York and trained as a nurse at Claverack College, Sanger's dismal experiences working in public-health facilities convinced her of the urgent need for family limitation. Seeking a forum in which to voice her radical ideas, Sanger founded a feminist magazine in 1914 called *Woman Rebels*. At the time, the practice of contraception was illegal, and dissemination through the mail of any information on the subject was a federal offense. Indicted for obscenity for her effort to establish the National Birth Control League, Sanger left the country in 1914.

She sought out birth control advocates in Europe, where the movement had already taken hold, and studied with the outspoken British psychologist HAVELOCK ELLIS. Inspired by her visits to the Jacobs Birth Control Clinics in Holland, Sanger returned to the United States with renewed conviction and commitment.

Continually harassed by federal authorities, Sanger was indicted in 1915 for sending information on contraception through the mails. The following year she opened a birth-control clinic in Brooklyn, New York, the first one of its kind in America. The clinic was shut down by the police, and Sanger was imprisoned.

Sanger's crusade gradually won support in public and political circles, eventually forcing amendment or repeal of anti-birth control legislation. In 1917 Sanger helped to establish the National Birth Control League, which, in 1921, evolved into the American Birth Control League, and then the Planned Parenthood Federation of American in 1942, eventually becoming the Planned Parenthood World Population Organization in 1961. Other birth-control clinics emerged, and these were allowed to remain open. In 1923 Sanger organized the National Committee on Federal Legislation for Birth Control. She served as director until 1937, when the group's goals were fulfilled: birth control under medical supervision was legalized in almost all the states.

Sanger was tireless in her campaign, traveling throughout the country to help open clinics and deliver lectures on family planning and contraception. In 1921 she organized the first American conference on birth control and launched the first international conference four years later. Traveling throughout Europe, Africa and Asia, Sanger launched the birth-control movement in India and Japan, founding the International Planned Parenthood Association in 1953.

Throughout her career Sanger wrote extensively on her life's work, including an autobiography published in 1938. Other written works include *The Case for Birth Control* (1917); *Woman and the New Race* (1920); *Happiness in Marriage* (1926); *Motherhood in Bondage* (1928); and *My Fight for Birth Control* (1931).

Andrew Victor Schally 1926–

Along with ROGER GUILLEMIN and ROSALYN YALOW, Andrew Schally is responsible for clarifying the function of the hypothalamus in hormone production and regulation of the pituitary gland and for recording the ensuing effects on the body's chemistry.

Schally left his native Poland for England at the age of 13 after the Nazi invasion of 1939. He studied at the National Institute for Medical Research and received a doctorate in biochemistry from McGill University in Montreal. Schally began his studies of brain chemistry in 1957 at Baylor Medical School in Texas. From 1962 he continued his work at the New Orleans Veterans' Hospital and at Tulane University.

The hypothalamus is a tiny structure situated in the core of the brain just under the thalamus. Although it weighs less than an ounce, it plays an enormous role in the interaction between the body and the mind. For years scientists gave the pituitary, a pea-sized structure dangling from the hypothalamus, the status of "master gland", but Schally discovered that the pituitary receives its instructions from the hypothalamus. Working primarily with pig brains, Schally discovered the hormone produced in the hypothalamus that signals the pituitary gland to release its hormones. This view of the hormonal hierarchy established the hypothalamus as the interpreter between the brain and the glands, and understanding of the relationship between body chemistry and emotions opened new doors in the field of psychosomatic medicine.

In recognition of his discovery and synthesis of hypothalmic hormones Schally, along with Guillemin and Yalow, were awarded the Nobel Prize for Physiology or Medicine in 1977.

Bela Schick 1877–1967

A prominent figure in modern pediatric medicine, Bela Schick is best known for his contribution to the conquest of diphtheria. In 1913 he devised a technique, now known as the "Schick test," that determines a patient's vulnerability to the disease. Once epidemic in many parts of the world, diphtheria is a highly contagious disease most commonly found in children. In the year that Schick introduced his diagnostic method deaths from the disease reached 1200 in New York City alone.

When the body has been infected by the bacterial agent *Corynebacterium diphtheriae* the entire system is attacked by a toxic substance causing chills, fever, severe inflammation of the throat and larynx and eventually impairment of heart and peripheral nerve functions. As the toxins destroy throat tissue a tough gray membrane is formed, often leading to strangulation of the victim.

Adapting a diagnostic method previously used to disclose other illnesses, Schick injected a minute quantity of diphtheria toxin into the subject's skin. He noted that if swelling and reddening occurs at the site of the injection, the patient does not have adequate immunity to the disease. A negative reaction, in which no irritation appears, indicates the presence of sufficient natural antitoxins to provide immunity.

Although a serum had been developed that was effective in the prevention and treatment of diphtheria, it was administered reluctantly because of a number of negative side effects. The Schick test enabled physicians to practice selective immunization with confidence. By 1923 an improved method of antitoxin immunization without threatening side effects had come into use, and it is now routinely given within the first year of a child's life. A passionate advocate for the health and welfare of children, Schick led the campaign for universal immunization. His test retained its value as a means of detecting the decrease or loss of immunity later in life, and in the immunization of allergic patients.

Aside from his study of diphtheria, Schick's medical contributions include advances in the understanding of scarlet fever, infantile tuberculosis, the biochemical and endocrinological aspects of infectious diseases and infant nutrition. Of particular note is his research in collaboration with celebrated Austrian physician CLEMENS VON PIRQUET on the subject of allergies. Based on their landmark findings, Schick published an article in 1905 entitled "*Serumkrankheit*" in which he presents the first description of serum sickness, as well as a discussion of the basic principles of allergy.

Born in Boglar, Hungary, Schick was educated in Graz, Austria, where he received a degree in medicine from the Karl Franz University in 1900. Two years later he joined the faculty at the University of Vienna, where he served successively as intern, clinical assistant in pediatrics, lecturer and, beginning in 1918, professor of pediatrics.

By that time his work had earned him international distinction. Among the many honors he received was an invitation to deliver the Harvey Lecture at the New York Academy of Medicine in 1923. During his stay he accepted the offer to join the staff at New York's Mt. Sinai Hospital as pediatrician-in-chief.

An indefatigable worker, Schick devoted most of his time and efforts to the care of children. During his 20-year tenure at Mt. Sinai he maintained a private practice and served as director of pediatrics at Sea View Hospital. He also acted as consulting pediatrician at Willard Parker and Beth Israel Hospitals, and at the New York Infirmary for Women and Children (see ELIZABETH BLACKWELL). A founder of the American Academy of Pediatrics, Schick joined the faculty of the Columbia University College of Physicians and Surgeons in 1936 as clinical professor of childhood diseases.

Children loved and trusted the gentle Dr. Schick, who was often found romping on the floor of the pediatrics ward, delighting young patients with his humor and frivolity. In an office furnished with his collection of toys and dolls Schick would ease the anxiety of a new patient by playing a song on the piano he kept in a corner of the room.

Considered by many to be the greatest pediatrician of his time, Schick treated more than one million patients in the course of his career. Hundreds of thousands of New York City schoolchildren expressed their appreciation for his tireless efforts by signing their names in a massive book that was presented to Schick in 1933. He considered it one of his prize possessions.

In addition to publishing a number of articles appearing in journals throughout the world, Schick cowrote *Child Care Today* in collaboration with William Rosenson. Advancing a highly unconventional approach for its time, the book emphasized honesty, tenderness and love as the most important tools in parenting. Despite his warning that "the bad influences brought to bear upon the child early in life have a lasting effect," Schick also commented that "many children must have developed an immunity to delinquency because too many of them grow up into nice adults."

Up until his death at the age of 90 Schick regarded his career as an adventure. "There is always something more to learn in medicine," he said. "To be a good pediatrician it helps to be a little childish."

Matthias Jakob Schleiden 1804–1881

As one of the founding fathers of cell theory, Matthias Schleiden contributed to one of the most important advances in the history of life sciences. Schleiden was the first to determine the cellular structure of plants, introducing the revolutionary notion of the cell as a basic unit of life. Although the term had been coined 175 years earlier by English physicist ROBERT HOOKE, it had always referred to an empty unit, or void, rather than an elementary living particle. Prevailing scientific doctrine had assumed that living organisms were made up of fibers or vessels, with a developmental mechanism similar to that of crystals. Much of the explosion of scientific progress in the nineteenth and twentieth centuries is ascribed to the concept of the living cell.

After completing a course of study in botany in his native Germany Schleiden presented a discussion of cell theory in a paper entitled *Beitrage zur Phytogenesis (Contribution to Phytogenesis)*, published in 1838. Although mistaken in some conclusions, the insightful work highlighted the importance of the nucleus in cellular structure and propagation. In the following year Schleiden joined the faculty at the University of Jena, where he was to remain as professor of botany for the next 25 years.

It was THEODOR SCHWANN who applied Schleiden's theory of plant structure to animal tissue. Schwann's cell theory also contained a number of fundamental misconceptions, to be corrected in the next decade by German pathologist RUDOLF VIRCHOW.

William Scholl 1882–1968

With a unique combination of skills in medicine, business and shoemaking, William Scholl established an entire industry devoted to the health and comfort of the feet. Better known by his professional title, Dr. Scholl became a familiar figure to millions by raising public "foot consciousness" and providing an extensive line of products designed to treat such common complaints as corns, blisters and fallen arches.

It is doubtful that Dr. Scholl would have achieved such phenomenal success had he not been inspired by a lifelong fascination with shoes and feet. One of thirteen children, William Scholl grew up on a dairy farm in Iowa, where he became interested in shoe construction and repair at a young age. He studied the latest techniques and materials, developing his own type of waxed thread that proved more durable than any of the brands then available. Having served for many years as the family cobbler, Scholl decided, when he was sixteen, to make the hobby his profession. After a year's apprenticeship at local shop he left his family to earn a living at his trade in Chicago.

Encountering a large and varied clientele there, Scholl was struck by the extent to which his urban customers neglected their feet, often causing painful blisters, bunions, knots, gnarls and other deviations. Even more startling, Scholl found, was the fact that neither the shoe industry nor the medical establishment had ever addressed these widespread problems.

Dedicating himself to the advancement of foot care and public consciousness, Scholl enrolled in the Chicago Medical School, where he attended night classes while working at a shoe store during the day. William Scholl became Dr. Scholl in 1904 when, at the age of 22, he was granted not only a medical degree but his first patent—for the invention of an arch support that became known as the "Foot-Eazer." Designed as an insert to fit in a variety of shoes styles and sizes, the "Foot-Eazer" was the first of his many simple and effective inventions for maintaining foot comfort.

In the interests of sales promotion as well as public health Scholl founded a correspondence course in podiatry for shoe salesmen, also establishing a network of spokesmen throughout the country who spread, through medical and public lecture circuits, the message of healthy, attractive feet.

In addition to a number of popular and medical articles Scholl published *The Human Foot: Anatomy, Deformities, and Treatment* in 1915, and a more general reference, appearing a year later, entitled *Dictionary of the Foot*.

Keenly aware of the power of advertising, Scholl launched a campaign that initially drew complaints from the more conservative areas of the United States for its brazen display of a human foot, nearly naked except for a scanty corn pad or heel insert. Despite the controversy Scholl doggedly followed his personal and professional credo: "Early to bed, early to rise, work like hell and advertise." Imaginative promotion and persistent advertising eventually established a powerful consumer identification for his yellow-and-blue packaging and logo. By the 1950s the display of Dr. Scholl's wide range of foot-care products had become a familiar sight in pharmacies, supermarket and department stores.

Theodor Schwann 1810–1882

In 1839 Theodor Schwann published a work entitled *Mikroskopische Untersuchungen (Microscopic Investigations)*, in which he formulated a momentous truth: "There exists a general principle of construction [*Bildunsprinzip*] for all organic products, and...this principle of construction is cell formation."

Expanding on the hypothesis of cellular structure in plants as expounded by MATHIAS SCHLEIDEN, Theodor Schwann introduced one of the pivotal ideas in biology—the cell theory. Schwann's generalization of Schleiden's botanic studies launched the study of cytology, which led to the scientific understanding of physiological development, genetics and the mechanism of many diseases.

In microscopic studies of embryonic tissue Schwann had recognized a parallel between an animal's notochord and plant parenchyma, a tissue of round, thin-walled cells. Relating animal and plant development, Schwann's cellular theory directly opposed prevailing physiological notions about the importance of blood in animal tissue formation.

Schwann's cell theory included a number of misconceptions, most notably the belief that new cells arise independently of existing cells out of a matrix he called the cytoblastema. By the 1850s the term had become defunct when it was determined by German biologist Robert Remak (1815–1865), that new cells generally arise by the process of cell division. Nonetheless, Schwann and Schleiden pioneered the notion of the cell as the basic unit of life, which stimulated microscopical research in a number of scientific disciplines.

Schwann's own research led him to an investigation of the organic nature of yeasts. Although fermentation had been relied upon commercially for centuries as a means of creating bread, yogurt, tofu and alcohol, the process was generally considered a magical phenomenon until the mid-nineteenth century, when Schwann suggested that fermentation depends on the activity of live organisms. Later confirmed by Louis Pasteur and others, this theory paved the way for the modern study of enzyme chemistry.

A native of Neuss, Germany, Schwann was educated at the Universities of Bonn and Wurtzburg before he went to the University of Berlin to study under the legendary physiologist and teacher Johannes Peter Müller. Schwann became professor of physiology at the University of Louvain in 1838, where he taught for ten years. He then joined the faculty at the University of Liege, where he spent the greater part of his career. In addition to teaching Schwann continued to conduct physiological and biological research until the end of his life. Other notable studies include an investigation of muscle contraction, the discovery of the enzyme pepsin, and a demonstration of the organic nature of putrefaction (enzymatic decomposition, especially of proteins). His name appears in a number of medical terms, most notably the "sheath of Schwann," a thin membrane surrounding large nerve fibers, and the "Schwann cell," one of the masses of protoplasm lining the inner surface of the "sheath of Schwann."

Roland Boyd Scott 1909–

As founding director of the Howard University Center for Sickle Cell Disease, Roland Scott for 40 years has helped to draw international attention to this hereditary blood disorder that affects populations in Greece, Italy, Africa, the Middle East, Central and South America, the Caribbean and the blacks in North America. In 1988 50,000 people in the United States alone were diagnosed with sickle cell anemia, and 2 million more were found to have the genetic trait for the disease.

While bearers of the sickle cell trait may not show symptoms, they can pass the genetic abnormality to their offspring, so that if both parents are carriers, there is a 25% probability that their child will be afflicted with the blood disorder. The disease is named for the characteristic crescent shape of the red blood cells, which is caused by the presence of an abnormal hemoglobin. Unlike normal doughnut-shaped red blood cells, sickle-shaped cells are fragile and easily destroyed. Because they cannot circulate smoothly, they tend to jam the circulatory system, particularly in the small blood vessels. This impedes oxygenation of the tissues and vital organs, causing pain, sensitivity or numbness in various parts of the body.

The onset of the disease usually occurs in infancy and is often marked by enlarged organs, painful swellings and poor resistance to infection. In adolescence an increasing number of complications occur, including poor muscle development, delayed sexual maturation, ulcers, gallstones and various growth aberrations such as jaw or skull malformations.

Although a cure is yet to be found, life expectancy has been increased as a result of the efforts of Scott and his colleagues at the Center for Sickle Cell Disease. Launching investigations of the clinical and pathological nature of the disorder in the early 1940s, he was among the first to report on the disease in the United States. After a technique was developed for detecting the condition at birth, Scott introduced early and continued treatment with prophylactic penicillin, a practice that has saved hundreds of thousands of infants by reducing their susceptibility to life-threatening bacterial infections.

Born in Houston, Texas, Scott received his medical degree from Howard University in 1934. He served as resident and fellow in pediatrics at the University of Chicago and held those same positions in immunology at Roosevelt Hospital. Returning to Howard University in 1939, he joined the faculty as assistant professor in pediatrics, later becoming professor and head of the department.

In 1971 Scott founded the Center for Sickle Cell Disease, which became one of the first national centers of its kind to be sponsored by the National Institutes of Health. In addition to establishing a comprehensive program for clinical and laboratory research, the center provides training for medical students and professionals as well as guidance counselors, social workers and educators. Recognizing the urgent need for increased public awareness of sickle-cell disease, Scott emphasized the development of public health programs for genetic screening, early diagnosis and social and psychological counseling for patients and their families. In 1975 the center launched its community outreach program, a mobile health and education unit that provides free blood screening and counseling services throughout the Washington, D.C. area.

The author of more than 200 published papers, Scott has received widespread recognition from professional and public organizations for his outstanding work. In 1985 the American Medical Association and the Academy of Pediatrics presented him with the Jacobi Award for his outstanding contribution to pediatric medicine and national public health.

Florence Seibert 1897–

Florence Seibert helped to perfect the diagnosis of tuberculosis by introducing a purified protein derivative of tuberculin that proved more reliable than the original tuberculin. Robert Koch had isolated the microorganism responsible for tuberculosis in 1882, later developing tuberculin, a nonlethal derivative of the tubercle bacillus. Intended for use in the diagnosis and treatment of tuberculosis, Koch's form of tuberculin was impure and therefore unreliable in detecting the disease.

Working with three strains of human tuberculosis produced in a protein-free medium, Seibert precipitated and concentrated the culture, then subjected the substance to her own specially designed filtration process. Successfully isolating the active tuberculin protein, Seibert produced a form of tuberculin that would become a manufacturing standard for purity. In patients with tuberculosis the substance causes inflammation where it is injected under the skin but causes no reaction in healthy subjects.

A native of Easton, Pennsylvania, Seibert was severely crippled by infantile paralysis at the age of three. She entered Yale University as a medical student but was convinced by a professor that she would be physically unable to meet the responsibilities of a career in medicine.

Following his advice, she turned to chemistry, winning her degree in that field from Yale in 1923.

Seibert left Connecticut at the invitation to participate in a study of tuberculin being conducted at the University of Chicago. Before developing her method of "ultrafiltration" to produce purified protein derivatives, Seibert investigated another problem of chemical impurities occurring in the clinical use of distilled water. As a part of some surgical procedures, the injection of distilled water would occasionally produce a violent reaction despite stringent and repeated sterilization. Seibert recognized that although bacteria were killed in the process of sterilization, some traces of bacteria remained, reentering the water in steam droplets. Seibert ensured the purity of the water by inventing a still containing a trap for any droplets of steam—a device that had the further advantage of simplifying and shortening the sterilization procedure.

Ignaz Philipp Semmelweis 1818–1865

The sensitive and intense nature that drove Ignaz Semmelweis to a brilliant career of medical discovery also led to his tragic death in a mental institution at the age of 47. Anticipating LOUIS PASTEUR'S revelations of disease-causing bacteria, Semmelweis realized that puerperal fever was transmitted to women during childbirth by the contaminated hands of the very doctors who tended them.

A cruel and common form of death among nineteenth-century women, puerperal or childbed fever was rampant in maternity wards throughout Europe. The disease is a bacterial infection and poisoning of the blood resulting in fever and inflammation of the uterus, followed, if untreated, with fatal renal failure.

Semmelweis deduced the source of the contamination and proposed a practical means of preventing it. Although infection by invisible organisms was not yet established, Semmelweis recommended that after every medical procedure a surgeon should rid himself of germs before moving on to the next patient. Foreshadowing the work of JOSEPH LISTER, Semmelweis for the first time attempted to impose conditions of asepsis. Blinded by personal and professional antagonisms, the medical establishment did not accept Semmelweis's discovery until decades after his death.

Born in Hungary of German ancestry, Semmelweis grew up in Budapest, where his parents owned a grocery store. The language of his Austrian schoolmasters was different from the mixture of Hungarian and German he heard at home and in the street, and this linguistic confusion led to a lifelong insecurity in the presence of an audience.

After graduating in philosophy at the University of Pest Semmelweis left for Vienna to study imperial law, dutifully pursuing his father's dreams, if not his own. At the invitation of a friend who was studying at the University of Vienna Medical School, Semmelweis sat in on an anatomy class and was immediately inspired to embark on a medical career. He enrolled at the University of Vienna but left after one semester, finding the atmosphere oppressive and intimidating, particularly among his fellow students, who scorned Hungarians as provincials in the Austrian Empire. However, Semmelweis developed long and enduring relationships with a few of his professors at Vienna, in particular with noted Austrian physician Joseph Skoda.

After two years of study at the New School of Medicine in Budapest Semmelweis returned to the University of Vienna, where he completed his doctorate under the gentle guidance of Skoda and other influential faculty members, including distinguished pathologist KARL ROKITANSKY and Jacob Kolletschka, a professor of forensic medicine.

After receiving his degree Semmelweis entered a graduate program in obstetrics and surgery. At a time when nine out of ten operations resulted in serious infection or death, Semmelweis found the study of surgical practice a demoralizing experience. "Everything they are trying to do here seems to me quite futile," wrote Semmelweis to a friend. "Deaths follow one another with regularity. They go on operating, however, without seeking to find out why one patient succumbs rather than another in identical circumstances."

After obtaining a degree in surgery and obstetrics Semmelweis was hired to serve as first assistant to Professor Johann Klein in the maternity wards of Allgemeines Krankenhaus Vienna's enormous general hospital. Moving into cell-like living quarters on the wards, Semmelweis was surrounded day and night with the agonized cries of women in labor.

A bitter antagonism quickly developed between Semmelweis and his superior, who managed one of the two sections of the Lying-in Hospital. Both maternity divisions provided seemingly identical conditions and treatment, though the section under Klein's supervision was used as a clinical training ground for medical students, while the other division was used in the training of midwives. It was therefore a curious yet confirmed phenomenon that among the patients treated in Klein's section the mortality was generally four times higher than among the patients treated in the other section. Semmelweis found the mystery compelling and was determined to solve it, although the hospital staff seemed indisposed to consider the disparity.

Semmelweis noted that even among women arriving at the hospital after giving birth—usually under highly unfavorable and unsanitary conditions—the mortality rate was lower than that of Klein's patients. Confirmed in his suspicion that the key to the mystery was to be found in Klein's ward, Semmelweis began by controlling and monitoring the women's birthing positions, but he found no change in the statistics. At the implication that his staff was to blame, Klein's irritation gave way to fury. After several months he fired Semmelweis.

In an effort mainly to quiet any protest, officials of the health ministry set up a commission to examine the situation, but after a cursory inquiry the commission concluded that the increased deaths in Klein's ward were due to the rough examination techniques of the male medical students.

After his dismissal Semmelweis was dealt another painful blow. His good friend Kolletschka had died due to an accidental wound from a scalpel he received while performing an autopsy. Examining his friend's cadaver, Semmelweis recognized a similarity between his fatal lesions and those of the many thousands of women who were still dying of childbed fever.

Skoda and other influential friends had arranged for Semmelweis's reinstatement at the Lying-in Hospital after a suitable period of detente. Armed with two important new clues, Semmelweis eagerly returned to his detective work in the maternity wards. He was convinced that Kolletschka's death was caused by something he had received from the point of his scalpel after it had been used on a cadaver. In addition, the commission's misguided conclusion had suggested another discrepancy between the two sections: a difference in personnel. Semmelweis deduced that the medical students, who frequently performed autopsies and examinations in the maternity ward on the same day, were transmitting the disease from cadaver to patient.

Based on the findings of Irish physician Robert Collins and others, Semmelweis determined that contamination could be removed with a solution of chlorinated lime. Arranging for the disinfectant to be made available at the entrance to the wards, he posted signs throughout the maternity hospital, requesting that all students and doctors wash their hands in this solution before every examination.

Dramatic results confirmed Semmelweis's theory, while further antagonizing Klein and many of the staff and student body. Semmelweis's critics seemed to be vindicated when, despite precautions, a fatal outbreak of puerperal fever killed twelve women in a particular row of beds. Klein and his co-workers were bitterly disappointed when Semmelweis found that infection could be transmitted from one patient to another. He expanded his antiseptic procedure to include washings between patient examinations.

Though he knew little about the invisible agents he suspected, Semmelweis continued to develop his theory of contamination, eventually recognizing the possibility of airborne transmission of infection. This discovery led him to institute a policy of isolation rooms for infectious patients.

The medical community was slow to respond to Semmelweis's findings. Klein, bent on revenge, plotted the systematic destruction of his career, which he effectively accomplished by a series of professional and political maneuvers. Unrecognized and in desperate financial straits, Semmelweis worked for a time as a clinical professor at the University of Pest while trying to establish a private practice. Slowly overcoming a number of personal and professional pitfalls, he began to regain his spirits, and in 1857, at the age of 39, he met and married 19-year-old Marie Weidenhofer.

After a brief respite from private and public agonies Semmelweis returned to his war with the medical world. Public acceptance of his controversial ideas was further hindered by his intense and high-strung nature. In 1861, 10 years after his original discoveries, he published *The Etiology, Concept and Prophylaxis of Puerperal Fever*. The work might have been more kindly received if Semmelweis had not included a fanatical and contemptuous section condemning all those who doubted his findings. As it was, the book was largely dismissed, leaving Semmelweis frustrated and enraged. Having finally lost his lifelong verbal inhibitions, he now lashed out in vituperative open letters, addressing real and imagined enemies. His ever-worsening obsession was only briefly suspended during a period in which he became interested in recent advances in gynecological surgery. In that time he performed the first ovariotomy in Hungary.

His wildly combative moods returned and grew more extreme. In July, 1865 he was brought to a mental hospital in Vienna, where he was restrained in a straitjacket. A month later Semmelweis was dead, the result, ironically, of an infected scalpel wound that led to fatal blood poisoning. The autopsy report, when finally released, suggested that his death may have been the result of beatings by members of the hospital staff.

Sir Charles Scott Sherrington 1857–1952

"It has been remarked," wrote Charles Sherrington, "that...to refrain from an act is no less an act than to commit one, because inhibition is coequally with excitation a nervous activity."

For more than half a century Charles Sherrington studied the complexities of mammalian nervous function. His landmark research describing the integrative action of the nervous system forms the basis of modern neurophysiology. Sherrington demonstrated that even a reflex—a seemingly simple physiological event—is the result of a concert of activities occurring at various levels of the nervous system. Noting that muscles are arranged to operate in mutually antagonistic pairs, Sherrington introduced the principle of "reciprocal inhibition," which states that the contraction of any muscle requires the simultaneous and equal relaxation of an opposing muscle.

Central to Sherrington's concept of a "double distribution" of incoming sensation was the synapse, a term he introduced based on earlier observations by SANTIAGO RAMON Y CAJAL. The synapse is a functional and morphological junction between nerve cells where the transmission of nerve impulses can take place. An incoming stimulus is distributed through a web of pathways, or sensory fibers, with multiple synaptic transmissions either interferring or combining to produce the final response. Sherrington described the nervous system as an "enchanted loom" that "weaves a dissolving pattern, always a meaningful pattern, though never an abiding one; a shifting harmony of subpatterns."

A native of London, Sherrington was educated at Cambridge, where he began studying nerve transmission between the brain and the spinal cord. He taught pathology for several years at the University of London before joining the faculty at the University of Liverpool, where he was professor of physiology rom 1895 to 1913. During that time he produced his major work, *Integrative Action of the Nervous System*. Published in 1906, the book outlined the cooperative and reciprocal process of nervous function, establishing the notion of a sensorimotor loop through the spinal cord.

Along with his description of synaptic function, Sherrington's discovery of sensory receptors in the muscles, joints and tendons led to a clear description of the mechanism of muscular reflexes and the phenomenon of "proprioceptive sensation," which occurs from moment to moment as the brain receives a flow of information from the skeletal muscles that allows it to continually monitor and correct muscular movement.

Sherrington accepted a professorship of physiology at Oxford University, which he held from 1913 until 1935. While continuing his experimental studies in neurophysiology he was also active in the search for cholera, diphtheria and tetanus antitoxins. Sherrington's clinical research was influential in raising the standards of industrial health and safety conditions in England during World War I. In recognition of these efforts he was awarded a knighthood in 1922, followed two years later by the Order of Merit.

Sherrington continued to develop his model of integrative nerve action, defining the neuron or nerve cell as its basic unit. For his enormous contribution to the understanding of neuron function Sherrington was awarded the 1932 Nobel Prize for Physiology or Medicine, which he shared with EDGAR D. ADRIAN.

Sherrington also maintained a distinguished reputation as a poet and philosopher. His many written works include *The Brain and Its Mechanism*, published in 1933, and *Man on His Nature*, first published in 1940, with a second edition in 1952.

William Shippen Jr. 1736–1808

Pioneering the establishment of medical education in America, William Shippen Jr. and John Morgan cofounded the College of Philadelphia Medical School, the first center for medical training in the colonies. Shippen became the country's first professor of anatomy and surgery and Morgan the first professor of medical theory and practice.

The son of a noted physician and Continental congressman, William Shippen Jr. served three years as an apprentice to his father before he was sent to Europe to obtain a formal medical education. He studied anatomy in London with the celebrated JOHN AND WILLIAM HUNTER and completed his medical training at the University of Edinburgh under the guidance of distinguished Scottish physician WILLIAM CULLEN. After receiving his degree in 1761 Shippen returned to America to promote the techniques of obstetrics and midwifery he had learned in Europe.

Facing no competition, Shippen quickly became Philadelphia's leading male midwife, attracting a following for his lectures on obstetrics and anatomy. The medical school at the College of Philadelphia opened its doors in the spring of 1765, providing not only the first American instruction in anatomy but also the first training course in the practice of obstetrics. Shipped invited male students to enroll, as well as any women who had "virtue enough to own their ignorance and apply for instruction."

In 1775 Morgan was appointed director-general and physician-in-chief of the army divisions east of the Hudson River, and the following year Shippen was named chief physician and director of the Continental Army west of the Hudson. Competitive hostility took hold of both men, setting in motion a feud that eventually escalated into a national scandal. When the medical department of the military was reorganized, Morgan was fired from his position and, to add to his humiliation, replaced by Shippen. Within months Shippen was accused of embezzling military funds and was court-martialed. He was initially acquitted, but in a second trial the verdict was less conclusive. Although not fully vindicated, he returned to Philadelphia to resume his academic career as professor of anatomy, surgery and midwifery.

James Marion Sims 1813–1822

American physician and surgeon James Sims was the first to establish gynecology as a separate branch of medicine, creating one of the first areas of surgical specialization. After four years of experimentation on black slave women in Alabama Sims developed the first successful treatment of a vesicovaginal fistula—an abnormal opening between the vagina and the bladder, usually the result of a mishap in childbirth. A key element in the success of Sims's operation was the position of the patient. He had found that the operation was greatly facilitated when the woman lay semi-prone on her left side with her right knee brought up to her chest. This position, still adopted in some gynecological procedures, is now referred to as "Sims's position." Sims also lent his name to two instruments of his own improved design, "Sim's catheter" and "Sims's speculum," also known as a double duck-billed vaginal speculum.

A native of South Carolina, Sims studied at Charleston Medical School and Jefferson Medical College in Philadelphia. He was later to declare that his medical schooling had taught him nothing about the practice of medicine. Sims began his career as a physician in Alabama, where his reputation soon spread as an innovative and effective surgeon.

In 1853 he left for New York, where two years later he established the State Hospital for Women, the first hospital in the world to specialize in gynecological medicine.

William Smellie 1697–1763

William Smellie, a pioneer in obstetrics, was a prominent midwife and teacher in eighteenth-century London. At that time male midwives were still a source of controversy, often enduring the scorn and ridicule of the female members of their profession.

Mrs. Elizabeth Nihell, a midwife practicing in the area of London's Hay Market, publicly taunted Smellie, calling him "a great horse-godmother of a he-midwife." She described his "figure softened by his pocket night-gown of flowered calico or his cap of office tied with silk and silver ribbon." He thought that the feminine touch in his clothing would forestall any alarm his patients might feel at the thought of such intimate treatment at the hands of a man.

A native of Lanark, Scotland, Smellie received a degree in medicine in 1745 from the University of Glasgow. Returning to Lanark, he established a general practice in which he performed pharmacological and surgical duties as well as the traditionally simpler chores of a country doctor. Nonetheless, Smellie felt limited by the scope of his practice and set out for London in 1738. The following year he left for Paris to attend a series of lectures given by the noted French obstetrician Jean Gregoire.

Returning to England in 1739, Smellie set up a midwifery practice in Pall Mall, London. Without connections or influence in London's medical community Smellie could not practice in association with any hospital or clinic. He attended pregnant, often impoverished women in their own homes, maintaining detailed records of any unusual cases. Smellie's documented observations of more than eleven hundred births provide the earliest detailed description of parturition.

In 1752 Smellie published a major work on obstetrical practice entitled *A Treatise on the Theory and Practice of Midwifery*, which included detailed anatomical descriptions and measurements but was most valuable for its sound advice for the safe and effective practice of midwifery. The *Treatise* also laid out a set of basic rules, still followed today, for the safe use of forceps.

Smellie rejected the use of the "cranioclast," an instrument used to crack the skull of an unborn baby when it could not be pulled through the pelvic opening. He favored the Chamberlens' midwifery forceps, although he altered their design to meet his own specifications. He also created several other types of forceps covered in leather, some shaped to fit a baby's head and others to follow the mother's pelvic structure. These redesigned forceps were quickly followed by many other variations and new devices, prompting the suggestion from the more traditional London midwives that there were as many different styles of forceps as there were male midwives.

Smellie's teaching career was an important part of his contribution to the development of obstetric medicine. As soon as he began his London practice Smellie took on students of midwifery, posting a sign outside his house proclaiming "Midwifery Taught for Five Shillings."

In addition to bringing his students along on house calls, Smellie devised a teaching aid that provided a clear and effective method of elucidating the birth process. Out of human bones and leather Smellie constructed an articulated model of the female reproductive system in pregnancy, containing an artificial fetus that could be pulled through the channels of the model to simulate the process of parturition.

With this device Smellie was able to demonstrate appropriate procedures in difficult births, where the fetus might present itself in various positions that made delivery difficult or impossible. In the worst case, when the baby lies transversely across the birth passage, Smellie recommended the "podalic method," a strenuous process (for both mother and doctor) whereby the midwife repositions the baby by reaching in and drawing the feet away so that the head can point toward the mouth of the uterus. Students of midwifery were far more likely to complete this extraordinary procedure successfully after several practice attempts with Smellie's teaching device. Over a ten-year period more than 900 pupils benefited from Smellie's innovative teaching methods, as well as his extensive practical experience and medical insight.

Hamilton Othanel Smith 1931–

A key figure in the development of recombinant DNA techniques, microbiologist Hamilton Smith discovered a new class of restriction enzymes that recognize particular sequences of nucleotides in a DNA molecule and break the genetic strands at a specific site.

Several years earlier WERNER ARBER and others had established the existence of restriction enzymes, but this first group, later termed Type I, will randomly sever the DNA molecule at an unpredictable point along the strand of genetic material. Smith's identification of Type II restriction enzymes, known as endonucleases, permitted geneticists an unprecedented opportunity to map the structure of DNA and develop methods of controlled recombination of genetic information.

A native of New York City, Smith graduated from the University of California at Berkeley , receiving a degree in medicine from Johns Hopkins University in 1956. After his tour of duty as a navy medical officer he joined the faculty at the University of Michigan, returning to Johns Hopkins as a research geneticist in 1967.

It was two years later, while studying the interaction of the bacterium *Haemophilus influenzae* with DNA, that Smith and his colleagues recognized the presence of a second type of site-specific restriction enzyme. Microbiologist DANIEL NATHANS elaborated Smith's findings in an independent but complementary research project also conducted at Hopkins.

Type II restriction enzymes were immediately recognized as a powerful tool in practical and theoretical genetics. Hoping to draw upon the "knowledge" of the endonuclease to grant access to particular fragments of nucleic acid for observation and analysis, scientists look forward to a form of "chemical surgery" for correcting genetic deformities.

Appointed professor of microbiology in 1973, Smith was honored for his outstanding discovery five years later with the award of the Nobel Prize for Physiology or Medicine, which he shared with Werner Arber and Daniel Nathans.

Homer Smith 1895–1962

Physiologist Homer Smith launched a new era in the study of renal physiology with his discovery of new uses for inulin, a form of glucose found in the Jerusalem artichoke. Because of the unique way in which inulin is processed by the kidney, Smith saw in it a valuable tool in the study of renal function. Although Smith never became a physician, his extensive investigation of the urinary system was an important contribution to the modern understanding of the critical role of the kidneys.

Functioning as a biochemical monitoring system for the blood, the kidneys regulate levels of water, mineral salts, urea and other elements. By orchestrating the chemical composition of the body's fluids the kidney maintains a stable and favorable internal environment for the living cells of the body. The blood, containing waste products along with essential substances, enters the kidney through a filtering system consisting of several million nephrons. A nephron, or filtering unit, is a tubule with a structure at one end called the glomerulus or renal corpuscle.

When blood passes through the glomerulus waste products are extracted into the tubule, while vital substances remain in the blood as it is recycled back into general circulation by way of the glomerulus. In order to accurately assess renal function Smith sought to obtain a precise measure of the glomerular filtration rate. This was made possible by inulin, a substance characterized by the fact that it is excreted by the glomerulus without being altered in any way by the tubules.

Born in Denver, Smith grew up in the Colorado goldmining camp of Cripple Creek. When, at the age of nine, Homer received his first chemistry set, he was immediately enchanted by the magic of chemical experiments. He soon progressed to the mysteries of anatomy, performing surgical experiments with animals under the supervision of a neighboring medical student.

After receiving his bachelor's degree from the University of Denver in 1917 Smith joined the army as a lieutenant, taking charge of a research facility located at American University in Washington, D.C. His first studies were in the area of chemical warfare. After the war he shifted his focus to chemotherapy research, working under William H. Howell at the Johns Hopkins University School of Hygiene and Public Health. After receiving his doctorate in 1921 Smith held research positions at the Eli Lilly Laboratories, the National Research Council at Harvard and the University of Virginia. In 1928 he was invited to head the New York University College of Medicine as director of the Physiological Laboratory. He was to retain the position for 31 years, helping to establish the laboratory as an internationally celebrated center for renal function research.

Smith dedicated his life to the study of kidney mechanism as a means of better understanding the broader principles of physiology, pathology, evolution and even philosophy. He went on an expedition to Kenya seeking the lungfish, a living relative of an ancient air-breathing fish. Fascinated by this "evolutionary experiment" with two respiratory resources, Smith was eager to study an animal that lived in the same way "as did his Devonian ancestors." Burying itself in mud for long periods of time, the lungfish is forced to burn its own tissues for fuel. Its kidneys must stop functioning for as long as it lives without water.

Smith published a number of written works, fictional and nonfictional, on subjects ranging from the concept of free will to the physiology of goosefish to the power of myth in human affairs. His philosophic novels include *Kamongo,* a best-seller of 1935, and *The End of Illusion.* His nonfiction works include *From Fish to Philosopher, Physiology of a Kidney, The Kidney: Structure and Function in Health and Disease* and *Man and His Gods.*

Theobald Smith 1859–1934

In demonstrating the spread of Texas cattle fever American pathologist Theobald Smith was among the first to emphasize the significance of animals as agents in the transmission of disease. Smith traced the disease to the parasite *Piroplasma bigeminum* and explained how it was passed from animal to tick to animal in a cycle of infection. He showed that the protozoon enters the red blood cells of an animal; ticks, feeding on the infected cattle, ingest the microorganism, passing it on to their own offspring. The young ticks in turn feed on other cattle, in the process transmitting the parasite.

Also recognized for his important contribution to theoretical immunology, Smith formulated a principle of antigen-antibody reaction in laboratory animals known as anaphylaxis or the "Theobald Smith phenomenon." The injection of a foreign protein or antigen may cause an exaggerated reaction, rendering the animal hypersensitive to a second injection of the same substance, Smith found. The violent reaction, which may include choking, loss of consciousness and possibly death, results from an overproduction of antibodies, causing the sudden neutralization of the antigen. Smith distinguished this "active" form of anaphylactic reaction from "passive anaphylaxis," which can be produced by injecting an animal with the blood of a sensitized donor.

Other significant research included a microbiological study of tuberculosis in which Smith first differentiated between human and bovine forms of tubercle bacilli. With DANIEL SALMON he helped establish the effectiveness of vaccines using killed microorganisms.

Smith was born in Albany, New York, where he earned his degree in medicine in 1883 from Albany Medical College. He taught bacteriology for nine years at Columbian University (now known as George Washington University) in Washington, D.C. In 1896 he left there to take the post of professor of comparative pathology at Harvard, where he remained until 1915. At the invitation of the Rockefeller Institute (now Rockefeller University) he accepted the directorship of the department of animal pathology, retaining that position until 1929.

George Davis Snell 1903–

In the 1940s pioneer immunologist George Snell launched an investigation of the genetic factor in immunological response, introducing the term "histocompatibility-gene-complex" to refer to a group of genetically determined antigens that control an individual's ability to recognize and react to a foreign substance.

Providing an explanation for the variations in individual resistance to disease and infection, Snell's discovery of histocompatibility genes in mice were later confirmed by noted French immunologist JEAN DAUSSET who established the existence of an analogous complex of genes in humans known as the HLA (human leucocyte antigen) complex. These systems are seen as two types of the "major histocompatibility complex" (MHC) found in all vertebrates.

In 1980 Snell, Dausset and fellow immunologist Baruj Benacerraf were recognized for their breakthrough discoveries in genetic immunology with the award of the Nobel Prize for Physiology or Medicine. Acknowledging the medical significance of Snell's biological research, the committee cited his discovery of "the genetic factors that determine the possibilities of transplanting tissue from one individual to another...With Snell's fundamental discoveries came the birth of transplantation immunology."

Although the function of HLA antigens is to help the body to defend itself against disease-causing organisms, an unfortunate by-product of their ability to recognize foreign cells is the rejection of transplanted organs. The HLA complex is thought to hold the key to successful organ transplants on a much broader scale than is now possible. By identifying the antigens that influence the immune response to transplanted organs, it may be possible to match donors and recipients more closely, thus reducing the risk of rejection.

Born in Bradford, Massachussetts, Snell completed graduate studies at Dartmouth in 1926 and received his doctorate in biology and immunology from Harvard four years later. At the University of Texas he trained under distinguished biologist HERMANN MULLER, who had been conducting genetics experiments with fruit flies for more than twenty years. After Muller's departure in 1932 Snell left for Bar Harbor, Maine to join the staff at the Jackson Laboratory.

In 1942 Snell launched a large-scale investigation of genetic variations in mice, carrying out a complex and tedious process of cross-breeding and back-cross-breeding in order to create strains with only the slightest genetic variations. Five years later his painstaking efforts were destroyed by a fire at the laboratory, but Snell took up the work again from the beginning, remaining at Jackson Laboratory until his official retirement in 1969.

A member of the National Academy of Sciences, the Genetic Society of America and the Transplantation Society, Snell has received worldwide recognition for his outstanding achievements and numerous honors, including the Bertner Foundation Award in Field Cancer Research in 1962, the Gregor Mendel Medal from the Czechoslovak Academy of Sciences in 1967 and the International Award of the Gairdner Foundation in 1976.

With Jean Dausset and Stanley Nathanson Snell published *Histocompatibility* in 1976. Other notable written works include *The Biology of the Laboratory Mouse* (1941).

By the time Snell was given the Nobel Prize in 1980 he had not conducted research for nearly seven years. "I retired at 70," he explained. "I could have gone back to the lab and done more work, but you can't do this sort of thing halfway."

John Snow 1813–1858

John Snow is best known for two remarkable achievements, one requiring a keen understanding of scientific method, the other requiring an equally keen grasp of political method. Snow was the first to demonstrate that cholera was caused by a contagion that might be communicated through drinking water. He is also credited with greatly advancing the science of anesthesiology, particularly as applied to childbirth.

Snow began his medical career as apprentice to a surgeon at Newcastle-on-Tyne in England during the great cholera epidemic of 1831–1832. He watched as patients endured the torments of this disease (or, as is now known, group of diseases). Symptoms might include acute diarrhea, vomiting, severe muscular cramps and intense thirst. Patients in the later stages of the disease would frequently sink into coma and possibly die of shock.

The young Snow was horrified at the devastation he observed. At the Hunterian School in London he began to systematically catalog all the most serious outbreaks of cholera. By careful investigation of dates and locations Snow observed a pattern in the "behavior" of the disease, which seemed to originate in India and travel westward over a period of centuries, eventually arriving in London and Paris, where by 1849 it had become a frightening epidemic. By paying attention to clues offered in every outbreak along the way Snow arrived at the ingenious conclusion that cholera was spreading by way of a contaminated water supply. The next wave of the disease, in 1858, allowed Snow the chance to prove his theory. He established that a public well in London known as the Broad Street Pump was being contaminated by leaks in a nearby sewer and that all those who drank that water came down with cholera. The etiology of the disease was determined twenty-five years later by celebrated bacteriologist Robert Koch, who discovered the villainous bacteria, known as *Vibrio cholerae*, or sometimes *Vibrio comma*, for its curved shape. The next giant steps in the study of bacterial infection were to be made by JOSEPH LISTER and LOUIS PASTEUR.

While Snow was still an apprentice, chemists in New York and Paris were independently creating a new solution that twenty years later would bring together the fates of Queen Victoria, pregnant woment in pain and the clever Dr. Snow. In addition to his interest in the spread of cholera Snow devoted a great part of his professional practice to administering anesthesia. He had followed the American experiments with ether and conducted many of his own in an effort to develop a reliable technique for administering the drug to patients. After a successful public demonstration his efforts were recognized by St. George's Hospital, and London's entire "ether practice" fell to Snow, who became the first English anesthetist.

Meanwhile the new spiritous solution of chloric ether, dubbed "chloroform" by Jean-Baptiste Dumas in 1835, had found its way to Scotland where noted obstetrician James Simpson became an enthusiastic proponent of this new and powerful drug. After experimenting on himself and his staff Simpson began using it on patients during childbirth, despite a tide of vehement public opinion against the interference, (in light of the biblical directive "In sorrow shalt thou bring forth"). Although Snow's expertise was in the administration of ether, he was eager to expand the scope of anesthesiology. After conducting his own experiments he recognized the tremendous value of chloroform for relieving the pain of childbirth. When he administered chloroform to the devout and revered Queen Victoria, first during her delivery of Prince Leopold in 1853 and again when Princess Beatrice was born in 1857, he instantly ensured its respectability. In fact, this method of relieving pain in childbirth became known as "chloroform a la reine." Since the nineteenth century our approach to relieving pain has evolved considerably, and chloroform is no longer used in childbirth due to its dangerous side effects, but Snow's work was vital to the progress of anesthesiology. He published the results of his findings in 1858 in a book entitled *On Chloroform and Other Anaesthetics*.

George Soulié de Morant 1878–1955

As a leading Western authority on Chinese medicine, George Soulié de Morant is largely responsible for introducing the practice of acupuncture into Occidental culture. Among the first to graduate from the newly established School of Oriental Languages in Paris, Soulié de Morant was hired to travel to China as the representative of a French bank. He was twenty when he arrived in Shanghai in 1899, and by the start of the new year and the new century he had been appointed French consul by the Ministry of Foreign Affairs.

Facing a major outbreak of cholera during his first year in office, he went on a tour of hospitals in the region of Yunnanfu, where the epidemic was particularly fierce. Soulié de Morant noted with some surprise that "treatment of patients by means of needles had better results than the medicines available at the time." Investigating the various applications of this mysterious medical practice, he became convinced of the enormous benefits of acupuncture and embarked on a formal study of the technique.

In 1908 he was granted the title of Master Physician by the Viceroy of Yunnan, later receiving the "Engraved Coral Button" from the government of China signifying the official rank of academician. His diploma was a long silk banner carrying one hundred signatures of distinguished citizens, each affirming that he had cured them "of an illness that does not cure itself."

Soulié de Morant remained in China for more than twenty years conducting an exhaustive study of ancient medical treatises. Recognizing the value of classic acupuncture techniques for Western medicine, he devoted much of his time to the translation of the major Chinese reference works. He also absorbed the subtle refinements of acupuncture technique from observing firsthand some of China's most noted practitioners.

Because of obstacles of geography, language, politics and culture, Eastern medical knowledge had been all but inaccessible to the rest of the world for many centuries. Interest in acupuncture began to emerge in France at the beginning of the nineteenth century, most notably with the attentions of RENÉ LAËNNEC, P.F. BRETONNEAU and physician Armand Trousseau (1801–1867). A European form of acupuncture bearing little relation to Chinese doctrines was practiced by a number of nineteenth-century French doctors, including Joseph Berlioz, the father of the composer.

In 1921 Soulié de Morant returned to France bearing his cargo of Oriental medical lore. He captured widespread attention with his first public demonstration of acupuncture, performed at the Hospital St. Antoine in Paris. Treating a patient with hemiplegia, a form of paralysis affecting only one side of the body, he inserted three needles at different points. In less than an hour he successfully cured a condition that had existed for several years. In the years that followed Soulie de Morant conducted clinical demonstrations at Bichat and other distinguished hospitals in and around Paris, attracting a devoted following of students and patients.

In 1928 he published a treatise on the examination of the pulse as a diagnostic method (see HUANG-TI), and six years later he produced the *Precis de la vraie acupuncture chinoise* (*Abstract on True Chinese Acupuncture*). He developed the ideas of the *Precis* in a two-volume reference work entitled *L'Acupuncture Chinoise*. Published in 1939, the book attracted interest throughout Europe and America, sparking a number of studies and published reports.

Despite increasing recognition for acupuncture, there remained considerable resistance among physicians, who actively opposed the practice of acupuncture in the West. In the mid-1940s the French Order of Physicians accused Soulie de Morant of practicing medicine illegally. Although they later agreed to drop the charge, he decided to emigrate to the United States. Named professor of acupuncture at several American universities, he was nominated for a Nobel Prize in 1950.

Soranus c. 98–117 A.D.

As one of earliest authorities on obstetric, gynecological and pediatric medicine, Soranus laid down clinical guidelines and practices that were to be followed for the next fourteen centuries. The skills of this astute clinician and surgeon have been celebrated by medical luminaries from Galen to AMBROISE PARÉ. It was Paré who rediscovered and revived the practice of "internal version," a technique developed by Soranus for use in cases of abnormal presentation of the fetus. To shift the fetus into a better position for delivery, Soranus inserted his hand through the vagina into the uterus, pushing the head away and drawing the feet toward the birth canal.

Soranus described many of his clinical observations and innovative techniques in an influential treatise entitled *On Midwifery and the Diseases of Women* (translated in 1882). In this enduring work Soranus not only offered important advances in medical knowledge of female anatomy and physiology but also emphasized a gentle and sensible approach to women in labor. Although he advised rupturing the membranes to hasten a slow and painful delivery, he rejected the use of force, invasive instruments or strong medication to speed the process. Soranus was a compassionate practitioner with a strong sense of responsibility to both mother and child. He asserted that "the fruit of conception is not to be destroyed at will because of adultery or of care for beauty, but is to be destroyed to avert danger appending to birth..."

In his book on midwifery, Soranus describes various conditions leading to complications in childbirth, including pelvic abnormalities and inflammation of the genital area. He was also the first to suggest emptying the bladder before delivery by means of a catheter. Although forbidden by law to perform dissections, Soranus made important observations on female reproductive anatomy. Clearly describing the structure of the uterus, Soranus demonstrated that the organ could be safely removed by surgery.

Soranus stressed kindness and reason in all areas of his practice, disdaining superstition and paying due attention to the psychological element in disease and pain. He used psychological methods of treatment for a number of physiological disorders, including menstrual difficulties. Soranus also introduced a system of classification for mental disorders that endured through the Middle Ages, based on a wide range of symptoms, including depression, agitation, hallucinations, etc.

Born at Ephesus in Asia Minor, Soranus studied at Alexandria, a celebrated center for medical education. He left to establish a practice in Rome, where he gained a distinguished reputation during the reigns of Trajan and Hadrian. In addition to his work in gynecology and obstetrics Soranus was a noted surgeon and general practitioner. His other written works include treatises on fractures, dislocations, vasomotor paralysis, pleurisy and various mental disorders.

Lazzaro Spallanzani 1729–1799

Lazzaro Spallanzani definitively resolved one of the great scientific controversies of the eighteenth century—the debate over the theory of "spontaneous generation," the fallacious belief that microorganisms develop from nonliving organic material.

Based on experiments with sealed containers of boiled broth, English bacteriologist J.T. Needham (1713–1781) staunchly defended the ancient concept of spontaneous generation, also known as abiogenesis. Demonstrating that microbes would "appear" only if heating had been insufficient or if air were inadvertently admitted to the container, Spallanzani discredited Needham's experiment and his findings. Spallanzani's work led the way for the enormous strides taken by bacteriologists of the next generation, including LOUIS PASTEUR and C.J. DAVAINE in France, J. Tyndall (1820–1893) in England and F.J. COHN in Silesia (Poland).

Born and educated in Italy, Spallanzani taught biology at the University at Reggio until 1763. He left to teach at the university in his native Modena until 1769, after which he joined the faculty at the University of Pavia where he served as professor for the next three decades.

In addition to his refutation of abiogenesis Spallanzani conducted further studies in the field of regeneration. Following Spallanzani's success in reanimating dried rotifers after long periods of dormancy, naturalists Jean-Baptiste Lamarck and MARIE FRANCOIS XAVIER BICHAT developed their influential theories on the nature and definition of the "life force."

Spallanzani was also a pioneer in the field of fertilization. Published in 1780, his writings accurately define the functions of spermatozoa and ovum and document his discovery of artificial insemination. Also documented are Spallanzani's studies on digestion, firmly establishing the chemical nature of this process. This understanding came with his discovery of the digestive action of saliva. Spallanzani's experimental work with gastric juice demonstrated its dissolving effect on food.

Hans Spemann 1869–1941

Hans Spemann's experiments with newt embryos revealed the complex feedback mechanisms involved in embryonic development. By transplanting pigmented tissues from one embryo to another Spemann was able to track their functions and interaction at each stage in the developmental process. For his discovery of "embryonic induction," the interactive process among tissues in the embryo, Spemann was awarded the Nobel Prize for Physiology or Medicine in 1935.

Educated in Stuttgart and Heidelberg, Spemann was named director of Berlin's Kaiser Wilhelm Institute of Biology in 1914. In 1919 he joined the faculty at the University of Freiburg as professor of zoology. It was there that he conducted his now- celebrated experiments in order to investigate the mechanism responsible for embryonic cell growth and differentiation.

Working with Hilde Mangold, Spemann found that cellular material is altered as it comes in contact with the dorsal lip of the blastopore, which serves as an "organizer" for the developmental process.

Noting that "organizers" influence various areas of the embryo to develop into differentiated organs and tissues, Spemann determined that cell differentiation is dependent on the relative positions of the cells and on various "organizer centers." These findings confirmed that each embryonic stage is necessary to induce the next stage.

Spemann's work conclusively overturned "pre-formation" theories of embryonic development based on the idea of an embryo expanding into a pre-existing form. In addition, his findings gave rise to a better understanding of congenital birth defects and fetal abnormalities.

Spemann outlined his research in *Embryonic Development and Induction*, published in German in 1936 and translated into English in 1938.

Roger Sperry 1913–

Roger Sperry's classic studies of "split-brain" individuals provided an alternative to what he considered science's demeaning and dehumanizing view of the human mind. These studies earned him the Nobel Prize for Physioloogy or Medicine in 1981 (shared with DAVID HUBEL and TORSTEN WIESEL) and transformed our understanding of left- and right-brain capabilities. Through his observations of mind-brain interaction Sperry established a scientifically acceptable context for the discussion of human consciousness.

Sperry's first neural experiments began while he was a graduate student at Oberlin College and were designed to challenge the theories of his mentor, PAUL WEISS. Sperry wanted to refute the idea that neural activity was determined solely by external causes. By experimenting with the vision of salamanders Sperry proved that the organization of neural networks is independent of the function they perform. His theory of predetermined nerve connections, based on an internal chemical code system, was developed over the next decade and became a vital step in the study of developmental neurobiology.

In the years that followed, Sperry's ideas met with great resistance, particularly from the growing ranks of behaviorists; but in 1954, after extensive animal studies, Sperry found a means of supporting and expanding his humanistic views in a powerful and dramatic way. He had been appointed Hixon Professor of Psychobiology at the California Institute of Technology, a post he was to hold for over thirty years. At the institute's hospital he encountered "split-brain" patients, individuals whose corpus callosa (the connecting cables between right and left hemispheres) had been severed surgically. At the time, the popular view was that the right brain was vastly inferior to the left brain, which had long been recognized as the site of linguistic ability. In his experiments Sperry found that a split-brain patient might deny the existence of an object placed out of view in his left hand (visual data from the left hand is sent to the right side of the brain). However, the same individual was able to correctly interpret information by nonverbal modes, such as searching by feel with the left hand for a matching object. Although Sperry's subjects would claim to be merely guessing, they would invariably make the proper selection from a group of items.

Through hundreds of experiments Sperry and his colleagues gleaned vital information about the heretofore mysterious right side of the brain. It is now widely recognized to be the seat of intuition and emotion as well as the center for processing visual and spatial information, or "mental images." The left side of the brain houses verbal, mathematical and logical skills.

Perhaps Sperry's most important contribution was his revolutionary presentation of the dual nature of human consciousness. In his observations of the effects of split-brain surgery Sperry found that each disconnected hemisphere could sustain an awareness and control of behavior that was independent of, and at times even contradictory to, the other. Sperry defined a new doctrine known as mentalism that holds that mental events can be viewed as physical properties of brain processes and can determine or explain behavior. Sperry stated:

> The key realization was that the higher levels in brain activity control the lower...They call the plays, exerting downward control over the march of nerve-impulse traffic. Our new model, mentalism, puts the mind and mental properties to work and gives them a reason for being and for having evolved in a physical system...Since each side of the surgically divided brain is able to sustain its own conscious volitional system...the question arises as to why, in the normal state, we don't perceive ourselves as a pair of separate left and right persons instead of the single, apparently unified mind and self that we all feel we are...Consciousness can be viewed as a higher emergent entity that supersedes the sum of its right and left awareness.

Sperry's attention to the nonmaterial aspects of human brain activity, its timing, spacing and holistic properties, allowed him to expand the scope of scientific observation and application to include consciousness, ethics and free will.

Benjamin McLane Spock 1903–

Perhaps the best-known pediatrician in history, Benjamin Spock has had a career that is almost as controversial as it has been influential. Spock's book *The Common Sense Book of Baby and Child Care,* presenting an approach to child-rearing that was a radical departure from the prevailing attitudes of the time, brought accusations that Spock had single-handedly produced the worldwide rebellion of youth in the 1960s. First published in 1946, Spock's guide has sold over 30 million copies, more than any other book published in the United States. With a reassuring tone and an emphasis on good judgment Spock suggested a rational, individualized approach to child-rearing, forgoing the more rigid methods generally recommended in America in the 1940s.

Born in New Haven, Connecticut, Spock was on the Yale crew team that won a gold medal at the Olympic Games of 1924. Graduating the following year, Spock went on to Columbia University College of Physicians and Surgeons, where he obtained his medical degree in 1929. He began pediatric practice in 1933, but it was his outspoken opinions on political issues as well as on child care that established Spock as a public figure of international prominence.

In 1955 he was named professor of child development at Western Reserve University in Ohio, where he remained until 1967. Spock resigned from teaching in order to fully devote his time and attention to the campaign against the Vietnam War. In 1968 he published a book, written with Mitchell Zimmerman, entitled *Dr. Spock on Vietnam.* In the same year he successfully overturned a conviction under the anticonscription law while running for president as the candidate of the People's Party, a liberal coalition of pacifists and populists.

Maintaining an active role in the nuclear disarmament movement, Spock was arrested more than a dozen times for acts of civil disobedience. In 1970 he published *Decent and Indecent: Our Personal Political Behavior.* As candidate for the People's Party, Spock ran for president again in the 1972 election, and for vice-president in 1976.

Other published works include *A Baby's First Year* (1954); *Feeding Your Baby and Child* (1955); and *Raising Children in a Difficult Time* (1972).

Wendell Meredith Stanley 1904–1971

"The viruses hold the key to the modification—for better or worse—of all life," Wendell Stanley stated in 1956. "They hold the key to the secret of life, to the solution of the cancer problem, to biological evolution, to the understanding and control of heredity, perhaps to the nature of all future life on earth."

As a college football star in the early 1920s Wendell Stanley was looking forward to a promising career as a sports coach when a chance encounter with a chemistry professor precipitated a series of momentous reactions.

That fortuitous conversation inspired Stanley to change the course of his life, leading him, in the decades that followed, to a Nobel Prize and world renown as a biochemist and virologist with a major influence on cancer research and immunology.

Subsequently hailed as a historic step in scientific research, Stanley's study of the tobacco masaic virus was launched in 1932 at the Princeton laboratory of Rockefeller Institute. Establishing that the virus is a protein substance, he isolated a pure concentrate of the infectious material in the form of dry, needlelike crystals. When the inert crystals were later dissolved in a water-based solution Stanley found that even after years of storage in an inert state the reproductive and infective functions of the virus were fully reactivated. In recognition of this revolutionary discovery, in addition to his detailed analysis of the molecular structure and characteristics of the virus, Stanley was awarded the 1946 Nobel Prize for Chemistry, which he shared with distinguished virologists John H. Northrop and James B. Sumner.

Born in Ridgeville, Indiana, Stanley was an undergraduate student at nearby Earlham College when he decided to pursue a career in science. He completed his education at the University of Illinois, receiving a doctorate in chemistry in 1929. Two years later he joined the faculty at the Rockefeller Institute for Medical Research, where he conducted the landmark investigation that would win international prominence for Stanley while he was still in his early thirties.

In the early 1940s Stanley conducted a series of investigations of various viral diseases, including, most notably, a study of influenza that led to the development of a vaccine, that was widely used to prevent influenza during World War ll.

In 1946 Stanley was en route to California when an unscheduled layover at a Wyoming airport set the stage for another fortuitous encounter with far-reaching consequences. Among the detained passengers was Robert Gordon Sproul, president of the University of California, who talked with Stanley for several hours as they waited for the weather to clear. Profoundly impressed with Stanley's ideas on the direction of virology research, Sproul subsequently offered him the opportunity to establish and preside over a virus laboratory at the Berkeley campus.

Opening its doors in 1948, the California Virus Laboratory was the largest research facility of its kind. An energetic and innovative director, Stanley led the center in investigations of the fundamental nature of life and the prevention of infectious disease, contributing significantly to the development of a number of vaccines, most notably the polio vaccine.

During the "red hunts" of Joseph McCarthy in the early 1950s Stanley joined a large segment of the Berkeley faculty in defying the university's request that he sign an oath of loyalty to the United States, condemning the demand as an abridgment of academic freedom.

Throughout his career Stanley was an outspoken advocate of the viral theory of cancer (see A.BORREL), most notably during the 1930s and 1940s, when the greater part of the medical research establishment challenged the relevance of virology in cancer research. Addressing a joint conference of the National Cancer Institute and American Cancer Society in 1956, Stanley declared:

> Evidence for the virus etiology of cancer has come from so many different laboratories and has been of such good quality that I find it very difficult to understand why so many investigators have continued to have such a firm blind spot...I continue to be amazed at the willingness of so many investigators to accept viruses as etiological agents for animal cancers and their unwillingness to consider them...in cancers in man (see PEYTON ROUS).

Another leading spokesman for the viral theory of cancer was noted surgeon and researcher Joseph W. Beard, who recalled the difficulties faced by the small circle of cancer-virologists in the 1940s: "We were as welcome as a bachelor at a family reunion," he said. "The virologists were not interested in tumours, and the animal cancer workers were not interested in viruses." By 1960 the tide had begun to turn in favor of the viral theory of cancer, and in the following decades conclusive evidence has confirmed the role of viruses in several forms of cancer.

Ernest Henry Starling 1886–1927

The word "hormone" is taken from the Greek and translates literally as "I arouse activity." The term was first used by E.H. Starling in 1905 to refer to a substance secreted by a particular organ, transported by the bloodstream and having a specific effect on another organ.

Although he prepared for a career in medicine, Starling joined the physiology department of London's University College as a researcher, where he embarked on studies that would revolutionize the field of biological science. He also taught physiology there and at Guy's Hospital, but his greatest commitment was to the pioneer research he achieved, much of it in collaboration with Sir William Bayliss. In 1902 they isolated secretin from the duodenum and showed that the substance traveled in the bloodstream to the pancreas, causing it to discharge digestive enzymes into the stomach. This discovery was an off shoot of William Beaumont's dramatic launching of the study of gastroenterology. Bayliss and Starling in turn launched the study of endocrinology with their remarkable findings. They began an investigation of the endocrine glands, which secrete their substances into the blood (as opposed to the exocrine glands, whose secretions are sent to their destination through a duct).

Starling was admired for his innovative experimental techniques that enabled him to explore the intricacies of intestinal, circulatory and coronary activity. His studies of the heart demonstrated that the energy of muscle contraction is a function of the length of muscle fiber. This correlation is known as Starling's law, which launched yet another important branch of medicine, the physiology of exercise. Another notable discovery was that of osmotic equillibrium in the capillaries, which governs the formation of lymph and the secretion of urine.

In World War I Starling turned his attentions to developing antidotes to poison gases. His many published works include *Principles of Human Physiology*, written in 1912.

Niels Stenson (var. Niels Stenson, Nicolaus Steno) 1638–1686

Niels Stenson led a conflicted life, torn between a deep scientific curiosity and an equally strong dedication to the Roman Catholic Church. He conducted innovative research in the fields of geology and anatomy but also converted from Lutheranism in 1667 to become a priest in 1675 and a vicar apostolic in 1677.

Born in Denmark, he lived and studied in Copenhagen, Paris, Amsterdam, Leyden and Florence. In addition to his observations of fossils, geologic strata and crystallization, Stenson studied the most vital areas of human anatomy—the heart, muscles, brain and glands. He confirmed the distinction between the glands and the lymph nodes (occasionally referred to as glands, but not part of the glandular system anatomically). He also confirmed MALPIGHI'S theories on the incubation of the ovum in humans and described the essential structure of the heart. He disproved the ancient belief that tears originate in the brain and in 1661 discovered the excretory duct of the parotid gland (one of two identical salivary glands). This is now known as the duct of Steno.

In the last decade of his life Stenson abandoned scientific pursuits and devoted himself exclusively to a life of missionary work.

Patrick Christopher Steptoe 1913–1988

Patrick Steptoe and his colleague Robert G. Edwards invented in vetro fertilization, revolutioning medical practice and raising pethora of philosophical, ethical and legal questions.

Fertilization normally takes place in the fallopian tubes, and natural conception is therefore difficult or impossible in a woman whose tubes are damaged or missing. Steptoe, a practicing obstetrician, established a way to remove the egg cells from the ovary, and Edwards, a specialist in female physiology, devised a system for controlling the ovulation cycle in order to have several egg cells available on demand. Together they developed a procedure in which human eggs can be fertilized by sperm in a glass container and then, after a brief period of development, reinserted into the uterus, where pregnancy would proceed in the usual fashion. The controversy that ensued was inevitable, no matter what name was given to this radical new procedure. Only a century before the idea of relieving the pain of childbirth had been severely criticized as unnatural and irreligious (see JOHN SNOW). Creating life outside the body was fraught with no less controversy.

Steptoe's daring medical career began at St. George's Hospital Medical School in London. He was licensed by the Royal College of Physicians in 1939 and also became a member of the Royal College of Surgeons. Serving as a naval surgeon in the Royal Volunteer Reserve during World War II, he was taken prisoner in 1941 and brought to Italy. His status as a physician allowed him a certain amount of freedom in the camp, and he used this privilege to help other prisoners escape. He was caught and put in solitary confinement and was not released until a prisoner exchange in 1943.

Back home in Manchester, England Steptoe completed medical studies in gynecology and began his practice, focusing on the problems of infertility. He developed his method of retrieving eggs from the ovary and perfected the use of the laparoscope, a tube that contains an optical-fiber light and is inserted in the abdominal cavity for medical examination or operation. In 1966 Steptoe and Edwards began their collaboration, and in 1978 they reached their goal when Lesley Brown gave birth to Louise Joy in Oldham, England on July 25 of that year. The birth of baby Louise brought international recognition to Steptoe and Edwards. They were both made Commanders of the British Empire, and in 1987 Steptoe was invited to join the fellowship of the Royal Society. Since the birth of baby Louise thousands more "test-tube babies" have been born to women with a variety of physiological problems, and the technique is now being offered in many clinics around the world.

In response to criticism based on fears of genetic manipulation, Steptoe compared the halting of his research to the banning of airplanes because they facilitated bombing.

Lina Solomonovna Stern 1878–1968

Distinguished Soviet physiologist Lina Solomonovna Stern pioneered the chemical investigation of physiological processes, most notably in the brain and central nervous system. The author of more than 400 works on medical and physiological topics,

Stern was the first to describe a membranous filter known as the "blood-brain barrier," which protects the nerves and spinal fluid from harmful substances in the blood.

Born in Latvia, Stern was raised in Switzerland, where she received a degree in medicine from the University of Geneva in 1903. As instructor and later professor of physiological chemistry, Stern remained at the university until 1925, when she emigrated to the Soviet Union. She was naturalized as a Soviet citizen and accepted a position at the Moscow Medical Institute, where she conducted the major portion of her research on the chemical foundation of physiological functions of the nervous system.

The first woman to be admitted to the Academy of Sciences in the Soviet Union, Stern took over directorship of the Moscow Institute. In 1943 she received the Stalin Prize for Scientific Research, but five years later a government purge found her guilty of "rootless cosmopolitanism," a code phrase generally used to stigmatize Jews. Stern was forced to resign from all academic positions.

After Stalin's death in 1953 Stern was "rehabilitated" and restored to a position of honor in the Soviet Union, where she remained until her death in 1968 at the age of 89.

Nettie Maria Stevens 1861–1912

In September, 1905 pioneer American cytologist Nettie Stevens published an article in the Carnegie Institution monograph series entitled "Studies in Spermatogenesis," which revealed the decisive difference in chromosomal patterns distinguishing male from female. Based on a detailed investigation of chromosomes in *Tenebrio molitor,* the common mealworm, she reported an astonishing discovery: "Since the somatic cells of the female contain twenty large chromosomes, while those of the male contain nineteen large ones and one small one, this seems to be a clear case of sex-determination, not by accessory chromosome, but by a definite difference in the character of the elements of one pair of chromosomes."

Stevens's unequivocal assertion that chromosomes of equal size determine the female sex while the presence of a single, smaller chromosome determines the male sex was a landmark achievement in the history of genetics, and yet during her lifetime and in the nearly eighty years since her death her status as the discoverer of this genetic distinction has been almost entirely ignored.

Credit for the discovery of X and Y chromosomes and their role in sex determination was given to by her former professor and mentor biologist Edmund B. Wilson (1856–1939), who published an article of his own one month before Stevens's article appeared in print but three months after he had read her manuscript. As a member of the Carnegie Institution's advisory board, Wilson reviewed Steven's report, returning it to her with his evaluation: "It is in every way a most admirable piece of work which is worthy of publication by any learned society, and I do not hesitate to recommend it to you for publication by the Institution."

Aside from the incidental timing of the two articles, there is no doubt that Stevens made her argument confidently while Wilson was hesitant. Wilson's article, which first appeared in the August, 1905 issue of the *Journal of Experimental Zoology,* cautioned the reader that

> great, if not insuperable, difficulties are encountered by any form of the assumption that these chromosomes are specifically male or female sex determinants. It is more probable...that the difference between eggs and spermatozoa is primarily due to differences in degree or intensity, rather than of kind, in the activity of the chromosome groups in the two sexes...The primary factor in the differentiation of the germ cells may, therefore, be a matter of metabolism, perhaps one of growth.

Nettie Stevens was born in Cavendish, Vermont, where her father worked as a carpenter. Described as modest and self-effacing, Nettie prepared for a career in teaching at the Westfield State Normal School in Massachussetts. For fifteen years she worked as a high school teacher and librarian, finally saving enough money to enroll at Stanford University in 1896. Entering as a freshman at the age of 35, she earned a master's degree in physiology within four years, and by 1901 she had published her first scientific article, on protozoan development. Later that year she entered the doctoral program at Bryn Mawr College, where she met Wilson as well as noted American biologist and future Nobel laureate T. H. Morgan, who would later defend Wilson's priority after his death.

By the time Stevens received her doctorate in 1903 she had already begun to explore the emerging theories of sex determination in chromosomes, with particular attention to the ideas of C. E. McClung, who suggested the possibility of an "accessory chromosome" bearing "those qualities which pertain to the male organism." Sponsored by a number of fellowship awards, she pursued chromosome studies at the Naples Zoological Station and at the University of Wurzburg until 1904, when she returned to Bryn Mawr as a postdoctoral research associate of the Carnegie Institution.

Although some of her theories on the dominant and recessive properties of X and Y chromosomes were later disproved, Stevens understood the fundamental significance of her discovery long before it was recognized by the scientific establishment. Wilson and Morgan are legitimately acknowledged as leading American geneticists of the twentieth century, but Nettie Stevens's name is still absent from nearly all historical record of scientific achievement.

Andrew Taylor Still 1828–1917

In 1892 Andrew Taylor Still founded a school of medicine known as osteopathy. Still, a country doctor from Jonesboro, Virginia, formulated a method of medical practice built on his theory that the human body possesses the capability to protect itself from disease. Maintaining that this function can only occur in a body where there is proper alignment of bones, muscles and nerves, Still defined health as the arterial circulation of the blood unimpeded by misalignment. With the idea that displaced vertebrae obstruct "the flow of life-forces through the nerves," Still developed the theory that all physiological disorders could be traced to "subluxations," his term for dislocations of the vertebrae.

Dismissing the therapeutic value of drugs, Still claimed to cure any illness by his own system of massage and manipulation of specific muscles and bones. In addition to many written works expounding his theories, Still's illustrated autobiography, published in 1897, included detailed descriptions of a number of specific cures.

Still based his findings on one year's study at the Kansas City School of Physicians and Surgeons and on his observation of the failure of orthodox medical care on the battlefields of the Civil War, in which he served as an officer. Originated as an alternative to conventional clinical practice, osteopathy met enormous resistance from the medical establishment. Over the years, however, osteopathic technique has evolved more and more in the direction of traditional medical methods, accepting the use of drugs and even surgery. Current schools of osteopathy maintain standards and curricula similar to those required in other medical schools.

Marie Charlotte Carmichael Stopes 1880–1958

Responsible for the establishment of the first birth-control clinic in Great Britain, Marie Stopes paved the way for a movement that, within decades, would be spread worldwide. With an impressive array of scientific and intellectual qualifications, combined with a commitment to political beliefs then considered radical, Marie Stopes was an influential if highly controversial figure of the early twentieth century.

Born near Dorking, in Surrey, England, Marie Stopes studied paleobotany at University College in London, obtaining her doctorate from the University of Munich in 1904. The first woman accepted to the science faculty at Manchester University, Stopes lectured for several years on paleobotany, with an emphasis on coal mining and fossil plants. In 1907 Stopes left Manchester to lecture in Japan. She remained in Tokyo for several years, collaborating with Professor Sakurai on an analytical treatise on the Japanese noh plays, published in 1913.

Married and divorced before she was 36, Stopes saw an urgent need to educate young men and women about sex and the realities of married life. Aware of the need for family planning, Stopes began to publicly express her views, publishing a book in 1918 entitled *Married Love.* Amid violent controversy the book, a best-seller in Britain, was banned in the United States until 1931.

Remarried to aircraft manufacturer Humphrey Verdon Roe, Stopes founded the first British birth-control clinic, in North London in 1921. Her desperate search for a simple and inexpensive contraceptive led her to recommend the use of a rubber sponge soaked in olive oil. She claimed a 100% success rate for the device.

A prolific writer, Marie Stopes authored seventy books, which include volumes of poetry, a play entitled *Our Ostriches,* studies of the sex cycle and works on paleobotany, eugenics and birth control, notably *Contraception: Its Theory, History and Practice* (1923).

Genpaku Sugita c. 600

Genpahu Sugita was instrumental in introducing the Western understanding of anatomy to Japan.

The first anatomical records in Japan date back to the sixth century. At that time Buddhist monks would often be sent to study with scholars in China and then be brought back to Japan to share all that they had learned. In this way the Japanese absorbed the Chinese understanding of anatomy, which went unchallenged until the eighteenth century. Although the government banned all contact with the West in 1603, some medical reference books did sneak through, and these works seriously contradicted the Chinese models of human anatomy. Japanese doctors became increasingly frustrated in their desire to establish a reliable standard. One physician, Genpaku Sugita, felt a strong professional obligation to his patients and was determined to find the truth. When he came across a copy of a Dutch translation of the German *Anatomische Tabellen(Antomical Tablets)* by J.A. Kulmus he was horrified at the discrepancies between Chinese and Western models of internal structures of the human body. At a public dissection Sugita invited two colleagues to help him put both versions to the test. The evidence clearly favored the Western descriptions. Sugita recalls in his journal his shame and embarrassement at having waited so long to question the erroneous Chinese model. The three physicians set about the arduous task of translating the Dutch version into Japanese. Since none of the three spoke Dutch, the translation took three years. When it was published as *Kaitai Shinso (A New Book of Anatomy)* it rocked the Japanese medical community and permanently altered their view of human anatomy. The five volumes of minutely detailed illustrations were nearly perfect copies of those in the Dutch book, with one obvious exception: Japanese faces had replaced all the European ones.

Earl Wilbur Sutherland Jr 1915–1974

Through chemical investigation of the way in which glycogen becomes glucose in the liver pharmacologist Earl Sutherland discovered the key to the process in a previously unknown substance, which he named cyclic AMP. Identifying cyclic AMP as a secondary messenger for epinephrine, Sutherland demonstrated that the compound plays an important role in the process by which various hormones control metabolism.

Structurally similar to the compound AMP, or adenosine monophosphate, cyclic AMP also contains adenine, a sugar ribose. Sutherland observed that epinephrine, a hormone secreted by the adrenal gland, alters the cellular structure of cyclic AMP, thereby regulating certain enzymatic reactions.

Sutherland received a medical degree in 1947 from Washington University in St. Louis, Missouri. It was there that he began research, in collaboration with noted biochemist CARL CORI, on the conversion of glycogen to glucose. Sutherland continued his investigation while teaching at Case Western Reserve University in Cleveland, Ohio. From 1963 until the year before his death Sutherland taught at Vanderbilt University in Tennessee.

In 1971 Sutherland's important work in hormone research was honored with the award of the Nobel Prize for Physiology or Medicine.

Thomas Sydenham 1624–1689

Known as "the English HIPPOCRATES," Sydenham took as his professional credo "What is useful is good" at a time when doctors, confusing medicine with philosophy,practiced on the basis of elaborately constructed theories. Sydenham was a "Roundhead" cavalry officer during the English Civil War and an amateur politician during the Cromwell years, but most significantly he was a practitioner of the art and science of medicine. Throughout his career Thomas Sydenham believed that medical training was not to be gained from books and university study but from careful and detailed observations of disease in living human beings.

Formal schooling was not a major factor in Sydenham's education. He spent just one year at Oxford, after which he found himself a bachelor of medicine as well as a full- fledged don due to political purges at the university. Sydenham's attention was drawn to the work of the chemist Robert Boyle, who inspired him to study the recurrent plagues ravaging London.

Sydenham left Oxford to set up a practice in Westminster and to raise a family with his new wife, Mary Gee. When the devastating epidemic of bubonic plague struck London in 1665 the Sydenhams retreated to the countryside. During this time he completed a book entitled *Methodus curandi febres (The Method of Treating Fevers)* which he dedicated to Boyle. It offered diagnostic tips, recipes for medications and suggestions for patient care.

The philosopher and political economist John Locke was impressed by Sydenham's practical approach to medicine and saw it as applicable to the science of government and economics. The two became friends, and Locke publicly defended Sydenham's controversial recommendations. Among these was his insistence that patients not be confined in airless rooms under heavy blankets. He opened the windows and spread the novel, even revolutionary gospel of fresh air and wholesome food. His commitment to treat venereal disease mostly by diet and hygiene outraged many moralists of the day, who considered sexually transmitted disease as a divine retribution for promiscuity. Sydenham taught that a physician should approach his task "not with the view of making men's minds more moral but for the sake of making their bodies sounder."

Albert Szent-Györgyi 1893–1986

Albert Szent-Györgyi summed up his goal as a scientist this way: "To see what everyone has seen and think what no one has thought."

This Nobel laureate, celebrated for isolating vitamin C, also advanced biochemistry in many other ways during a career that spanned more than 65 years.

In the course of his investigation of ascorbic acid, or vitamin C, for which he was awarded the 1937 Nobel Prize for Physiology or Medicine, Szent-Györgyi discovered flavone, or vitamin P, an active ingredient in paprika. Szent-Györgyi found the substance to be effective against purpura, a group of disorders in which the blood escapes into the tissues below the skin causing red or purplish spots. He also described the mechanism of plant respiration.

In pioneer studies of the chemistry of muscle contraction he discovered the protein actin and described its role in muscular movement when combined with myosin and adenosine triphosphate (ATP). After many years of biochemical research Szent-Györgyi shifted his focus to submolecular biology to explore the roots of cancer, a passionate pursuit that lasted until his death at 93.

In addition to his work as a scientist Szent-Györgyi devoted much of his time and energy to the cause of peace and nuclear disarmament. He worked courageously for the Hungarian anti-fascist resistance in

World War II and actively opposed political and scientific tyranny throughout his life.

Albert Szent-Györgyi was born in Budapest, Hungary, where he attended the University of Budapest Medical School. The outbreak of World War II was the first of several interruptions in his academic career. He was awarded the Silver Medal of Valor for his service in the medical corps but later extricated himself from service by shooting himself in the arm so that he could be sent home to complete his studies in Budapest.

After graduation he worked briefly at a pharmacological factory until accepting a position at the University of Groningen.

By 1926 Szent-Györgyi had begun his pioneering work on the catalytic activity involved in biological combustion and oxidation, but his studies were as yet inconclusive. A small scientific journal published his paper on the mechanism of cellular respiration in the potato, but the article brought little initial response. Already evaluating alternative career opportunities, Szent-Györgyi attended the International Physiological Congress of 1926 in Stockholm. Delivering the presidential address was the distinguished physiologist SIR FREDERICK GOWLAND HOPKINS, and, much to Szent-Györgyi's astonishment, Hopkins referred to the potato paper several times in his speech. When introduced, Hopkins offered to arrange a Rockefeller fellowship that would permit Szent-Györgyi to accept a position at Cambridge, where Hopkins was head of the department of physiology.

It was in his Cambridge laboratory that Szent-Györgyi finally crystallized the catalytic agent he had isolated in cabbages, oranges, lemons and adrenal glands. In an article submitted to the *Biochemical Journal* he identified the agent by the formula $C_6H_8O_6$, humbly admitting the limitations of his findings by referring to the substance as "ignose." The *Journal's* editor accepted the article provided that Szent-Györgyi give the discovery a more dignified name. Szent-Györgyi's counteroffer was "Godnose," but he grudgingly settled for "hexuronic acid." Several years later, when it was determined that the substance was identical to vitamin C and thereby effective against scurvy, Szent-Györgyi and noted English chemist Norman Haworth formally changed the name to ascorbic acid.

After receiving his doctorate from Cambridge in 1927 Szent-Györgyi left to spend a year at the Mayo Clinic in Minnesota at the invition of EDWARD KENDALL, who headed the clinic's department of biochemistry. By now Szent-Györgyi had gained considerable stature in the international scientific community. At the request of the Hungarian minister of education he returned to Hungary to help stimulate the scientific development of his homeland, still suffering from the war's devastation. He accepted the chair of medical chemistry at the University of Szeged, where, in the course of cellular research, he discovered a substance of bright yellow pigment that he named "cytoflave." The protein later came to be known as vitamin B_2 He also organized an academy of science where Hungarian scientists were offered food as well as laboratory equipment and intellectual support.

Despite his heroic anti-fascist activities in the underground during World War II, United States officials were reluctant to grand Szent-Györgi a visa in view of the Soviet Union's enthusiastic support for his efforts during the war. It was the intervention of American scientists that convinced government authorities to allow Szent-Györgyi to enter the country. Naturalized as a citizen in 1955, he settled in Woods Hole, Massachussetts, where he continued to write and research while remaining politically vocal and active until his death in 1986.

His extensive writings on a variety of subjects include a book for young people entitled *The Crazy Ape* (1970). Other published works include *On Oxidation, Fermentation, Vitamins, Health and Disease* (1940), *The Chemistry of Muscular Contraction* (1951), *Bioenergetics* (1957), *Introduction to Submolecular Biology* (1960), *Bioelectrics* (1968), *The Living State with Remarks on Cancer* (1972) and *Electric Biology and Cancer* (1976).

T

Edward Lawrie Tatum 1909–1975

For his contribution to the formulation of the one-gene-one-enzyme theory American biochemist and geneticist Edward Tatum shared the 1958 Nobel Prize for Physiology or Medicine with his protege JOSHUA LEDERBERG and his collaborator GEORGE BEADLE.

Tatum and Beadle had begun working together eighteen years earlier at Stanford University, where they studied the genetic mechanism of the simple red bread mold *Neurospora.* Recognizing that chemical reactions in living cells are catalyzed by enzymes, Tatum and Beadle explored the possibility that genes cause the cell to carry out specific chemical reactions.

Using X rays to induce mutations, they discovered that by altering the genetic makeup of an organism they could change its nutritional requirements. By 1944 Tatum and Beadle had formulated their "one-gene-one-enzyme theory," which states that each gene initiates the synthesis of an enzyme, which in turn mediates a specific chemical reaction. When the one-to-one relationship between gene and reaction was studied at a molecular level two decades later Tatum and Beadle's theory was amended to a "one-gene-one-polypeptide theory".

Born in Denver, Colorado, Edward Tatum was educated at the University of Wisconsin, where he received his doctorate in 1934. From 1937 to 1957 he taught at Stanford University, and then at Yale for three years. It was at Yale in 1946 that Joshua Lederberg became his student and collaborator in a student of molecular genetics using the bacterium *E. coli.* Noting. that genetic material could be passed on to succeeding generations of the bacterium, they defined that genetic recombination as a form of sexual reproduction.

In 1957 Tatum left Stanford to join the research staff at Rockefeller Institute for Medical Research, where he continued genetic studies of mold, yeast and bacteria until his death in 1975.

Helen Brooke Taussig 1898–1986

Credited with saving the lives of many thousands of children, Helen Taussig was co-inventor of a surgical procedure devised to treat the condition known as "blue baby" syndrome. With this congenital heart defect, also called pulmonary stenosis, an infant's pulmonary artery is constricted, preventing an adequate amount of blood from being carried from the heart to the lungs, where it can receive fresh oxygen. The lack of oxygen in the blood, bringing a blue cast to the skin, frequently led to brain damage and death.

With surgeon ALFRED BLALOCK Taussig developed the "blue baby operation," a surgical method of rerouting the unoxygenated blood back into the lungs, bypassing the defective artery. Known as the Blalock-Taussig operation, this invention kept thousands of infants alive until research cardiologists achieved an effective means of correcting these defects through open-heart surgery.

Graduating from the University of Berkeley in 1921, Taussig, at her father's suggestion, applied to the Harvard School of Public Health. Harvard, no exception to the prevailing opposition to women in medicine, begrudgingly accepted her as a student, though with a number of provisos. When attending lectures she was to sit apart from the male students; when studying tissue culture slides she was to do her work in a separate room; and, regardless of her ability, she would not be permitted to graduate.

Taussig remained at Harvard until the affront was too great. When she was barred from all anatomy classes she transferred to Boston University Medical School. Although her work was exemplary, the dean and the faculty urged her to leave, recommending Johns Hopkins Medical School, which was known for its tolerant attitude toward women. In its inception Johns Hopkins had been largely financed by a committee of women who insisted on the admission of female students as a pre-condition to receiving funds. Johns Hopkins Medical School did grant Taussig a degree in 1927, although they informed her that she could not do her internship in internal medicine, her chosen specialization, because there was already one female intern in that department.

Undaunted, Taussig transferred to the pediatrics department, winning a fellowship from the university's cardiology clinic. As head of the children's department of that clinic, Taussig often encountered pulmonary stenosis, a condition poorly understood and considered untreatable. Taussig's studies led her to develop a bypass procedure for diverting the blood.

It was not until 1941 that she found a surgeon willing to collaborate on the idea. After several years of animal experimentation Taussig and Blalock successfully performed the first "blue baby operation" in 1944, proving not only that the technique was effective, but that newborn infants could survive cardiac surgery. Paving the way for the remarkable advances in cardiology and open-heart surgery that lay ahead, Taussig and Blalock were widely recognized for their breakthrough. Among Taussig's honors were the U.S. Medal of Freedom, the Legion d'Honneur, awarded by the French government and, ironically, an honorary degree from Boston University. Taussig also became the first woman president of the American Heart Association. In addition to her work on pulmonary sterosis Taussig conducted important research on rheumatic fever, an inflammatory disease found mostly in children.

In 1962, when a former student called her attention to the disturbingly large number of serious birth defects occurring in Europe, Taussig, then 64, felt compelled to investigate the phenomenon. Examining the many seriously deformed patients in pediatric clinics throughout England and Germany, Taussig deduced that the common cause was Thalidomide, a sedative that had yet to be legalized in the United States. Returning to America, she met with Dr. Frances Kelsey, a medical officer with the U.S. Food and Drug Administration, who shared Taussig's suspicion that the drug was responsible for birth defects. Thalidomide was never allowed to be sold in the United States and was banned throughout the world in 1962.

Taussig's book *Congenital Malformations of the Heart* first appeared in 1947, with a second edition published in 1960.

Warren Tay 1843–1927

When London-born surgeon Warren Tay was brought in for consultation on a case of "Tay's choroiditis" he asked his colleague, "Incidentally, why do they call it "Tay's choroiditis?" Reminded that he had been the first to describe the disease, the retiring—and absentminded—Dr. Tay replied, "Oh, so I did, but Mr. Hutchinson gave it a name."

Distinguished for his acute diagnostic and clinical insights, Tay collaborated for many years with fellow British surgeon Jonathan Hutchinson (1828–1913). "Tay's choroiditis," a degenerative disease of the eye marked by irregular yellow spots around the retina, is also occasionally referred to as "Hutchinson's disease." As eminent Fellows of the Royal College of Surgeons in London, both men contributed important observations in ophthalmology, dermatology and syphilology, the study of syphilis.

However, Tay's name is most widely known in association with "Tay-Sachs disease," an inherited degenerative condition found mainly among Jews. The result of a dominant chromosomal abnormality, the disease is usually evident in the first six months of life, and its victims rarely live beyond the age of four. Although credit goes to American neurologist BERNARD SACHS for the first comprehensive clinical description of the disease, Tay observed and noted its distinguishing characteristics.

Obtaining his medical training at London Hospital, Tay qualified in 1866 as a physician and in 1869 as a surgeon. Serving more than 30 years as attending surgeon at London Hospital, he earned a distinguished reputation, most notably in the field of ophthalmic surgery. For most of his career the unassuming Tay lived alone in a modest house at Finsbury Square, dividing his time between patients at London Hospital, Moorfields Hospital, the Hospital for Skin Diseases at Blackfriars and North-Eastern Hospital for Children (now Queen's Hospital). In 1902 he slowed his pace to that of consulting surgeon, and a decade later he withdrew from practice to live quietly in the village of Croydon until his death at 84.

Max Theiler 1899–1972

Max Theiler, the man who developed the first effective vaccine against yellow fever, had first to establish the fact that the agent of the disease was a virus and not a bacterium, as was commonly supposed. Once the target was identified, the long, painstaking research had to be shifted from prohibitively expensive rhesus monkeys to mice and chick embryos before a successful vaccine could be provided against a scourge that had claimed thousands of lives.

Once thought to be confined to tropical jungles, yellow fever soon proved highly exportable. Ships fannings out from tropical ports transported in their water casks the larvae of the mosquito *Aedes aegypti*, which carried the yellow fever virus and which brought epidemics to any port hospitable to the mosquitoes. Though most victims survived yellow fever, about 15% died exhibiting a raging temperature, jaundice and black vomit caused by internal bleeding.

The ravages of yellow fever, called "yellowjack," had been curbed in Cuba and Panama by an attack on the breeding grounds of *Aedes aegypti* led by Walter Reed and the Cuban physician Carlos Finlay following the Spanish-American War. However, the unknown microorganisms responsible for the disease were still at large when Max Theiler arrived at Harvard University in 1922.

He had been taking a brief postgraduate course at the London School of Tropical Medicine and Hygiene when he was spotted by a Harvard bacteriologist who was looking for an assistant to work in the Department of Tropical Medicine at Harvard Medical School. At loose ends after his medical education in London, and with a pronounced antipathy to a career as a practicing physician, Max Theiler at the age of 23 was ready for a career in medical research.

He had come to London from South Africa, where he was born the son of distinguished veterinary scientist

Sir Arnold Theiler, who had found his native Switzerland too confining and opted for pioneering in the rugged hinterland of South Africa. Though handicapped by the loss of one hand, Arnold Theiler became noted as an innovative leader in protecting South Africa's horses, cattle and swine against the numerous diseases that afflicted them, including one caused by a protozoan parasite that bears his name.

When Max was born the family was living in the village of Daspoort, near Pretoria. His father inculcated in his children—two boys and two girls—a taste for scientific observation whether of humans or animals. At seventeen Max was sent to take whatever medical courses were available at the Cape of Good Hope University. When the flu epidemic of 1918 left corpses lying in the streets because coffins could not be made fast enough, Max joined other students and physicians at work in the slums of Cape Town.

A year after the end of World War I Max sailed for London to complete his medical education but found that his Cape Town experience yielded him no credentials. He would have to spend two years repeating courseshehad already taken in order to qualify for entrance into a British medical school. He chose instead to undertake a four-year program at St. Thomas's Hospital that could not give him a medical degree but would offer him a certification for practice. It would later seem ironic that, though he was laden with honors, including the Nobel Prize, Theiler never obtained the simple medical degree accorded most practitioners.

Under Andrew Watson Sellards, head of the Department of Tropical Medicine at Harvard, Theiler learned the basics of scientific research in an assignment to study dysentery and rat-bite fever. In 1928, however, Sellards returned from East Africa with the frozen liver of a rhesus monkey that had died of yellow fever after being bitten by mosquitoes that had previously fed on a human yellow fever patient. It was the first indication of the possibility that yellow fever might be studied in a laboratory animal.

At the 1928 price of $7 per chimpanzee, it was important to Theiler that a cheaper laboratory animal be found. Mice were discovered to be invulnerable to abdominal or intradermal injections of blood tainted by yellow fever, but Theiler recalled that both LOUIS PASTEUR and KARL LANDSTEINER had successfully injected test material directly into the brains of their laboratory animals.

It was during this time that Theiler discovered a poliolike viral disorder in his mice that he termed "spontaneous encephalomyelitis" but that has since come to be called "Theiler's disease."

When in the course of his experiments he became convinced that the agent of yellow fever was a virus, he met the disapproval of Sellards, who had posited a bacterial etiology for the disease. He also earned Sellards's disapproval by marrying, an act his chief regarded as a dilution of his devotion to science. However, Theiler's wife, the former Lillian Graham, a laboratory technician, quickly became a collaborator of her husband's.

After he published a brief report in *Science* suggesting that the yellow fever virus could be rendered safe by successive passage through the brains of mice he was invited to join the Yellow Fever Laboratory at the International Health Division of the Rockefeller Foundation. There Theiler succeeded in culturing the yellow fever virus in chick embryo cells, thereby creating a limitless supply ofthe virus for experimental use.

The process of developing a vaccine was laborious until Theiler's team found that somewhere between the 89th and 114th cultures of a particular strain of the virus a mutation had occurred that rendered it capable of producing enough antibodies in test animals to confer an immunity.

Theiler tested it on himself, though he had already acquired some protection when he recovered from an attack of yellow fever several years earlier. He then tested it on his wife and those colleagues who had never been exposed to yellow fever. The vaccine did indeed confer an immunity against the disease; which he reported in *The Journal of Experimental Medicine* of June, 1937.

Demand for the vaccine was worldwide. More than 1,300,000 doses were shipped to Brazil, and after entry of the United States into World War II some 8,000,000 service personnel were vaccinated. Theiler was given the Chalmers Medal by the Royal Society of Tropical Medicine as well as the Lasker Award by the American Public Health Association. Though, in his characteristic shyness, he evaded public appearances on those occasions, he could not hide from the publicity attendant on the award of the Nobel Prize for Physiology or Medicine in 1951, when he and his family traveled to Stockholm for the presentation.

Subsequently Thelier became laboratory director of the Division of Medicine and Public Health in the Rockefeller Foundation. Later he served on the Yale faculty until he retired to become professor emeritus, continuing to lecture there up to his death from heart disease in 1972.

Axel Hugo Teodor Theorell 1903–1982

Swedish biochemist Hugo Theorell was awarded the 1955 Nobel Prize for Physiology or Medicine for his significant contribution to the study of oxidation enzymes. Theorell's work constituted the first detailed description of enzyme activity in which the mechanisms and interaction of "coenzymes" and "apoenzymes" were clearly outlined. Produced by living cells, enzymes are complex proteins capable of mediating specific chemical reactions in other substances without being altered themselves.

In 1934 Theorell isolated the yellow enzyme responsible for converting sugar, discovering that it consisted of two components. The "apoenzyme," consisting of pure protein, is capable of recognizing the substance being acted upon by the enzyme but is unable to perform the catalytic function until it is activated by the other enzyme component, the "coenzyme."

A native of Linköping, Sweden, Theorell received a medical degree in 1930 from the Karolinska Institute in Stockholm. A crippling attack of polio forced him to abandon practice as a physician, however, and he became a professor and researcher at the University of Uppsala. It was there that he embarked on the biochemical studies of enzymes that would eventually lead to the Nobel Prize. In 1937 Theorell took over as director of the Nobel Institute for Biochemistry—a department of the Karolinska Institute.

Also recognized for his earlier research on proteins, Theorell was the first to isolate a pure, crystalline form of myoglobin, a red-colored variety of hemoglobin found in muscle fibers. His other notable achievements include the invention of a blood test for drunkenness.

Hugh Owen Thomas 1834–1891

Recognized as the founder of modern orthopedic medicine, Hugh Owen Thomas belonged to four generations of what the Welsh call *meddygon esgyrn*—"bone setters." His father Evan, without benefit of formal medical training, was the first of the Thomases to earn his living as a "manipulator," but it was Hugh Thomas who developed the principles and techniques of orthopedics.

After studying medicine and surgery in Edinburgh, London and Paris Hugh Thomas practiced orthopedic medicine in Liverpool for more than thirty years, treating fractures and dislocations with his own innovative methods. Rejecting the prevalent use of immobilizing plaster casts, Thomas pointed out that this technique "did not allow frequent inspection, was much labour at first, and little afterwards, and provided no opportunity for the display of skill." Thomas recognized the need to rest an injured limb but strongly urged his patients to avoid constraining devices and to continue normal activities as much as possible, asserting that "A man who understands my principles will do better with a bandage and a broomstick than another can do with an instrument-maker's arsenal."

Appalled at the inefficiency of wooden contrivances commonly used to support broken limbs, Thomas designed a variety of metal splints to accomodate a wide range of fractures and deformities. Employing a full-time blacksmith, a saddler and several mechanical assistants, Thomas produced sophisticated splints forged in iron and padded with leather that are the forerunners of modern orthopedic appliances.

Several splints bearing his name are still used today; Thomas's knee splint removes pressure from the knee joint by redistributing body weight to the hips and pelvic area. Thomas's posterior splint is designed to provide support for patients with diseased or damaged hip joints.

In the 1870s, however, the French army rejected Thomas's design for a splint for femur injuries, despite the frequency of such injuries in war. In his *Memoirs*, published fifty years later, Thomas's nephew Robert Jones, who carried on the tradition of orthopedic medicine, remarked on the irony of that refusal: "The Great War afforded the most convincing proof of the mishandling of complicated, and even simple fractures. Fractures of the femur serve as a notable example...In 1916 the mortality from these fractures amounted to 80 percent...later when the Thomas splint was applied almost exclusively...the mortality in 1918 was reduced to 20 percent."

Born on the island of Anglesey in Wales, Hugh Thomas grew up in Liverpool, where his father was well reputed as a master of "limb manipulation." As an adolescent Hugh was apprenticed to his uncle, a successful physician in St. Asaph. At the age of 21 Thomas entered medical college at the University of Edinburgh, where he completed three years of study. He spent the following year studying surgery at University College Hospital in London and at a number of surgical clinics in Paris. Thomas returned to Liverpool in 1858, intending to join his father's practice, but by then the two generations had become professionally incompatible. The conservative-minded Evan Thomas was skeptical of his son's unorthodox ideas and fearful of trying new methods that might provoke distrust in his patients or suspicion in the medical establishment.

Within a year Hugh was practicing on his own in premises where he could begin to develop equipment to suit his orthopedic theories. His reputation was soon established among patients and medical professionals as a skillful and effective practitioner. Thomas was also recognized for his diligence and generosity, providing his services free of charge to those patients who could not afford his care. He often saw as many as two hundred patients on a Sunday, when he would open his offices to the public as a "free clinic."

Thomas's written works include a treatise on orthopedic methods entitled *Hip, Knee, and Ankle*, published in 1872.

Nikolaas Tinbergen 1907–1988

Ethology, a species-specific approach to the study of animal behavior, was established and defined in the

1930s by Nikolaas Tinbergen and Konrad Lorenz. By observing animals in their natural settings Tinbergen sought to present clear and conclusive theories of behavior by examining the control mechanisms and biological function, or survival value, of specific behavior patterns. A pioneer in the experimental study of function, Tinbergen demonstrated the protective or defensive value of a wide range of behaviors.

Born into an illustrious Dutch family, Nikolaas's eldest brother Jan was a Nobel Prize-winning economist, and his younger brother Lukas an important research biologist. Watching herring gulls along the Dutch coastline, young Niko developed a passion for natural history at an early age. This introduction to the animal kingdom in its own environment may account for Tinbergen's lifelong emphasis on the importance of field observation rather than studies of animals in captivity.

Studying biology at the University of Leiden, Tinbergen retained a particular interest in ornithology. In 1930 he collaborated on a book entitled *Het Vogeleilland (The Bird Island)*, a collection of photographs and observations of bird behavior and physiology.

A proficient and versatile athlete, Tinbergen was a hockey player of international standing. Although in the midst of graduate studies, he leapt at the chance to join an expedition to Greenland in 1930. In addition to enjoying the cultural and physical aspects of the adventure, Tinbergen studied two local bird species, the northern phalarope and the snow bunting.

Returning to the University of Leiden, Tinbergen received his doctorate in 1932 and remained as professor of zoology. His early research focused on the description and documentation of species-specific natural behavior. To examine the internal and external causes of behavior, Tinbergen conducted studies on a wide variety of animals, including gulls, wasps, butterflies and foxes. At the University of Leiden he encountered noted Austrian ethologist Konrad Lorenz, and the two were invited to establish a separate school of animal behavior. They collaborated briefly, but their partnership was cut short by the onset of World War II. Among the many intellectuals incarcerated for protesting the Nazi regime, Tinbergen spent most of the war in prison.

After the war Tinbergen visited the United States on a brief lecture tour, but his ethological theories were poorly received. Encouraged by the presence of Sir Alister Hardy, Tinbergen joined the faculty at Oxford University in 1949 and has remained there ever since. At Oxford Tinbergen shifted his attention to the evolution of behavior, attempting to reconstruct it experimentally. His studies crystallized the notion of "ritualization," the evolutionary process whereby signals and behaviors are exaggerations or distortions of their original pattern.

Over the years Tinbergen's work has gained worldwide acclaim. He served as scientific advisor to the Serengeti Research Institute and was named a fellow of the Royal Society in 1962 and a foreign fellow of the Netherlands Academy of Science in 1964. In recognition of his great contribution to the advancement of biological science Tinbergen received the Nobel Prize for Physiology or Medicine in 1973, with Konrad Lorenz and Karl von Frisch.

Throughout his career Tinbergen wrote of the relevance of ethology to human behavior, although he did not begin to apply ethological methods to human study until late in life. Through clinical observation of children with a form of autism known as Kanner's syndrome Tinbergen proposed an interpretation based on ethological theory. Tinbergen suggests that this form of autism, an illness characterized by extreme withdrawal from social intercourse and external reality, results from a conflict between the child's fears and his frustrated desire for human contact.

Tinbergen's many written works include *Eskimoland* (1930), *The Study of Instinct* (1951), *Social Behavior in Animals* (1953); *The Herring Gull's World* (1953) and *Signals for Survival* (a book and a film by the same name were both produced in 1967).

Alexander Robertus Todd, Baron Todd of Trumpington
1907–

In recognition of his landmark analysis of the chemical structure and composition of nucleotides, nucleosides and nucleotide coenzymes, Scottish biochemist Alexander Robertus Todd was awarded the Nobel Prize for Chemistry in 1957. Establishing the fundamental chemical structure of the nucleic acids, Todd's research provided vital clues in the investigation of genetic mechanisms and the structure and function of nucleic acids.

Born in Glasgow, Todd was granted the first of several doctoral degrees in 1931 from the University of Frankfurt, receiving a second doctorate in science two years later from Oxford University. A leading authority on biochemistry, medical chemistry and preventive medicine, Todd conducted research at the Lister Institute of Preventive Medicine and the University of Edinburgh, later serving as professor of chemistry at London, Manchester and Cambridge Universities as well as visiting professor at colleges throughout the United States, Europe and Australia.

In the 1930s Todd began a series of pharmacological studies at the University of Edinburgh, with particular attention to the structure and synthesis of vitamins B_1, B_{12}, and E. In the following decade he completed a comprehensive investigation of those substances as well as detailed analyses of the chemical constituents of plant and insect coloring matters, various mold products and hashish, a species of *Cannabis*. In 1938 he was appointed professor and head of the department of chemistry at Manchester University, and it was there that his research on the function of vitamins led him to examine the chemical structure of coenzymes.

Defined as essential factors to the growth and development of an organism, vitamins are not synthesized by the body and must therefore be obtained from food. Only small amounts are required, however, because vitamins do not function as a source of fuel, but rather as vital factors in the metabolic activity of the cell. Intracellular metabolism also relies on the catalytic action of enzymes, a group containing hundreds of different protein compounds produced in the cells that induce chemical changes in specific substances. To detect and recognize its own particular substrate, the enzyme relies on a specific component called an apoenzyme; and to perform its catalytic function, a second component known as a coenzyme acts as a trigger. Coenzymes are nonprotein organic substances that are not produced by the body, so that a vitamin may function as a coenzyme or contribute to its formation.

Contained within some coenzymes is a compound of phosphate, sugar and an organic base known as a nucleotide. As the basic building block of nucleic acid, nucleotides link together to form two complementary chains of DNA. Along the length of each chain bases jut out perpendicularly to connect to their complementary bases on the opposite chain, joining the two strands in the configuration of a double helix. Elucidating the general chemical structure of the subunits of RNA and DNA, Todd played a key role in advancing scientific understanding of the physical structure and biological function of the nucleic acids.

During World War II Todd supervised a number of government research projects, serving as chairman of Britain's Advisory Council on Scientific Policy from 1952 to 1964. Recognized as a distinguished member of Britain's scientific community, he was granted a knighthood in 1954 and a baronetcy in 1962. In 1975 he was elected president of the Royal Society, retaining the post for five years in succession. A foreign associate of the National Academy of Sciences of United States, Todd was recognized throughout the world for his outstanding contribution to science. In addition to publishing hundreds of scientific papers he produced an autobiography in 1983 entitled *A Time to Remember*.

Susumu Tonegawa 1939–

Susumu Tonegawa unraveled an immunological mystery that had baffled scientists since the nineteenth century.

As biologists came to understand the function of the immune system they observed a phenomenon that seemed to defy logical explanation. When a foreign substance, or antigen, is introduced into the body, the plasma cells of the immune system respond by producing a specific protein molecule capable of attacking that particular antigen. The body, it seemed, could produce a specific defensive antibody against any of the millions of antigens, even those it had not yet encountered. In what appeared to scientists to be a paradox, the vast number of individual antibody types exceeds the number of cells responsible for their production.

It was suggested that individual genes might perform structural modifications within the antibody molecule, but this hypothesis was abandoned when it became clear that even the number of genes did not come close to the antibodies' enormous range of diversity. Refining the theory of genetic involvement, some scientists conjectured that different types of antibodies might be produced at various stages of the development of the individual.

In experimental studies using laboratory-bred mice Tonegawa studied the antibodies produced by B lymphocytes, a type of white blood cell known to produce only its own particular antibody. Demonstrating his findings in what was later described by the Nobel Committee as "a convincing and elegant manner," Tonegawa established that the genes involved in the formation of antibodies are broken down into separate components so that they may be shuffled and recombined into billions of permutations, accommodating the system's requirements of both enormous diversity and unique response.

In an article published in *Scientific American* leading immunologist Philip Leder described the antibody's genetic mechanism: "Rather than harboring a set of complete and active antibody genes, these cells contain bits and pieces of the genes: a kit of components."

In honor of his outstanding achievement Tonegawa was awarded the Nobel Prize for Physiology or Medicine in 1987, becoming the first Japanese scientist to be recognized in that category.

Born in the city of Nagoya, Tonegawa studied chemistry at the University of Kyoto and then left for the United States to enter the doctoral program in biology at the University of California in San Diego. After receiving his degree in 1969 Tonegawa remained to pursue postdoctoral research at the university and at the Salk Institute, also in San Diego.

In 1971 Tonegawa embarked on his investigation of the genetics of the immune system, serving for ten years as assistant professor at the Basel Institute for Immunology in Switzerland. It was there between 1974 and 1981 that he conducted the major part of his Nobel prize-winning research. Returning to the United States, he accepted a professorship at the Massachussetts Institute of Technology, where he currently runs a small biological laboratory. Described by one colleague as "very focused and very intense," Tonegawa is known as a single-minded and brilliant scientist.

Frederick Treves 1853–1923

British surgeon and anatomist Frederick Treves introduced important advances in operative technique, most notably in the treatment of appendicitis; but the mythic quality of his reputation arises from his relationship with Joseph Carey Merrick, his most celebrated patient, better known as the Elephant Man.

Merrick suffered from a condition that has been tentatively diagnosed as acute neurofibromatosis, a rare congenital disorder marked by tumorous growths covering much of the surface of the skin and bones and developmental abnormalities of bone, muscle and internal organs. The disfiguring effects of the disease began to emerge when he was five years old, and from that point on Merrick was trapped inside a body so deformed that he could barely speak or walk, and so grotesque that people recoiled in horror at the sight of him. His head was more than three feet in circumference, with hanging pockets of discolored skin and and a grossly misshapen jaw.

After four years of confinement in a workhouse Merrick escaped into the bowels of London's back alleys, where he was exploited by hustlers and charlatans and displayed in freak shows. Locked in a cage, he was treated like a subhuman creature until he made the acquaintance of Dr. Treves in 1886.

Treves brought him to the protective environment of London Hospital, where Merrick was admitted as a permanent patient. Four years later he died in his sleep from accidental suffocation.

Treves was born in Dorchester, England and at the age of eighteen was admitted to the London Hospital Medical School. Three years later he obtained his degree in medicine as well as appointments as house surgeon at London Hospital and anatomy lecturer at the college.

In 1876 Treves accepted a position as medical officer at the Royal National Hospital for Scrofula at Margate, where he began research on scrofula, a form of tuberculosis characterized by the formation of abscesses, usually in the lymph nodes. Establishing private surgical practice in Derbyshire, Treves gained national distinction in 1883 as the founding chairman of the British Red Cross.

While serving as Hunterian professor in anatomy and Wilson professor of pathology at London's Royal College of Surgeons Treves was named surgeon extraordinary to Queen Victoria in 1900. Awarded a knighthood the following year, he became sgt.-surgeon to Edward VII and later to George V. In 1905 he was appointed president of the Medical Board of the War Office.

Throughout his career Treves contributed advances in surgical technique as well as a number of important anatomical observations. Among these is the first description of a ridge in the peritoneum, located between the ileum and the appendix, which is now known as the "bloodless fold of Treves."

A prolific author, Treves produced a number of valuable medical texts, but his writings were not limited to scientific subjects. His notable published works include: *Scrofula and its Gland Diseases* (1882), *Surgical Applied Anatomy* (1883), *A Manual of Operative Surgery* (1891), *The Students' Handbook of Surgical Operations* (1892), *A System of Surgery* (2 vols., 1895), *Intestinal Obstruction and Its Varieties, With their Pathology, Diagnosis and Treatment* (1899, 1902), *Tale of a Field Hospital* (1900), *Highways and By-Ways of Dorest* (1906), *Uganda for a Holiday* (1910), *The Riviera of the Corniche Road* (1921) and *The Elephant Man and Other Reminiscences* (1923).

Trotula c. 1050

Trotula, also referred to as "Maestra Trotula" and "Dame Trot," is reputed to have been a brilliant and successful physician specializing in gynecologic, obstetric and pediatric care. There is some debate as to whether this legendary eleventh-century midwife was a historic figure or merely the creation of an imaginative historian. There is evidence on both sides of that argument, and the question remains unresolved.

Said to have graduated from the renowned Medical College of Salerno, Trotula is reported to have practiced medicine there, following a doctrine of practical and sensible care largely in accord with the teachings of Galen. Although her patients were for the most part women and children, Trotula is also credited with advances in the treatment of epilepsy and of various diseases of the eye, ear and mouth.

Those who claim that Trotula is a myth insist that she stems from a mistaken interpretation of a compilation of documents entitled "The Trotula." This collection of medical articles, it is charged, is the work of Trottus, a male physician who once practiced in Salerno. "Maestra Trotula" is merely a personification of these writings, these debunkers maintain.

Others credit an actual woman named Trotula with *De Morbis Mulierum et Eorum Cura*, an impressive treatise on the diseases of women and their remedies. In addition to chapters on various diseases of the reproductive system, the book, whether by Trotula or Trottus, includes discussions on nutrition and hygiene for pregnant women and newborns and a description of a child's normal dental development. There is also a chapter devoted to early education, including recommendations for teaching a child language skills.

Edward Livingston Trudeau 1848–1915

At the age of twenty-six physician Edward Livingston Trudeau was informed by his doctors that he would be dead within six months from advanced tuberculosis. Trudeau had contracted the disease several years earlier while nursing his older brother, whose resignation in the face of death exemplified the romantic tradition of "consumption," as pulmonary tuberculosis was then called. Less suited to the role of a sensitive, doomed victim, Edward Trudeau regained his health and dedicated the next forty years to an enthusiastic crusade against tuberculosis.

Born in New York City, Trudeau was raised in Paris, where he was educated until the age of eighteen. Returning to New York to attend Columbia University, he ministered to his dying brother before enrolling in the College of Physicians and Surgeons. He received his medical degree in the spring of 1871, and within the year he had married and entered into partnership practice.

When he learned of his "terminal" condition Trudeau sought the advice of New York physician Alfred Loomis, who recommended that he rest at a friend's cabin in the Adirondack mountains. Nearly incapacitated by the effects of the disease, Trudeau was brought to a shack in the wilderness forty miles from the nearest railway station at Ausable Forks, New York, and over the next three years he gradually rid himself of the disease.

This he is supposed to have done by conditioning his body to the rigors of the environment by "living constantly out of doors." Wrapped in blankets, he would brave temperatures of –40° F, becoming a living testament to the virtues of "open-air treatment" for tuberculosis. As his recovery advanced Trudeau began to explore the surrounding area, where he soon became known as "the Beloved Physician." In addition to providing gentle and effective medical care to local residents and summer visitors, he frequently attended to the various ailments of his neighbors' cows, horses and dogs.

In 1877 Trudeau took over a saw mill and six cabins on the shore of Saranac Lake as the first step toward the establishment of a sanitarium "that should be the everlasting foe of tuberculosis." Five years later, when celebrated English bacteriologist Robert Koch announced his discovery of the tubercle bacillus, Trudeau was among the first Americans to obtain a pure culture of the infecting agent for research purposes.

The cluster of houses on Saranac Lake was attracting considerable attention by then as doctors in New York and elsewhere began to recognize Trudeau's therapeutic methods, which were based mainly on the restorative effects of rest and fresh air. Patients with advanced cases of tuberculosis were sent to Trudeau, often as a last resort, and in many cases their condition was reversed.

In 1885 Trudeau built a "little red shack" on Mount Pisgah near Saranac Lake, establishing the celebrated central office for the Adirondack Cottage Sanitarium. Unlike the luxury spas of Europe, the sanitarium operated as a nonprofit clinic in which patients paid what they could afford, and donations were solicited to cover the costs of maintaining the institution.

Among the many distinguished patients who sought treatment at the sanitarium, Robert Louis Stevenson spent several months at Saranac Lake, writing, among other works, a treatise in defense of FATHER DAMIEN. Stevenson developed a lasting friendship with Trudeau and later presented the doctor with a collection of his published works in which he inscribed a couplet at the beginning of each volume. On the flyleaf of the personalized volume of *Dr. Jekyll and Mr. Hyde* he wrote:

> Trudeau was all the Winter at my side,
> I never saw the nose of Mr. Hyde.

Internationally acclaimed as a pioneer of the open-air treatment for tuberculosis, Trudeau was granted honorary degrees from a number of distinguished medical institutions, including Columbia, Yale, McGill and the University of Pennsylvania.

As president of the Eighth Congress of Physicians and Surgeons at Washington, D.C., he appeared in public for the last time in 1910, plainly a victim of tuberculosis, which was taking its toll, however long delayed. Barely able to stand, he spoke in a thin, quavering voice as he addressed his colleagues on "The Value of Optimism in Medicine":

"So let us not quench the faith nor turn from the vision which we carry, whether we own it or not; and thus inspired, many will reach the goal."

Finally succumbing to tuberculosis at the age of 67, Trudeau was succeeded by his son as director and head physician at the Adirondack Cottage Sanitarium. His grandson, also a physician, set up a practice in the village after the sanitarium closed. Trudeau's great-grandson, Garry, gained recognition as a Pulitzer Prize-winning cartoonist.

William Tuke 1732–1822
Henry Tuke 1755–1814
Samuel Tuke 1784–1857
James Hack Tuke 1819–1896
Daniel Hack Tuke 1827–1895

For more than a century the Tuke family was in the vanguard of the crusade for individual and humane treatment of the mentally ill. Four generations of Tukes dedicated themselves to eradicating the insensitive and often brutal approach that generally prevailed in insane asylums both in Europe and in America in the eighteenth and nineteenth centuries. Believing in the curability of mental disease, the Tukes proposed a therapy of reeducation, resocialization and reward for individual progress.

In 1796 William Tuke established the York Retreat, an institute dedicated to intelligent and humane treatment of mental disease. The ideals and therapeutic philosophy followed at the York Retreat were gradually adopted by others in the field of psychiatric care and much later influenced modern behavior therapy.

William Tuke was born in York to a prominent family of tea and coffee merchants that included some of the earliest English Quakers. As an adult William looked after the company but was more active as a Quaker and a philanthropist. When a fellow member of the Society of Friends was found dead in the county asylum Tuke strongly suspected that mistreatment had contributed to the man's death.

Seeing the urgent need for a facility "for the care and proper treatment of those labouring under that most afflictive dispensation—the loss of reason," Tuke set out to raise money for the establishment of an institute that would offer an alternative method of treating the insane. Rejecting the use of corporal punishment or unnecessary restraining measures, Tuke proposed a quiet and civilized environment, offering opportunities for paid employment to patients competent enough to work.

With the help of his son Henry, William Tuke realized his goal in 1796 when the York Retreat was formally established. A Latin inscription on the foundation stone of the home read *Hoc fecit amicorum caritas in humanitatis argumentum* (The caring of friends gives proof of humanity).

Henry Tuke carried on his father's tradition, developing the retreat into a respected institution. His son Samuel was also dedicated to the reform of mental health care, making a lifelong study of the historical and medical aspects of mental diseases and treatments. In 1811 Samuel Tuke published two papers describing his observations and theories. Entitled *On the State of the Insane Poor* and *On the Treatment of Those Labouring under Insanity*, these documents are among the first to call for humane treatment of the mentally ill. Two years later he published an influential though controversial book on his family's philosophy for the treatment of insanity entitled *Description of the Retreat*.

The fourth generation of Tukes produced perhaps the most widely recognized member of the family, Daniel Hack Tuke. A certified physician and member of the Royal College of Surgeons, Daniel Hack Tuke's contribution to his family's cause was honored with the award of the Association for Improving the Condition of the Insane in 1854. Four years later he published *A Manual of Psychological Medicine*, an authoritative and sensitive treatment of the subject. His brother James Hack Tuke assisted in the management of the York Retreat while maintaining the family's still-profitable tea and coffee business.

In the course of his travels Daniel Hack Tuke met with other advocates of mental health reform, including PHILIPPE PINEL and JEAN-MARTIN CHARCOT at the Salpetriere in Paris, and he visited a number of mental asylums in North America. Published in 1885, his treatise entitled *The Insane in the United States and Canada* was a scathing account of what he considered the cruel and immoral treatment of the mentally ill, particularly in Benjamin Rush's hospital in Philadelphia and in many of the facilities in Quebec, Canada. His detailed descriptions of physical restraint and coercion were so shocking that they brought about investigations that eventually led to the improvement of conditions in some of the institutions mentioned in Tuke's expose.

V

John Robert Vane 1927–

In recognition of his biochemical research on prostaglandins British pharmacologist and chemist John Robert Vane was awarded the 1982 Nobel Prize for Physiology or Medicine, which he shared with SUNE K. BERGSTROM and BENGT I. SAMUELSSON.

After receiving his doctorate from Oxford University in 1953 Vane taught at Yale University in the United States, then returned to England to teach at the Institute of Basic Medical Sciences, a part of the University of London. In 1973 Vane left teaching to join the Wellcome Research Laboratories in Beckenham, England. It was there that he focused his attention on the study of prostaglandins, a group of powerful substances produced as needed by cell membranes in all parts of the body.

Different prostaglandins carry out various functions essential for protection from disease and pain. Some compounds may raise or lower blood pressure, stimulate defense against infection or regulate metabolism. Noting the participation of prostaglandins in inflammation and body temperature regulation (initiated in the hypothalamus), Vane was the first to recognize (in 1971) that aspirin and other analgesics reduced fever and inflammation by blocking prostaglandin synthesis.

In 1976 Vane discovered a prostaglandin subtype that proved a valuable tool in preventive medicine. Known as prostacyclin, the substance inhibits blood clots that might otherwise lead to a stroke or heart attack.

Andreas Vesalius 1514–1564

Andreas Vesalius is known primarily for his authorship, at the age of 29, of the remarkable anatomical text *De humani corporis fabrica (The Structure of the Human Body)*. Familiarly known as *De fabrica,* the book was an annotated collection of woodblock prints depicting more or less accurately the bones, muscles, ligaments, organs, veins and and arteries and the skeletal structure of the human body. The most spectacular illustrations are the three skeletons, 14 "muscle men" and 24 "nerve men," all portrayed as living Renaissance gentlemen posing elegantly, though stripped of skin and flesh. Providing a detailed commentary on the artwork Vesalius' accompanying text was printed in type elaborately interwoven with illustrative initials and decorations that inject a dark humor into the work. Twined around the first letter of chapters or paragraphs are cupids engaged in various nefarious pursuits. They leap into graves, haul off corpses, perform a Caesarean section on a dog, play the stomach of a corpse like a bagpipe and pore over the excrement of an aging man.

The illustrations are considered to be the most remarkable part of the book (most of Vesalius's Latin text has never been translated into English), and it is perhaps a clue to the author's entrepreneurial integrity that no credit for the art was given. Much of it has been attributed to John Stephen of Calcar, who is also credited with introducing Vesalius to the great painter Titian. A number of artists from Titian's atelier in Venice were probably also anonymous contributors to *De fabrica*. It is not known how many copies were printed in 1543, but there are 100 copies still extant in libraries around the world. The original printing woodblocks were preserved up until the twentieth century. Some were destroyed in Louvain in World War I, and others were lost in Munich during World War II.

Vesalius was born Andreas van Wesel on December 31, 1514 in a house on a Brussels street called Hell's Lane. As was the academic custom, his name was Latinized during his medical studies, and he became Andreas Vesalius. While still a student at the University of Paris he gained widespread reputation for his public dissections. He continued this anatomical research after he returned to Louvain in 1536. The following year he entered the University of Padua and, bypassing many of the usual requirements, was offered the chair of surgery and anatomy by the end of the year. His duties included daily lectures on anatomy, and in the spring he was expected to perform several public dissections.

Vesalius himself drew extensive illustrations to clarify his lectures. Though many of these sketches were incorrect, they were copied, plagiarized and sold at great profit. This prompted the publication of *Tabulae anatomicae sex (Six Anatomic Drawings)*, whose illustrations were credited to Joannes Stephanus and were accompanied by a multilingual text. The Greek and Latin sections were written by Vesalius, but the Hebrew and Arabic sections most likely were written by Lazarus de Frigel. Other published works followed, including a monograph on bloodletting known as *The Venesection Letter*. Vesalius's fame grew, and Padua officials went out of their way to support his work, going so far as to time executions so that he might have a fresh corpse when he needed one. At 26 Vesalius embarked on his masterwork and recalled the difficulties of production:

"The bad tempers of artists...made me more miserable than did all the bodies I was dissecting."

Mysteriously, Vesalius chose to use a printer 400 miles away in Switzerland, although there were many publishers closer at hand. It may have been the political climate in Venice or the local copyright laws, or simply the brilliant reputation of Johannus Oporinus of Basel that prompted Vesalius to seek him out.

Response to *De Fabrica* was mixed. Shortly after publication Vesalius changed course and applied for the position of staff physician to the emperor Charles V. He got the job and developed a reputation as a clever prognosticator, being among the first to recognize and describe an aneurysm, a saclike widening in a blood vessel. He also revived the HIPPOCRATIC technique of draining the thorax of pus. Vesalius as the first to challenge the ARISTOTELIAN correlation between heart and personality, recognizing instead the role of the brain and nervous system.

As the authority of Charles V began to fade so did Vesalius's position in the empire. Asked to perform an autopsy on a Spanish nobleman, he found after the first incision that the "corpse" was still alive. This resulted in charges of murder and, worse still, impiety. Vesalius was ordered to make a pilgrimage to the Holy Land to atone for his sin. He undertook the trip with his wife and child but abandoned them during a quarrel at Sete, on the Gulf of Lyon. After reaching Jerusalem he set sail to return to Europe but died in a storm near the Greek island of Zante.

Rudolf Ludwig Karl Virchow 1821–1902

It is probably impossible to define Rudolf Virchow by the professions he followed. As a pathologist he was the first to describe leukemia; as a histologist and biologist he demonstrated that cells develop only from other cells—a notion that was shockingly novel in the mid-nineteenth century; as an epidemiologist he found a connection between disease and hunger and poverty.

He tackled many of the problems of a turbulent society—disease, antiquated sewers, an overly bureaucratic medical system and menacing racist doctrines (which he sought to refute on anthropological expeditions). In his many-sided career Virchow found himself a rebel on the barricades, a member of national, state and city legislatures, a teacher and, above all, a scientist in his laboratory. Wherever he worked he was always exuberantly engaged in the vital questions of his day.

Rudolf Virchow was born to a moderately prosperous family in the town of Schivelbein in Pomerania, a province of Prussia. At the age of 18 he indicated his omnivorous appetite for learning when he defined his life's goal as an "all-round knowledge of nature from the Deity down to the stone." When he applied to the Friedrich-Wilhelms Institute for a free medical education the examining officer noted in his recommendation, "This young man is gifted for everything but catching a disease."

From the institute Virchow went to the University of Berlin, where he won his medical degree in 1843 at the age of 22. He immediately embarked on what today might be called a rotating internship at the Charité in Berlin, a teaching hospital that was open to all the new ideas then bubbling and bursting in the European medical world. One of his fellow students at the Charité, THEODOR SCHWANN, stimulated Virchow's interest in cellular theory, and the wife of one of the obstetricians at the Charité ran a salon that introduced Virchow to the newest currents in political, economic and scientific thought.

At 24 this extraordinary intern was preaching to his elders at the Friedrich-Wilhelms Institute, urging them to give up venerated philosophic systems that held few medical answers. One prevalent answer that Virchow found to be wrong was the notion that phlebitis, the inflammation of a vein, lay at the root of most if not all pathology. Virchow began by analyzing fibrin, the protein found in blood clots, and coined the term fibrinogen to correctly define its function as the essential factor in coagulation. He then refuted the common explanation of an obstructed pulmonary artery as due to a "local phlebitis." He convincingly demonstrated that thrombi found in a patient's lung did not arise locally but were carried from other sites by the blood. He named these clots fragments "emboli" and the process "embolism." "Thrombosis" was another word coined by Virchow to designate the condition in which an artery may be obstructed by an embolus.

The "inflammation cells" postulated by his fellow student Schwann turned out to be merely degenerated epithelia, according to Virchow's probing investigations. Similarly "pus cells," he showed, were no more than leukocytes—white blood cells. Step by step he was immersing himself ever more deeply in the cell as a key to medical mysteries. His probing of the leukocytes led him to identify and name a disease that had not been recognized up to that time—leukemia, a disordered proliferation of leukocytes.

"I vindicate for leukocytes a place in pathology," Virchow wrote, as if he were hurling a revolutionary challenge. Indeed, revolutionary challenges seemed to be in the wind over Europe whether the establishment being confronted was political or scientific. Doctors tended to favor reformism out of humane as well as economic considerations. Virchow's motivations sprang from both. Not only were his sensibilities outraged by the social ills of the time, but he himself worked at the Charité on a salary about one third that of a carpenter.

Though his pay increased modestly after he was given the post of assistant professor, his liberalism never faltered and was evident even in the *Archives for*

Pathological Anatomy and Physiology and Clinical Medicine, a widely acclaimed journal that he helped to found. Despite Virchow's critical view of the government, he was named to investigate a typhus epidemic in Upper Silesia. While his report described the outbreak and suggested medical measures, it also designated hunger, miserable housing and lack of sanitation as prime causes. To his strictly medical recommendations he added this prescription: "Democracy, education, freedom, and prosperity."

He returned to Berlin on the eve of the 1848 revolutions that seemed to be sweeping most of Europe. Virchow took his turn briefly on the barricades, where, by all accounts, he was singularly ineffectual. He was elected to the Prussian Diet but could not serve because at 27 he was considered too young. He investigated a rampaging epidemic of cholera in outlying areas of Prussia and again found its etiology in social miseries.

He had more gratifying results when he and two colleagues founded a weekly, *Die Medizenische Reform (Medical Reform)*. In it he wrote: "Physicians are the natural attorneys of the poor, and social problems fall to a large extent within their jurisdiction."

By the end of the year, however, the euphoria of liberals had given way to defeat as everywhere hard-won democratic freedoms were canceled. In March, 1849 Virchow was suspended from his post at the Charité, though protests by students and faculty subsequently forced his reinstatement. The administration of the hospital balked, however, at giving the vanquished rebel his room and board.

In the last issue of *Die Medizenische Reform*, which appeared in June 1849, Virchow wrote: "We must wander through the desert and struggle. Our task is an educational one. We must raise men able to fight the battle of humanism." Privately he wrote: "I did not push my way into politics. Events pushed me into it." It seemed a definitive farewell to politics, but his rejection of that recourse was to prove temporary.

He accepted the offer of a professorship at the University of Wurzburg and returned to Berlin only to marry Rose Mayer, whose mother had conducted the intellectually stimulating salon where Virchow, as a student, had encountered the ideas that did so much to mold him. The Berlin bureaucracy, uneasy at the return of the firebrand, expelled him from the Prussian capital as soon as the wedding ceremony was concluded.

At Wurzburg he resumed his exploration of the cell and the phenomenon of inflammation, which he depicted as a nutritional disturbance. It was in an 1852 paper entitled *Nutrition Units and Disease Foci* that he outlined the process of cell replication by division, refuting theories advanced by a friend from his student days, Theodor Schwann, who had postulated a substance he called blastema as the source of cells.

Though earlier scientists such as Francois Raspail had suggested the possibility of cell division, Virchow had convincingly proved it. "There is no life but through direct succession," he wrote, and he fashioned his theory into a Latin slogan: *Omnis cellula a cellula* (Everything [grows] from cell to cell).

So far-reaching were the implications of Virchow's findings and so widely acclaimed were his papers that in 1856 he was invited to return to Berlin, where a Pathological Institute was to be designed to his specifications. The government, feeling less threatened, had changed, but Virchow had not. When he was dispatched to study famine in a Bavarian district he added to his strictly medical report his usual prescription for education, freedom and socioeconomic betterment. In 1859 his medical prestige had grown so impressively that he was elected to the Berlin city council and to the Prussian council of scientific advisors.

Two years later he was serving in the Prussian Diet, rallying the remnants of liberalism against the "Iron Chancellor," Otto von Bismarck. While active in the parliament he continued to teach and to research his favorite subject—the cell. He extended his cellular studies to oncology in an 1800-page work, *Die Krankhaften Geschwulste (The Tumor Sickness)*, which was a striking achievement for the time but has since been outdated by the progress in oncology.

When the Franco-Prussian War broke out in 1870 Virchow opposed it but nevertheless organized a hospital train and rode with it (along with two of his sons) to the front. When peace came he was elected to the Reichstag, where he continued to oppose Bismarck on most issues. Disturbed by the idea of Papal infallibility, he sided with Bismarck's anti-Catholic campaign, for which Virchow invented the word *Kulturkampf* (culture clash). He bitterly fought the anti-Semitic Christian Social Party and its leader, Adolf Stocker, whom Adolf Hitler was subsequently to hail as hero.

Virchow had taken time away from his other work to dig for skulls and skeletons in Pomerania in order to disprove the racist theories proclaiming an alleged biological superiority of pure Germans. When he was in his sixties Virchow joined the expeditions in which anthropologist Heinrich Schliemann found the glories of Egypt and ancient Troy. Virchow delighted to humble his countrymen by reports of civilizations that existed when the ancestors of Germans had lived in caves.

On a January day in 1902, when he was over 80 but still at work, he jumped from a streetcar and suffered a fractured femur. Rudolf Virchow died on September 5 of that year, not from the injury to the bone, which had healed long before, but, it was said, from the enforced rest, which proved fatal to that obsessively active scientist-statesman-anthropologist-humanist.

W

Julius Wagner-Juaregg (or Wagner von Juaregg) 1857–1940

Julius Wagner-Juaregg was awarded the Nobel Prize for Physiology or Medicine in 1927 in honor of his development of "fever therapy" as a treatment for dementia paralytica, a condition of rapidly progressing general paralysis. Accounting for 15% of all patients in mental institutions, "creeping paralysis," as it was then called, attacked the central nervous system and generally led to death within a period of three to four years.

In clinical studies begun in 1887 Wagner-Juaregg observed that the mental condition of his psychiatric patients showed a marked improvement following an attack of febrile diseases, such as typhus or malaria. Seeking to adapt this phenomenon to a controlled form of therapy, he experimented over a period of twenty years using tuberculosis, typhus, staphylococci and streptococci vaccines. Significant results were achieved in only a minority of patients until Wagner-Juaregg decided to try an injection of blood taken from a patient with tertian malaria. Emboldened by the recent success with quinine as treatment for malaria, he decided to risk this dangerous procedure in June, 1917. The treatment led to dramatic improvements and, in some cases, total remission of the paresis.

A precursor to subsequent forms of shock treatment, malarial fever therapy was widely used for several decades until it was replaced by the use of antibiotic drugs, most notably penicillin.

Austrian-born Julius Wagner-Juaregg studied at the University of Vienna Medical School, receiving his doctoral degree in 1880. As a student he worked at the Institut fur Allgemeine und Experimentelle Pathologie (Institute for General and Experimental Pathology), where he established a lifelong friendship with Sigmund Freud. Despite fundamental differences on various scientific and psychiatric issues, the two maintained a mutual respect and professional admiration for one another.

In 1883 Wagner-Juaregg joined the staff at the university's psychiatric clinic, where he served under Max von Leidesdorf. It was there that he focused his attention on the two areas that would dominate his research—the study of the thyroid gland and the treatment of dementia paralytica. Within four years he was certified as a teacher of neurology and psychiatry.

Based on experimental animal studies of the effects of thyroidectomy, Wagner-Juaregg published an article in 1894 demonstrating the relationship between cretinism and defective thyroid function. His study of goiter, a disease characterized by enlargement of the thyroid gland, revealed that the condition could be controlled by a regular intake of iodine. Based on his findings the Swiss and Austrian governments arranged for the distribution of iodized salt in areas where cases of goiter commonly occurred.

As the director of Vienna's Psychiatric and Neurological Clinic and a member of the Austrian Board of Health, Wagner-Juaregg was an influential figure in mental health care reform. His work on fever therapy not only yielded an effective treatment for paresis but contributed significantly to scientific understanding of the mechanism of malaria. Retiring from the clinic in 1928, Wagner-Juraegg left behind a legacy of innovative and influential work reflected in the distinguished careers of his students.

Selman Abraham Waksman 1888–1973

For his discovery of streptomycin, the mainstay of modern tuberculosis therapy, Selman Waksman was awarded the Nobel Prize for Physiology or Medicine in 1952. Produced by soil bacteria, streptomycin is an antibiotic, a term coined by Waksman to denote a substance that inhibits the growth of certain microorganisms. Waksman found that bacteria of the genus *Streptomyces* provided the first effective means of controlling tuberculosis, a highly contagious disease that was considered a major threat to public health.

Selman Waksman was born in Priluka in the Ukraine, emigrating to the United States in 1910. Five years later he was an American citizen and a graduate of Rutgers University, with a degree in microbiology. He received his doctorate from the University of California at Berkeley in 1918 and returned to Rutgers to begin a career of teaching and research that would span four decades.

In 1921 Waksman became associated with the New Jersey State Agricultural Experiment Station, where he began his first studies of the origin and nature of humus, the organic matter created as microorganisms break down animal and vegetable matter in the soil. Observing this decomposition of organic material, Waksman noted the destructive effect of these microorganisms on certain bacteria. In 1939 Waksman formally began his search for antibiotics among these microbes, discovering streptomycin in 1943. He recognized its value in treating tuberculosis as well as a number of other bacterial infections.

Among a great many scientific articles and papers Waksman's published work includes *Enzymes* (with W.C. Davison, 1926); *Principles of Soil Microbiology* (1927); *The Soil and the Microbe* (with R.L. Starkey, 1931); *Humus* (1936); *Microbial Antagonisms and Microbiotic Substances* (1945); *Streptomycin* (1949); the autobiographical *My Life with the Microbes* (1954); *The Actinomycetes* (3 vols., 1959–1962); and *The Conquest of Tuberculosis* (1964).

George Wald 1906–

In acknowledgment of his important contribution to the understanding of color blindness George Wald received the 1967 Nobel Prize for Physiology or Medicine, which he shared with Ragnar Granit and HALDAN HARTLINE. With his colleague Paul K. Brown, Wald identified the yellow-green pigment in the color receptor cells of the eye as a component in color perception.

Born to immigrant parents at the turn of the century, Wald grew up on the Lower East Side of New York City. He graduated from New York University in 1927 and received his doctoral degree in zoology from Columbia University in 1932. Invited to Berlin to work as a fellow in the laboratory of distinguished chemist OTTO WARBURG, Wald conducted pioneering studies on the relationship between vision and nutrition. His findings include the discovery of vitamin A in the retina, the area of the eye where the light receptors are located.

After two years in Berlin Wald returned to the United States to continue his work at Harvard University, where he remained until 1977. Investigating the complex biochemical processes involved in vision, Wald uncovered the chemical reactions occurring during the activity of the rods, the low-light receptors of the retina.

His opposition to the Vietnam War early in the 1960s is thought to have been a factor in his early retirement from Harvard University. Since then he has lectured extensively on the threat of nuclear war and the dangers of the arms race.

Wald's published writings include *General Education in a Free Society* (1945) and *Twenty-six Afternoons of Biology: An Introductory Laboratory Manual* (1962).

Lillian D. Wald 1867–1940

Dedicated to the cause of public health, Lillian Wald was responsible for establishing important social reforms to meet the needs of the growing immigrant population of New York City at the turn of the century.

After receiving her nursing degree in 1888 from New York Hospital Training School for Women, Wald moved to the Lower East Side of New York City to better understand the pressures and demands of the impoverished immigrant community. She began by establishing a visiting nurse service in 1893. This program soon evolved into the Henry Street Settlement, a neighborhood center providing opportunities for recreation and artistic expression as well as medical services. Under her directorship, which lasted until 1933, the Henry Street Settlement gained worldwide attention and respect.

Committed to improving inner-city conditions, Wald instituted important social reforms, many of them inspired by her ongoing involvement with the settlement. A pioneer in the field of child welfare, Wald introduced the notion that it was the responsibility of the community to see that children were provided for. In 1902 she launched the first program to provide nursing service in the public schools. Her recommendation of a United States Children's Bureau was adopted in 1912.

Enlisting the cooperation of the Red Cross and the Metropolitan Life Insurance Company, Wald established a large-scale home nursing organization. An active member in many charity organizations and reform groups, Wald played an important part in the founding of the National Organization for Public Health Nursing, becoming its first president in 1912.

Wald produced two autobiographical works, *The House on Henry Street*, published in 1915, and *Windows on Henry Street*, published in 1934.

Wilhelm von Waldeyer-Hartz 1836–1921

Distinguished German anatomist Wilhelm von Waldeyer-Hartz is noted for his investigations in morphology, pathology and anthropology, and most notably for his role in establishing the fundamental mechanism of the nervous system. His many contributions to medical nomenclature include the introduction of the words "neuron" (from the Greek meaning cord or nerve) and "chromosome" (derived from the Greek words *khroia*, meaning color, and *soma*, meaning body or structure) to describe the dark-staining strands in the cell nucleus. In addition, Waldeyer's name identifies a great many anatomical structures, including a set of glands in the inner skin of the eyelid ("Waldeyer's glands"), the vascular layer of the ovary ("Waldeyer's layer"), a pair of spiral-shaped cavities within the cochlear duct of the ear ("Waldeyer's sulci"), and a circular set of tissues surrounding the pharynx ("Waldeyer's tonsillar ring").

Influenced by the neurohistological studies of pioneer Spanish physiologist SANTIAGO RAMON Y CAJAL, Waldeyer provided morphological evidence to support the concept of an anatomically and physiologically autonomous nerve cell or "neurone" as the fundamental unit of the nervous system. As a result of the combined efforts of Waldeyer, Cajal, WILHELM HIS, Edward Sharpey-Schafer, Swiss physician and psychiatrist August Forel (1848–1904) and others, the "neurone doctrine" was firmly established by the end of the nineteenth century, superseding Camillo Golgi's view of the nervous system as a net of interlocked and interdependent nerves.

Born in Hehlen, Germany, Waldeyer was drawn to a career in biological science as a student of celebrated German anatomist Friedrich Henle at the University of Gottingen. Completing his doctoral studies under Karl Reichert at the University of Berlin, Waldeyer taught physiology and histology at Konigsberg and at Breslau, where he initiated important research in pathology, most notably the early diagnosis of cancer. Based on an investigation of the cellular mechanisms in various forms of cancer, Waldeyer pinpointed the origin of tumor growth in the cells of the outer layer of the skin.

At the age of 29 he was named professor of pathology and director of Breslau's newly founded department of postmortem research, and within three years' time he was appointed to the university's chair of pathology. In 1872 he was offered the chair of anatomy at the University of Strasbourg, where Germans were being recruited to replace the French faculty following the Prussian takeover of Alsace.

Waldeyer remained at Strasbourg until 1883, when he returned to the University of Berlin to succeed his former mentor, Karl Reichert, as director of the department of anatomy as well as professor of pathology, embryology and anatomy. Widely recognized for his diagnostic insight as well as for his advanced knowledge of the anatomy and pathology of the throat, Waldeyer was among the physicians called in to examine Emperor Frederick III when he was afflicted with a tumor of the vocal cords.

A distinguished administrator and an influential teacher at the University of Berlin, Waldeyer also published a number of important papers, including studies of the urogenital system, the anatomy of the pelvis and the spinal cord of the gorilla. He retired at the age of eighty and five years later suffered a fatal stroke at his home in Berlin.

Owen Harding Wangensteen 1898–1981

An influential figure in twentieth-century surgical medicine, Owen Wangensteen made important contributions to the surgical treatment of cancer, appendicitis, ulcers and gastrointestinal disease. His invention of an aspiration device, since called the "Wangensteen tube," offered surgeons a valuable tool in abdominal surgery for the removal of gas from the intestine.

Wangensteen's lifelong association with the University of Minnesota led to the development of an internationally distinguished department of surgery. Recognizing the importance of physiology training in the study of surgery, Wangensteen's efforts to combine those two disciplines led the University of Minnesota to become a center for the development of open-heart surgery. Wangensteen's skills as a clinician, researcher and educator contributed to the training of the most outstanding practitioners in the field, notably CHRISTIAAN BARNARD, John Lewis, Norman E. Shumway, C. WALTON LILLEHEI and Vincent Gott, among others.

Born and raised on a farm in Minnesota, Owen was encouraged by his father to become a doctor. After graduating from the University of Minnesota Wangensteen studied in Europe for a year, visiting surgical clinics in England, France, Italy, Germany, Holland, Switzerland and Denmark. Appalled at the lack of experimental work being done in surgical research, Wangensteen said he "became convinced of the importance of physiology training to the surgeon and that this would be the stepping-stone for the surgeon in the twentieth century as anatomy had been in the nineteenth century."

Returning to the University of Minnesota in the fall of 1928, Wangensteen was chairman of the department of surgery by the time he was 31. He was to retain that position until 1967, establishing the strength and reputation of his department while continuing to pursue his own clinical and experimental research.

Primarily interested in intestinal obstruction, Wangensteen introduced the use of a catheter smaller than the one currently favored for draining enterocolostomies the operative formation of a passage between the colon and the small intestine. As a result, the incidence of potentially fatal damage during such procedures was greatly reduced. His introduction in 1932 of a suction apparatus for treatment of acute bowel obstruction further contributed to the tremendous drop in mortality rate from obstruction- related conditions.

In addition to pioneering advances in the surgical treatment of appendicitis when accompanied by peptic ulcers, inflammation of the peritoneum, and other disorders, Wangensteen initiated a two-part testing program for cancer at the university in 1948. Noting a disparity in recurrence rates depending on whether the lymph nodes had or had not been involved with the cancer, Wangensteen instituted the "second-look program," requiring return checkups for those patients with nodal involvement and therefore at greater risk of recurrence. At the same time Wangensteen introduced a screening program for early detection of the disease.

With the collaboration of his wife, Sarah, managing editor of *Modern Medicine*, Wangensteen produced a monumental study of medical history entitled *The Rise of Surgery, Emergence from Empiric Craft to Scientific Discipline.* Proceeds from the book, published in 1979, were donated to the University of Minnesota. In addition, Wangensteen has authored or co-authored nearly 900 published articles.

Otto Heinrich Warburg 1883–1970

German physiologist and biochemist Otto Warburg is celebrated for his pioneering research in cellular respiration and metabolism, particularly in cancer cells. For his discovery of the nature and mechanism of a crucial respiratory enzyme, now known as Warburg's enzyme, he was awarded the Nobel Prize for Physiology or Medicine in 1931.

Born in Frieburg, Warburg embarked on his training in physiology and chemistry at the University of Berlin in 1901. Twelve years later, after completing doctoral studies at the University of Heidelberg, he returned to Berlin to accept a research position at the Kaiser Wilhelm Institute for Cell Physiology (later renamed the Max Planck Institute). Warburg was 30 when he launched what was to be a lifelong association with the institute. A significant influence for more than half a century, he served as director at the Max Planck from 1953 until his death in 1970.

Warburg's outstanding contribution to medical research includes innovations in experimental methodology as well as important advances in the chemistry of cellular metabolism and respiration, photosynthesis and the formation and growth of tumors. Isolating and identifying an organic iron compound found in all tissues, he established the substance as a primary factor in cell respiration. Hailed as a significant breakthrough in the study of cell metabolism, the discovery of "Warburg's enzyme" was awarded the Nobel Prize in 1931. Three years later his work was again honored by the Nobel Committee, but, because he was a Jew, Warburg was prevented from accepting the prize by decree of Nazi leader Adolf Hitler.

A prolific author, Warburg published five books and more than 500 articles and monographs. Notable writings include *The Metabolism of Tumours* (Eng. trans. 1931), *Heavy Metal Prosthetic Groups and Enzyme Action* (Eng. trans. 1949), *New Methods of Cell Physiology* (Eng. trans. 1962).

August Paul von Wassermann 1866–1925

August Wassermann lent his name to a diagnostic blood-serum test designed to detect the presence of syphilis. The first reliable method for diagnosing syphilis, the Wassermann test was also the first effective means of determining whether or not the disease had been cured. The general application of Wasserman's discovery exposed many of the misconceptions surrounding syphilis and indicated to medical professionals that the disease was far more persistent and widespread than had been believed. In addition, widespread use of the test revealed the ineffectiveness of mercury, the prevailing treatment for syphilis, encouraging PAUL EHRLICH'S discovery of a definitive cure five years later.

Positive test results in patients who had been given mercury demonstrated that the "cure" was generally incomplete. Misinterpreted symptoms, such as partial paralysis, lack of muscle coordination and certain types of heart disease were shown to be the disguised effects of syphilis.

Born in Bamberg, Germany, Wassermann studied bacteriological medicine at the universities of Erlangen, Vienna, Munich and Strasbourg. After obtaining a medical degree in 1898 he joined the staff of the Robert Koch Institute for Infectious Diseases in Berlin. Wassermann conducted investigative research in bacteriology and chemotherapy, a term coined by Erlich to refer to a method of treatment using drugs to act selectively against the microorganisms causing a disease.

Working with Albert Neisser and Carl Bruck, Wassermann developed his method for detecting syphilis in 1906. Also known as the "Wassermann reaction," the test is based on the discovery that sera taken from patients with syphilis contain an element that destroys red corpuscles in the blood of sheep. The test is considered highly reliable even in asymptomatic cases, although a few other diseases (including leprosy) may occasionally produce a false positive reaction.

In 1906 Wassermann was named director of the department of experimental therapy and serum research at the Koch Institute, and he remained there until 1913. In addition to his pioneer work on syphilis Wassermann developed an antitoxin treatment for diphtheria and inoculations against cholera, typhoid and tetanus. He left the Koch Institute to head the department of experimental therapy at the Kaiser Wilhelm Institute, also in Berlin, serving as director until his death in 1925. Wassermann's serum research conducted at Kaiser Wilhelm produced a reliable diagnostic test for tuberculosis.

James Dewey Watson see FRANCIS HARRY COMPTON CRICK.

John Broadus Watson 1878–1958

John Watson introduced the psychological school known as behaviorism in 1913 in an article called "Psychology as a Behaviorist Views It." Dismissing the notions of soul, consciousness, subjective states and introspection as irrelevant to the study of psychology, Watson launched a movement that was to radically affect all aspects of psychology.

Born in Greenville, South Carolina, Watson was teaching psychology at the University of Chicago by the time he was twenty-five and in 1908, at the age of thirty, he was named director of the psychology laboratory at Johns Hopkins University. His original 1913 paper on behaviorism was refined and expanded within a year into what is considered his most important work, *Be-*

havior-An Introduction to Comparative Psychology. Defining behavior as a physiological response to stimuli, Watson maintained that the purpose of psychology was to predict and control human behavior. He rejected all but empirical evidence in his experimental work, repudiating the testimony of conscious or unconscious mental activity.

The doctrine of behaviorism stressses the influence of learning and environment, while de-emphasizing the effects of heredity and instinct. Watson performed extensive experimental research on birds, rats, and monkeys, and in 1918 he began his now-famous study of human infants. Based on experimental observation of newborns, Watson conceded only three "unconditioned" or unlearned responses: fear, rage, and love.

Calling attention to the practical applications of psychology, behaviorism has been an influential force in child-rearing since its inception. In 1925, Watson wrote *Behaviorism*, a book intended for popular audiences, in which he claimed that if he were given a dozen healthy infants and a free hand to create the proper environment, he could turn any one of them into anything that might be ordered: "doctor, lawyer, artist, merchant chief, and yes even beggarman and thief, regardless of his talents, penchants, tendencies, abilities, vocations, and race of his ancestors."

Behaviorism's laboratory-based theories declined in popularity over the years, although, mainly through the work of B.F. Skinner*, "descriptive behaviorism" and techniques of conditioning remain important in modern psychology.

In 1920 Watson became embroiled in a divorce scandal that forced his resignation from Johns Hopkins University. Leaving behind his life as an academic, Watson went on to become an advertising executive.

Watson's other published works include *Psychology from the Standpoint of a Behaviorist* (1919) and *Psychological Care of Infant and Child* (1928).

August Weismann 1834–1914

August Weismann was a key figure in the heated controversies over the mechanism of evolution in the late nineteenth century. Insisting that acquired characteristics cannot be inherited, Weismann, along with fellow evolutionists Alfred Russel Wallace (1823–1894) and Wilhelm Roux, launched a long and fierce debate that extended beyond biology to include philosophical, political and moral principles, pitting "neo-Darwinists" against "neo-Lamarckists."

Even though he had described natural selection as the primary agent of evolution, Darwin believed in the "inherited effects of the use and disuse of parts." "Weismannism," a form of neo-Darwinism or ultra-Darwinism, was a materialistic theory stating that the material of heredity is contained in an immutable form set aside in the germ cells during the parent's own development. Referring to this protoplasmic material as "germ plasm," Weismann asserted that the hereditary information it contained was not subject to changes in the environment or circumstances of the parent's life.

Based partly on the ideas of Dutch geneticist Hugo de Vries (1848–1935), Weismann's theory stated that the nuclei, and particularly the chromosomes, contain all the necessary information for determining the development and particular characteristics of plants and animals. In the decades that followed Weismann's studies genetic research revealed chromosomes to be simply strands of genes, the fundamental units of inheritance. For a time the role of the nucleus was disregarded, until later studies in molecular biology and biochemistry revealed the chemical aspect of the genetic mechanism.

Weismann entered into further controversy with his theories on the mechanism of inheritance in sexual reproduction. A debate raged around the question of how offspring resemble their parents while still retaining their own individuality. In his book *Das Keimplasm (The Germ Plasm)*, published in 1892, Weismann asserted that the two sets of chromosomes always retain their integrity, repudiating the notion that fertilization is a process of blending or fusion of male and female hereditary material. Weismann's theory was confirmed several decades later with the full acceptance of Mendelian laws of heredity and variation.

A native of Frankfurt, Germany, Weismann became professor of zoology at the University of Freiburg in 1866. Among his first published works was an article on the development of the *Diptera*, the zoological order of flies. In the decade that followed he published a series of papers, translated in 1882 as *Studies in the Theory of Descent*. His theories of inheritance are expounded in a collection of his works appearing in translation in two volumes entitled *Essays upon Heredity and Kindred Biological Problems* (1889–1892).

Thomas Huckle Weller 1915–

Distinguished virologist and parasitologist Thomas Weller participated in the first experimental cultivation of the poliovirus in human tissue. This achievement, accomplished in 1949, faciliated the mass production of the virus, which in turn enabled the development of JONAS SALK's poliomyelitis vaccine. In addition, laboratory cultivation of the virus permitted effective and widespread diagnosis of the disease at a time when polio was still taking many thousands of lives every year.

Weller did much of his work as a member of a distinguished collaborative trio that also included JOHN F. ENDERS and FREDERICK C. ROBBINS. The three shared the 1954 Nobel Prize for Physiology or Medicine.

The son of the chief of the pathology department at the University of Michigan, Weller grew up in Ann

Arbor surrounded by his father's colleagues and students. Weller's grandfather, a general practitioner, contributed further inspiration for young Thomas's medical career. Weller became intrigued with parasitology during his undergraduate years at the University of Michigan, where he obtained a master's degree in 1937. He entered Harvard Medical School in that same year, receiving his doctorate in 1940.

Before graduating Weller received a Rockefeller Foundation fellowship that led to a tour of duty in Florida, where poverty, malnutrition and malaria combined to create severe community health problems. Firmly committed to the service of public health, Weller returned north to complete his studies at Harvard with an increased interest in virology. He began work as an intern in Enders's laboratory, but their work together was interrupted by the war.

Weller trained in the army's school for medics and in the fall of 1942 was assigned to a parasitology laboratory in Puerto Rico. Before the end of the war Weller had taken over as chief of the parasitology, biology and virology divisions of the army's Antilles Department laboratory.

Weller returned to Boston to complete his residency at the Children's Hospital, where Enders had been invited to head the new Research Laboratory for Infectious Diseases. Weller and Enders were planning studies of mumps and chicken pox when they were joined by Robbins, who was being supported by a fellowship in viral research from the National Foundation for Infantile Paralysis. After successfully cultivating the mumps virus in embryonic tissue Weller attempted to perform the same experiments with the virus for chicken pox, or varicella.

Also available in the laboratory was a strain of poliovirus, and a last-minute decision was made to use the technique with both types of virus. Although the varicella failed to grow, the poliovirus was successfully cultured, leading to further experimentation with various types of human tissue and different strains of the virus. In the years that followed Enders, Weller and Robbins successfully isolated and cultivated thirteen different strains of poliovirus.

After receiving the Nobel Prize Weller returned to the study of tropical diseases later isolating the varicella and rubella viruses as well as the cytomegalovirus, also known as the salivary gland virus. As a faculty member at Harvard's School of Public Health Weller devoted his time to research, teaching and clinical practice in the field. He later became head of the university's Department of Tropical Health.

George Hoyt Whipple 1878–1976

Studying the effects of diet on blood formation, American pathologist George Whipple demonstrated the therapeutic effects of kidney, beef and, most notably, liver in the treatment of anemia.

Characterized by an abormally low blood level of hemoglobin, anemia can be caused by blood loss, by increased destruction of red blood cells, the carriers of hemoglobin, or by a defect in hemoglobin production, resulting in pernicious anemia. In this last form of the disease severe atrophy of the stomach leads to a deficiency in gastric secretions, particularly of the proteins needed for the absorption of vitamin B_{12}.

For several decades researchers had considered the role of nutrition in anemia, but it was not until Whipple systematically evaluated the effects of various foods on the process of blood formation that the significance of diet was revealed. Using dogs as experimental subjects, Whipple induced anemia by bleeding the animals, then established a stable blood level of hemoglobin as a baseline. A comparative analysis of blood level fluctuations in response to various foods showed that a great increase in blood level follows the ingestion of liver.

In 1922 physicians GEORGE RICHARDS MINOT and William Parry Murphy traveled to the University of Rochester to visit Whipple's laboratory. Intrigued by Whipple's experimental findings, Murphy remarked that although diet had previously been used therapeutically, a specific food "had often been selected because it appeared to be easily digested or because it seemed particularly nutritious or strength-giving. Rarely have diets been chosen for some assumed direct effect on the blood."

Empowered by Whipple's conclusive results, Minot and Murphy went on to develop a cure for pernicious anemia based on the therapeutic value of liver. Acknowledging the final achievement as well as Whipple's considerable contribution at the earliest stages of the research, the Nobel Prize for Physiology or Medicine was awarded jointly to all three scientists in 1934.

Born in New Hamsphire, Whipple graduated from Yale in 1900, receiving his medical degree five years later from Johns Hopkins University. The newly founded medical school had just begun to establish its distinguished reputation as the first American institution to rival the celebrated medical colleges of Europe. Strongly influenced by noted pathology professor William H. Welch, a member of the school's original faculty, Whipple was to carry on the traditions and high standards of Hopkins as a professor of medicine at the University of California, and later as the first dean of the medical school at the University of Rochester.

An influential figure in the American scientific establishment, Whipple served as director of the Hooper Foundation for Medical Research. As a trustee of the Rockefeller Foundation and the General Education Board, he also served for seventeen years on the board of scientific directors at the Rockefeller Institute for Medical Research.

Charles White 1728–1813

Charles White is credited with elevating the art of midwifery from a brutal practice distorted by superstition to a humane and scientifically based form of medicine. One of the leading obstetricians of his century, White was an early proponent of antisepsis, anticipating by more than a century the discoveries of LISTER, PASTEUR and SEMMELWEIS. White wrote extensively on his clinical observations of puerperal fever, asserting that he had discovered the means of curing and even averting the disease.

With remarkable insight White wrote, "In hospitals if separate apartments cannot be allowed every patient, at least as soon as the fever has seized one, she ought immediately to be removed into another room, not only for her immediate safety, but for that of the other patients."

White and his contemporary Alexander Gordon (1752–1799) recognized the phenomenon of transmitted infection, but although both published articles strongly recommending the disinfection of maternity wards and personnel, the medical establishment paid little attention. White's tremendous success as an obstetrician did receive notice, however, as did his masterful work entitled *Treatise on the Management of Pregnant and Lying-In Women, and the means of Curing, but more especially of Preventing the Principle Disorders of which they are Liable.* Published in 1773, the book was translated into French and German and reprinted in America in 1793. At a time when cleanliness was rarely considered in the practice of medicine, White's book called for hygienic conditions for the patient, the practitioners and even the medical instruments.

In addition to discussions of fever and infection White described a condition of venous thrombosis that occurs in some women after childbirth, causing massive swellings of the legs, though without inflammation—a symptom known as "white leg," " milk leg," or *phlegmasia alba dolens puerperarum.*

Born in Manchester, England, White received his earliest medical training from his father, who served as physician and midwife to the poor of Manchester. After studying anatomy with the celebrated WILLIAM HUNTER in London Charles White attended the newly established school of obstetrics at Edinburgh, finally returning to Manchester in 1749 to join his father's practice.

In 1757 White's financial condition improved dramatically due to a strange and unpredictable piece of luck. One of his patients died, leaving him £25,000 in her will on condition that he embalm her body and ensure that it remain above ground for 100 years. The will further stipulated that White visit her corpse once every year and, in the presence of two witnesses, lift the veil from her face. White fulfilled the requirements of the will, keeping the cadaver in his anatomical museum for several years. He later bought an estate with part of his peculiarly earned fortune, moving his benefactress into the attic of his new mansion.

The balance of White's inheritance went to the development of obstetrics, a goal that led him to help found the Manchester Lying-In Hospital in 1790.

Paul Dudley White 1886–1973

Paul Dudley White was a major figure in the development of twentieth-century cardiology. Internationally respected as a physician and researcher, White gained public recognition in 1955 when he treated President Eisenhower for a myocardial infarction.

In addition to his distinguished reputation as a clinician, White is celebrated for his investigation of the causes of heart disease. During a career that spanned more than half a century White made important contributions to the prevention and diagnosis of coronary disease. Among the first cardiologists to call attention to the relationship between heart disease and diet, exercise and stress, White was also one of the earliest to use an electrocardiograph, a device for evaluating the action of the heart muscle by measuring and recording the electric current produced by contraction.

As a promising young physician at Massachussetts General Hospital, White was sent to London in 1924 to study cardiology under Welsh physiologist Sir Thomas Lewis, a leading authority on heart disease. Lewis was an early advocate of the electrocardiograph, recognizing its enormous potential for early detection and diagnosis of cardiac disorders.

White served on the staff of Massachussetts General Hospital throughout his career. In 1914 he joined the faculty at Harvard Medical School, where for 40 years he remained an influential and much-admired figure.

In 1922 White founded the American Heart Association. His writings include the widely respected *Heart Disease.* Published in 1931, White's work has become a standard reference text for medical practitioners.

Torsten Nils Wiesel 1924–

Torsten Wiesel conducted pioneering research exploring the brain's mechanism for processing visual information. After receiving his medical degree in 1954 from the Karolinska Institute in his native Sweden Wiesel was invited to conduct neurological research at Johns Hopkins Medical School. His work there brought him together with DAVID HUBEL, launching a long and productive collaboration. In 1959 the two transferred to Harvard Medical School, where they pursued their study of the system of information processing between brain and visual input.

Experimenting with cats and monkeys, Wiesel and Hubel set out to decipher the visual interpretation process one cell at a time. For more than two decades they charted the functions of the cells of the visual cortex, determining that individual neurons or nerve cells perform specific functions in the complex process of creating a coherent picture from visual information.

In 1981 Wiesel and Hubel were awarded the Nobel Prize for Physiology or Medicine, which they shared with Roger Sperry, for their important work in mapping the complex neurological mechanism of visual processing.

William Robert Wilde 1815–1876

William Wilde would have been better known, perhaps, for his achievements in aural and ophthalmic surgery if his prominence had not been overshadowed by the talent and notoriety of his son, Oscar Wilde.

William Wilde was born in the tiny Irish village of Castlerea, where his father served as general medical practitioner. At 17 Wilde left for Dublin to train for a career in surgery at Steeven's Hospital, obtaining his qualifying degree in 1837. Seizing the opportunity for a change of scene, Wilde accepted a position as personal physician to a wealthy invalid and for the next nine months lived on board a private yacht as he and his patient sailed around the Mediterranean. His account of the trip, entitled *The Narrative of a Voyage to Madeira, Teneriffe, and along the shores of the Mediterranean* (sic), appeared in 1840 as his first published work.

After this fling at travel he resumed his medical training, studying advanced surgical techniques for the treatment of eye and ear disorders at the Universities of London, Berlin and Vienna. In 1841 he settled in Dublin to establish a surgical practice specializing in eye and ear surgery. Soon recognized as a highly skilled practitioner, Wilde also gained distinction throughout the country for providing his services free of charge to impoverished patients. Ireland's generous "aurist" and "oculist," as such specialists were then known, contributed his first earnings to the establishment of St. Mark's Ophthalmic Hospital, the first such institution in Dublin.

Firmly committed to the advancement of all branches of medicine, Wilde was founding editor of the *Dublin Quarterly Journal of Medical Science* as well as a versatile and prolific author of books and monographs on a wide range of medical topics. As medical commissioner for the Irish census he wrote a reference manual entitled *The Epidemics of Ireland*, which provides a medical and historical account dating back to ancient times.

Wilde contributed most significantly to the elevation and expansion of his specialties with the publication of *Epidemic Ophthalmia* in 1851 and *Aural Surgery* in 1853. By then his reputation, already distinguished at home, had begun to extend beyond the boundaries of Ireland. In 1853 he was commissioned "surgeon-oculist in ordinary to the Queen of Ireland," a royal appointment created in his honor.

Wilde's marriage to Jane Francesca Elgee, the daughter of an Episcopalian minister, a popular writer and the center of a literary circle, had by then produced a first child, also named William. A noted London journalist, he died at the age of 46. The Wildes became parents for the second time in 1854 with the birth of Oscar O'Flahertie Wills Wilde.

William Wilde's scholarship extended beyond medical science to natural history, ethnology, archeology and topography. He was a considered a leading authority on Irish antiquities and achieved his greatest literary success with the publication of his *Catalogue of the Contents of the Museum of the Royal Irish Academy*, a masterpiece of archeological theory and detailed description presented in three volumes, the first of which appeared in 1858. For his work on the Irish census Wilde was knighted in 1864 by the Irish Viceroy, acting for Queen Victoria.

Maurice High Frederick Wilkins see FRANCIS HARRY COMPTON CRICK

Thomas Willis 1621–1675

Thomas Willis helped to formulate our modern understanding of the mind and the functioning of the brain. Before the concept of cerebral localization defense was understood and accepted, the idea of a "sensorium commune" was the generally accepted model for the mind. The theory depicted a brain that was a catch-all for every sensory message of input. This idea first appeared at the end of the fourth century and managed to hold until its first serious challenges nearly 1200 years later. Descartes expanded this ancient notion, maintaining that all mental activity took place in the pineal gland and could occur only in beings with a "non-material soul."

Thomas Willis rejected the idea of non-human animals as machines incapable of experiencing sensation, and referred to the "soul of a brute" or corporeal soul. Willis treated perception and even imagination as organic activities, leaving only the powers of judgment and reason to the rational soul. He carefully described and distinguished a wide range of thought processes and responses, situating them in various areas of the brain. In Willis's model, involuntary motion originated in the cerebellum, voluntary motion in the cerebrum, and both were the result of "reflected activity." He located the power of memory in the cortex.

Willis also developed an enlightened system of animal classification that clearly differentiated the respiratory, circulatory and nervous systems. His anatomical and physiological descriptions led to the use of his name to identify a circle of arteries at the base of the brain, the eleventh cranial nerve and a particular form of deafness. He also christened the pineal gland *pineus* (pine cone), although he misinterpreted its function. These ideas were published in Latin in 1664 as *De Cerebri Anatome* (*On the Anatomy of the Brain*; illustrated by Sir Christopher Wren). In 1672 he published *De Anima Brutorum (The Soul of a Brute)*.

Willis was born and educated in England and spent the first six years of his career as a professor of natural philosophy at Oxford. In 1666 he established what was to be a highly successful private medical practice in London. He continued to study and write about the nervous system and examined other aspects of clinical medicine as well. Willis is credited as the first physician to note the presence of sugar in the urine of diabetic patients, which he discovered by testing the specimens. He developed theories of animal heat and fermentation and wrote about his investigations of the plague.

As a logical extension of his view of human mental activity, Willis understood insanity and mental derangement as a disease and offered the first clear description of paresis (a partial paralysis), although he did not recognize it as a symptom of syphilis. Many of his theories and conclusions have long been disproven. Nevertheless, his discussion of the faculties of insight and imagination as functions of the brain were of profound importance, although he wrongly situated such activity in the corpus callosum, the bundle of nerve fibres connecting the two hemispheres of the brain.

Almroth Wright 1861–1947

The practice of vaccination was introduced in the late 1800s by EDWARD JENNER, but it was not until the beginning of the twentieth century that vaccines were used to cure or prevent bacterial diseases. This advance, which required investigation of the immune system, is owed in large part to the work of Almoth Wright in the area of pathological bacteriology.

Wright was born in Yorkshire, England and pursued a well-rounded medical education at Dublin, Leipzig, Strasbourg and Marburg in Germany. He began teaching pathology in 1892 at the Army Medical School in Netley, England. After ten years there he left to teach experimental pathology at the University of London. In 1902 he became principal of the Institute of Pathology and Research at St. Mary's Hospital. A number of people had already begun studying the mysteries of the immune system, notably ELIE METCHNIKOFF, who had noticed that white blood cells engulf bacteria in a process known as phagocytosis. Generally bacteria would be digested and killed, but occasionally the bacteria would kill the white cells. In 1903, enlarging on these studies, Wright described the activities of opsonins, substances in the blood that coat the white cells to aid in the phagocytosis of bacteria. In showing the serum factors necessary for this process he demonstrated a combined involvement of cell tissue and body fluids. These findings enabled Metchnikoff and Alexis Carrel to develop the ideas that led to organ and tissue transplants.

His authority in the field of vaccine therapy was widely recognized. ALEXANDER FLEMING, the noted microbiologist, became one of Wright's pupils in the early days of his tenure at St. Mary's. Wright introduced the first antityphoid inoculation, and in 1906 he received a knighthood, mainly for his brilliant work on parasitic diseases. He remained at St. Mary's until the end of his life. His published works include *Pathology and the Treatment of War Wounds* (1942), *Researches in Clinical Physiology* (1943) and *Studies on Immunization* (1943–1944).

Y

Rosalyn S. Yalow 1921–

Rosalyn Yalow helped devise the method of measurement known as "radioimmunoassay," or RIA, a technique designed to detect and measure extremely small amounts of biologically active substances. By means of radioactive "tracers," the system recognizes minute concentrations of hormones, vitamins, enzymes, toxins and other materials previously undetectable.

The daughter of first-generation Jewish immigrants, Yalow grew up in the Bronx during the Depression. Her scientific ambitions took hold in childhood, and by 1941, at the age of nineteen, she became the first student to receive a degree in physics and chemistry from Hunter College in New York. In the 1940s there was still considerable resistance to the candidacy of a woman for a graduate school assistantship. To get around that hurdle she took a job as secretary for a biochemist at Columbia University in the hope of gaining admission to graduate lectures.

When the entry of the United States into World War II began to drain the male student population, the physics department of the University of Illinois in desperation accepted Yalow as its first female graduate assistant since 1917. She received her doctorate in 1945 and two years later began research in the field of nuclear medicine. She returned to the Bronx as a part-time consultant at the Veterans Administration Hospital. Anticipating the potential of radioisotopes as a powerful tool in medical diagnosis, therapy and research, Yalow designed and constructed equipment with which to conduct experimental research with these radioactive elements.

In 1950 Yalow joined forces with a young internist, Solomon A. Berson, in a fruitful and rewarding scientific collaboration that would last until Berson's death in 1972. Together Yalow and Berson created the RIA, a valuable resource in many different areas of medicine. Useful in diagnosing a wide range of conditions, including diabetes, hepatitis, sterility and some forms of cancer, it has also proved an important tool in blood banks and in forensic medicine.

After Berson's death Yalow was widely acclaimed for her role in the invention of RIA. In 1976 she became the first woman to receive the Albert Lasker Basic Medical Research Award. This prestigious honor was followed by many others, culminating in the Nobel Prize for Physiology or Medicine in 1976, which she shared with ROGER GUILLEMIN and ANDREW V. SCHALLY. As the prize is never awarded posthumously, the Nobel committee could not recognize Berson's contribution. Yalow honored Berson by giving his name to her research laboratory.

James Yearsley 1805–1869

A pioneer in aural surgery, British physician and surgeon James Yearsley established the connection between deafness and nasopharyngeal disease.

Born in northern Scotland, Yearsley began his professional training in Gloucester as an apprentice to eminent surgeon Ralph Fletcher. After completing clinical requirements at St. Bartholomew's Hospital in London Yearsley was accepted as a member of England's Royal College of Surgeons and as a licentiate of the Society of Apothecaries in 1827. After several years in Cheltenham as a general practitioner Yearsley left for London, where, in 1837, he became the city's first aural surgeon.

In the decade that followed he investigated various treatments for deafness, most notably the implantation of an artificial tympanic membrane. Commonly known as the eardrum, the tympanic membrane separates the middle ear from the inner end of the external ear canal, creating a cavity called the tympanum. Sound waves resonating in the auditory canal cause the thin membrane of the eardrum to vibrate against the malleus, a hammer-like structure in the middle ear. To treat cases of deafness or hearing impairment due to a malfunction of the eardrum, Yearsley developed a procedure for replacing the defective membrane with a delicate film that approximated the sensitivity of eardrum response.

Establishing clinical and research facilities on Sackville Street, Picadilly, Yearsley created the first institution dedicated to the advancement of otological disorders. Appointed surgeon to the Royal Society of Musicians in 1846, he contributed important advances in the study and treatment of speech defects and throat disease.

In 1852 Yearsley founded the *Medical Circular*, a respected journal that merged with the *Dublin Medical Press* in 1866. He is also noted as one of the originators of the distinguished *Medical Directory*, a classic reference guide for physicians. Other notable writings include *Contributions to Aural Surgery* and *Stammering* (both published in 1841), *A Treatise on Enlarged Tonsils* (1842), *On Throat Deafness* (1853) and *Deafness Practically Illustrated* (1854).

Alexandre Émile Jean Yersin 1863–1943

As the study of immunology increased its momentum toward the end of the nineteenth century bacteriologist Alexandre Yersin contributed significantly to the advancement of preventive medicine with his work on antitoxins.

Once a student of LOUIS PASTEUR, Yersin conducted landmark studies with P.P.E. Roux at the Pasteur Institute in Paris on diphtheria antitoxin. Demonstrating that the diphtheria bacillus produces a substance that causes the disease, Yersin and Roux showed that the diphtheria toxin can be separated from the integral structure of the bacillus. This discovery led to a formal distinction between "exotoxins," poisons emitted by bacterial cells in diseases like diphtheria and botulism, and "endotoxins," poisons that are an inherent part of the bacterial structure. Endotoxins are released as the cell itself disintegrates.

In the 1890s Yersin and Japanese bacteriologist SHIBASABURO KITASATO conducted independent studies of the bacillus of the bubonic plague. Both scientists isolated the causative agent *Pasteurella pestis*, paving the way for an effective method of immunization against this ancient and deadly disease.

Born of Swiss parentage in Rougemont, France, Yersin was educated at the universities of Lausanne, Marburg and Paris. He went on to study at the newly founded Pasteur Institute in Paris, where Louis Pasteur himself was serving as director in the last years of his life.

After completing his work with Roux Yersin left for Hong Kong, where he discovered the plague bacillus in 1893, later developing a serum to combat the disease. After establishing two Pasteur Institutes in China Yersin went on to head the Pasteur Institute at Nhatrang in southeast Annam. In addition to serving as inspector general of the Pasteur Institutes at Saigon, Hanoi and Dalat, Yersin is noted for having introduced the rubber tree into Indochina.

Thomas Young 1773–1828

The versatile English physician Thomas Young is best known for his important advances in the study of optics and vision. He was considered a leading authority of his time in a number of diverse fields, distinguishing himself in the areas of physics, perception, medicine and Egyptology. Young is still credited for his contributions to the theory of tides, the establishment of a coefficient of elasticity, the deciphering of the Rosetta stone and the introduction of modern science's concept of energy.

Born at Milverton, Somerset, Thomas Young began practicing as a physician in London in 1799 after studying medicine at the universities of London, Edinburgh, Gottingen and Cambridge. Within two years Young gave up medical practice to pursue his own scientific research. As professor of natural philosophy at London's Royal Institution, Young expounded many of his developing theories on light and light perception.

His extensive medical education had familiarized Young with the physiology of the ear and the eye, and his studies of physics had emphasized the science of acoustics. Referring to Newton's discussion of the oscillatory nature of light, Young performed a series of now-famous experiments in which separate sources of light combine in patterns similar to those observed in overlapping waves of water. Young's "interference patterns" of light were designed to demonstrate his theory that every color of light is characterized by a particular frequency and wavelength.

Young's association of light color to wave variation led him to understand the mechanism of color perception. In 1807 he introduced the idea of trichromatic sensitivity of the retina, according to which the retina contains nerve fibers differentially sensitive to red, green and violet, the three primary colors of light. HERMANN VON HELMHOLTZ corroborated and expanded Young's ideas on color perception, along with those of Scottish physicist J.C. Maxwell (1831–1879). The concept of color vision as a result of three sets of retinal nerve fibers is now known as the Young-Helmholtz theory.

Young's ophthalmological investigations contributed to an advanced understanding of the physiological structure of the eye and the mechanics of various disorders, including color blindness and astigmatism. His experimental work demonstrated that visual accomodation occurred when the curvature of the refractive surfaces of the eye was altered or defective.

Young's scientific contribution also includes a physical of capillarity—the effect of a solid vessel on the surface of a liquid. In 1807 Young published *A Course of Lectures on Natural Philosophy and the Mechanical Arts*, where, in addition to his ideas on vision and optics, Young coined the word "energy," presenting the first modern physical interpretation of that concept.

Z

Hans Zinsser 1878–1940

Hans Zinsser was considered the world's leading authority on typhus and rickettsial disease, but he was also widely honored for his outstanding work in bacteriology, immunology and epidemiology. His wide-ranging interests produced important studies of syphilis, rheumatic fever, the mechanism of the antigen-antibody reaction and the phenomenon of delayed hypersensitivity and allergy, particulary in tuberculin reaction.

By the 1920s the causative agent for murine (or endemic) typhus had been established as *Rickettsia mooseri.* At the time, "Brill's disease" was considered another form of typhus, but Zinsser established that disease as a clinically distinct entity. Isolating the etiologic agent as *Rickettsia prowazekii,* Zinsser suggested that the outbreak of "Brill's disease" occurs in patients who have recovered from an initial case of epidemic typhus. When this theory was later confirmed the condition was renamed "Brill-Zinsser's" disease.

Born in New York City, Zinsser was nevertheless raised in the cultural traditions of a European heritage. His father, August Zinsser, was a German immigrant who had established a successful business in selling chemical products, ensuring young Hans a fashionable education at private schools in New York, supplemented by frequent trips to Europe during vacations.

Enrolled at Columbia College in 1895, Hans pursued literature and science with equal enthusiasm. His professional life in biology and medicine never detracted from his commitment as a serious poet.

Following graduation from the Columbia College of Physicians and Surgeons in 1903 Zinsser completed his internship at Roosevelt Hospital and established a private practice that proved to be short-lived. In 1923, after serving as professor of immunology and bacteriology at Stanford and Columbia universities, Zinsser joined the staff at Harvard Medical School. Appointed Charles Wilder Professor of Bacteriology and Immunology in 1925, he spent the remaining fifteen years of his life as an esteemed member of the Harvard faculty. Working with colleagues M. Ruiz Castaneda, S.H. Zia, Harry Plotz and Nobel prize-winning virologist JOHN ENDERS, Zinsser introduced advanced methods of staining and culturing *Rickettsia,* facilitating the subsequent development and mass production of the typhus vaccine.

Greatly admired by students and colleagues, Zinsser was an influential if unconventional figure at the university, approaching the study of science by way of literature, art, music, history, philosophy and politics. His unpretentious and joyful manner is fondly recalled by many of his former students, including John Enders, who stated simply, "He was my master." Among other distinguished associates was noted microbiologist and Nobel laureate MAX THEILER, who was profoundly inspired by Zinsser's work but who fondly recalls a personal friendship as well, during which the two Harvard scientists exchanged recipes for homemade beer during Prohibition.

Concerned with the issues of sanitation and the epidemiological mechanism of infectious disease, Zinsser took part in a number of research expeditions around the world. In 1915, as a member of the American Red Cross Sanitary Commission, he visited Serbia to investigate a typhus epidemic. He later studied outbreaks of the disease in the Soviet Union, Mexico and China. These experiences are recounted in a popular and engaging work, decribed by Zinsser as a "biography of the life of typhus." First published in 1935, *Rats, Lice, and History* combined personal references and wide-ranging remarks on history, philosophy and bacteriology.

In addition to numerous papers on a variety of bacteriology and immunological subjects, Zinsser also published several internationally acclaimed reference texts. First appearing in 1910, *A Textbook of Bacteriology* has been translated into a number of foreign languages, including Chinese. *Infection and Resistance,* still widely recognized, was published in 1914.

Zinsser's final work, *As I Remember Him,* is autobiographical. Written in the third person, the book is presented in the form of a memior recalling "R.S." (Zinsser's "Romantic Self"). Presenting a moving account of his struggle with lymphocytic leukemia, *As I Remember Him* was published in 1940, the year of Zinsser's death.

Chronology

B.C.

c. 2838	Shen Nung writes the *Pen-Tsao,* first medical herbal text
c. 2600	*Nei Ching (Canon of Medicine),* by Huang Ti, establishes principles of yin and yang and introduces poppy juice used as sleep-inducing drug
c. 800	Homer describes a drug brought from Egypt (thought to be opium) that has the power to rob grief and anger of their sting and extinguish painful memories
c. 700	*Atharva-Veda*—Indian medical text
	Ayurvedic medicine
c. 530	Philosophic medical center of Pythagoras
c. 500	First healing temples of Asclepios
493–438	Empedocles
c. 500–400	Hippocrates
430	Plague epidemic in Athens—earliest record of plague in Europe
384–322	Aristotle
c. 310–250	School of Alexandria marks begining of medical education
c. 300	Herophilus dissects bodies, studies brain
c. 250	Erasistratus notes cirrhosis of the liver
c. 160	First record of practicing woman doctor in China

A.D.

c. 30	*De Re Medicina* by Celsus
c. 60	Dioscorides's *De Materia Medica*
c. 130	Soranus of Ephesus
131–201	Galen
c. 300	Plague epidemic in Rome kills 5,000
860–932	Rhazes
	Chemical principles applied to pharmacology
980–1036	Avicenna writes medical *Canon* and alchemical *De Anima*
1126–1198	Averroës
1137	St. Bartholomew's hospital founded in London
1215	St. Thomas Hospital, London
1250	Arsenic discovered
1280	Eyeglasses invented
1334–1350	Black Death—bubonic and pulmonary plague epidemic; from one to three quarters of the population in Europe and uncounted millions in Asia are killed
1493–1541	Paracelsus
1496–1500	Syphilis epidemic in Europe
1505	Charter of Royal College of Surgeons of Edinburgh
1510–1573	John Caius contracts with government for two bodies a year for study

1514–1564	Vesalius
1518	College of Physicians established in London
1533–1619	Fabricius ab Acquapendente
1536	*Chirurgia Magna* by Guy de Chauliac
1540	Guild of Barber-Surgeons established
	Ambroise Paré abandons biling-oil cautery
1543	*De humanis corporis fabrica* ("On the Structure of the Human Body") by Vesalius
1546	*De Contagione* by Fracastoro
1550	Establishment of anatomy theaters
1561	*Observationes Anatomicae* by Fallopio
	Eustachius writes on anatomy
1578–1657	William Harvey
1580	*Schlafkrankheit* epidemic throughout Europe (febrile and lethargic illness later identified as a version of Parkinson's disease)
1596–1650	René Descartes
1590	Introduction of compound microscope by Jansen
1601–1680	Athanasius Kircher suggests microorganisms as a cause of infectious disease
1609	Invention of clinical thermometer by Sanctorius
1617	Society of Apothecaries founded
1624–1689	Thomas Sydenham
1627–1691	Robert Boyle
1642–1727	Isaac Newton
1628	*De Motu Cordis et Sanguinis* by Harvey
1635–1703	Robert Hooke
c. 1650	Microorganisms seen under microscope
	Obstetrics emerges as medical discipline
1661	Boyle's *The Sceptical Chymist*
	Malpighi demonstrates capillaries
1664	Willis studies anatomy of the brain
1665	Bubonic plague epidemic in London kills 75,000
1667	Discovery of cellular structure in plants
1668–1738	Hermann Böerhaave
1672	Leeuwenhoek observes spermatozoa
1672–1675	*Schlafkrankheit* epidemics in London
1681	Royal College of Physicians in Edinburgh
1708	*Institutiones Medicae* by Böerhaave
1714	Fahrenheit's mercury thermometer
1718–1783	William Hunter
1721	Zabdiel Boylston conducts first inoculation against smallpox in Boston
1726	First university department of obstetrics, chaired by Gibson
1733	*Osteographia* by Cheselden
	First description of obstetric forceps by Chapman Hales measures blood pressure
1734	William Bull is first American to graduate from a medical school (University of Leiden)
1735	*Systema Naturae* by Linnaeus
1742	Celsius creates scale for temperature
1743–1794	Antoine Lavoisier
1752	Benjamin Franklin and Dr. Thomas Bond found first hospital in U.S.
1761	*De Sedibus et Causis Morborum* by Morgagni
1763	Linnaeus introduces his classification of diseases
1765	First Medical College founded in U.S. (now University of Pennsylvania School of Medicine)
1770	William Hunter establishes school of anatomy at Windmill Street, London
1771	Galvani discovers electric properties of the nervous system
1774	*Kaitai Shinso* (*A New Book of Anatomy*) by Genpaku Sugita published in Japan
	The Anatomy of the Human Gravid Uterus by William Hunter
1776	Oxygen discovered by Joseph Priestley, named by Lavoisier

1778	Franz Mesmer studies hypnotism
	Introduction of modern water closet
1781–1826	René Laënnec
1785	Benjamin Franklin invents bifocal eyeglasses
1790	James Derham becomes first black to practice medicine in U.S.
1798	Jenner introduces vaccination
	Pinel removes the insane from prisons
1799	Humphry Davy discovers intoxicating properties of laughing gas (nitrous oxide)
1800	Royal College of Surgeons in England
	Bichat studies histology
1806	Isolation of morphine by Friedrich Serturner
1808	Corvisart develops modern clinical medicine
1809	McDowell performs ovariotomy
1812	Charles Bell studies motor and sensory nerves
1816	Laënnec's monaural stethoscope
1820–1910	Florence Nightingale
1822–1884	Gregor Mendel
1822–1895	Louis Pasteur
1823	First publication of *Lancet* medical journal
1824	Preservation of meat in cans
1827	Von Baer observes ovum
1827–1912	Joseph Lister
1828	Synthesis of urea by Wohler
1829	Dr. John Dix Fisher founds first school for the blind (Perkins School in Boston)
1832	Cholera epidemic in New York City
1842	Anaesthesia used during surgery in U.S. for the first time by Crawford W. Long
1843–1910	Robert Koch
1844	Nitrous oxide first used as an anesthetic by American dentist Horace Wells
1845–1922	Alphese Laveran
1846	American Medical Association establishes code of ethics declaring a physician's obligation to treat victims of epidemic diseases even at risk to his own life
	Establishment of the American Association for the Advancement of Science
	William Morton introduces ether as surgical anesthetic
1847	Experiments with chloroform by Simpson
1848	First Public Health Act, in England
	First medical school for women
	Mass. School for the Idiotic founded (first school for the mentally retarded)
1849	Addison studies adrenal glands
	Elizabeth Blackwell becomes first woman in U.S. to receive a medical degree
1851	Opthalmoscope introduced by Helmholtz
1852	Establishment of American Pharmaceutical Association
1852–1934	Santiago Ramon y Cajal
1854–1915	Paul Ehrlich
1856–1939	Sigmund Freud
1855	Dr. Emmeline R. Jones becomes first woman dentist
1858	*Cellular Pathology* by Virchow
	General Medical Act founded in England
	Pasteur disproves theory of spontaneous generation
	James Young Simpson publishes *On Chloroform and Other Anaesthetics*, introducing the use of drugs for relieving pain during childbirth
1859–1906	Pierre Curie
1860	*On the Origin of Species* by Charles Darwin
	Pierre-Paul Broca discovers speech center in the brain
	Binaural stethoscope introduced by George P. Cammann
1861	Semmelweis studies puerperal fever

1863	Helmholtz studies hearing
	National Academy of Sciences chartered in U.S.
1864	International Red Cross founded
	Lister uses carbolic spray, introduces antiseptic surgery
1866	Gregor Mendel announces fundamental principles of genetics and is generally ignored
1867–1934	Marie Curie
1869–1939	Harvey Cushing
1869	Mendeleev introduces periodic table
1873	Yellow fever, cholera and smallpox epidemics sweep the southern United States
1875–1965	Albert Schweitzer
1876	*The Aetiology of Anthrax* by Koch
	Alexander Graham Bell invents the telephone
1878	Yellow fever epidemic in New Orleans
1879	First hearing aid patented in U.S. by R.S. Rhodes
1881	Clara Barton organizes American Red Cross in Washington, D.C.
1882	Tuberculosis bacillus isolated by Robert Koch
1884	Cocaine is discovered and isolated by Pierre Robiquet
1885	Pasteur cures nine-year-old Joseph Meister of rabies
1886	*Psychopathia Sexualis* by Krafft-Ebbing
1887	First successful removal of a tumor from the neural substance in the spinal cord
1888	First incubator for infants constructed by Dr. William C. Deming in U.S.
1889	Pasteur Institute founded
	Use of surgical gloves by Halsted
1889–90	Influenza epidemic in Italy
	American Psychological Association founded
1893	Cardiac conducting system by His
1894	Electrical heart activity studied by Einthoven
	First free hospice for terminal cancer patients established in U.S. by Rose Lathrop
1895	Röntgen discovers X rays
1896	Riva-Rocci introduces sphygmomanometer
	Babinski reflex discovered
1898	Marie and Pierre Curie isolate radium
1899	Aspirin is introduced on the market by Farbenfabriken Bayer, a German pharmaceutical firm
1900	Mechanism of heredity rediscovered by Correns, DeVries and Tschermak
	Wertheim operates on uterine cervical cancer
	Bordet and Gengou discover antibodies
	The Interpretation of Dreams by Freud
1901	Army Nurse Corps established as a branch of U.S. Army
	Landsteiner studies blood types
	Mosquito implicated in transmission of yellow fever
	Rockefeller Institute for Medical Research founded (became Rockefeller Institute in 1958)
1902	International Sanitary Bureau established by 21 countries in North and South America (later known as Pan American Health Organization)
	Hormone studies by Bayliss and Starling
	Carrel develops tissue transplants
	Midwives' Act enacted in England
1906	*Integrative Action of the Nervous System* by Sherrington
	Wassermann introduces test for syphilis
	Pekelharing, Hopkins, Eijkman, and Funk discover vitamins and demonstrate nutritional deficiency as a cause of disease
	William Bateson introduces the term "genetics"
1907	Ross Granville Harrison develops technique for tissue culture
	L'Office International d'Hygiene Publique (International Office of Public Health) established in Paris
1909	Bateson publishes *Mendel's Principles of Heredity*

	Dale studies endocrinology
	Kocher studies thyroid
1910	Ehrlich uses salvarsan to treat syphilis
	Flexner produces poliomyelitis experimentally
1911	Russell Hibbs introduces spine fusion operation
	Flexner report on medical education
	Medical Research Council founded in England
	Biochemical Society of London founded
1912	First description of myocardial infarction (heart attack) by James B. Herrick
	AMA amends 1846 Epidemic Code of Ethics, allows physicians to refuse a patient except under emergency situations
1913	American College of Surgeons founded
1915	Irrigation of wounds performed by Carrel and Dakin
	Tetanus prophylactic shot introduced
1916	Gaskell identifies involuntary nervous system
1916	Poliomyelitis epidemic in New York City
1916–1927	*Encephalitis lethargica* pandemic afflicts 5 million
1917	Vitamin B isolated
1918	Influenza pandemic kills 22 million
	Rehabilitation medicine introduced
1919	J.B. Watson presents theory of behaviorism
1921	Banting and Best discover use of insulin for treatment of diabetes
	First attempts at microsurgery
	American Birth Control League founded
1922	Carrel discovers leucocytes
	Evans discovers Vitamin E
1922	Vitamin D isolated
1923	Isolation of insulin by Banting and Best
	Carlos Williamson describes rejection phenomenon
	League of Nations institutes Health Organization
	Chemical physiology of muscle contraction is described
1925	Florence Sabin becomes first woman member of the National Academy of Science
	Whipple, Minot, and Murphey discover active principle in liver affecting blood formation
1926	*Conditioned Reflexes* by Pavlov
1927	First use of iron lung, by Drinker and Agassiz
1928	Fleming discovers penicillin
	Hormonal test for early pregnancy introduced by Ascheim and Zondek
	Pap test developed by Papanicolaou
1929	Fleming reports observations on anti-bacterial effects of penicillin
1932	First use of sulfa drugs
1933	First blood bank founded by Flosdorf and Mudd in U.S.
1935	Domagk discovers sulphanilamide
	Cortisone isolated
	First lobotomy performed by Egas Moniz
1938	Florey and Chain study antibiotics
	Synthetic estrogen developed by Dodds
	Fenestration operation introduced by Lempert
1939	Discovery of the RH factor by Landsteiner and Wiener
	Paul Müller develops DDT
1940	Discovery of Rh factor in blood
1941	Gregg studies rebulla and birth defects
	Penicillin used to treat pneumonia
1943	Hoffman develops LSD-25
1944	Oswald Avery establishes the existence of DNA
	Scatz, Bugie and Waksman develop streptomycin

1945	First kidney dialysis machine invented by Kolff in the Netherlands
	Introduction of streptomycin
1948	Merging of Health Organization of the League of Nations and United Nations Relief and Rehabilitation Administration to form the World Health Organization (soon joined by Pan American Health Organization)
	Initiation of National Health Service in Great Britain
1949	Gastric suction tube invented by I.J.Wood
1951	Discovery of double-helical structure of DNA
	Study of chromosome numbers
	Introduction of oral contraceptive drugs by G. Pincus
	Artificial heart-lung machine
1953	Chemical configuration of DNA is described
	Polio virus cultured
	Pump-oxygenator for cardiac by-pass by Gibbon
	Cryosurgery
1954	First successful kidney and tissue transplants
1955	Polio vaccine made commercially available
	Open-heart surgery performed for first time
	Chlorpromazine and lithium treat psychiatric disorders
1957	A.M.A. drops 1846 Epidemic Code of Ethics, but retains 1912 provision
1958	Intestinal biopsy tube invented by Margot Shiner
	Dopamine identified as a neurotransmitter
1960	Beginning of "community psychiatry"
	Theodore H. Maiman demonstrates the first laser
	Kendrew and Perutz describe structure of protein myoglobin
	Pacemakers for human hearts are introduced
	Asbestos identified as carcinogenic
1961	Genetic code is deciphered
	Human Tissues Act enacted
1963	First liver transplant performed by Starzl
	Measles vaccine perfected
1965	Medicare begins
1966	First artificial heart implanted
1967	First heart transplant performed by Christiaan Barnard in South Africa
	DNA virus is synthesized
	Nirenberg establishes that mammals, amphibians, and bacteria share common genetic code
	Amniocentesis developed
1968	Ribonuclease molecule is synthesized
1969	Isolation of a single gene (of bacterium *E. coli*)
	Enzyme synthesized
1970	Test-tube babies (Steptoe and Edwards)
	CAT-SCANS (computerized axial tomography)
	Identification of 17 amino acids
1971	Human growth hormone is synthesized
1973	Identification of neuro-receptors for opiate drugs
1974	International group of molecular biologists call for temporary ban on gene-splicing until potential dangers of recombinant DNA technology are more fully understood and safety guidelines can be established
	Research experiments with cancer vaccinations show success with animal subjects
1976	First synthetic gene introduced
	National Institutes of Health issues guidelines for genetic engineering research
	Legionnaire's disease is discovered when 26 die at American Legion convention in Philadelphia
1977	Development of genetic engineering for curing disease
1978	First test-tube baby is born
	Smallpox is eliminated

1979	Interferon research conducted
1981	First clinical description of AIDS
1982	First brain tissue transplants, used for Parkinsonism
1984	First successful gene-therapy in a mammal
1984	First baby born from frozen embryo
1985	A.H. Robbins spends $615 million to settle claims against Dalkon Shield I.U.D.
1986	I.U.D.s banned
	World Health Organization declares AIDS "a health disaster of pandemic proportions."
	AIDS virus is isolated
1987	Defective genes linked to colon cancer and hereditary form of Alzheimer's disease
	Artificial chromosomes are produced
	FDA approves Azidothymidine (AZT) for treatment of AIDS
	Vatican condemns test-tube fertilization
	Gene-altered bacteria tested on California strawberry plants to prevent frost damage
1988	Scanning-tunneling microscope produces first clear image of molecular structure
	First patent issued for a "transgenic non-human mammal"—a genetically-altered mouse
	Fetal cell research brought into question by U.S. Public Health Service
	National Institutes of Health approves injection of genetically altered cells into humans.

Bibliography

Blake J.B., ed. *Education in the History of Medicine.* New York and London: Hafner Publishing Co., 1968.

Brock, Arthur J. *Greek Medicine: Extracts of Medical Writers from Hippocrates to Galen.* London and Toronto: J.M. Dent and Sons, 1929.

Burroughs, Wellcome & Co. *The History of Inoculation and Vaccination.* London, 1913.

Bynum, W.F., Browne, E.J., and Porter, Roy, eds. *Dictionary of the History of Science.* Princeton, N.J.: Princeton University Press, 1981.

Cartwright, F.F. *The English Pioneers of Anaesthesia.* Bristol: John Wright and Sons, 1952.

Clendening, Logan. *Source Book of Medical History.* New York and London. Paul B. Hoeber, 1942.

Comrie, John D. *History of Scottish Medicine.* New York: AMS Press, 1976.

Cumston, Charles Greene. *An Introduction to the History of Medicine from the Time of the Pharaohs to the End of the Eighteenth Century.* New York: Alfred A. Knopf, 1926.

Dorland's Illustrated Medical Dictionary. 26th ed. Philadephia and London: W.B. Saunders Company, 1981.

Duffy, J. *The Rise of American Medicine.* New York: McGraw Hill, 1976.

Dictionary of Scientific Biography, 1975.

Encyclopaedia Brittanica, 1988.

Freud, Sigmund. *An Outline of Psychoanalysis.* Trans. by James Strachey. New York: W.W. Norton and Co., 1949.

Garrison, F.H. *An Introduction to the History of Medicine.* 4th Ed. Philadelphia: W.B. Saunders and Co., 1929.

Gordon, B.L. *Medicine Throughout Antiquity.* Philadelphia: F.A. Davis Co., 1949.

Harris, William H. and Levey, Judith S., eds. *The New Columbia Encyclopedia.* New York and London: Columbia University Press, 1975.

Huard, P. and Wong, M. *Chinese Medicine.* New York: McGraw Hill, 1968.

Hunter, John. *Lectures on Anatomy.* 1837. Reprint. Amsterdam, London, and New York: Elsevier Publishing Co., 1972.

Jenner, E. *An Inquiry into the Causes and Effects of the Variolae Vaccinae.* 1798. Reprint. London: Dawsons of Pall Mall, 1966.

Keys, Thomas E. *The History of Surgical Anesthesia.* New York: Dover Publications, 1963.

Leake, C.D. *An Historical Account of Pharmacology to the Twentieth Century.* Springfield, Illinois: Charles C. Thomas, Publisher, 1975.

Long, E.R. *Selected Readings in Pathology from Hippocrates to Virchow.* Springfield, Illinois: Charles C. Thomas Publisher, 1929.

Lyons, Albert S. and Petrucelli, R. Joseph II. Medicine: *An Illustrated History.* New York: Harry N. Abrams Inc., Publishers, 1978.

Medawar, P.B. and Medawar, J.S. *Aristotle to Zoos: A Philosophical Dictionary of Biology.* Cambridge, Massachussetts: Harvard University Press, 1983.

Metchnikoff, Elie. *The Founders of Modern Medicine: Pasteur—Koch—Lister.* 1939. Reprint. CNY: Books for Libraries Press, 1971.

Osler, Sir William. *The Evolution of Modern Medicine.* New Haven: Yale University Press, 1921.

Pare, Ambroise. *The Collected Works of Ambroise Pare.* Trans. from the Latin by T. Johnson. Pound Ridge, N.Y.: Milford House, 1948.

Pinel, P. *A Treatise on Insanity.* Trans. from the French by D.D. Davis. New York: New York Academy of Medicine and Hafner Publishing Co., 1962.

Shryock, R.H. *The Development of Modern Medicine.* Madison, Wisconsin: University of Wisconsin Press, 1979.

Sigerist, Henry. *The Great Doctors: A Biographical History of Medicine.* Trans. by Eder and Cedar Paul. Garden City, N.Y.: Doubleday and Co., Anchor Books, 1958.

Singer, Charles. *The Evolution of Anatomy and Physiology: From the Greeks to Harvey.* New York: Dover Publications, 1957.

Williams, Greer. *Virus Hunters.* New York: Alfred A. Knopf, Inc., 1967.

Zinsser, H. *Rats, Lice, and History.* London: George Routledge and Sons, 1937.

Name Index

(Names within parentheses denote cross-references)

Subject Index